ROLE OF THE ADIPOCYTE IN DEVELOPMENT OF TYPE 2 DIABETES

Edited by **Colleen Croniger**

Role of the Adipocyte in Development of Type 2 Diabetes
Edited by Colleen Croniger

Published by InTech
Janeza Trdine 9, 51000 Rijeka, Croatia

Publishing Process Manager Mirna Cvijic

Technical Editor Teodora Smiljanic

Cover Designer InTech Design Team

Additional hard copies can be obtained from orders@intechopen.com

Role of the Adipocyte in Development of Type 2 Diabetes, Edited by Colleen Croniger
p. cm.
ISBN 978-953-307-598-3

For EU product safety concerns:
IN TECH d.o.o., Prolaz Marije Krucifikse Kozulić 3, 51000 Rijeka, Croatia,
info@intechopen.com or visit our website at intechopen.com.

Meet the editor

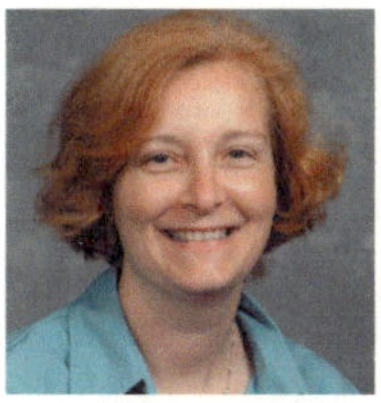

Dr. Colleen Croniger received her graduate degree in Molecular Biology from Case Western Reserve University in Cleveland, Ohio. After completing her graduate studies, she studied and learned metabolism from her post-doctoral mentor, Dr. Richard Hanson at Case Western Reserve. In 2002, Dr. Croniger joined the faculty of the Nutrition Department at Case Western Reserve as an Siistant Professor. Her research is focused on obesity, diabetes, nonalcoholic steatohepatitis (NASH) and alcoholic steatohepatitis (ASH) using genetically modified mouse models. She also teaches graduate and medical students nutrition and metabolism. Dr. Croniger has received Scholarship in Teaching award for her teaching, and for the design and implementation of the current medical school curriculum. In addition Dr. Croniger is a member of American Diabetes Association (ADA) and American Society for Biochemistry and Molecular Biology (ASBMB). Finally Dr. Croniger is the Metabolic Core director for the Case Western Reserve University Mouse Metabolic Phenotyping Core (MMPC). The Case MMPC is one of six centers that are NIH-NIDDK funded.

Contents

Preface

Adipocytes are important in the body for maintaining proper energy balance by storing excess energy as triglycerides. However, efforts of the last decade have identified several molecules that are secreted from adipocytes, such as leptin, which are involved in signaling between tissues and organs. These adipokines are important in overall regulation of energy metabolism and can regulate body composition as well as glucose homeostasis. Excess lipid storage in tissues other than adipose can result in development of diabetes and nonalcoholic fatty liver disease (NAFLD). In this book we review the role of adipocytes in development of insulin resistance, type 2 diabetes and NAFLD. Because type 2 diabetes has been suggested to be a disease of inflammation we included several chapters on the mechanism of inflammation modulating organ injury. Finally, we conclude with a review on exercise and nutrient regulation for the treatment of type 2 diabetes and its co-morbidities.

Colleen Croniger
Department of Nutrition
Case Western Reserve University
School of Medicine
Cleveland,Ohio
USA

Part 1

Adipocyte Function

1

The Sick Adipocyte Theory: The Forces of Clustering at Glance

Valmore Bermúdez et al.*
Endocrine and Metabolic Diseases Research Center, The University of Zulia, Maracaibo, Venezuela

1. Introduction

The concept and repercussions of Obesity have evolved alongside Humankind. First seen as an advantageous trait in the beginning of time, it´s now a double edged sword definition that shows how slowly genometabolic traits are acquired and how quickly can environmental factors turn it around. Being obese is not only a matter of Body Mass Index (BMI) and adiposity, its influence stretches out to include type 2 Diabetes Mellitus (T2DM), Psychological disorders like depression, anxiety disorders, and other eating disorders, Osteoarticular problems, Metabolic Syndrome, Cardiovascular Diseases (CVD) like hypertension, stroke, and myocardial infarction, Neurological disorders, Cancer, and even Immunity-related issues, such as low grade inflammation (Must, 1999; Oster, 2000; Thompson, 2001; Marchesini, 2003; Adami, 2003; Niskanen, 2004; Panagiotakos, 2005).

Obesity has been rising slowly yet steadily ever since the Industrial revolution and its pace has increased since the dawn of the 20th Century. Even though nutritional disorders have plagued Man, it was common to see that undernutrition and malnourishment were the higher numbers around the globe. Yet, the tables were turned when Gardner & Halweil published in 2000 that the number of excess-weight patients surpassed the number of the underweight population, welcoming Humanity to the supersized phase of the *land of milk and honey* (O´Dea, 1992). In 2006, the World Health Organization reported that by 2005 1.6 billion above 15 years of age would be overweight and at least 400 million would be obese, while it is predicted to reach 2.3 billion of overweight and over 700 million of obese adults by the year 2015 (World Health Organization [WHO], 2006). The figures published by Kelly et al, 2008 darken the scope, predicting that by 2030 1.12 billion individuals will be obese and 2.16 million will be overweight.

There are many factors that have influenced the increasing prevalence of obesity worldwide, and have influenced the scientific community to coin the term *obesogenic* environment (Egger & Swinbum, 1997) as the external factors that act as "second hit" triggers in the

*Joselyn Rojas[1,2], Miguel Aguirre[1,3], Clímaco Cano[1], Nailet Arraiz[1], Carlos Silva Paredes[1], Marcos Lima[3], Raquel Cano[1,4],Eneida Fonseca[1] and Manuel Velasco[1,5]
1 Endocrine and Metabolic Diseases Research Center, The University of Zulia, Maracaibo, Venezuela
2 Institute of Clinical Immunology, University of Los Andes, Mérida, Venezuela.
3 Endocrinology Service, I.A.H.U.L.A, Mérida, Venezuela
4 Endocrinology and Metabolic Diseases Unit, University Hospital of Caracas, Venezuela
5 Clinical Pharmacologic Unit, Vargas Medical School, Central University of Venezuela, Venezuela

multifactorial theory of obesity (see Figure 1). Many factors have been nominated and proven key to the etiology of obesity, such as dietary energy intake, physical activity, intrauterine environment (fetal programming), and other comorbidities like alcohol intake, physical disabilities, endocrine disorders, drug treatments, among others (Pi-Sunyer, 2002; Caballero, 2007). Physical activity has become fundamental in the intervention strategies for primary (Pate et al., 1995) and secondary prevention (Thompson, 2003) in obese patients, since it has been portrayed as a major independent risk factor for coronary artery disease (Fletcher et al., 1992). It can be defined as any voluntary skeletal muscle movement that consumes energy, usually measured by at least 30 minutes of physical activity that consumes at least 4 METs (*i.e.* brisk walk) (Dunn et al., 1998). On the contrary, physical *in*activity (sedentarism) is the lack of these ~ 30 minutes of energy consumption a day (Dunn et al., 1998), resulting in positive energy balance.

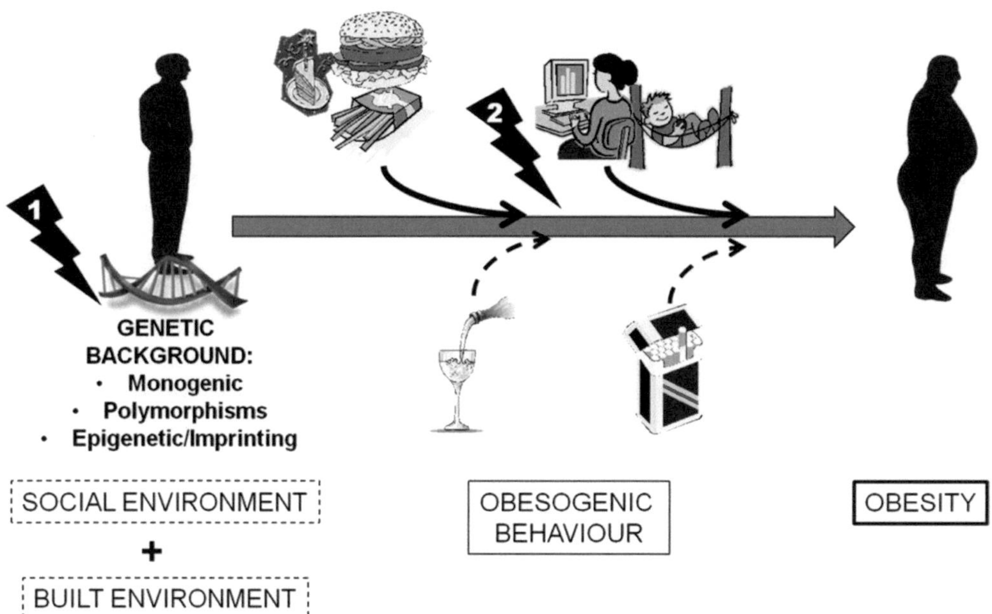

Fig. 1. The Two Hit proposal of obesity. A subject who is genetically-prone to obesity – either due to a monogenic syndrome, associated polymorphisms or imprinting (as seen *in utero*) have the first hit intrinsically. If he is subject to an obesogenic environment and subsequently develops an obesogenic behaviour (second hit), the end result will be progressive weight gain till obesity values are achieved. The obesogenic factors include high fat/carbohydrate diet, low physical activity, alcohol and smoking habits.

One of the interesting aspects about the term "physical activity" is that it´s used as an interchangeable term between "cardiorespiratory fitness", but they aren´t defined equally nor do they have the same impact on the patients. Physical activity relates to energy expenditure while cardiorespiratory fitness relates to oxygen supplition by the heart. However, both terms can relate to the same definition but they don´t explain the same aspects. In a meta-analysis by Williams, 2001 concludes that these terms should be treated as different and independent risk factors, findings that are similar to those reported by Hein et al., 1992 concerning 4,999 men who were followed for 17 years in the Copenhagen Male Study, using physical fitness and leisure time physical activity as risk factors for ischemic heart disease (IHD). This team reported that being very fit offers no protection to IHD when sedentary, and being unfit and sedentary offers higher risk for this disease. Other studies have examined the relationship between fitness and sedentarism [Fletcher et al., 1996; Rosengren et al., 1997; Pollock et al., 2000; Blair et al., 2001) demonstrating without a doubt that sedentarism has been underestimated for a long time (Saltin, 1992).

2. Set

A sedentary patient is a real conundrum, and each one is unique especially if overweight/obese. Adiposity varies in degree and distribution, being classified according to anatomical location as subcutaneous and visceral adipocytes, each with a different metabolic profiling.

2.1 Adipocytes

Classically, white adipose tissue - adipocytes are recognized as the lipid-storing professional cells, and we remark professional because other types of cells can accumulate lipids yet it is not their main objective, as can be seen with myocytes, β-cells and neurons. The key feature of the mature adipocyte is that it can store fat without compromising its integrity or anatomy. The ontogeny of the adipocytes is still poorly understood, yet the process is being researched relentlessly (Gregoire et al., 1998; Darlington et al., 1998; Godínez-Gutiérrez et al., 2002)]. Mesenchymal stem cells differentiate into adipoblasts, which subsequently express early transcription markers and enter the preadipocyte I phase; the markers for the preadipocytes are α2Col6, Lipoprotein lipase, IGF-1 and Krox20. Once the cell´s fate has been decided, mitosis and clonal expansion begins entering the pre-adipocyte II phase, characterized by active C/EBPβ/γ, SREBP-1, PPARγ2 and KLF5. Maturity of the cell cannot begin until it leaves the cell cycle and starts differentiation in coordination with upregulation of late markers which induce cell arrest and begin lipid accumulation: C/EBPα, GLUT4, Perilipin, TNF-α, TGF-β, lipogenic and lipolytic enzymes. The mature adipocyte develops when the markers include the expression and adipocyte-related hormones, cytokines and enzymes related lipid storage and release towards blood circulation. Perhaps the most interesting aspect of adipocyte differentiation is how preadipocytes are driven towards adipocyte profile (Fu et al., 2004; Simons et al., 2005; Sethi et al., 2007), which is all a gameplay of members of the Peroxisome-Proliferator-Activated-Receptors and the CCAAT-enhancer-binding protein (C/EBP) families. The first step is the short-term expression of C/EBPβ and C/EBPγ2, followed closely by C/EBPα which activates PPARγ2, responsible for the adipogenesis genetic program. The sterol-response-element-binding-protein-1c (SREBP1c) activates the lipogenic program through PPARγ, finalizing the accomplishment of the differentiated phenotype; see Figure 2.

The mature adipocyte (Gregoire, 2001; Kershaw et al., 2004; Halberg et al., 2008) is a very specialized cell which is the center of energy storage and provision mechanisms, which is under a very tight central and peripheral control. Besides the basic anatomical role, the adipocytes are also endocrine cells which secrete several factors including leptin, adipsin, angiotensinogen, adiponectin, TNF-α, acylation stimulation protein, SPARC (secreted protein acidic and rich in cysteine), and PGAR/FIAF (PPARγ, Angiopoietin related/fasting-induced adipose tissue). This adipocyte secretome incorporates adipose tissue to immunologic processes with low grade inflammation phenomena and autoimmunity-related diseases, and angiogenesis due to synthesis of angiogenic factors, various effects from macrophagic-related substances, extracellular matrix deposition and metalloproteinase remodeling (Frünbeck et al., 2001; Kershaw, et al., 2004). Given these features is not unusual to find that adipose tissue is part of several axes such as the adipo-insular axis (Kieffer et al., 2000; Vickers et al., 2001) [36-37], the adipocyte-vessels-brain axis (Elmquist et al., 2004; Guzik et al., 2007; Mietus-Snyder et al., 2008), and the adipocyte-myocyte axis (Sell et al., 2006; Taube et al., 2009).

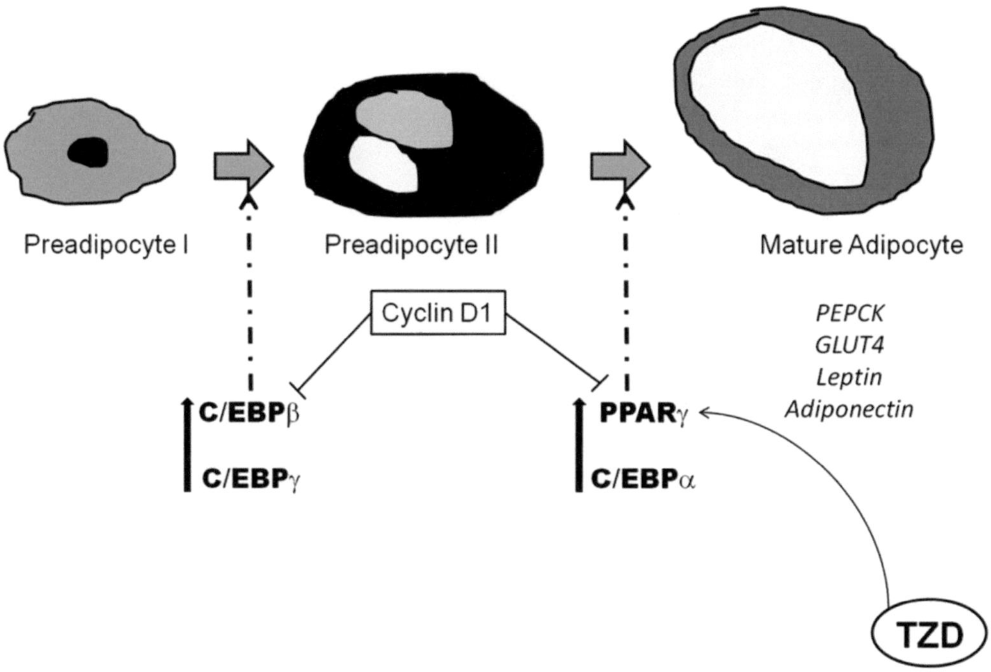

Fig. 2. Adipogenesis. The mature adipocyte goes through several stages of maturation until the professional lipid-storing profile is achieved. The interplay between CCAAT-enhancer binding protein (C/EBP) isoforms with Peroxisome-Proliferator-Activated Receptor-γ (PPARγ) ensures the progression towards final differentiation once the preadipocyte II has left the cell cycle. As long as Cyclin D1 is active, progression to a G_0 phase will be difficult – almost impossible – since this factor inhibits the differentiation transcription factors. Thiazolinilediones (TZD) are known agonists of the PPARγ enhancing the adipogenic program.

2.2 Myocytes

Sarcomeres are the functional elements of muscles cells. The contractile unit is composed of myosin fibers and actin, whose interaction allows the shortening of itself, displaying as a contracted myocyte. There are several classifications for muscle cells (Scott et al., 2001), yet the biochemical differentiation is discussed here. Muscle fibers are classified (Pette & Staron, 1997; Bassel-Budy & Olson, 2006) in Type I, Type IIa, Type IId/x, and Type IIb, having

particular metabolic properties, a) fast-twitch glycolytic fibers (types IIx and IIb), b) fast-twitch oxidative fibers (type IIa), and c) the slow-twitch oxidative fibers (type I). Dynamically, muscle fibers are classified as slow-twitch and fast-twitch motor units, and the fast fibers are subdivided in fast-twitch fatigue-resistant, fast-twitch fatigue-intermediate, and fast-twitch fatigable. Humans have a mixture of these muscle fibers and the number changes as the weight/metabolic profile is modified throughout life. Obese subjects are known to have few type I fibers and more type IIb fibers compared to lean subjects (Hickey et al., 1995). Tanner et al., 2001 reported that obese African-American women had low levels of type I fibers, and lower levels compared to obese Caucasian women, which reflects that fiber content also varies according to ethnicity.
Skeletal muscle is more than just the motor unit which gives us the possibility of movement, it´s also the most important tissue for glucose disposal, making it an essential part in energy metabolism (DeFronzo et al., 1985) and the primary target for insulin-resistance related disturbances (Lillioja et al., 1987). The disposal of glucose into skeletal muscle is fiber-specific, being greater in type I fibers compared with type IIa and IIb (Song et al., 1999) [50]. Type I/slow twitch oxidative myocytes are more efficient in regards of insulin binding, enhanced insulin receptor and post-receptor cascade activities, and higher GLUT4 translocation, compared to Type II/fast-twitch glycolytic myocytes; this suggests that insulin´s actions are more *oxidative than glycolytic*. Type II muscle fibers are insulin resistant (Henriksen et al., 1990; Henriksen & Holloszy, 1991) giving a partial explanation to the insulin resistance observed in obesity, which is also associated with abnormal lipid partitioning and intramuscular lipid accumulation.

2.3 The sick and the dying

In obesity, myocytes are sick while adipocytes die slowly due to asphyxiation. The interaction of both is what makes the adipocyte-myocyte axis so important in obesity and related diseases including Type 2 Diabetes; see Figure 3.
Plasticity - the ability to non-reversibly adapt to external load/pressure - can be seen in adipocytes, expressed as hypertrophy and hyperplasia (Arner et al., 2010). In overfed states, adipose tissue´s capacity to store excessive energy safely reaches its limit, causing a "spill-over" effect all over the body. This nutritional overload mechanism and subsequent damage can be seen in models for catch-up growth (Dulloo et al., 2009; Summematter et al., 2009), where refeeding states are associated with hyperinsulinemia, lipogenesis, plasma membrane switching from polyunsaturated fatty acids to saturated fatty acids, increased triglyceride production, ending in adipocyte hypertrophy and glucose intolerance. How plasticity can be associated to insulin-resistance is a very complex scenario. Genetic background - *thriftiness* - is a strong influential factor (Lindsay et al., 2001; Kadowaki et al., 2003; Prentice et al., 2005). Thrifty related genes and metabolic profiles ensure that all excess energy ingested will be "efficiently" stored, reminiscing those famine/feast days of the hunter-gatherers or the postnatal days of intrauterine-growth-restricted newborns. Thrifty traits have many targets (Prentice et al., 2005), yet 2 are essential: metabolic thrift, which is focused on mitochondrial electronic transport, protein turnover, fuel channeling, and substrate cycling, and adipogenic thrift, which relates to proneness of fat gain.
The physiological adaptation to overnutrition is not without intricacy, since 2 theories have been proposed. The *adipokine dysregulation* conveys the fact that overfed states triggers changes in the quantum and quality of the substances expressed in the adipocyte, for example, adiponectin secretion is lowered in obesity (Arita et al., 1999; Weyer et al., 2001),

while resistin´s is enhanced (Steppan et al., 2002; Vendrell et al., 2004). The second theory is based on *ectopic fat accumulation* of lipids in myocytes, hepatocytes and β-cells, where intramyocellular lipids correlates to insulin resistance (Virkamäki et al., 2001; Moro et al., 2008).

The continued stimulus and lipid accumulation makes the adipocyte (140 - 180 µm in diameter [Brook et al., 1972]) hypertrophy but the size of the cell is limited by the oxygen supply. Hypoxia (Hosogai et al., 2007) and increase synthesis of secretory proteins (Marciniak & Ron, 2006) are the main cause for adipocyte´s endoplasmic reticulum (ER) stress via the unfolded protein response (UPR) pathway. The latter proposal is quite simple to grasp since never-ending signals for secretion goes awry when the unfolded protein in the ER lumen surpasses the folded proteins quota due to a) lack of necessary components for the synthetized molecule, b) frequency of the secretion signal, and 3) shortage of chaperone proteins due to "sequestration" within the abnormal proteins accumulated within the lumen. This traffic alteration has been linked to several diseases including Type 2 diabetes (Scheuner & Kaufman, 2008), Tumor hypoxia and prognosis (Koumenis & Wouters, 2006), Alzheimer´s (Kudo et al., 2006) and Parkinson´s Disease (Ryu et al., 2002).

In 2004, Trayhurn & Woods suggested for the first time that it was hypoxia the culprit for low-chronic inflammation of obesity, conveying that as the adipose tissue advances and the outer sectors become hypoxic, inflammatory cytokines and acute phase proteins are locally secreted to enhance angiogenesis and stop the vicious cycle. Hypoxia in adipose tissue is due to hypoperfusion, especially after the 100 µm diameter phase of the hypertrophic adipocyte, suggesting that achieving 180 µm is a hypoxic state (Ye et al., 2007). In adipose tissue, low oxygen levels can alter gene expression, being related to decreased adiponectin mRNA, which is controlled by C/EBP and is inhibited by UPR-induced CHOP (C/EBP homologous protein) (Hosogai et al., 2007). It also can modify adipocyte secretome (Wang et al., 2007), resulting in enhanced expression of Hypoxia Induced Factor-1α (inducing GLUT1 mRNA), IL-6, leptin, Plasminogen activator inhibitor 1 (PAI-1), and Vascular Endothelial growth factor (VEGF), while haptoglobin and adiponectin are markedly decreased. Taking this one step further, hypoxia inhibit insulin post-receptor cascade though HIF-1α and HIF-2, which is thought to be crucial for the insulin resistance state observed in obese patients (Regazzetti et al., 2009); this is mediated by lowered autophosphorylation of the insulin receptor by means yet to be understood, but apparently it involves the mTOR (mammalian target of rapamycin) (Dann et al., 2007), S6K pathway (Um et al., 2006) and subsequent activation of NF-κB (Michiels et al., 2002). Almost 6 years later, hypoxia is now known to be a glucose metabolism modulator, which at first can induce glucose uptake - via GLUT1 synthesis and export - but can later decreased due to IRS-1 and insulin receptor phosphorylation, while at the same time, it can induce free fatty acid (FFA) release, leading to adipocyte dysfunction and worsening of peripheral insulin resistance (Yin et al., 2009; Copps et al., 2009).

To finally dissect adipocyte´s cyanotic life, macrophages enter the picture. Adipose tissue is not a homogenous organ, in fact is very heterogeneous and is populated with adipocytes, fibroblasts, vascular endothelia and immunologic cells. One of these, are the macrophages, who contribute significantly to the inflammatory array of signals being sent from the adipocyte (Weisberg et al., 2003). Insulin resistance depends of the abdominal adipose tissue distribution and plasticity, rather than pre-adipocyte and small adipose cells (Hauner, 2010). Adipose tissue macrophages are responsible perpetuating pre-adipocyte state and differentiation signal (Lacasa et al., 2007), by secreting TNF-α and IL-1, known suppressors of the adipogenic program via NF-κB which quashes PPARγ dependent genes. Macrophage´s secretome include VEGF, TNF-a, IL-1b, IL-6, reactive oxygen species (ROS), and prostaglandins. Monocyte recruitment towards the adipose tissue is regulated by many molecules, but C-C motif chemokine ligand 2 (CCL2) and its receptor (CCR2) are perhaps the most important ones (Bruun et al., 2005), so importantly that blocking macrophage infiltration surrounding dead/dying adipocytes is a proper therapeutic goal (Bruun et al., 2005).

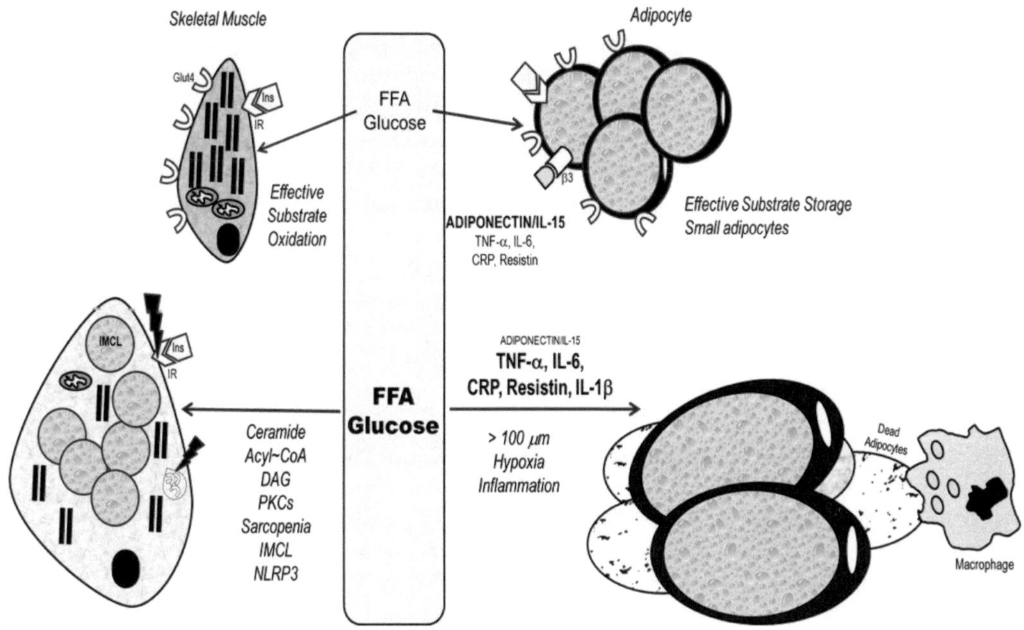

Fig. 3. The Sick and the Dying. This diagram depicts the effects of elevated free fatty acids (FFA) and hyperglycemia on adipocytes and myocytes, as it is observed in obese patients. Once the injury is fixed and has reach a point of no return, both cells begin plasticity to cope with the hostile environment. The sick myocyte loses sarcomeres at the expense of intramyocellular lipid droplets, which are source of acyl~CoAs, diacylglycerol (DAG) and ceramides, who in turn focus on serine/threonine phosphorylation of Insulin receptor and IRS-1, blunting the insulin pathways - becoming insulin resistant- Meanwhile, the growing adipocyte becomes hypoxic, releasing several cytokines who in turn affect myocyte´s already weaken metabolism, perpetuating the metabolic disturbance. As the adipocytes die in the sidelines of the adipose tissue, macrophages are recruited, worsening the inflammatory microenvironment.

The progressive growth and demise of adipocytes have collateral damage - a very sick insulin resistant skeletal myocyte. The sick myocyte not only has impaired insulin signaling, but also decreased expression of myogenin (muscle-specific transcription factor involved in myogenesis), IL-6, IL-8 and MCP-1 (monocyte chemotactic protein), with higher ceramides levels and lower mitochondrial capacity (Sell et al., 2008). How the muscle becomes insulin resistant is (still) a matter of debate, even though several mechanisms have been proposed.

Sir Phillip Randle (1963) was the first one to formulate a theory trying to explain how fuel substrates changed in muscle and how this would explain skeletal muscle insulin resistance (Randle et al., 1963). The Randle´s Hypothesis (glucose-fatty acid cycle) proposes that FFA compete with glucose as fuel substrate for mitochondrial oxidation, increasing β-oxidation within the myocyte. The consumption of FFA would in turn inhibit pyruvate dehydrogenase and phosphofructokinase, acting as barriers in the glycolytic pathway and reduced glucose uptake and oxidation. Over 30 years later, Shulman, 2000 singlehandedly dethroned Randle´s hypothesis, by stating that low FFA intramyocellular metabolism or enhanced lipid uptake leads to cytosolic accumulation of metabolites such as diacylglycerol, ceramides and acyl~CoA, which in turn activate serine/threonine kinase (PKC) cascade that end with the phosphorylation and inhibition of Insulin Receptor and IRS-1, blunting insulin post-receptor pathways, decreasing PI3-k activation and glucose uptake via GLUT4.
Beyond the glucose utilization bluntering, others morphological changes occur within the sick myocyte. Skeletal muscle also shows plasticity traits, anatomical and functional. It can use glucose or lipids for fuel production; however, in obesity lipid oxidation is decreased due to diminished enzyme capacity and reduced carnitine-palmitoyl transferase 1 (CPT1) activity (Kelley et al., 1999). Triglyceride (TAG) accretion in muscle can be attributed to 2 causes: reduced fatty acid oxidation (Kim et al., 2000) or enhance TAG synthesis (Hulver et al., 2003). Intramyocellular lipids (IMCL) are a far better predictor of muscular insulin resistance than BMI or waist-hip ratio (Pan et al., 1997), and it inversely correlates to visceral visfatin levels (Varma et al., 2007). IMCL turnover determines the amount of accumulation inside the myocyte, which modulates the level of lipid metabolites that can alter the PI3K pathways, via activation of PKC isotypes. Breakdown of the IMCL results in acyl~CoAs which can be readily oxidized in mitochondria (Guo, 2007), but it has been reported that obese mitochondria are slow oxidizers (mitochondrial dysfunction [Rabøl et al., 2010; Pagel-Langenickel et al., 2010]) and are positioned in different parts of the cytosol, slowing oxidation and increasing the cytosolic lipid droplet, making this lipid handling alteration a metabolic risk for insulin resistance (Koonen et al., 2010). There is a paradox in this whole IMCL issue: highly trained athletes use IMCL as a source for energy during exercise (Klein et al., 1994), so it makes for quite a riddle. Since from a sports point of view IMCL is advantageous, then the harm is not whether the IMCL are formed or not, it´s the availability of toxic lipid intermediates.
Now, how does a dying adipocyte, full of TAG and choking on ER stress, can make the susceptible myocyte sick? Since adipose tissue is considered an endocrine organ, then cross-talks with other organs is plausible. The first evidence of this dialogue was published by Dietze et al., 2002 using skeletal myocytes cultured in the same medium as adipocytes. They reported a profound disturbance in insulin signaling, characterized by nulled insulin-stimulated phosphorylation of IRS-1, reduced Akt activation, inducing an insulin resistant state. Several of the adipokines have been implicated in the process, including TNF-α (Hotamisligil, 1999), resistin (de Luis et al., 2009), IL-6 (Rotter et al., 2003), leptin (Shimomura et al., 1999), adiponectin (Yamauchi et al., 2001), MCP-1 (Sartipy et al., 2003) and RBP-4 (Graham et al., 2006), among others. One important feature between adipose-induced muscle insulin resistance is the role of the macrophages, which are slowly becoming pivotal for (adipose) and skeletal muscle insulin resistance. Macrophages cultured with palmitate serum medium secrete major proinflammatory cytokines that lower insulin action (Samokhvalov et al., 2009) via JNK mediated decreased phosphorylated Akt (Varma et al., 2009). SIRT1, a member of the Sirtuin family of NAD-dependent deacetylases, is able

to blunt macrophages capacity for inducing insulin resistance in Zucker fatty rats, shedding light to the complex axis (Yoshizaki et al., 2010). All in all, adipokine mediators are able to induce reversible (regeneration of myotubes and IL-6 secretion) and irreversible (IL-8 and MCP-1 secretion and myogenin expression) changes in the muscle proteome promoting insulin resistance in the myocyte (Sell et al., 2008; Kewalrami et al., 2010).

3. Go

3.1 Glycemic control

Physical activity and diet are the primary tools to intervene and modify lifestyle in the obese patient, yet it's not exclusive, since these strategies can also be applied to type 2 diabetics, hypertensive patients, and other insulin-disturbances related diseases. Physical activity can be defined as any daily activity undertaken for at least 30 minutes a day that ends in caloric consumption, and it´s deficiency is considered an individual risk factor for cardiovascular disease (Carnethon, 2009). It has been proposed the basic etiology of complex diseases is associated with disturbances of oxygen metabolism (Koch & Britton, 2008), making cardiorespiratory fitness a fine predictor for health risk (Lee et al., 2005), metabolic syndrome (LaMonte et al., 2005) and type 2 diabetes (Sawada et al., 2010). Regular exercise improves glycemic control, weight reduction and manages metabolic risks associated with adiposity. The molecular basics for this improvement have been extensively reviewed somewhere else (Hayashi et al., 1997; Hamilton et al.; 2000, Rose et al., 2005) and are shown in Figure 4. The mechanisms that are at play to ensure glucose uptake and consumption seem redundant since it centers on the translocation of GLUT4 towards the membrane, enhanced by AMPK, Ca^{++}/Calmodulin dependent protein kinase , and Nitric Oxide, and act as insulin mediators during and after exercise mediating increases glucose and fatty acid oxidation (Turcotte & Fisher, 2008). The main destination of glucose uptake is to replenish the glycogen stores in the skeletal muscle, and it does not depend on insulin signaling, since there is no increase IRS-1, IRS-2 or PI3K activation.

Focusing on the muscle fibers, constant exercise is known to induce a switch of muscle fibers towards the type I ones. Fiber shifts are thought to be the end result of fast myosin chain induction, with concomitant reduction of slow type I myosine. This muscle functional plasticity can be induced by any type of exercise, endurance, sprint or heavy resistance (Andersen et al., 1994; Fitts, 2003). The basic changes of fibers is characterized by reduction of type IIb percentage with slow increase of type IIa and type I, turning muscle metabolism into an oxidant kind over time, and become resistant to fatigue since the myocyte recovers from "metabolic stunnedness" and efficiently synthetizes ATP during and after exercise. The mechanisms underlying these adaptations are still poorly understood, but it is possible that AMPK and calcineurin activate parallel pathways that control myocyte adaptation (Röckl et al., 2007).

AMP-activated protein kinase (AMPK) is a pivotal regulator of intracellular energy during stressful states like starvation, hypoxia, exercise, among others, and it is central in the hormonal control of metabolic processes that consume or produce ATP (Lim et al., 2010). AMPK is active when AMP/ATP ratio rises, inhibiting ATP consuming pathways and enhancing ATP producing processes like glucose and FFA oxidation. During exercise, AMPK is activated and immediately phosphorylates and inhibits acetyl~CoA carboxylase (ACC), the key enzyme that synthetizes malonyl~CoA – negative allosteric modulator of

CPT1. Once CPT1 is released from control, β-oxidation continues full force (Musi et al., 2001). AMPK also modulates glycogen synthesis by increasing glucose availability inside the cell via phosphorylation and inhibition of Akt-Substrate 160 (AS160), main break for translocation of GLUT4 vesicles, and, regulates IMCL breakdown via phosphorylation of Hormone sensitive lipase (Jørgensen et al., 2006). And on a final note, AMPK can modulate the expression of GLUT4 by regulating GLUT4 enhancer factor (GEF) and myocyte enhancer factor 2 (MEF2) (Holmes et al., 2005) guaranteeing an appropriate glucose-uptake phenotype. Calcineurin - cyclosporine-sensitive, calcium-regulated serine/threonine phosphatase - is an enzyme that controls the signaling pathway for myogenic processes by modulation of the MyoD and MEF2 transcription factors (Chin et al., 1998), considered fundamental for fiber remodeling (Schiaffino et al., 2002; Bassel-Duny et al., 2003) with PPARδ as downstream effector (Wang et al., 2004).

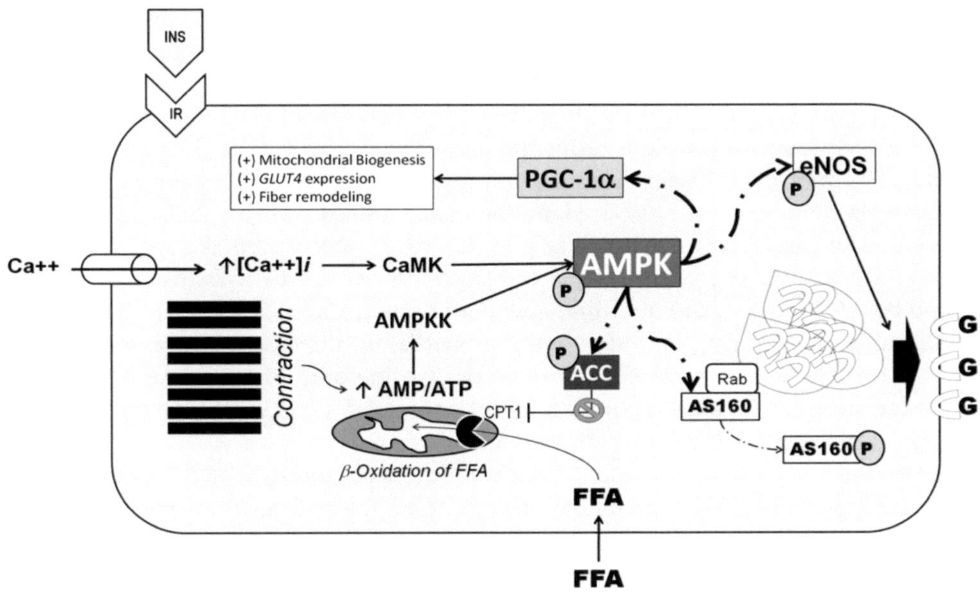

Fig. 4. Molecular basics of exercise. Once the AMP/ATP rises continuously according to muscle workout, AMPK kinase (AMPKK) is activated, alongside Ca++/calmodulin dependent Kinase (CaMK), both known to phosphorylate the a-subunit of AMPK, activating it. AMPK then inhibits by phosphorylation Acetyl~CoA Carboxilase, enzyme known to synthetize malonyl~CoA, main negative modulator of carnitine-palmitoyl transferase 1 (CPT1); blocking malonyl~CoA synthesis, β-oxidation is enhanced, using free fatty acids (FFA) from circulation and from lipid storage inside the myocyte. Secondly, AMPK activates PPARγ coactivator 1α (PGC-1α) which co-induces the PPARγ adipogenic program. Next, AMPK phosphorylates and activates endothelial Nitric Oxide Synthetase, which generates nitric oxide which serves as a vasodilator (increasing and maintaining blood flow) and is also an enhancer of GLUT4 translocation. Finally, AMPK phosphorylates Akt Substrate 160 (AS160), who is blocking Rab-GTPase molecule from initiating the movements of the GLUT4 vesicles towards the membrane. Once AS160 is "neutralized", GLUT4 are exported to the plasma membrane, increasing glucose uptake.

Insulin sensitivity restoration is a bit more complicated. Muscle straightening activity has been known to enhance sensitivity among adults, serving as proper program to reduce insulin resistance (Cheng et al., 2007). Glucose uptake and IMCL turnover have been implicated, yet there is paradox lingering around, endurance athletes have higher intramuscular lipids but are highly insulin sensitive (Goodpaster et al., 2001; Meex et al., 2010). Now, this beneficial effect can be obtained whether acutely - daily muscle contraction inducer energy flux - and by chronic modifications - mitochondrial oxidative capacity and induced GLUT4 expression (Thyfault, 2008; Jiang et al., 2010).

3.2 Thriftiness

As we have formerly mentioned, exercise is associated with modification of gene expression, specially affecting genes that control energy deposit and consumption, even in high training statuses. The Thrifty genotype theory published in 1962 (Neel, 1962) proposed that genes that favored energy saving during feast/famine cycles in the Late Paleolithic Era were incorporated into the human genome, because they were advantageous during famine phases. Exercise can modify gene expression according to the type of activity exerted, for example, aerobic exercise (endurance) is not associated with increased phosphorylated $p70^{S6K}$, but high resistance work-out is indeed related (Sherwood et al., 1999). Wendorf & Goldfine, 1991 proposed that during those hunter-gatherers years a selective insulin resistance in muscle had to be imposed, to avoid hypoglycemia during fasting and allow energy storage during feeding, traits that would turn disastrous in a sedentary individual, such as the obese patient. Evidence of this theory can be seen in different racial groups all around the world. The Arizona Pima Indians have the highest prevalence of diabetes in the world with increased sedentarism, compared to the Mexican Pimas (Valencia et al., 1999) and the scenario is similar with the Pacific Islanders in Asia (Zimmet et al., 1990). Needless to say, physical inactivity is then associated with insulin resistance and the genetic implications of exercise and its mediators are an important aspect of the whole concept, and in desperate need of continuous investigation (Abate et al., 2003; Chakravarthy et al., 2004).

3.3 Inflammation

Other metabolic changes are observed during physical training in obese patients, such as anti-inflammatory effects. In previous sections, the low-grade inflammation characteristically seen in obesity was discussed. Pedersen et al., 2007 reported that since the muscle was able to release cytokines under exercise conditions, these signaling molecules should be named *myokines* and the para/endocrine effects should be separated from their usual physiological profile.

Interleukin-6 is perhaps the most important of these myokines, yet the muscle is known to secrete IL-8, IL-15, IL-10 and IL-1ra, and very intense exercise can induce TNF–α secretion (see Table 1) (Petersen et al., 2005; Marini et al., 2010). The IL-6 expression and release patter is astounding, with a 100-fold level in response to exercise. The dilemma lies in this: how does a known insulin resistance-mediating molecule can exert protective effects? The answer lies in the true inflammatory levels and profiles. It has been suggested that IL-6 plays a villain role in the metabolic syndrome, alongside TNF-α. Nevertheless, Kubaszek et al., 2003 reported that the risk genotypes for metabolic disturbances (including obesity and type 2 diabetes) are characterized by increased transcription of TNF-α with decreased expression of IL-6. Now, the reader needs to me reminded that TNF-α triggers the release of

IL-6, not the other way around, so it´s logical to conclude that adipocyte derived TNF-α induces local expression of IL-6 in the adipose tissue (Pedersen et al., 2007), which correlates with the fact that IL-6 is not overtly elevated in diabetic patients and is not highly expressed in lean patients with insulin resistance (Carey et al., 2004). The insulin-sensitizing effects of IL-6 are still controversial, yet it has been reported that the myokine enhances glucose uptake and glycogen synthesis in the myocyte, via activation of AMPK while reducing TNF-α levels (Pedersen et al., 2007).

Myokine	Locus	Effect
IL-6	7p21	Anti-inflammatory when secreted before TNF-α (Carey et al., 2004; Pedersen et al., 2007).
IL-8	4q12-q13	Angiogenesis and neutrophil chemoatraction thru the CXCR2 (Freydelund et al., 2007).
IL-15	4q31	Reduction of body fat, especially visceral body fat (Carbó et al., 2001; Acharyya et al., 2004)
IL-10	1q31-q32	Downregulation of Proinflammatory cytokines and chemokines (de Vries, 1995; Acharyya et al., 2004)
IL-1ra	2q14.2	Restriction and modulation of the inflammatory response during exercise (Ostrowski et al., 1999; Opal et al., 2000; Suzuki et al., 2000)

Table 1. Myokines and their effects concerning Obesity and Metabolic Syndrome.

Parallel to IL-6 effects, IL-15 has progressively risen as a major modulator of fat metabolism and muscle accretion in skeletal muscle over the past 15 years, which have been discussed elsewhere (Carbó et al., 2000; Quinn et al., 2008; Argilés et al., 2009), yet the following aspects need to be discussed. IL-15 is a cytokine which is related to NK cell maturation, which actions are not reserved for the immunology universe. This protein is synthetized also by placenta, muscle and other tissues, supporting the idea of non-immune functions in such organs. Muscle hypertrophy at the expense of myotube accretion by inhibition of protein degradation is observed in animal models (Quinn et al., 2002), and this has been proposed as a therapeutic option for wasting syndromes such as cancer (Carbó et al., 2000) . This effect is probably due to induction of PPAR-δ which mediates protein synthesis in such cells. As for adipose tissue, the cytokine has been related to reduce lipid accumulation in pre-adipocytes enhancing their differentiation, and inducing adiponectin secretion in matured adipocytes (Quinn et al., 2005). These findings were further confirmed, when it was proven that IL-15 effect also reached brown adipose tissue, with an acute induction of thermogenesis via upregulation of Uncoupling Proteins 1 and 3, PPAR-δ and -α and a final association with reduction of white adipose tissue mass (Almendro et al., 2008). The evidence pointed to a more multifaceted muscle-adipose axis with IL-15 as remote modulator (Quinn et al., 2009) when secreted from skeletal muscle, inducing GLUT4, enhancing glucose utilization, reducing adipose deposition and adipocyte size. Further studies have linked polymorphisms of IL-15 and metabolic syndrome propensity, including the following protein SNPs: rs1589241, rs1057972 (Pistilli et al., 2008), with a unique relation to metabolically obese normal weight patients (Di Renzo et al., 2006).

On a final note, a new twist in the *metainflamamtion phenomena* (Hotamisligil, 2006) observed in obesity has been described. The innate receptors members of the Pattern Recognition

Receptor Family, the NLRPs, are part of an ancestral detection system which recognizes danger associated molecules, resulting in the recruitment of Caspase-1 and the activation of IL-1β and IL-18, known proinflammatory cytokines (Lamkanfi & Dixit, 2009). Receptor NLRP3 has been associated to lipotoxicity sensing by recognizing ceramides production in macrophages and adipocytes, contributing to obesity-related inflammation by synthesis of IL-1β and blunted insulin signaling in liver and adipose tissue (Vandanmagsar et al., 2011). Moreover, IL-1β has been proven to regulate adipogenesis towards a more insulin resistance phenotype (Stienstra et al., 2010), which renders fundamental in a proinflamatory and toxic environment which is seen around the hypoxic and pre-adipocyte rich areas of adipose tissue.

4. Conclusions

Obesity is a multifactorial disease, characterized by adiposity-related consequences and disease, such as type 2 diabetes, cardiovascular disease, obstructive sleeping apnea, osteoarthritis, and cancer. Understanding the molecular dialogue between the 2 principally affected cells - adipocyte and skeletal myocyte - serves as the underlying scientific platform to understand why physical activity is beneficial and mandatory in these patients. The very notion that glucose uptake is enhanced in skeletal muscle during and after exercise provides a great glycemic control strategy, lowering the effects of excessive glucose in circulating plasma, like glycosylated hemoglobin levels (Andrade-Rodríguez et al., 2007; Sigal et al., 2007), increases plasma glutamine and arginine levels for the production of NO and glutathione not only improving vasodilation properties but also increasing antioxidant defenses (Krause & de Bittencourt,, 2008), and myocyte-derived IL-6 enhances glucose induced insulin secretion (Newsholme et al., 2010).

The application of a proper exercise program in obese patients, along with diet and lifestyle modification, ensures that the obese myocyte will get in shape, with a dynamic IMCL turnover, improved glucose and fat oxidation, genetic modulation of fiber remodeling, ending in progressive and sustained metabolic control. The dying myocytes will stop being so stressed with external stimuli and over-availability of substrates, decreasing in size and in oxygen requirements, modulating macrophage recruitment and inflammatory signals derived from them. The application of therapeutic drugs to improve the effects of exercise and act synergistically has been reported.

Thiazolidinediones (TZD) are a group of drugs that activate PPARγ, modulating all the downstream genes regulated by the transcription factor, including acyl~CoA synthetase, phosphoenolpyruvate carboxykinase and lipoprotein lipase, inducing FFA capture and storage in de novo adipocytes, lowering FFA levels in plasma at the cost of fast redistribution ("Lipid-steal" phenomenon) (Bermúdez et al., 2010). In insulin resistant models, TZD correct impaired myocyte insulin action (Zierath et al., 1998), normalize muscular insulin sensitivity and GLUT4 synthesis in conjunction with exercise (Hayener et al., 2000), lower waist-hip ratio due to a selective increase in lower body fat (Shadid et al., 2003), improve exercise capacity in type 2 diabetic patients (Regensteiner et al., 2005), and increase adiponectin levels (Yang et al., 2002) just as exercise does (Kriketos et al., 2004; Højbjerre et al., 2007); which is why the combination of a TZD and exercise are self-complementary in the treatment of insulin resistance (Lessard et al., 2007). The world-famous biguanide, Metformin, is the other pharmacological candidate to enhance exercise effects on the insulin resistance milieu. Exercise has been known to improve metformin effects (Tang et al., 2001), acting as co-adjuvants in the reduction of the incident of diabetes (Doggrell, 2002), increasing vascular function and lowering Ischemia Coronary Artery Disease patients (Jadhay et al., 2006), and finally, both can reduce the expression of the fat transporter FAT/CD36, blunting the progression of ceramides-mediated insulin resistance in myocyte (Smith et al., 2007). The insulin sensitizing effect of metformin are carried out via activation of AMPK (Hawley et al., 2002), simulating the very first effects on physical activity in skeletal muscle. Finally, Exercise is an ideal lifestyle intervention suitable and rightful to all obese patients, due to its counteracting measures against the molecular derangements observed in obesity, modulating local and systemic metabolic disturbances.

5. References

Abate N. & Chandalia M. (2003). The impact of ethnicity on type 2 diabetes. *Journal of Diabetes and its Complications* Vol. 17, No. 1 (January - February 2003), pp. 39-58.

Acharyya S, Ladner K, Nelsen LL, Damrauer J, Reiser PJ, et al. (2004). Cancer cachexia is regulated by selective targeting of skeletal muscle gene products. *Journal of Clinical Investigation* Vol. 114, No. 3 (August 2004), pp. 370-78.

Adami HO &Trichopoulos D. (2003). Obesity and mortality from cancer. *New England Journal of Medicine* Vol. 348, No.17 (April 2003), pp.1623-24.

Almendro V, Fuster G, Busquets S, Ametller E, Figueras M, et al. (2008). Effects of IL-15 on rat brown adipose tissue: uncoupling proteins and PPARs. *Obesity* Vol. 16, No. 2 (February 2008), pp. 285-89.

Andersen JL, Klitgaard H & Saltin B. (1994). "Myosin heavy chain isoforms in single fibers from m. vastus lateralis of sprinters: influence of training". *Acta Physiologica Scandinavica* Vol. 151, No. 2 (June 1994), pp. 135-42.

Andrade-Rodríguez HJ, Valadez-Castillo FJ, Hernández-Sierra JF, Gordillo-Moscoso AA, Dávila-Esqueda ME, et al. (2007). Effectiveness of supervised aerobic exercised in alternating weekdays associated with glycosilated hemoglobin levels among type 2 sedentary diabetic patients. *Gaceta Medica de Mexico* Vol. 143, No. 1 (January-February 2007), pp. 11-5.

Argilés JM, López-Soriano FJ & Busquets S. (2009). Therapeutic potential of interleukin-15: a myokine involved in muscle wasting and adiposity. *Drug Discovery Today* Vol. 14, No. 3-4 (February 2009), pp. 208-13.

Arita Y, Kihara S, Ouchi N, Takahashi M, Maeda K, et al. (1999). Paradoxical decrease of an adipose-specific protein, adiponectin, in obesity. *Biochemical and Biophysical Research Communications* Vol. 257, No. 1 (April 1999), pp.79-83.

Arner E, Westermark PO, Spalding KL, Britton T, Rydén M, et al. (2010). Adipocyte turnover: relevance to human adipose tissue morphology". *Diabetes* Vol. 59, No. 1 (January 2010), pp. 105-09.

Bassel-Duby R & Olson E. (2006). Signaling pathways in skeletal remodeling. *Annual Review of Biochemistry* Vol. 75, pp. 19-37.

Bassel-Duny R & Olson EN. (2003). Role of calcineurin in striated muscle: development, adaptation and disease. *Biochemical and Biophysical Research Communications* Vol. 311, No. 4 (November 2003), pp. 1133-1141.

Bermúdez V, Finol F, Parra N, Parra M, Pérez A, et al. "PPAR-γ agonists and their role in type 2 diabetes mellitus management". *American Journal of Therapeutics* Vol. 17, No. 3 (May-June 2010), pp. 274-283.

Blair SN, Cheng Y & Holder JS. (2001). Is physical activity or physical fitness more important in defining health benefits?. *Medicine Science in Sports and Exercise* Vol.33, No.6 (June 2001), pp.S379-S399.

Brook CG, Lloyd JK & Wolf OH. Relation between age of onset of obesity and size and number of adipose cells. *British Medical Journal* Vol. 2, No. 5804 (April 1972), pp. 25-27.

Bruun JM, Lihn AS, Pedersen SB, Richelsen B. (2005). Monocyte chemoattractant protein-1 release is higher in visceral than subcutaneous human adipose tissue (AT): implication of macrophage resident in the AT. *Journal of Clinical Endocrinology and Metabolism* Vol. 90, No. 4 (April 2005), pp. 2282-89.

Caballero B (2007). The global epidemic of obesity: an overview. *Epidemiologic Reviews* Vol.29, (June 2007), pp.1-5.

Carbó N, López-Soriano J, Costelli P, Alvarez B, Busquets S, et al. (2001). Interleukin-15 mediates reciprocal regulation of adipose and muscle mass: a potential role in body weight control. *Biochimica et Biophysica Acta* Vol. 1526, No. 1 (April 2001), pp. 17-24.

Carbó N, López-Soriano J, Costelli P, Busquets S, Alvarez B, et al. (2000). Interleukin-15 antagonizes protein waste in tumour-bearing rats. *British Journal of Cancer* Vol. 83, No. 4 (August 2000), pp. 526-31.

Carey AL, Bruce CR, Sacchetti M, Anderson MJ, Olsen DB, et al. (2004). Interleukin-6 and tumor necrosis factor-alpha are not increases in patients with type 2 diabetes: evidence that plasma IL-6 is related to fat mass and not insulin responsiveness. *Diabetologia* Vol. 47, No. 6 (June 2004), pp. 1029-37.

Carnethon MR. (2009). Physical activity and cardiovascular disease: how much is enough?. *American Journal of Lifestyle Medicine* Vol. 3, No. 1 (July 2009), pp. 44S-49S.

Chakravarthy M. &Booth FW. (2004). Eating, exercise and 'thrifty' genotypes: connecting the dots toward an evolutionary understanding of modern chronic disease. *Journal of Applied Physiology* Vol. 96, No. 1 (January 2004), pp. 3-10.

Cheng YJ, Gregg E, De Rekeneire N, Williams DE, Imperatore G, et al. (2007). Muscle-strengthening activity and its association with insulin sensitivity. *Diabetes Care* Vol. 30, No. 9 (September 2007), pp. 2264-70.

Chin E, Olson EN, Richardson JA, Yang Q, Humphries C, et al. (1998). A calcineurin - dependent transcriptional pathway controls skeletal muscle fiber type. *Genes & Development* Vol. 12, No. 16 (August 1998), pp. 2499-2509.

Copps K &White M. (2009) Breathing room: the (un)natural history of adipose michrohypoxia and insulin resistance. *Diabetes* Vol. 58, No. 1 (January 2009), pp.26-27.

Dann SG, Selvaraj A & Thomas G. mTOR complex1-S6K1 signaling: at the crossroads of obesity, diabetes and cancer. *Trends in Molecular Medicine* Vol. 13, No. 6 (June 2007), pp. 252-59.

Darlington G, Ross S & MacDougald O. (1998). The role of C/EBP genes in adipocyte differentiation. *Journal of Biological Chemistry* Vol.273, No.46 (November 1998), pp. 30057-060.

de Luis DA, Gonzalez Sagrado M, Conde R, Aller R, Izaola O, et al. (2009). Relation of resistin levels with cardiovascular risk factors and insulin resistance in non-diabetes obese patients. *Diabetes Research and Clinical Practice* Vol. 84, No. 2 (May 2009), pp.174-8.

de Vries J. (1995). Immunosuppressive and anti-inflammatory properties of interleukin 10. *Annals of Medicine* Vol. 25, No. 5 (October 1995), pp. 537-41.

DeFronzo RA, Gunnarsson R, et al. (1985). Effect of insulin on peripheral and splanchnic glucose metabolism in noninsulin-dependent (type II) diabetes mellitus. *Journal of Clinical Investigation* Vol.76, No. 1 (July 1985), pp. 149-155.

Di Renzo L, Bigioni M, Bottini FG, Del Gobbo V, Premrov MG, et al. (2006). Normal weight obese syndrome: role of single nucleotide polymorphism of IL-15Ralpha and MTHFR 677C—T genes in the relationship between body composition and resting metabolic rate. *European Review for Medical Pharmacological Sciences* Vol. 10, No. 5 (September-October 2006), pp. 235-45.

Dietze D, Koenen M, Röhrig K, Horikoshi H, Hauner H, et al. (2002). Impairment of insulin signaling in human skeletal muscle cells by co-culture with human adipocytes. Diabetes Vol. 51, No. 8 (August 2002), pp. 2369-76.

Doggrell S. (2002). Metformin & lifestyle intervention prevent type 2 diabetes: lifestyle intervention has the greater effect. *Expert Opinion on Pharmacotherapy* Vol. 3, No. 7 (July 2002), pp. 1011-13.

Dulloo AG, Jacquet J, Seydoux J, Montani JP. (2006). The thrifty 'catch-up fat' phenotype: its impact on insulin sensitivity during growth trajectories to obesity and metabolic syndrome. *International Journal of Obesity (London)* Vol.30, No. S4 (December 2006), pp. S23-S35.

Dunn A, Andersen R, Jakicic JM. (1998). Lifestyle physical activity interventions. History, short- and long-term effects, and recommendations. *American Journal of Preventive Medicine* Vol.15, No.4 (November 1998), pp.398-412.

Egger G & Swinburn B (1997). An ecological approach to the obesity pandemic. *British Medical Journal* Vol.315, No.7106 (August 1997), pp.477-80.

Elmquist JK & Flier J. (2004). The fat-brain axis enters a new dimension. Science Vol. 304, No. 5667 (April 2004), pp. 63-64.

Fitts R. (2003). Effects of regular exercise training on skeletal contractile function". *American Journal of Physical Medicine & Rehabilitation* Vol. 82, No. 4 (April 2003), pp. 320-31.

Fletcher GF, Balady G, Blair SN, Blumenthal J, Caspersen C, et al. (1996). A statement for Health Professionals by the Committee on Exercise and Cardiac rehabilitation of the Council on Clinical Cardiology, American Heart Association.. *Circulation* Vol.94, No.4 (August 1996), pp.857-62.

Fletcher GF, Blair SN, Blumenthal J, Caspersen C, Chaitman B, et al. (1992). Statement on exercise. Benefits and recommendations for the physical activity programs for all Americans. A statement for health professionals by the Committee on Exercise and Cardiac Rehabilitation of the Council on Clinical Cardiology, American Heart Association. *Circulation* Vol.86, No.1 (July 1992), pp.340-44.

Frühbeck G, Gómez-Ambrosi J, Muruzábal FJ, Burrell MA. (2001). The adipocyte: a model for integration of endocrine and metabolic signaling in energy metabolism regulation. *American Journal of Physiology Endocrinology and Metabolism* Vol. 280, No. 6 (June 2001), pp. E827-E847.

Frydelund-Larsen L, Penkowa M, Akerstrom T, Zankari A, Nielsen S, et al. (2007). Exercise induces interleukin-8 receptor (CXCR2) expression in human skeletal muscle. *Experimental Physiology* Vol. 92, No. 1 (January 2007), pp. 233-40.

Fu M, Wang C, Li Z, Sakamaki T, Pestell RG. (2004). Cyclin D1: normal and abnormal functions. *Endocrinology* Vol.145, No. 12 (December 2004), pp.5439-47.

Gardner G & Halweil B (2000). "Hunger, escaping excess". World Watch Vol.13,No4 (July 2000), pp.25-35.

Godínez-Gutiérrez S, Marmolejo-Orozco G, Marquez-Rodríguez E, Siordia-Vázquez JJ & Baeza-Camacho R. (2002). La grasa visceral y su importancia en obesidad. *Revista de Endocrinología y Nutrición* Vol. 10, No. 3 (July-September 2002), pp.121-27.

Goodpaster B, He J, Watkins S, Kelley D. (2001). Skeletal muscle lipid content and insulin resistance: evidence for a paradox in endurance-trained athletes. *Journal of Clinical Endocrinology and Metabolism* Vol. 86, No. 1 (December 2001), pp. 5755-5761.

Graham T, Yang Q, Blüher M, Hammarstedt A, Ciaraldi TP, et al. (2006). Retinol-binding protein 4 and insulin resistance in lean, obese, and diabetic subjects. *New England Journal of Medicine* Vol.354, No. 24 (June 2006), pp.2552-63.

Gregoire F, Smas C & Sul HS (1998). Understanding adipocyte differentiation. *Physiological Reviews* Vol.78, No.3 (July 1998), pp.783-809.

Gregoire F. (2001). Adipocyte differentiation: from fibroblast to endocrine cell. *Experimental Biology and Medicine* Vol.226, No. 11 (December 2001), pp.997-1002.

Guo Z. (2007). Intramyocellular lipid kinetics and insulin resistance. Lipids in Health and Disease Vol. 6 (July 2007), pp.18-25.

Guzik TJ, Marvar PJ, Czesnikiewicz-Guzik M, Korbut R. (2007). Perivascular adipose tissue as a Messenger of the brain-vessel axis: role in vascular inflammation and dysfunction". *Journal of Physiological Pharmacology* Vol.58, No. 4 (December 2007), pp.591-610.

Halberg N, Wernstedt-Asterholm I, & Scherer PE. (2008). The adipocyte as an endocrine cell. *Endocrinology and Metabolism Clinics of North America* Vol. 37, No. 3 (September 2008), pp. 753-68.

Hamilton M & Booth F. (2000). Skeletal muscle adaptation to exercise: a century of progress. *Journal of Applied Physiology* Vol. 88, No. 1 (January 2000), pp. 327-331.

Hauner H. (2010). Adipose tissue inflammation: are small or large fat cells to blame?. *Diabetologia* Vol. 53, No. 2 (February 2010), pp. 223-225.

Havener A, Reichart D & Olefsky J. (2000). Exercise and thiazolidinedione therapy normalize insulin action in the obese Zucker fatty rat. *Diabetes* Vol. 49, No. 12 (December 2000), pp. 2154-59.

Hawley S, Gadalla AE, Olsen GS, Hardie DG. (2002). The antidiabetic drug metformin activates the AMP-activated protein kinase cascade via an Adenine Nucleotide-independent mechanism. *Diabetes* Vol. 51, No. 8 (August 2002), pp. 2420-25.

Hayashi T, Wojtaszeski J & Goodyear L. (1997). Exercise regulation of glucose in skeletal muscle. *American Journal of Physiology Endocrinology and Metabolism* Vol. 273, No. 6 pt1 (December 1997), pp. E1039-E1051.

Hein HO, Suadicani P, Gyntelberg F. (1992). Physical fitness or physical activity as predictor of ischemic heart disease? A 17-year follow-up in the Copenhagen Male Study. *Journal of Internal Medicine* Vol.232, No.6 (December 1992), pp.471-79.

Henriksen EJ & Holloszy JO. Effect of diffusion distance on measurement of rat skeletal muscle glucose transport in vitro. *Acta Physiologica Scandinavica* Vol.143, No. 4 (December 1991), pp. 381-86.

Henriksen EJ, Bourey RE, Rodnick KJ, Koranyi L, Permutt MA, Holloszy JO. (1990). Glucose transport protein content and glucose transport capacity in rat skeletal muscle: *American Journal of Physiology Endocrinology and Metabolism* Vol. 259, No. 4(pt 1) (October 1990), pp. E593-E598.

Hickey MS, Carey JO, Azevedo JL, Houmard JA, Pories WJ, Israel RG, Dohm GL. (1995). Skeletal muscle fiber composition is related to adiposity and in vitro glucose transport rate in humans. *American Journal of Physiology Endocrinology and Metabolism* Vol. 268, No. 3(pt 1) (March 1995), pp. E453-E457.

Højbjerre L, Rosenzweig M, Dela F, Bruun JM, Stallknecht B. (2007). Acute exercise increases adipose tissue interstitial adiponectin concentration in healthy overweight and lean subjects. *European Journal of Endocrinology* Vol. 157, No. 5 (November 2007), pp. 613-23.

Holmes B, Sparling DP, Olson AL, Winder WW, Dohm GL. (2005). Regulation of muscle GLUT4 enhancer factor and myocyte enhancer factor 2 by AMP-activated protein kinase. *American Journal of Physiology Endocrinology and Metabolism* Vol. 289, No. 6 (December 2005), pp. E1071-E1076.

Hosogai N, Fukuhara A, Oshima K, Miyata Y, Tanaka S, et al. (2007). Adipose tissue hypoxia in obesity and its impact on adipocytokine dysregulation. *Diabetes* Vol. 56, No. 4 (April 2007), pp. 901-11.

Hotamisligil GS. (1999). Mechanism of TNF-alpha induced insulin resistance. *Experimental and Clinical Endocrinology & Diabetes* Vol. 107, No. 2, pp.119-125.

Hotamisligil GS. (2006). Inflammation and metabolic disorders. *Nature* Vol. 4444, No. 7121 (December 2006), pp. 860-67.

Hulver MW, Berggren JR, Cortright RN, Dudek RW, Thompson RP, et al. (2003). Skeletal muscle lipid metabolism with obesity. *American Journal of Physiology Endocrinology and Metabolism* Vol. 284, No. 4 (April 2003), pp. E741-E747.

Jadhav S, Ferrel W, Greer I, Petrie JR, Cobbe SM, et al. (2006). Effects of metformin on microvascular function and exercise tolerance in women with angina and normal coronary arteries. *Journal of the American College of Cardiology* Vol. 48, No. 5 (September 2006), pp. 956-96.

Jiang LQ, Garcia-Roves PM, de Castro Barbosa T, Zierath JR. (2010). Constitutively active calcineurin in skeletal muscle increases endurance performance and mitochondrial respiratory capacity. *American Journal of Physiology Endocrinology and Metabolism* Vol. 298, No. 1 (January 2010), pp. E8-E16.

Jørgensen S, Richter EA & Wojtaszewski J. (2006). Role of AMPK in skeletal muscle metabolic regulation and adaptation in relation to exercise. *Physiology* Vol. 574, No. pt 1 (July 2006), pp. 17-31.

Kadowaki T, Hara K, Yamauchi T, Terauchi Y, Tobe K, et al. (2003). Molecular mechanism of insulin resistance and obesity. *Experimental Biology and Medicine* Vol.228, No. 10 (November 2003), pp. 1111-1117.

Kelley DE, Goodpaster B, Wing RR, Simoneau JA. (1999). Skeletal muscle fatty acid metabolism in association with insulin resistance, obesity and weight loss. *American Journal of Physiology Endocrinology and Metabolism* Vol. 277, No.6 pt 1(December 1999), pp. E1130-E1141.

Kelly T, Yang W, Chen CS, Reynolds K, He J. (2008). Global burden of obesity in 2005 and projections to 2030. *International Journal of Obesity (London)* Vol.32, No.9 (September 2008), pp.1431-37.

Kershaw E & Flier J. (2004). Adipose tissue as an endocrine organ. *Journal of Clinical Endocrinology & Metabolism* Vol 89, No. 6 (June 2004), pp. 2548-56.

Kewalrami G, Bilan OJ & Klip A. (2010). Muscle insulin resistance: assault by lipids, cytokines and local macrophages". *Current Opinion in Clinical Nutrition and Metabolic Care* Vol. 13, No. 4 (July 2010), pp.382-90.

Kieffer TJ & Habener JF. (2000). The adipoinsular axis: effects of leptin on pancreatic β-cells. *American Journal of Physiology Endocrinology and Metabolism* Vol. 278, No. 1 (January 2000), pp.E1-E14.

Kim JY, Hickner RC, Cortright RL, Dohm GL, Houmard JA. (2000). Lipid oxidation is reduced in obese human skeletal muscle. *American Journal of Physiology Endocrinology and Metabolism* Vol. 279, No. 5 (November 2000), pp. E1039-E1044.

Klein S, Coyle EF & Wolfe RR. (1994). Fat metabolism during low-intensity exercise in endurance-trained and untrained men. *American Journal of Physiology Endocrinology and Metabolism* Vol. 267, No. 6 pt 1 (December 1994), pp. E934-E940.

Koch LG & Britton SL. (2008). Aerobic metabolism underlies complexity and capacity. *Journal of Physiology* Vol. 586, No. 1 (January 2008), pp. 83-95.

Koonen D, Sung M, Kao C, Dolinsky VW, Koves TR, et al. (2010). Alterations in skeletal muscle fatty acid handling predisposes middle-aged mice to diet-induced insulin resistance. *Diabetes* Vol. 59, No. 6 (June 2010), pp. 1366-75.

Koumenis C & Wouters B. (2006). Translating tumor hypoxia: unfolded protein response (UPR)—dependent and UPR—independent pathways. *Molecular Cancer Research* Vol.4, No. 7 (July 2006), pp. 423-36.

Krause Mda S & de Bittencourt PI. (2008). Type 2 diabetes: can exercise impair autoimmune event? The L-arginine/glutamine coupling hypothesis. Cell Biochemistry and Function Vol. 26, No. 4 (June 2008), pp. 406-33.

Kriketos A, Gan SK, Poynten AM, et al. (2004). Exercise increases adiponectin levels and insulin sensitivity in humans. *Diabetes Care* Vol. 27, No. 2 (February 2004), pp. 629-30.

Kubaszek A, Pihlajamaki J, Komarovski V, Lindi V, Lindström J, et al. (2003). Promoter polymorphism of the TNF-alpha (G-308A) and IL-6 (C-174G) genes predict the conversion from impaired glucose tolerance to type 2 diabetes: the Finnish Diabetes Prevention Study. *Diabetes* Vol. 52, No. 7 (July 2003), pp. 1872-76.

Kudo T, Katayama T, Imaizumi K, Yasuda Y, Yatera M, et al. (2002). The unfolded protein response is involved in the pathology of Alzheimer´s disease. *Annals of the New York Academy of Sciences* Vol. 977,pp.349-55.

Lacasa D, Taleb S, Keophiphath M, Miranville A, Clement K. (2007). Macrophage-secreted factors impair human adipogenesis: involvement of proinflammatory state in preadipocytes. *Endocrinology* Vol. 148, No. 2 (February 1007), pp. 868-77.

Lamkanfi M & Dixit VM. (2009). Inflammasomes: guardians of cytosolic sanctity. *Immunological Reviews* Vol. 227, No. 1 (January 2009), pp. 95-105.

LaMonte M, Barlow C, Jurca R, Kampert JB, Church TS, et al. (2005). Cardiorespiratory fitness is inversely associated with incident of metabolic syndrome. A prospective study of men and women. *Circulation* Vol. 112, No. 4 (July 2005), pp. 505-12.

Lee SJ, Kuk J, Katzmarzyk PT, Blair SN, Church TS, et al. (2005). Cardiorespiratory fitness attenuates metabolic risk independent of abdominal subcutaneous and visceral fat in mean. *Diabetes Care* Vol. 28, No. 4 (April 2005), pp. 895-901.

Lessard S, Rivas D, Chen ZP, Bonen A, Febbraio MA, et al. (2007). Tissue-specific effects of rosiglitazone and exercise in the treatment of lipid-induced insulin resistance. *Diabetes* Vol. 56, No. 7 (July 2007), pp. 1856-64.

Lillioja S, Young A, Culter C, Ivy JL, Abbott WG, et al. (1987). "Skeletal muscle capillary density and fiber type are possible determinants of in vivo insulin resistance in man. *Journal of Clinical Investigation* Vol. 80, No.2 (August 1987), pp. 415-24.

Lim CT, Kola B & Korbonits M. (2010). "AMPK as a mediator of hormonal signaling. *Journal of Molecular Endocrinology* Vol. 44, No. 2 (February 2010), pp. 87-97.

Lindsay RS & Bennett PH. (2001). Type 2 diabetes, the thrifty phenotype - an overview. *British Medicine Bulletin* Vol. 60, pp. 21-32.

Marchesini G, Natale S, Tiraferri F, Tartaglia A, Moscatiello S, et al (2003). The burden of obesity on everyday life: a role for osteoarticular and respiratory diseases. *Diabetes Nutrition and Metabolism* Vol.16, No.5-6 (October-December 2003), pp.284-90.

Marciniak SJ & Ron D. (2006). Endoplasmic reticulum stress signaling in disease. *Physiological Reviews* Vol. 86, No. 4 (October 2006), pp. 1133-1149.

Marini M & Veicsteinas A. (2010). The exercised skeletal muscle: a review". E*uropean Journal of Translational Myology – Myology Reviews* Vol. 10, No. 3, pp. 105-120.

Meex R, Schrauwen-Hinderling V, Moonen-Kornips E, Schaart G, Mensink M, et al. (2010). Restoration of muscle mitochondrial function and metabolic flexibility in type 2 diabetes by exercise training is paralleled by increased myocellular fat storage and improved insulin sensitivity. *Diabetes* Vol. 59, No. 3 (March 2010), pp. 572-79.

Michiels C, Minet E, Mottet D, Raes M. (2002). Regulation of gene expression by oxygen: NF-kappaB and HIF-1, two extremes. *Free Radical Biology and Medicine* Vol. 33, No. 9 (November 2002), pp.1231-42.

Mietus-Snyder M & Lustig RH. (2008). Childhood obesity: adrift in the limbic triangle. *Annual Review Medicine* Vol. 59, pp.147-62.

Moro C, Bajpeyi S & Smith SR. (2008). Determinants of intramyocellular triglyceride turnover: implications for insulin sensitivity. *American Journal of Physiology Endocrinology and Metabolism* Vol. 294, No. 2 (February 2008), pp.E203-E213.

Musi N, Fujii N, Hirshman M, Ekberg I, Fröberg S, et al. (2001). AMP-activated protein kinase (AMPK) is activated in muscle of subjects with type 2 diabetes during exercise. *Diabetes* Vol. 50, No. 5 (May 2001), pp. 921-27.

Must A, Spadano J, Coakley E, Field AE, Colditz G, Dietz WH. (1999). The disease burden associated with overweight and obesity. *Journal of the American Medical Association* Vol. 282, No.16 (October 1999), pp.1523-29.

Neel JV. (1962). Diabetes mellitus: a 'thrifty' genotype rendered detrimental by 'progress'?. *American Journal of Human Genetics* Vol. 14 (December 1962), pp. 353-62.

Newsholme P, Homem de Bittencourt P, O'Hagan C, De Vito G, Murphy C, et al. (2010). Exercise and possible molecular mechanism of protection from vascular disease and diabetes: the central role of ROS and nitric oxide. *Clinical Science* Vol. 118, No. 5 (November 2010), pp. 341-49.

Niskanen L, Laaksonen D, Nyyssönen K, et al. "Inflammation, abdominal obesity, and smoking as predictors of hypertension". *Hypertension* 2004;44:859-65

O'Dea K (1992). Obesity and diabetes in "the land of milk and honey. *Diabetes Metabolism Review* Vol.8, No.4 (December 1992), pp. 373-88.

Opal SM & DePalo VA. (2000). Anti-inflammatory cytokines. *Chest* Vol. 117, No. 4 (April 2000), pp. 1162-72.

Oster G, Edelsberg J, O'Sullivan AK, Thompson D. (2000) The clinical and economic burden of obesity in a managed care setting. *American Journal of Managing Care* Vol. 6, No.6, (June 2000), pp. 681-89.

Ostrowski K, Rohde T, Asp S, Schjerling P, Pedersen BK. (1999). Pro- and anti-inflammatory cytokine balance in strenuous exercise in humans. *Journal of Physiology* Vol. 515 (February 1999), pp. 287-91.

Pagel-Langenickel I, Bao J, Pang L, Sack M. (2010). The role of mitochondria in the pathology of skeletal muscle insulin resistance. *Endocrine Reviews* Vol. 31, No. 1 (February 2010), pp. 25-51.

Pan DA, Lillioja S, Kriketos AD, Milner MR, Baur LA, et al. (1997). Skeletal muscle triglycerides levels are inversely related to insulin action. *Diabetes* Vol. 46, No. 6 (June 1997), pp. 983-88.

Panagiotakos DB, Pitsavos C, Yannakoulia M, Chrysohoou C, Stefanadis C. (2005). The implication of obesity and central fat on markers of chronic inflammation: the ATTICA study. *Atherosclerosis* Vol.183, No.2 (December 2005), pp.308-15.

Pate RR, Pratt M, Blair SN, Haskell WL, Macera CA, et al. (1995). Physical activity and public health - A recommendation from the Centers for Disease Control and Prevention and the American College of Sports Medicine. *Journal of the American Medical Association* Vol.273, No.5 (February 1995), pp.402-07.

Pedersen BK, Åkerström TC, Nielsen AR, Fischer CP. (2007). Role of myokines in exercise and metabolism. *Journal of Applied Physiology* Vol. 103, No. 3 (September 2007), pp. 1093-98.

Pedersen BK, Febbraio M & Mooney R. (2007). Interleukin-6 does/does not have a beneficial role in insulin sensitivity and glucose homeostasis. *Journal of Applied Physiology* Vol. 102, No. 2 (February 2007), pp. 814-16.

Petersen AM & Pedersen BK. (2005). The anti-inflammatory effect of exercise. *Journal of Applied Physiology* Vol. 98, No. 4 (April 2005), pp.1154-62.

Pette D & Staron RS. (1997). Mammalian skeletal muscle fiber type transitions. *International Review of Cytology* Vol. 170, pp.143-223.

Pistilli EE, Devaney JM, Gordish-Dressman H, Bradbury MK, Seip RL, et al. (2008). Interleukin-15 and Interleukin-15Ra SNPs and association with muscle, bone and predictors of metabolic syndrome. *Cytokine* Vol. 43, No. 1 (July 2008), pp. 45-53.

Pi-Sunyer FX. (2000). The obesity pandemic: pathophysiology and consequences of obesity. *Obesity Research* Vol.10, No.10, pp.97S-104S.

Pollock M, Franklin B, Balady G, Chaitman BL, Fleq JL, et al. (2000). AHA Science Advisory. Resistance exercise in individuals with and without cardiovascular disease. *Circulation* Vol.101, No.7 (February 2000), pp.28-33.

Prentice A, Rayco-Solon P & Moore S. (2005). Insights from the developing world: thrifty genotypes and thrifty phenotypes. *Proceedings of the Nutrition Society* Vol.64, No. 2 (May 2005), pp.153-161.

Quinn LS, Anderson BG, Drivdahl RH, Alvarez B, Argilés JM. (2002). Overexpression of interleukin-15 induces skeletal muscle hypertrophy in vitro: implications for treatment of muscle wasting disorders. *Experimental Cell Research* Vol. 280, No. 1 (October 2002), pp. 55-63.

Quinn LS, Anderson BG, Strait-Bodey L, Stroud AM, Argilés JM. (2009). Oversecretion of interleukin-15 from skeletal muscle reduces adiposity. *American Journal of Physiology Endocrinology and Metabolism* Vol. 296, No. 1 (January 2009), pp. E191-E202.

Quinn LS, Strait-Bodey L, Andersen BG, Argilés JM, Havel PJ. (2005). Interleukin-15 stimulates adiponectin secretion by 3T3-L1 adipocytes: evidence for a skeletal muscle-to-fat- signaling pathway. *Cell Biology International* Vol. 29, No. 6 (June 2005), pp. 449-57.

Quinn LS. (2008). Interleukin-15: a muscle-derived cytokine regulating fat-to-lean body composition. Journal of Animal *Science* Vol. 86, No. 14 Suppl (April 2008), pp. E75-E83.

Rabøl R, Larsen S, Højberg PM, Almdal T, Boushel R, et al. (2010). Regional anatomic differences in skeletal muscle mitochondrial respiration in type 2 diabetes and obesity. *Journal of Clinical Endocrinology and Metabolism* Vol.95, No. 2 (February 2010), pp.857-63.

Randle PJ, Garland PB, Hales CN, Newsholme EA. (1963). The glucose fatty acid cycle: its role in insulin sensitivity and the metabolic disturbances of diabetes mellitus". *Lancet* Vol.13, No.1 (April 1963), pp.7285-89.

Regazzetti C, Peraldi P, Grémeaux T, Najem-Lendom R, Ben-Sahra I, et al. (2009). Hypoxia decreases insulin signaling pathways in adipocytes. *Diabetes* Vol.58, No.1 (January 2009), pp. 95-103.

Regensteiner J, Bauer T & Reusch J. (2005). Rosiglitazone improves exercise capacity in individuals with type 2 diabetes. *Diabetes Care* Vol. 28, No. 12 (December 2005), pp. 2877-83.

Röckl K, Hirshman MF, Brandauer J, Fujii N, Witters LA, et al. (2007). Skeletal muscle adaptation to exercise training. AMP-activated protein kinase mediates muscle fiber type shift. *Diabetes* Vol. 56, No. 8 (August 2007), pp. 2062-69.

Rose AJ & Richter EA. "Skeletal muscle glucose uptake during exercise: how is it regulated?. *Physiology* (Bethesda) Vol. 20 (August 2005), pp. 260-70.

Rosengren A &Wilhelmsen L. (1997). Physical activity protects against coronary death and deaths from all causes in middle-aged men. Evidence from a 20-year follow-up of the primary prevention study in Göteborg. *Annals of Epidemiology* Vol.7, No.1 (January 1997), pp.69-75.

Rotter V, Nagaev I & Smith U. (2003). Interleukin-6 (IL-6) induces insulin resistance in 3T3-L1 adipocytes and is, like IL-8 and Tumor Necrosis Factor-α, overexpressed in human fat cells from insulin-resistant subjects. *Journal of Biological Chemistry* Vol. 278, No. 46 (November 2003), pp. 45777-784.

Ryu E, Harding H, Angelastro JM, Vitolo OV, Ron D, et al. (2002). Endoplasmic reticulum stress and the unfolded protein response in cellular models of Parkinson´s disease. *Journal of Neuroscience* Vol. 22, No. 24 (December 2002), pp. 10690-698.

Saltin B (1992). Sedentary lifestyle: an underestimated health risk. *Journal of Internal Medicine* Vol.232, No.6 (December 1992), pp. 467-69.

Samokhvalov V, Bilan P, Schertzer JD, Antonescu CN, Klip A. (2009). Palmitate-and lipopolysaccharide-activated macrophage evoke contrasting insulin responses in muscle cells. *American Journal of Physiology Endocrinology and Metabolism* Vol. 296, No. 1 (January 2009), pp.E37-E46.

Sartipy P & Loskutoff D. (2003). Monocyte chemoattractant protein 1 in obesity and insulin resistance. *Proceedings of the National Academy of Sciences of the United States of America* Vol. 100, No. 12 (June 2003), pp.7265-70.

Sawada S, Lee IM, Naito H, Noguchi J, Tsukamoto K, et al. (2003). Long-term trends in cardiorespiratory fitness and the incidence of type 2 diabetes. *Diabetes Care* Vol. 33, No. 6 (June 2010), pp. 1353-57.

Scheuner D & Kaufman R. (2008). The unfolded protein response: a pathway that links insulin demand with β-cell failure and diabetes. *Endocrine Reviews* Vol. 29, No. 3 (may 2008), pp.317-33.

Schiaffino S & Serrano AL. (2002). Calcineurin signaling and neural control of skeletal muscle fiber type and size. *Trends in Pharmacological Sciences* Vol. 23, No. 12 (December 2002), pp. 569-75.

Scott W, Stevens J & Binder-Macleod SA. (2001). Human skeletal muscle fiber type classifications. *Physical Therapy* Vol. 81, No. 11 (November 2001), pp. 1810-16.

Sell H, Dietze-Schroeder D & Eckel J. (2006). The adipocyte-myocyte axis in insulin resistance. *Trends in Endocrinology and Metabolism* Vol. 17, No. 10 (December 2006), pp. 416-22.

Sell H, Eckardt K, Taube A, Tews D, Gurqui M, et al. (2008). Skeletal muscle insulin resistance induced by adipocyte-conditioned medium: underlying mechanisms and reversibility. *American Journal of Physiology Endocrinology and Metabolism* Vol. 294, No. 6 (June 2008), pp. E1070-E1077.

Sethi JK &Vidal-Puig AJ. (2007). Adipose tissue function and plasticity orchestrate nutritional adaptation. *Journal of Lipid Research* Vol. 48, No. 6 (June 2007), pp.1253-62.

Shadid S & Jensen M. (2003). Effects of pioglitazone versus diet and exercise on metabolic health and fat distribution in upper body obesity. *Diabetes Care* Vol. 26, No. 11 (November 2003), pp. 3148-52.

Sherwood DJ, Dufresne SD, Markuns JF, Cheatham B, Moller DE, et al. (1999). Differential regulation of MAP kinase, p70(S6k) and Akt by contraction and insulin in rat skeletal muscle. *American Journal of Physiology* Vol. 276, No. 5 pt 1 (May 1999), pp. E870-E878.

Shimomura I, Hammer R, Ikemoto S, Brown MS, Goldstein JL. (1999). Leptin reverses insulin resistance and diabetes mellitus in mice with congenital lipodystrophy. *Nature* Vol. 401, No. 6748 (September 1999), pp.73-76.

Shulman G. (2000). Cellular mechanisms of insulin resistance. *Journal of Clinical Investigation* Vol.106, No2 (July 2000), pp.171-76.

Sigal RK, Kenny GP, Boulé NG, Wells GA, Prud´homme D, et al. (2007). Effects of aerobic training, resistance training, or both on glycemic control in type 2 diabetes: a randomized trial. *Annals of Internal Medicine* Vol. 147, No. 6 (September 2007), pp. 357-69.

Simons PJ, van de Pangaart P, van Roomen CP, Aerts JM, Boon L. (2005). Cytokine-mediated modulation of leptin and adiponectin secretion during in vitro adipogenesis: evidence that tumor necrosis factor-α- and interleukin-1β treated human preadipocytes are potent leptin producers. *Cytokine* Vol. 32, No. 2 (October 2005), pp.94-103.

Smith AC, Mullen KL, Junkin KA, Nickerson J, Chabowski A, et al. (2007). Metformin and exercise reduce muscle FAT/CD36 and lipid accumulation and blunt the progression of high-fat diet-induced hyperglycemia. *American Journal of Physiology Endocrinology and Metabolism* Vol. 293, No. 1 (July 2007), pp. E172-E181.

Song, XM, Ryder JW, Kawano Y, et al. (1999). Muscle fiber type specificity in insulin signal transduction. American Journal of Physiology Regulatory Integrative Comparative Physiology Vol. 277, No. 6 (December 1999), pp. R1690-R1696.

Steppan C & Lazar MA. (2002). Resistin and obesity-associated insulin resistance". *Trends in Endocrinology and Metabolism* Vol. 13, No. 1 (January-February 2002), pp. 18-23.

Stienstra R, Joosten LA, Koenen T, van Tits B, van Diepen, et al. (2010). The inflammasome-mediated caspase-1 activation controls adipocyte differentiation and insulin Sensitivity. *Cell Metabolism* Vol. 12, No. 6 (December 2010), pp. 593-605.

Summermatter S, Marcelino H, Arsenijevic D, Buchala A, Aprikian O, et al. (2009). Adipose tissue plasticity during catch-up growth fat driven by thrifty metabolism. *Diabetes* Vol. 58, No. 10 (October 2009), pp. 2228-37.

Suzuki K, Yamada M, Kurakake S, Okamura N, Yamaya K, et al. (2000). Circulating cytokines and hormones with immunosuppressive but neutrophil-priming potentials rise after endurance exercise in humans. *European Journal of Applied Physiology* Vol. 81, No. 4 (March 2000), pp. 281-87.

Tang T & Reed MJ. (2001). Exercise adds to metformin and acarbose efficacy in db/db mice. *Metabolism* Vol. 50, No. 9 (September 2001), pp. 1049-53.

Tanner CJ, Bakarat H, Dohm L, Pories WJ, MacDonald KG, Cunnigham PR, et al. (2001). Muscle fiber type is associated with obesity and weight loss. *American Journal of Physiology Endocrinology and Metabolism* Vol. 282, No. 6 (June 2001), pp.E1191-E1196.

Taube A, Eckardt K & Eckel J. (2009). Role of lipid-derived mediators in skeletal muscle resistance. *American Journal of Physiology Endocrinology and Metabolism* Vol. 297, No. 5 (November 2009), pp. E1004-E1012.

Thompson D, Wolf A. (2001) The medical-care cost burden of obesity. *Obesity Reviews* Vol.2 No.3 (August 2001), pp. 189-97.

Thompson P. (2003). "Exercise and. physical activity in the prevention and treatment of atherosclerotic cardiovascular disease. *Arteriosclerosis Thrombosis and Vascular Biology* Vol.23, No.8 (August 2003), pp.1319-21.

Thyfault JP. (2008). Setting the stage: possible mechanisms by which acute contraction restores insulin sensitivity in muscle. *American Journal of Physiology Regulatory Integrative and Comparative Physiology* Vol. 294, No. 4 (April 2008), pp. R1103-R1110.

Trayhurn P & Woods IS. (2004). Adipokines: inflammation and the pleiotropic role of white adipose tissue. *British Journal of Nutrition* Vol. 92, No. 3 (September 2004), pp. 347-55.

Turcotte L & Fisher J. (2008). Skeletal muscle insulin resistance: roles of fatty acid metabolism and exercise. *Physical Therapy* Vol. 88, No. 11 (November), pp. 1279-96.

Um SH, D´Alessio D & Thomas G. Nutrition overload, insulin resistance and ribosomal protein S6 kinase 1, S6K1. *Cell Metabolism* Vol. 3, No. 6 (June 2006), pp.393-402.

Valencia ME, Bennett PH, Ravussin E, Esparza J, Fox C, et al. (1999). The Pima Indians in Sonora, Mexico. *Nutrition Reviews* Vol. 57, No. 5 pt 2 (May 1999), pp. S55-S57.

Vandanmagsar B, Youm YH, Ravussin A, Galgani JE, Stadler K, et al. (2011). The NLRP3 inflammasome instigates obesity-induced inflammation and insulin resistance. *Nature Medicine* Vol. 17, No. 2 (February 2011), pp. 179-88.

Varma V, Yao-Borengasser A, Rasouli N, Nolen GT, Phanavanh B, et al. (2009). Muscle inflammatory response and insulin resistance: synergistic interaction between macrophages and fatty acid leads to impaired insulin action. *American Journal of Physiology Endocrinology and Metabolism* Vol. 296, No. 6 (June 2009), pp. E1300-E1310.

Varma V, Yao-Borenhasser A, Rasouli N, Bodles AM, Phanavahn B, et al. (2007). Human visfatin expression: relationship to insulin sensitivity, intramyocellular lipids, and inflammation. *Journal of Clinical Endocrinology and Metabolism* Vol. 92, No. 2 (February 2007), pp.666-72.

Vendrell J, Broch M, Vilarrasa N, Molina A, Gómez JM, et al. (2004). Resistin, adiponectin, ghrelin, leptin, and proinflammatory cytokines: relationships in obesity. *Obesity Research* Vol. 12, No. 6 (June 2004), pp.962-71.

Vickers MH, Reddy S, Ikenasio BA, Breier BH. (2001). Dysregulation of the adipoinsular axis - a mechanism for the pathogenesis of hyperleptinemia and adipogenic diabetes induced by fetal programming. *Journal of Endocrinology* Vol. 170, No. 2 (August 2001), pp. 323-332.

Virkamäki A, Korsheninnikova E, Seppälä-Lindroos A, Vehkavaara S, Goto T, et al. (2001). Intramyocellular lipid is associated with resistance to in vivo insulin actions on glucose uptake, antilipolysis, and early insulin signaling pathways in human skeletal muscle. *Diabetes* Vol. 50, No. 10 (October 2001), pp.2337-43.

Wang B, Wood IS & Tryhurn P. (2007). Dysregulation of the expression and secretion of inflammation related adipokines by hypoxia in human adipocytes. *European Journal of Physiology* Vol.455, No. 3 (December 2007), pp. 479-92.

Wang YX, Zhang CL, Yu RT, Cho HK, Nelson MC, et al. (2004). Regulation of muscle fiber type and running endurance by PPARδ. *PLoS Biology* Vol. 2, No. 10 (October 2004), pp. 1532-39.

Weisberg S, Hunter D, Huber R, Lemieux J, Slaymaker S, et al. (2006). CCR2 modulates inflammatory and metabolic effects of high-fat deeding. Journal of Clinical Investigation Vol. 116, No. 1 (January 2006), pp.115-124.

Weisberg SP, McCann D, Desai M, Rosenbaum M, Leibel RL, et al. (2003). Obesity is associated with macrophage accumulation in adipose tissue. *Journal of Clinical Investigation* Vol. 112, No. 12 (December 2003), pp. 1796-1808.

Wendorf M & Goldfine ID. (1991). Archaeology of NIDDM. Excavation of the 'thrifty' genotype. *Diabetes* Vol. 40, No. 2 (February 1991), pp. 161-65.

Weyer C, Funahashi T, Tanaka S, Hotta K, Matsuzawa, et al. (2001). Hypoadiponectinemia in obesity and type 2 diabetes: close association with insulin resistance and hyperinsulinemia. *Journal of Clinical Endocrinology and Metabolism* Vol. 86, No. 5 (May 2001), pp. 1930-35.

Williams PT. (2001). Physical fitness and activity as separate heart disease risk factors: a meta-analysis. *Medicine and Science in Sports and Exercise* Vol.33, No. 5 (May 2001), pp.754-61.

World Health Organization (September 2006). Obesity and Overweight. In: WHO, January 2011, available from http://www.who.int/mediacentre/factsheets/fs311/en/print.html

Yamauchi T, Kamon J, Waki H, Terauchi Y, Kubota N, et al. (2001). The fat-derived hormone adiponectin reverses insulin resistance associated with both lipoatrophy and obesity. *Nature Medicine* Vol. 7, No. 8 (August 2001), pp.941-46.

Yang WS, Jeng CY, Wu TJ, Tanaka S, Funahashi T, et al. (2002). Synthetic peroxisome prolifetator-activated receptor-gamma agonist, rosiglitazone, increases plasma levels of adiponectin in type 2 diabetes patients. *Diabetes Care* Vol. 25, No. 2 (February 2002), pp. 376-80.

Ye J, Gao Z, Yin J, He Q. (2007). Hypoxia is a potential risk factor for chronic inflammation and adiponectin reduction in adipose tissue of ob/ob and dietary obese mice. *American Journal of Physiology Endocrinology and Metabolism* Vol. 293, No. 4 (October 2007), pp. E1118-E1128.

Yin J, Gao Z, He Q, Zhou D, Guo Z, Ye J. (2009). Role of hypoxia in obesity-induced disorders of glucose and lipid metabolism in adipose tissue. *American Journal of Physiology Endocrinology and Metabolism* Vol. 296, No. 2 (February 2009), pp. E333-E342.

Yoshizaki T, Schenk S, Imamura T, Babendure JL, Sonoda N, et al. (2010). SIRT1 inhibits inflammatory pathways in macrophages and modulates insulin sensitivity. *American Journal of Physiology Endocrinology and Metabolism* Vol. 298, No. 3 (March 2010), pp. E419-E428.

Zierath J, Ryder J, Doebber T, Woods J, Wu M, et al. (1998). Role of skeletal muscle in thiazolidinedione insulin sensitizer (PPARγ agonist) action. *Endocrinology* Vol. 139, No. 12 (December 1998), pp. 5034-41.

Zimmet P, Dowse G, Finch C, Serjeantson S, King H. (1990). The epidemiology and natural history of NIDDM – lessons from the South Pacific. *Diabetes/Metabolism Reviews* Vol. 6, No. 2 (March 1990), pp. 91-124.

2

Lipid Droplets and Very Low Density Lipoproteins; Their Relation to Insulin Resistance

Sven-Olof Olofsson et al.*
Department of Molecular and Clinical Medicine and the Wallenberg laboratory Sahlgrenska University Hospital/S, University of Gothenburg Sweden

1. Introduction

1.1 Organization of the lipid droplet

Lipid droplets are organelles involved in the storage of neutral lipids, such as triglycerides or cholesterol esters. These molecules are neither soluble in water nor in the amphipathic monolayers that build up intracellular membranes, and are therefore stored in a separate hydrophobic "oil phase", which is the core of the lipid droplet. Since this is a general process, the ability to form lipid droplets is preserved throughout evolution and is present in most mammalian cells (Martin and Parton, 2006; Murphy and Vance, 1999; Olofsson et al., 2008; Olofsson et al., 2009).
The core of the lipid droplets is surrounded by a monolayer of amphipathic lipids, such as phospholipids and unesterified cholesterol (Martin and Parton, 2006; Olofsson et al., 2008; Olofsson et al., 2009). The monolayer is also associated with a number of different proteins, of which the best described and quantitatively most important are the PAT domain proteins (Dalen et al., 2007; Londos et al., 1999) (reviewed in (Brasaemle, 2007)), named after the first discovered members of the family i.e. perilipin, adipocyte differentiation-related protein (ADRP) and tail interacting protein 47 (TIP47). They are characterized by an amino-terminal PAT domain with a high degree of homology between the family members. Recent additions to the list of known PAT proteins include lipid storage droplet protein 5 (LSDP5; also known as OXPAT), myocardial lipid droplet protein (MLDP; also known as PAT-1) (Dalen et al., 2007; Wolins et al., 2006) and S3-12 (Dalen et al., 2004; Wolins et al., 2003).

1.1.1 Perilipin

Perilipin, which is mainly expressed in adipocytes and steriogenic cells (Londos et al., 1995), exists in three isoforms (perilipin A, B and C), which are formed from a single gene through

*Linda Andersson, Jeanna Perman, Mikael Rutberg, Lilliana Håversen, Li Lu, Emma Lu, Reza Mobini, Marcus Ståhlman, Susanna Myhre, Christina Olsson, Rosie Perkins,Thomas Larsson, Jan Borén and Martin Adiels.
Department of Molecular and Clinical Medicine and the Wallenberg laboratory Sahlgrenska University Hospital/S , University of Gothenburg, Sweden.

alternative splicing (Lu et al., 2001). Perilipin A is by far the most abundant and well-investigated isoform (Londos et al., 1999).
Perilipin has an important dual role in the turnover of triglycerides in lipid droplets It protects against triglyceride degradation when expressed in cells that lack natural expression of the protein (Brasaemle et al., 2000). Moreover, perilipin A-knockout mice show a substantial increase in basal lipolysis and reduction in adipose mass, and are resistant to diet-induced obesity (Martinez-Botas et al., 2000; Tansey et al., 2001). Perilipin also promotes triglyceride degradation: β-adrenergic stimulation does not promote lipolysis in perilipin A-knockout mice, and cells derived from these mice fail to show translocation of hormone-sensitive lipase (HSL) to the lipid droplet (Martinez-Botas et al., 2000; Tansey et al., 2001) (reviewed in (Londos et al., 2005)). A proposed model, based on these and more direct results (Granneman et al., 2007), states that concomitant phosphorylation of perilipin and HSL results in translocation of HSL to the lipid droplet where it catalyzes the hydrolysis of triglycerides (Granneman et al., 2007).
Perilipin also has an important role in the activation of adipose triglyceride lipase (ATGL), which catalyzes the first step in the degradation of triglycerides. Perilipin A interacts with CGI-58, the activator of ATGL (Lass et al., 2006). Phosphorylation of perilipin A promotes its dissociation from CGI-58, which will then associate with ATGL on lipid droplets to allow lipolysis (Granneman et al., 2007; Miyoshi et al., 2007).

1.1.2 ADRP

ADRP seems to play a central role in the assembly of lipid droplets even in perilipin-expressing cells such as the adipocyte. It is expressed in increasing amounts early in adipocyte differentiation, but is replaced by perilipin at later stages (Brasaemle et al., 1997).
In contrast to perilipin, ADRP is expressed ubiquitously (Brasaemle et al., 1997). The expression is highly related to the amount of neutral lipids in the cell (Heid et al., 1998), and overexpression of ADRP results in an increased formation of droplets (Imamura et al., 2002; Magnusson et al., 2006; Wang et al., 2003). The regulation of ADRP levels in the cell is complex. It is regulated at the transcriptional level by peroxisome proliferator-activated receptor α (PPARα) (Dalen et al., 2006; Edvardsson et al., 2006; Targett-Adams et al., 2003), but also through post-translational degradation by the proteasomal system (Masuda et al., 2006; Xu et al., 2005), which occurs when there are low levels of lipids in the cell. Thus, accumulation of intracellular triglycerides appears to stabilize ADRP and prevents it from being sorted to degradation.

1.1.3 TIP47

TIP47 was initially described as a ubiquitously expressed cytosolic and endosomal 47 kDa protein involved in the intracellular transport of mannose 6-phosphate receptors between the trans-Golgi and endosomes (Diaz and Pfeffer, 1998; Krise et al., 2000). TIP47 is believed to act as an effector for the Rab9 protein in this process, causing budding of vesicles directed to lysosomes (Carroll et al., 2001). TIP47 is also present on lipid droplets (Wolins et al., 2001). In contrast to ADRP, which is always associated with droplets and is degraded in the absence of neutral lipid, cytosolic TIP47 is shifted to lipid droplets in the presence of increased levels of fatty acids (Wolins et al., 2001).

1.1.4 LSDP5 (OXPAT)

LSDP5 is mainly expressed in tissues with high rates of β-oxidation, such as muscle, heart, liver, and brown adipose tissue (Wolins et al., 2006). Overexpression of LSDP5 in cultured cells results in a substantial increase in the accumulation of triglycerides in response to fatty acid treatment (Wolins et al., 2006), which might be explained by a decrease in both basal and stimulated lipolysis (Dalen et al., 2007). Thus, LSDP5 seems to protect the triglyceride core of lipid droplets from degradation in a similar manner to perilipin. LSDP5 is transcriptionally regulated by PPARα in striated muscle and liver, and by PPARγ in white adipose tissue (Dalen et al., 2007; Wolins et al., 2006; Yamaguchi et al., 2006).

1.1.5 S3-12

S3-12 is mainly expressed in white adipose tissue, and it shares only a weak sequence homology with the PAT proteins (Wolins et al., 2003). S3-12 expression is transcriptionally regulated by PPARγ (Dalen et al., 2004).

1.1.6 Other lipid droplet-associated proteins

Several other proteins have also been described on lipid droplets (Brasaemle et al., 2004; Cermelli et al., 2006; Liu et al., 2004). They are involved in processes such as sorting/transport (e.g. RABs, ARFs, SNARE proteins and motor proteins), lipid biosynthesis [e.g. acyl-CoA synthetase, diacylglycerol acyltransferase (DGAT), acyl-CoA synthase and lanosterol synthetase] and lipid turnover [e.g. ATGL and its co-activator CGI-58, HSL, and cytosolic phospholipase A_2 ($cPLA_2$)] (reviewed in (Olofsson et al., 2009).

Caveolin and vimentin have been proposed to be present on lipid droplets (Brasaemle et al., 2004; Franke et al., 1987; Liu et al., 2004), but their function is not understood. One suggestion is that the presence of caveolin reflects an involvement of caveolin-rich plasma membranes in the assembly of lipid droplets (Ost et al., 2005). Caveolin has also been linked to triglyceride lipolysis in the droplets (reviewed in (Martin and Parton, 2006)). There are several other lipid droplet-associated proteins with functions that are yet to be elucidated.

1.2 Assembly of lipid droplets

Lipid droplets are formed from microsomal membranes (Brown, 2001). The main driving force in the assembly process is the formation of triglycerides (Marchesan et al., 2003; Stone et al., 2009) and all stimuli that promote triglyceride biosynthesis will therefore also promote the formation of lipid droplets. Other factors important for the assembly process include phospholipase D_1 (PLD_1) (Andersson et al., 2006; Marchesan et al., 2003), which catalyzes the formation of phosphatidic acid, a lipid that is essential for lipid droplet assembly (Andersson et al., 2006; Marchesan et al., 2003). PLD_1 contains a pleckstrin homology (PH) domain that is targeted by phosphatidylinositol (4,5) bisphosphate (PI(4,5) P2), which is essential for PLD_1 activity (McDermott et al., 2004; Powner and Wakelam, 2002). Additional targets for PI(4,5)P_2 that have been identified as important for lipid droplet formation include ARF1 (and proteins involved in the regulation of its activity) (Guo et al., 2008) and $cPLA_2$ (Gubern et al., 2008).

We have shown that lipid droplet formation also requires extracellular regulated kinase 2 (ERK2), which phosphorylates the motor protein dynein and thereby sorts it to lipid droplets (Andersson et al., 2006). The lipid droplets are then able to contact microtubules and are thus transported towards the center of the cell (Bostrom et al., 2005). Movement in both directions has been demonstrated (Bostrom et al., 2005; Welte et al., 1998). Our results clearly show that dynein is essential for lipid droplet fusion (see below), but also indicate that dynein is involved in the initial formation of the droplet (Andersson et al., 2006). The details of this latter process have not been elucidated, but one possibility is that dynein provides a "pull force" that is necessary for the budding of droplets from the microsomal membrane.

The mechanism for the creation of cytosolic lipid droplets from the ER is not fully elucidated. One mechanism that was proposed several years ago (but without substantial experimental evidence) suggests that, upon formation, triglycerides are 'oiled out' between the leaflets of the microsomal membranes to form a lens that will become the core of the primordial lipid droplet. The rationale behind this model is that whereas the triglyceride precursors (diglycerides and acylCoA) are highly soluble in the cytosolic leaflet of the microsomal membrane, triglycerides have limited solubility in this leaflet and are therefore forced into the hydrophobic part of the membrane (Figure 1) (Brown, 2001; Olofsson et al., 2008).

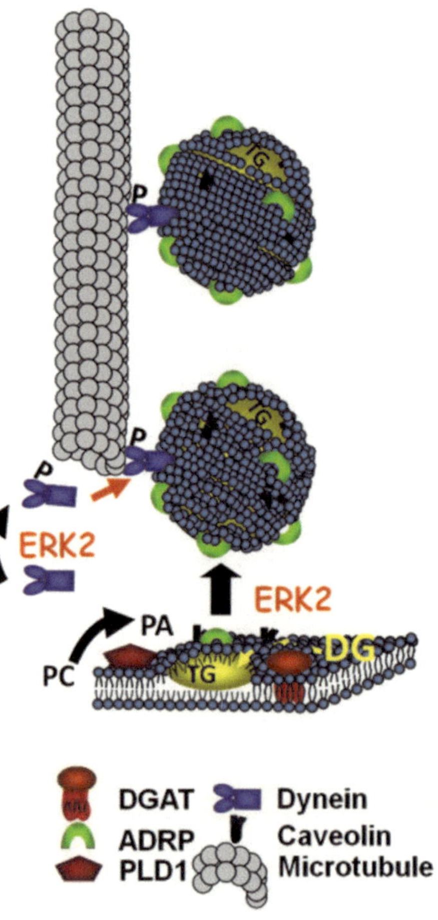

Fig. 1. Lipid droplets are formed from microsomal membranes. The assembly is driven by triglyceride formation from diglycerides, which is catalyzed by DGAT. The assembly process also requires PLD_1 and the formation of phosphatidic acid and ERK2. ERK2 phosphorylates dynein, which is then sorted onto droplets allowing them to migrate on microtubules.

1.3 Growth of lipid droplets

Newly synthesized lipid droplets are only 0.2 μm in diameter (Brown, 2001). However, mature lipid droplets are much larger (1-20 μm in diameter), indicating that they are able to grow after their formation. DGAT, which catalyzes the conversion of diglycerides to triglycerides, and the ongoing biosynthesis of triglycerides are essential for this process. It has been suggested that the surface of lipid droplets contains DGAT2, and thus the droplets may acquire triglycerides by direct biosynthesis (Kuerschner et al., 2008). However, because DGAT2 is known to span a bilayer twice (Stone et al., 2006), substantial adaptation of the enzyme would be required if it were to fit into the monolayer surface of the lipid droplet.

We demonstrated that lipid droplets can grow by fusion (Figure 2), and that approximately 15% of all droplets are engaged in the fusion process at a given time (Bostrom et al., 2005). The importance of this process, however, cannot be completely understood until we establish methods to follow the smallest lipid droplets by time lapse studies. Our very preliminary observations indicate that the fusion rate is highest among these primordial droplets. An interesting implication of fusion is that it likely involves droplets at all stages, and thus the larger droplets could have a relatively rapid connection with the DGAT2-dependent formation of the primordial lipid droplets in the microsomal membrane (Figure 3)

In addition to its dependence on dynein (Andersson et al., 2006; Bostrom et al., 2005), we have shown that lipid droplet fusion also involves the SNARE proteins synaptosomal-associated protein of 23 kDa (SNAP23), syntaxin-5 and vesicle-associated protein 4 (VAMP4) (Bostrom et al., 2007) and proteins involved in their regulation, namely the ATPase N-ethylmaleimide-sensitive factor (NSF) and α-soluble NSF adaptor protein (α-SNAP) (Bostrom et al., 2007). Recent results demonstrate that the ARF-like GTPase ARFRP1 is involved in determining the size of the droplets by sorting SNAP23 to lipid droplets (Hommel et al., 2010).

The role of the SNARE proteins, NSF and α-SNAP in fusion processes has primarily been investigated in the fusion between transport vesicles and target membranes. Central to this process is the formation of a four-helix bundle between α-helical domains present in the SNAREs (SNARE domains), which forces the membranes together promoting their fusion. A detailed molecular model of this process has recently been proposed (Giraudo et al., 2009; Sudhof and Rothman, 2009). The stable four-helix bundle present after the completed fusion is unwound by NSF and α-SNAP (for reviews, see (Hong, 2005; Jahn and Scheller, 2006; Malsam et al., 2008; Sudhof and Rothman, 2009)).

It is important to note that the presence of SNARE proteins on lipid droplets and the described fusion process open up the possibility for interactions with other organelles. Thus, fusion between a lipid droplet and the outer monolayer of the bilayer around a peroxisome may theoretically result in a structure very similar to that suggested to be formed between these two organelles (Binns et al., 2006). Further investigation is required to determine whether fusion accounts for the relatively tight interaction between lipid droplets and other organelles such as mitochondria (Shaw et al., 2008), peroxisomes (Binns et al., 2006) and the endoplasmic reticulum (ER) (Ozeki et al., 2005).

1.4 Lipid droplets and insulin resistance

Systematic insulin resistance is highly related to ectopic lipid accumulation, i.e. the accumulation of triglycerides in non-adipocytes such as liver, skeletal muscle and macrophages. Here, we focus on skeletal muscle, which is the tissue with the highest insulin-dependent consumption of glucose and thus of major importance in the development of insulin resistance.

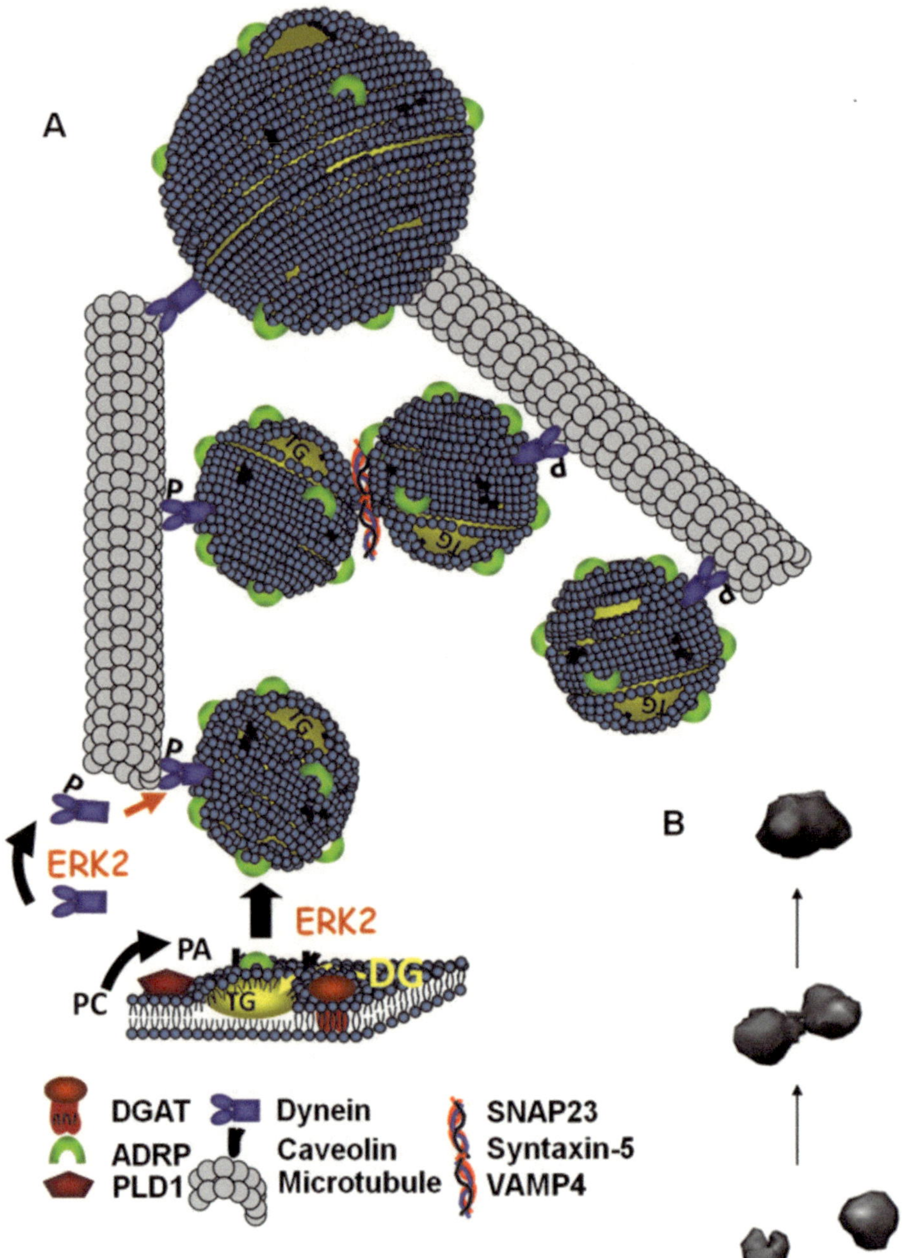

Fig. 2. The migration of lipid droplets on microtubules is important for the fusion between the droplets. This fusion is catalyzed by the SNARE proteins SNAP23, syntaxin-5 and VAMP4. (A) A schematic view of the fusion process. (B) A time lapse study of the fusion between two droplets. The process was viewed by confocal microscopy and three dimensional structures of the droplets were constructed as described in (Andersson et al., 2006).

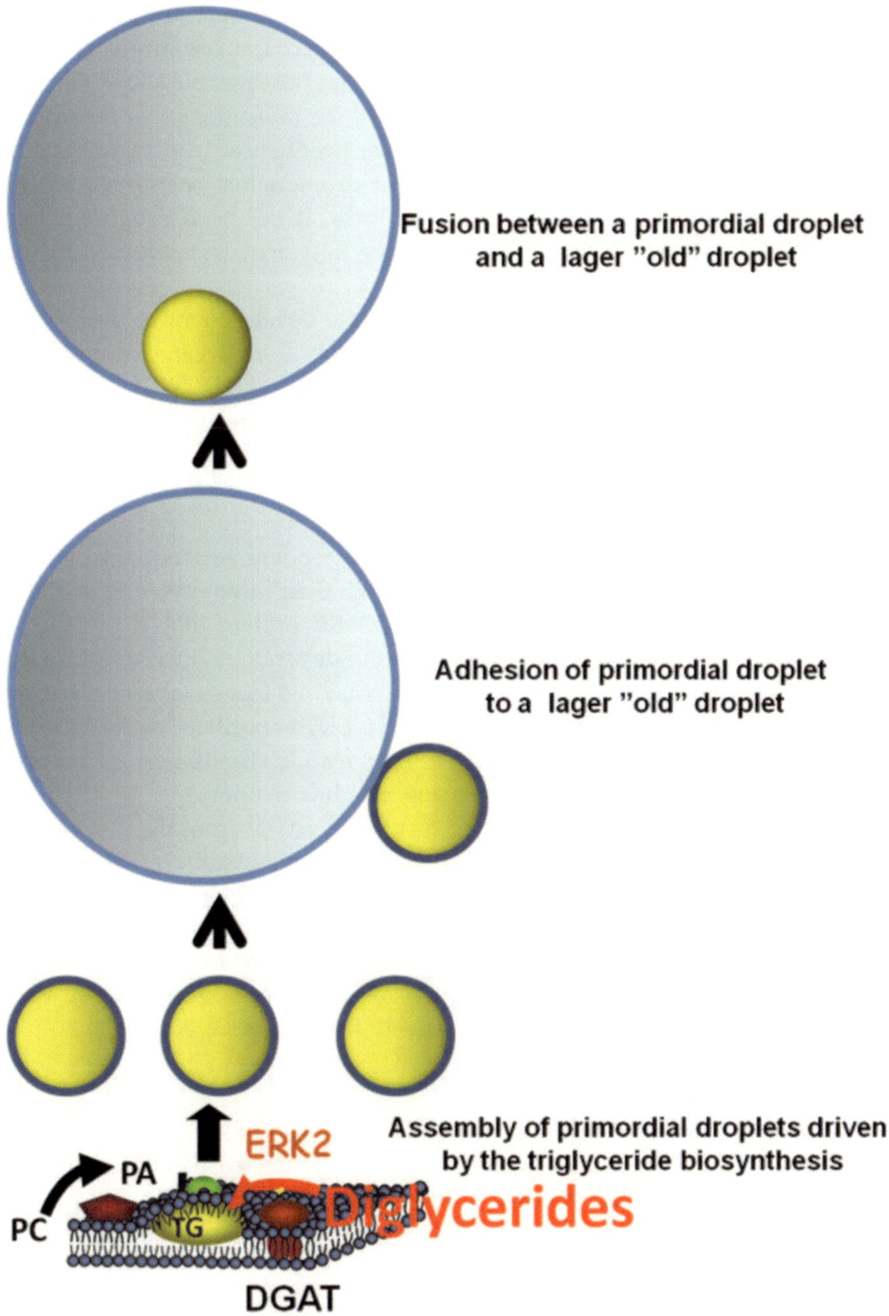

Figure 3. The fusion process allows small droplets to fuse with larger droplets. The primordial droplets formed by triglyceride biosynthesis in the microsomal membrane can fuse with larger "old" droplets and thus provide these droplets with newly synthesized triglycerides.

The strong correlation between lipid droplet accumulation in skeletal muscle and insulin resistance was for many years used as evidence that such accumulation causes insulin resistance. However, endurance-trained athletes also accumulate triglycerides in their skeletal muscle but are extremely insulin sensitive. This "athletes paradox" (Goodpaster et al., 2001; van Loon and Goodpaster, 2006) was one of the indications that the accumulation of triglycerides per se was not the problem but rather products of triglycerides such as fatty acids. Indeed, the accumulation of triglycerides in droplets has been regarded to be the result of a surplus of fatty acids in the cell. Moreover, it has been proposed that insulin resistance and inflammation are prevented by forcing fatty acids into droplets by increasing the levels of DGAT (Koliwad et al., 2010).

Several products of fatty acids have been linked to the development of insulin resistance, including partially oxidized fatty acids (Koves et al., 2008), ceramides (reviewed in (Summers, 2006)) and diglycerides (reviewed in (Samuel et al., 2010). The mechanism behind the influence of the two first is not known in detail, but diglycerides are known to impair insulin signaling through activation of protein kinase C θ (PKCθ). PKCθ phosphorylates insulin receptor substrate I, thus preventing the phosphorylation involved in the insulin signal for details, see (Samuel et al., 2010).

Fatty acids can also directly influence the insulin-dependent recruitment of the glucose transporter 4 (GLUT4) to the plasma membrane though their influence on SNAP23 (Bostrom et al., 2007). As described above, SNAP23 is a SNARE protein that is involved in lipid droplet fusion, but it also plays a central role in insulin-dependent glucose uptake in skeletal muscle and adipose tissue. SNAP23 together with syntaxin-4 form a target SNARE complex, which interacts with the vesicle SNARE VAMP2 on GLUT4-specific vesicles (GSV) and thus allows GSV to fuse with the plasma membrane upon insulin stimulation. GLUT4 is thereby directed to the plasma membrane, thus increasing the glucose uptake.

We demonstrated first in cells that fatty acids displace SNAP23 from the plasma membrane (and the fusion of GSV) to the interior of the cell, resulting in insulin resistance (Bostrom et al., 2007). We translated these results into humans by studying skeletal muscle biopsies from patients with type 2 diabetes and lean and obese controls (Bostrom et al., 2010). In agreement with our results in cells, we observed that triglyceride accumulation in human skeletal muscle is accompanied by both insulin resistance and redistribution of SNAP23 from the plasma membrane to the interior of the cell (Bostrom et al., 2010).

1.5 Lipid droplets in hypoxia/ischemia

Both human macrophages and heart muscle cells that are exposed to hypoxia accumulate lipid droplets. In both cell types, lack of oxygen results in a decrease in the oxidation of fatty acids, an increase in glycolysis and lactate production and increased triglyceride biosynthesis. Thus, the accumulation of lipid droplets seems to be part of a mechanism that adapts the metabolism to minimize oxygen consumption.

Macrophages are exposed to hypoxia in both atherosclerotic lesions (Bjornheden et al., 1999) and adipose tissue (Donath and Shoelson, 2011; Trayhurn et al., 2008; Ye, 2009). Thus, the described mechanism may be of importance for creating lipid-loaded macrophages (foam cells) in atherosclerotic lesions and in the adipose tissue of obese individuals. It is well known that cholesterol from low-density lipoproteins (LDL) contributes to the lipid droplet formation in macrophages in the arterial wall. The mechanism involving modified LDL and scavenger receptor(s) has been described in detail elsewhere (see for example (Greaves and Gordon, 2005). However, it should be noted that macrophages from atherosclerotic lesions contain high levels of triglycerides (Mattsson et al., 1993). Adipose tissue hypoxia results in macrophage recruitment and has a role in the inflammation seen in the adipose tissue during insulin resistance/type 2 diabetes (Donath and Shoelson, 2011; Trayhurn et al., 2008; Ye, 2009).

We have shown that accumulation of lipid droplets in hypoxic macrophages promotes the formation and secretion of eicosanoids and chemokines by recruiting $cPLA_2$ to the lipid droplet surface (Bostrom et al submitted). $cPLA_2$ catalyzes the production of arachidonic acid, which is the precursor of eicosanoids. Thus, triglyceride accumulation in hypoxic macrophages induces inflammation. By contrast, triglyceride accumulation caused by increased expression of DGAT1 in macrophages prevents insulin resistance and inflammation (Koliwad et al., 2010). This difference suggests that the triglyceride storage seen in hypoxia may be accompanied by a surplus of lipotoxic fatty acids, ceramides and diglycerides that have not been metabolized. Because DGAT1 promotes the conversion of diglycerides to triglycerides, increased levels of DGAT1 will likely promote the conversion of lipotoxic lipids to a hydrophobic, inert lipid that is safely stored in lipid droplets.

We have also shown that the hypoxia/ischemia-induced accumulation of triglyceride-containing lipid droplets in heart muscle cells is completely dependent on the VLDL receptor, which promotes the endocytosis of triglyceride-rich lipoproteins (Perman et al., 2011). Hypoxia-induced VLDL receptor expression is dependent on hypoxia-inducible factor 1α through its interaction with a hypoxia-responsive element in the promoter of the VLDL receptor (Perman et al., 2011). We also observed an increased accumulation of lipid droplets and a parallel increase in expression of the VLDL receptor in biopsies from ischemic left ventricle from human hearts compared with biopsies from non-ischemic left ventricles (Perman et al., 2011).

The VLDL receptor induced accumulation of lipid droplets during hypoxia/ischemia is accompanied by increases of both ER stress (which is at least partly caused by increased formation of long chain ceramides) and apoptosis in mouse hearts (Perman et al., 2011). Importantly, VLDL receptor knockout mice have improved survival in response to an acute myocardial infarction than wildtype mice (Perman et al., 2011). Thus, the VLDL receptor and the accumulation of lipid droplets seen in hypoxia/ischemia are potential targets for treatment against early death following an acute myocardial infarction.

2. The secretion of triglycerides

Triglycerides are mostly secreted from the intestine and liver as triglyceride-rich lipoproteins, which have an organization that is very similar to the lipid droplets. Thus, they consist of a core of the neutral lipids surrounded by a monolayer of phospholipids, cholesterol and proteins (known as apolipoproteins). The primary apolipoprotein is apoB, which is required for the formation of lipoproteins. It exists in two forms: apoB48 on chylomicrons (the lipoproteins formed in the intestine); and apoB100 on very low-density lipoproteins (VLDL; the lipoproteins formed in the liver). Here we focus on the formation of VLDL.

The secretory pathway

As for other secretory proteins, apoB is synthesized on ribosomes attached to the surface of the ER (Figure 4) and the 'nascent' polypeptide is translocated through a channel (reviewed in (Johnson and Haigh, 2000; Johnson and van Waes, 1999)) to the lumen of the ER, where it is folded into its correct structure with the help of chaperone proteins. When folded correctly, the secretory proteins are sorted into exit sites to leave the ER by transport vesicles. Failure to fold results in retention in the ER and retraction through the membrane channel followed by sorting to proteasomal degradation (Ellgaard and Helenius, 2001; Ellgaard and Helenius, 2003; Ellgaard et al., 1999; Johnson and Haigh, 2000; Johnson and van Waes, 1999; Kostova and Wolf, 2003; Lippincott-Schwartz et al., 2000).

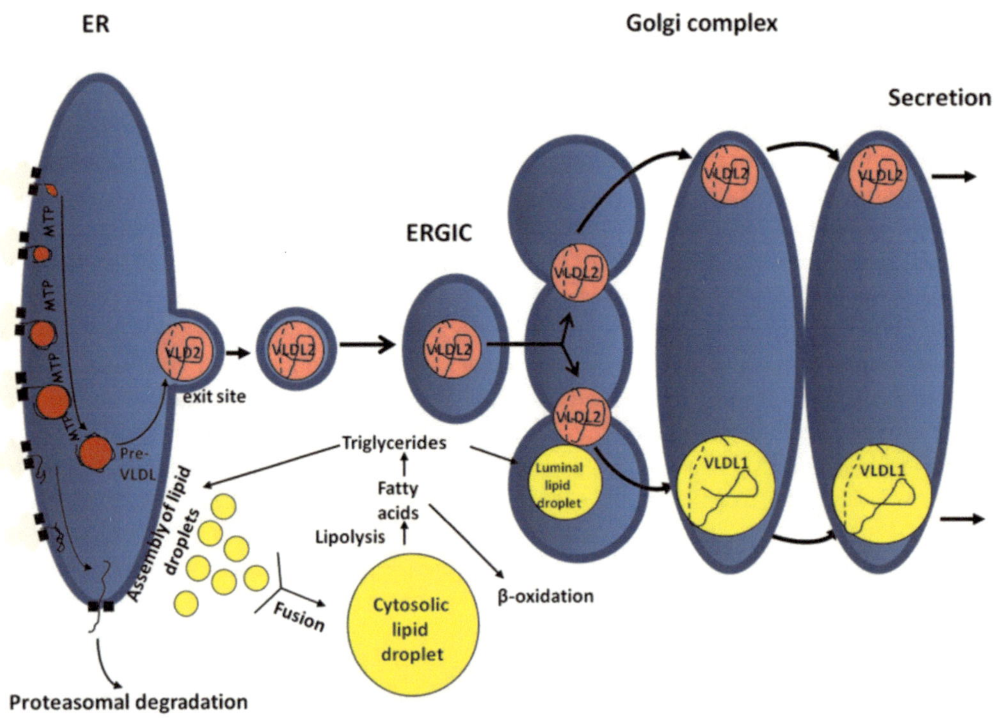

Fig. 4. The formation of VLDL1 and VLDL2. ApoB is formed on ribosomes attached to the ER and translocated to the lumen of the ER. During this translocation, the protein is lipidated by the microsomal triglyceride transfer protein (MTP) to form pre-VLDL. If this lipidation is inadequate, apoB is sorted back to the cytosol to be degraded by proteasomes. By post-translational lipidation, the pre-VLDL forms VLDL2, which is allowed to leave ER through exit sites. Pre-VLDL that is not converted to VLDL2 will be sorted to degradation (most likely by autophagocyty). VLDL2 is translocated through the secretory pathway and is either secreted or converted to VLDL1 in the Golgi apparatus by bulk lipidation, a process that is highly dependent on the amount of triglycerides that is stored in the cell.

The vesicles that bud off from the ER exit sites form the ER Golgi intermediate compartment (ERGIC), which is involved in protein sorting. ER-specific proteins are returned to the ER from the ERGIC and are thereby prevented from entering the later part of the secretory pathway. The ERGIC matures into cis-Golgi, which undergoes 'cisternal maturation' to form the medial- and trans-Golgi apparatus. During this maturation, proteins that will be secreted are transferred through the Golgi stack. Finally, the proteins are transported from the trans-Golgi to the plasma membrane for secretion (reviewed in (Elsner et al., 2003; Kartberg et al., 2005)).

2.1 The assembly of VLDL

The assembly of VLDL involves three types of particles: a primordial lipoprotein (pre-VLDL), a triglyceride-poor form of VLDL (VLDL2) and a triglyceride-rich atherogenic form of VLDL (VLDL1) (Stillemark-Billton et al., 2005).

2.1.1 The primordial lipoprotein

The assembly process starts when the growing apoB100 is cotranslationally lipidated by MTP in the lumen of the ER (Figure 4), resulting in the formation of a dense, partially lipidated form of apoB100 that is retained in the cell (Boström et al., 1988; Stillemark-Billton et al., 2005). This product, which we refer to as primordial lipoprotein (or pre-VLDL), is a precursor to VLDL2 and VLDL1.

The appearance of the apoB100 primordial lipoprotein is highly dependent on the C-terminal region of apoB100 (Stillemark-Billton et al., 2005). Moreover, the particle is highly associated with chaperone protein such as binding proteins (BiP) and protein disulfide isomerase (PDI). A potential explanation is that regions in the C-terminal of apoB100 sense the degree of lipidation and anchor the partially lipidated particle to chaperones, which retain the particle in the ER. Once the level of lipidation is sufficient to allow apoB100 to fit on the particle and the C-terminal to fold correctly, the chaperones dissociate and the particle can transfer out of the ER. Thus, the primordial lipoprotein is either retained in the cell and degraded (if not sufficiently lipidated) or further lipidated to form VLDL2 (Figure 4) (Olofsson and Asp, 2005; Olofsson et al., 1999; Olofsson et al., 2000; Stillemark-Billton et al., 2005).

2.1.2 VLDL2

VLDL2 formation is highly dependent on the length of apoB, and truncated forms of apoB result in the formation of denser particles (Stillemark et al., 2000). Indeed, there is an inverse relation between the density of the lipoproteins formed and the length of apoB. *Bona fide* VLDL2 is only formed with apoB100. The lipoprotein formed by apoB48 (which is produced only in the intestine in humans but in both the intestine and liver in mice) has the same density as high-density lipoprotein (HDL) (Stillemark-Billton et al., 2005). However, despite having the same density as apoB100 pre-VLDL (which is retained in the cell unless further lipidated), the dense lipoprotein formed by apoB48 is secreted and behaves in the same way as a VLDL2 particle formed by apoB100. We therefore propose that it is a VLDL2 analog. Thus, both *bona fide* VLDL2 and VLDL2 analogs can be either secreted or further lipidated to form VLDL1 (Fig 4).

2.1.3 VLDL1

VLDL1 is formed from VLDL2 by a second type of lipidation in which the VLDL2 particle receives a bulk load of lipids in the Golgi apparatus (Stillemark-Billton et al., 2005). We have detected a precursor-product relationship between VLDL2 and VLDL1 both in cell cultures (Stillemark-Billton et al., 2005) and turnover experiments in humans (Adiels et al., 2007).

In contrast to the formation of VLDL2, apoB only needs to have a minimum size of apoB48 to allow the conversion to VLDL1 (Stillemark-Billton et al., 2005). We have recently demonstrated that the sequence close to the C-terminal of apoB48 is essential for the VLDL1 formation. We have identified a protein (BAP31) that interacts with this sequence and promotes the formation of VLDL1 (Beck et al. Manuscript in revision).

The formation of VLDL1 is dependent on the GTPase ARF1, a protein that is required in the anterograde transport from ERGIC to cis-Golgi (Asp et al., 2000). This is consistent with results showing that VLDL1 formation occurs in the Golgi apparatus (Stillemark et al., 2000), and indicates that the formation of VLDL1 requires a transfer of apoB100 from the ER to the Golgi apparatus (Figure 4). Thus, one would expect a time delay of approximately 15 min between the biosynthesis of apoB100 and the major addition of lipids to form the VLDL1 particle. Indeed, in turnover studies in humans, we confirmed the presence of two steps in the assembly of VLDL1 with a 15 min difference between the secretion of newly formed apoB100 and newly formed triglycerides (Adiels et al., 2005b).

It has been suggested that the formation of lipid droplets in the lumen of the secretory pathway plays a central role in VLDL assembly, i.e. lipid droplets fuse with apoB to form VLDL (Alexander et al., 1976). This is an interesting hypothesis that still remains to be tested, particularly in terms of elucidating the mechanism by which a luminal lipid droplet is formed and how it fuses with VLDL2. The proposed mechanism may link the assembly of the core of VLDL1 to the process by which the core of a cytosolic lipid droplet is assembled. It has been proposed that the assembly of a droplet starts in the hydrophobic portion of the microsomal membrane with the formation of a triglyceride lens, which is then released into the cytosol. A triglyceride lens may also bud into the lumen of the secretory pathway, thereby giving rise to a luminal droplet that becomes the core of VLDL. This hypothesis remains to be tested experimentally (Brown, 2001; Murphy and Vance, 1999; Olofsson et al., 1987).

Several authors have demonstrated that fatty acids used for the biosynthesis of VLDL triglycerides are derived from triglycerides stored in cytosolic lipid droplets (Gibbons et al., 2000; Salter et al., 1998; Wiggins and Gibbons, 1992), and that enzymes involved in the release of such fatty acids have an influence on the formation of VLDL (Dolinsky et al., 2004a; Dolinsky et al., 2004b; Gilham et al., 2003; Lehner and Vance, 1999; Trickett et al., 2001).

2.2 VLDL assembly in type 2 diabetes

A major factor in the development of the dyslipoproteinemia seen in type 2 diabetes is the increased secretion of VLDL1 (Taskinen, 2003). This secretion has important implications for the formation of small dense LDL and the low levels of HDL. Below, we will discuss possible mechanisms for the increased secretion of VLDL1 during type 2 diabetes.

Using stable isotope techniques, we and others (Adiels et al., 2006; Fabbrini et al., 2009; Fabbrini et al., 2008) have repeatedly shown a relationship between liver fat content and secretion of VLDL particles. Thus, the major determinant for the secretion of VLDL1 is the amount of triglycerides in the liver. An accumulation of ectopic triglycerides in the liver is a major event in the development of insulin resistance/type 2 diabetes. Thus, lipids in the liver link type 2 diabetes to increased secretion of VLDL1.

Another factor of importance is insulin. Although insulin inhibits the assembly of VLDL1 in individuals with low liver lipid levels, insulin does not have a similar effect in patients with

high liver lipid levels (Adiels et al., 2007). These findings are in agreement with lipid accumulation in the liver being the most important regulator of VLDL1 assembly.
Several possibilities to explain why insulin inhibits VLDL1 formation have been summarized previously (Taskinen, 2003). One potential reason is that insulin inhibits lipolysis in adipose tissue and thereby decreases the inflow of fatty acids to the liver. Support for an influence on the lipolysis in the adipose tissue was obtained from studies using nicotinic acid analogs (reviewed in (Taskinen, 2003)).
Insulin is also known to promote the formation of lipid droplets (Andersson et al., 2006). Thus, it is possible that insulin diverts triglycerides from the bulk lipidation of VLDL2 to the formation of lipid droplets. Indeed, we have observed other situations where promoting the formation of lipid droplets inhibits VLDL1 assembly. For example, increased levels of ADRP in the cell result in increased storage of neutral lipids in lipid droplets and reduces their entry into the assembly pathway (Magnusson et al., 2006). Such a manipulation results in decreased VLDL1 production, despite increased levels of triglycerides in the cell. In addition, increasing the rate of fusion between droplets results in decreased VLDL secretion and an increased number of droplets in the liver cell (Li et al., 2005).

2.3 ApoB100 degradation

It has long been known that apoB100 undergoes intracellular degradation (reviewed in (Davidson and Shelness, 2000; Olofsson et al., 1999; Shelness and Sellers, 2001)). The degradation is dramatically reduced when the supply of fatty acids (and the biosynthesis of triglycerides) is increased (Borén et al., 1993; Boström et al., 1986) and it is known that post-translational degradation is important for the regulation of the secreted apoB. The intracellular degradation of apoB100 occurs at three different levels (Fisher and Ginsberg, 2002; Fisher et al., 2001): (i) close to the biosynthesis of apoB (co- or post-translationally) by a mechanism that involves retraction of the apoB molecule from the lumen of the ER to the cytosol (through the same channel as it entered during its biosynthesis), ubiquitination and subsequent proteasomal degradation (Fisher et al., 2001; Liang et al., 2000; Mitchell et al., 1998; Pariyarath et al., 2001); (ii) post-translationally by an unknown mechanism that seems to occur in a compartment separate from the rough ER, and is referred to as post-ER presecretory proteolysis (PERPP) (Fisher et al., 2001); (iii) by reuptake from the unstirred water layer around the outside of the plasma membrane (Williams et al., 1990) via the LDL receptor. The LDL receptor has been shown to have an important role in regulation of the secretion of apoB100-containing lipoproteins (Horton et al., 1999; Twisk et al., 2000).
Interestingly, the PERPP has been linked to the autophagocytic pathway (Pan et al., 2008). Contrary to post-translational degradation which targets proteins, the autophatocytic pathway allows the degradation of particles, such as pre-VLDL and VLDL.
The intracellular degradation of apoB seems to be a consequence of a failure to form the correct particle. To avoid degradation, apoB100 needs to form pre-VLDL during translation and the pre-VLDL must be converted to VLDL2 (see above: The primordial lipoprotein). Both steps are dependent on the amount of lipids that are loaded on to apoB. The formation of VLDL1 is not necessary for apoB100 secretion but allows increased secretion of triglycerides from the liver.

2.4 The turnover of VLDL in the circulation

Lipid changes in metabolic diseases such as insulin resistance, the metabolic syndrome and type 2 diabetes, commonly known as diabetic dyslipidemia, consist of elevated triglycerides, low HDL cholesterol and formation of small dense LDL. The formation of small dense LDL may occur without an increase in total LDL cholesterol, but is often connected to an increase in total apoB100.

The secreted apoB100 lipoproteins are hydrolyzed in the circulation. Because protein has a higher density than lipids, removal of the core lipids will result in the formation of smaller and denser particles. In a sequential order, hydrolysis of VLDL1 will result in first VLDL2, then intermediate-density lipoprotein (IDL) and finally LDL. The initial steps are carried out by lipoprotein lipase (LPL), which is present at the luminal side of endothelial cells in peripheral tissues such as adipose tissue, skeletal muscle and the heart. The liberated fatty acids are then taken up by different mechanisms in the target tissue (including the CD36 receptor-mediated pathway), and are re-esterified for storage or used as energy through mitochondrial oxidation. LPL has several modulators in the circulation, such as apoC-II and apoC-III, which enhance and inhibit lipolysis, respectively. New evidence also suggests that apoA-V, angiopoietin-like proteins 3 and 4, lipase maturation factor 1 and glycosylphosphatidylinositol-anchored HDL binding protein 1 (GPIHBP1) may be important for LPL function (Dallinga-Thie et al., 2010). The later steps in the removal of triglycerides are carried out by hepatic lipase. Of importance for the formation of the end product i.e. LDL is also the cholesterol ester transfer protein (CETP) (Chapman et al., 2010). IDL and LDL are removed from the circulation by the LDL receptor uptake or heparin sulphate proteoglycan mechanisms in the liver.

The triglyceride content of circulating VLDL1 has been estimated to be ~10500 molecules per particle (i.e. per apoB100 molecule), whereas VLDL2, IDL and LDL have ~3500, ~1200 and ~180-280 molecules per particle (Kumpula et al., 2008). Thus, although only 10% of the total apoB100 are in the VLDL1 and VLDL2 fractions, the majority of triglycerides are in the VLDL1 fraction and, to a lesser extent, the VLDL2 fraction (Hiukka et al., 2005). The cholesteryl ester content of lipoprotein particles increases with increasing density: VLDL1, VLDL2, IDL and LDL have ~500, ~950, ~1400 and ~1000-1500 molecules of cholesterol ester per particle (Kumpula et al., 2008). This compositional change reflects the action of cholesterol ester transfer protein, which transports cholesterol esters from HDL and LDL to VLDL particles in exchange for triglycerides (Chapman et al., 2010). This transport is increased when triglyceride levels are increased and thus type 2 diabetic subjects have lower relative amount of triglycerides in VLDL1 but higher relative amount of cholesterol esters in VLDL1 and VLDL2 compared with control subjects (Hiukka et al., 2005).

2.5 *In vivo* studies of VLDL secretion and turnover in humans

Circulating levels of apoB100, triglycerides and cholesterol are thus dependent on many different mechanisms: the rate of secretion of apoB100 and triglycerides as VLDL1 and VLDL2 particles, the rate of lipolysis by LPL and hepatic lipases (and the impact of regulating molecules on these enzymes) and the rate of removal from the circulation by uptake mechanisms. To fully understand the contribution of these mechanisms to the final plasma concentration, in particular how these different processes contribute to the development of dyslipidemia, it is necessary to quantify these within humans.

Today, most studies indirectly calculate the rates of these processes using stable isotope labeling techniques, either by *in vivo* labeling of protein content using labeled amino acids as precursors or labeling of triglycerides using labeled glycerol as precursor or by *ex vivo* labeling (Magkos and Sidossis, 2004). The methods differ in the choice of molecules to study (i.e. triglcyerides or apoB100) and consequently in the choice of tracer molecules, but also in the choice of detail (i.e. VLDL, VLDL1 and VLDL2, or VLDL, IDL and LDL) and in the modeling approach.

Our approach is a combined experiment where the kinetics of both apoB100 and triglycerides are determined in VLDL1 and VLDL2 using a combined model (Adiels et al., 2005b). Briefly, stable isotope labeled leucine and glycerol are simultaneously injected as a bolus and blood is drawn repeatedly for 10 hours. Enrichment of leucine is measured free in plasma as well as in apoB100 protein from VLDL1 and VLDL2 particles separated by ultracentrifugation. Enrichment of glycerol is measured in the triglyceride content of the VLDL1 and VLDL2 particles. Enrichment is measured using sensitive gas-chromatograph/mass-spectrometry equipment. The time series data are used as input in a mathematical model in which the different rates of transfer and synthesis can be calculated.

The kinetics of apoB100 and triglycerides have been well studied in type 2 diabetes. Most studies have revealed an increased secretion of VLDL (Cummings et al., 1995; Kissebah et al., 1982; Ouguerram et al., 2003; Sorensen et al., 2011)) and VLDL1 (Adiels et al., 2005a; Taskinen et al., 1990). Several studies have also shown impaired suppression of VLDL secretion by insulin in type 2 diabetes (Adiels et al., 2007; Lewis et al., 1993; Malmstrom et al., 1997; Sorensen et al., 2011). Some studies also suggest that diabetic subjects have slower clearance of VLDL particles (Duvillard et al., 2000; Kissebah et al., 1982; Taskinen et al., 1986) but these results are less conclusive, which may reflect the importance of other factors such as genetic background and the progress of diabetes.

3. Acknowledgement

This work was supported by grants from the Swedish Research Council, the Swedish Foundation for Strategic Research, the Swedish Heart and Lung Foundation, Söderbergs Foundation, the Swedish Diabetes association, and the EU projects LipidomicNet. .

4. References

Adiels, M., J. Boren, M.J. Caslake, P. Stewart, A. Soro, J. Westerbacka, B. Wennberg, S.O. Olofsson, C. Packard, and M.R. Taskinen. 2005a. Overproduction of VLDL1 driven by hyperglycemia is a dominant feature of diabetic dyslipidemia. *Arterioscler Thromb Vasc Biol*. 25:1697-1703.

Adiels, M., C. Packard, M.J. Caslake, P. Stewart, A. Soro, J. Westerbacka, B. Wennberg, S.O. Olofsson, M.R. Taskinen, and J. Boren. 2005b. A new combined multicompartmental model for apolipoprotein B-100 and triglyceride metabolism in VLDL subfractions. *J Lipid Res*. 46:58-67.

Adiels, M., M.R. Taskinen, C. Packard, M.J. Caslake, A. Soro-Paavonen, J. Westerbacka, S. Vehkavaara, A. Hakkinen, S.O. Olofsson, H. Yki-Jarvinen, and J. Boren. 2006. Overproduction of large VLDL particles is driven by increased liver fat content in man. *Diabetologia*. 49:755-765.

Adiels, M., J. Westerbacka, A. Soro-Paavonen, A.M. Hakkinen, S. Vehkavaara, M.J. Caslake, C. Packard, S.O. Olofsson, H. Yki-Jarvinen, M.R. Taskinen, and J. Boren. 2007.

Acute suppression of VLDL1 secretion rate by insulin is associated with hepatic fat content and insulin resistance. *Diabetologia*. 50:2356-2365.

Alexander, C.A., R.L. Hamilton, and R.J. Havel. 1976. Subcellular localization of B apoprotein of plasma lipoproteins in rat liver. *J. Cell Biol.* 69:241–263.

Andersson, L., P. Bostrom, J. Ericson, M. Rutberg, B. Magnusson, D. Marchesan, M. Ruiz, L. Asp, P. Huang, M.A. Frohman, J. Boren, and S.O. Olofsson. 2006. PLD1 and ERK2 regulate cytosolic lipid droplet formation. *J. Cell. Sci.* 119:2246-2257.

Asp, L., C. Claesson, J. Borén, and S.-O. Olofsson. 2000. ADP-ribosylation factor 1 and its activation of phospholipase D are important for the assembly of very low density lipoproteins. *J. Biol. Chem.* 275:26285 - 26292.

Binns, D., T. Januszewski, Y. Chen, J. Hill, V.S. Markin, Y. Zhao, C. Gilpin, K.D. Chapman, R.G. Anderson, and J.M. Goodman. 2006. An intimate collaboration between peroxisomes and lipid bodies. *J Cell Biol*. 173:719-731.

Bjornheden, T., M. Levin, M. Evaldsson, and O. Wiklund. 1999. Evidence of hypoxic areas within the arterial wall in vivo. *Arterioscler Thromb Vasc Biol*. 19:870-876.

Borén, J., S. Rustaeus, M. Wettesten, M. Andersson, A. Wiklund, and S.-O. Olofsson. 1993. Influence of triacylglycerol biosynthesis rate on the assembly of apoB-100–containing lipoproteins in Hep G2 cells. *Arterioscler. Thromb.* 13:1743–1754.

Bostrom, P., L. Andersson, M. Rutberg, J. Perman, U. Lidberg, B.R. Johansson, J. Fernandez-Rodriguez, J. Ericson, T. Nilsson, J. Boren, and S.O. Olofsson. 2007. SNARE proteins mediate fusion between cytosolic lipid droplets and are implicated in insulin sensitivity. *Nat Cell Biol*. 9:1286-1293.

Bostrom, P., L. Andersson, B. Vind, L. Haversen, M. Rutberg, Y. Wickstrom, E. Larsson, P.A. Jansson, M.K. Svensson, R. Branemark, C. Ling, H. Beck-Nielsen, J. Boren, K. Hojlund, and S.O. Olofsson. 2010. The SNARE protein SNAP23 and the SNARE-interacting protein Munc18c in human skeletal muscle are implicated in insulin resistance/type 2 diabetes. *Diabetes*. 59:1870-1878.

Bostrom, P., M. Rutberg, J. Ericsson, P. Holmdahl, L. Andersson, M.A. Frohman, J. Boren, and S.O. Olofsson. 2005. Cytosolic lipid droplets increase in size by microtubule-dependent complex formation. *Arterioscler Thromb Vasc Biol*. 25:1945-1951.

Boström, K., J. Borén, M. Wettesten, A. Sjöberg, G. Bondjers, O. Wiklund, P. Carlsson, and S.-O. Olofsson. 1988. Studies on the assembly of apo B-100-containing lipoproteins in HepG2 cells. *J. Biol. Chem.* 263:4434–4442.

Boström, K., M. Wettesten, J. Borén, G. Bondjers, O. Wiklund, and S.-O. Olofsson. 1986. Pulse-chase studies of the synthesis and intracellular transport of apolipoprotein B-100 in Hep G2 cells. *J. Biol. Chem.* 261:13800-13806.

Brasaemle, D.L. 2007. Thematic review series: Adipocyte Biology. The perilipin family of structural lipid droplet proteins: stabilization of lipid droplets and control of lipolysis. *J Lipid Res*. 48:2547-2559.

Brasaemle, D.L., T. Barber, N.E. Wolins, G. Serrero, E.J. Blanchette-Mackie, and C. Londos. 1997. Adipose differentiation-related protein is an ubiquitously expressed lipid storage droplet-associated protein. *J Lipid Res*. 38:2249-2263.

Brasaemle, D.L., G. Dolios, L. Shapiro, and R. Wang. 2004. Proteomic analysis of proteins associated with lipid droplets of basal and lipolytically stimulated 3T3-L1 adipocytes. *J Biol Chem*. 279:46835-46842.

Brasaemle, D.L., B. Rubin, I.A. Harten, J. Gruia-Gray, A.R. Kimmel, and C. Londos. 2000. Perilipin A increases triacylglycerol storage by decreasing the rate of triacylglycerol hydrolysis. *J Biol Chem*. 275:38486-38493.

Brown, D.A. 2001. Lipid droplets: Proteins floating on a pool of fat. *Curr Biol*. 11:R446-449.

Carroll, K.S., J. Hanna, I. Simon, J. Krise, P. Barbero, and S.R. Pfeffer. 2001. Role of Rab9 GTPase in facilitating receptor recruitment by TIP47. *Science*. 292:1373-1376.

Cermelli, S., Y. Guo, S.P. Gross, and M.A. Welte. 2006. The lipid-droplet proteome reveals that droplets are a protein-storage depot. *Curr Biol*. 16:1783-1795.

Chapman, M.J., W. Le Goff, M. Guerin, and A. Kontush. 2010. Cholesteryl ester transfer protein: at the heart of the action of lipid-modulating therapy with statins, fibrates, niacin, and cholesteryl ester transfer protein inhibitors. *Eur Heart J*. 31:149-164.

Cummings, M.H., G.F. Watts, A.M. Umpleby, T.R. Hennessy, R. Naoumova, B.M. Slavin, G.R. Thompson, and P.H. Sonksen. 1995. Increased hepatic secretion of very-low-density lipoprotein apolipoprotein B-100 in NIDDM. *Diabetologia*. 38:959-967.

Dalen, K.T., T. Dahl, E. Holter, B. Arntsen, C. Londos, C. Sztalryd, and H.I. Nebb. 2007. LSDP5 is a PAT protein specifically expressed in fatty acid oxidizing tissues. *Biochim Biophys Acta*. 1771:210-227.

Dalen, K.T., K. Schoonjans, S.M. Ulven, M.S. Weedon-Fekjaer, T.G. Bentzen, H. Koutnikova, J. Auwerx, and H.I. Nebb. 2004. Adipose tissue expression of the lipid droplet-associating proteins S3-12 and perilipin is controlled by peroxisome proliferator-activated receptor-gamma. *Diabetes*. 53:1243-1252.

Dalen, K.T., S.M. Ulven, B.M. Arntsen, K. Solaas, and H.I. Nebb. 2006. PPARalpha activators and fasting induce the expression of adipose differentiation-related protein in liver. *J Lipid Res*. 47:931-943.

Dallinga-Thie, G.M., R. Franssen, H.L. Mooij, M.E. Visser, H.C. Hassing, F. Peelman, J.J. Kastelein, M. Peterfy, and M. Nieuwdorp. 2010. The metabolism of triglyceride-rich lipoproteins revisited: new players, new insight. *Atherosclerosis*. 211:1-8.

Davidson, N.O., and G.S. Shelness. 2000. Apolipoprotein B: mRNA editing, lipoprotein assembly, and presecretory degradation. *Ann. Rev. Nutr*. 20:169-193.

Diaz, E., and S.R. Pfeffer. 1998. TIP47: a cargo selection device for mannose 6-phosphate receptor trafficking. *Cell*. 93:433-443.

Dolinsky, V.W., D.N. Douglas, R. Lehner, and D.E. Vance. 2004a. Regulation of the enzymes of hepatic microsomal triacylglycerol lipolysis and re-esterification by the glucocorticoid dexamethasone. *Biochem J*. 378:967-974.

Dolinsky, V.W., D. Gilham, M. Alam, D.E. Vance, and R. Lehner. 2004b. Triacylglycerol hydrolase: role in intracellular lipid metabolism. *Cell Mol Life Sci*. 61:1633-1651.

Donath, M.Y., and S.E. Shoelson. 2011. Type 2 diabetes as an inflammatory disease. *Nat Rev Immunol*. 11:98-107.

Duvillard, L., F. Pont, E. Florentin, C. Galland-Jos, P. Gambert, and B. Verges. 2000. Metabolic abnormalities of apolipoprotein B-containing lipoproteins in non-insulin-dependent diabetes: a stable isotope kinetic study. *Eur J Clin Invest*. 30:685-694.

Edvardsson, U., A. Ljungberg, D. Linden, L. William-Olsson, H. Peilot-Sjogren, A. Ahnmark, and J. Oscarsson. 2006. PPARalpha activation increases triglyceride mass and adipose differentiation-related protein in hepatocytes. *J Lipid Res*. 47:329-340.

Ellgaard, L., and A. Helenius. 2001. ER quality control: towards an understanding at the molecular level. *Curr Opin Cell Biol*. 13:431-437.

Ellgaard, L., and A. Helenius. 2003. Quality control in the endoplasmic reticulum. *Nat Rev Mol Cell Biol*. 4:181-191.

Ellgaard, L., M. Molinari, and A. Helenius. 1999. Setting the standards:Quality control in the secretory pathway. *Science*. 286:1882 - 1888.

Elsner, M., H. Hashimoto, and T. Nilsson. 2003. Cisternal maturation and vesicle transport: join the band wagon! (Review). *Mol Membr Biol*. 20:221-229.

Fabbrini, E., F. Magkos, B.S. Mohammed, T. Pietka, N.A. Abumrad, B.W. Patterson, A. Okunade, and S. Klein. 2009. Intrahepatic fat, not visceral fat, is linked with metabolic complications of obesity. *Proc Natl Acad Sci U S A*. 106:15430-15435.

Fabbrini, E., B.S. Mohammed, F. Magkos, K.M. Korenblat, B.W. Patterson, and S. Klein. 2008. Alterations in adipose tissue and hepatic lipid kinetics in obese men and women with nonalcoholic fatty liver disease. *Gastroenterology*. 134:424-431.

Fisher, E.A., and H.N. Ginsberg. 2002. Complexity in the secretory pathway: the assembly and secretion of apolipoprotein B-containing lipoproteins. *J Biol Chem*. 277:17377-17380.

Fisher, E.A., M. Pan, X. Chen, X. Wu, H. Wang, H. Jamil, J.D. Sparks, and K.J. Williams. 2001. The triple threat to nascent apolipoprotein B. Evidence for multiple, distinct degradative pathways. *J Biol Chem*. 276:27855-27863.

Franke, W.W., M. Hergt, and C. Grund. 1987. Rearragement of vimentin cytoskeleton durin adipose conversion: formation of an intermediate filament cage around lipid globules. *Cell*. 49:131-141.

Gibbons, G.F., K. Islam, and R.J. Pease. 2000. Mobilisation of triacylglycerol stores. *Biochim. Biophys. Acta*. 1483:37-57.

Gilham, D., S. Ho, M. Rasouli, P. Martres, D.E. Vance, and R. Lehner. 2003. Inhibitors of hepatic microsomal triacylglycerol hydrolase decrease very low density lipoprotein secretion. *Faseb J*. 17:1685-1687.

Giraudo, C.G., A. Garcia-Diaz, W.S. Eng, Y. Chen, W.A. Hendrickson, T.J. Melia, and J.E. Rothman. 2009. Alternative zippering as an on-off switch for SNARE-mediated fusion. *Science*. 323:512-516.

Goodpaster, B.H., J. He, S. Watkins, and D.E. Kelley. 2001. Skeletal muscle lipid content and insulin resistance: evidence for a paradox in endurance-trained athletes. *J Clin Endocrinol Metab*. 86:5755-5761.

Granneman, J.G., H.P. Moore, R.L. Granneman, A.S. Greenberg, M.S. Obin, and Z. Zhu. 2007. Analysis of lipolytic protein trafficking and interactions in adipocytes. *J Biol Chem*. 282:5726-5735.

Greaves, D.R., and S. Gordon. 2005. Thematic review series: the immune system and atherogenesis. Recent insights into the biology of macrophage scavenger receptors. *J Lipid Res*. 46:11-20.

Gubern, A., J. Casas, M. Barcelo-Torns, D. Barneda, X. de la Rosa, R. Masgrau, F. Picatoste, J. Balsinde, M.A. Balboa, and E. Claro. 2008. Group IVA phospholipase A2 is necessary for the biogenesis of lipid droplets. *J Biol Chem*. 283:27369-27382.

Guo, Y., T.C. Walther, M. Rao, N. Stuurman, G. Goshima, K. Terayama, J.S. Wong, R.D. Vale, P. Walter, and R.V. Farese. 2008. Functional genomic screen reveals genes involved in lipid-droplet formation and utilization. *Nature*. 453:657-661.

Heid, H.W., R. Moll, I. Schwetlick, H.R. Rackwitz, and T.W. Keenan. 1998. Adipophilin is a specific marker of lipid accumulation in diverse cell types and diseases. *Cell Tissue Res*. 294:309-321.

Hiukka, A., J. Fruchart-Najib, E. Leinonen, H. Hilden, J.C. Fruchart, and M.R. Taskinen. 2005. Alterations of lipids and apolipoprotein CIII in very low density lipoprotein subspecies in type 2 diabetes. *Diabetologia*. 48:1207-1215.

Hommel, A., D. Hesse, W. Volker, A. Jaschke, M. Moser, T. Engel, M. Bluher, C. Zahn, A. Chadt, K. Ruschke, H. Vogel, R. Kluge, H. Robenek, H.G. Joost, and A. Schurmann. 2010. The ARF-like GTPase ARFRP1 is essential for lipid droplet growth and is involved in the regulation of lipolysis. *Mol Cell Biol*. 30:1231-1242.

Hong, W. 2005. SNAREs and traffic. *Biochim Biophys Acta*. 1744:493-517.

Horton, J.D., H. Shimano, R.L. Hamilton, M.S. Brown, and J.L. Goldstein. 1999. Disruption of LDL receptor gene in transgenic SREBP-1a mice unmask hyperlipidemia resulting from production of lipid-rich VLDL. *J.Clin.Invest*. 103:1067-1076.

Imamura, M., T. Inoguchi, S. Ikuyama, S. Taniguchi, K. Kobayashi, N. Nakashima, and H. Nawata. 2002. ADRP stimulates lipid accumulation and lipid droplet formation in murine fibroblasts. *Am J Physiol Endocrinol Metab*. 283:E775-783.

Jahn, R., and R.H. Scheller. 2006. SNAREs--engines for membrane fusion. *Nat Rev Mol Cell Biol*. 7:631-643.

Johnson, A.E., and N.G. Haigh. 2000. The ER translocon and retrotranslocation: is the shift into reverse manual or automatic? *Cell*. 102:709-712.

Johnson, A.E., and M.A. van Waes. 1999. The translocon: a dynamic gateway at the ER membrane. *Annu Rev Cell Dev Biol*. 15:799-842.

Kartberg, F., M. Elsner, L. Froderberg, L. Asp, and T. Nilsson. 2005. Commuting between Golgi cisternae-mind the GAP! *Biochim Biophys Acta*.

Kissebah, A.H., S. Alfarsi, D.J. Evans, and P.W. Adams. 1982. Integrated regulation of very low density lipoprotein triglyceride and apolipoprotein-B kinetics in non-insulin-dependent diabetes mellitus. *Diabetes*. 31:217-225.

Koliwad, S.K., R.S. Streeper, M. Monetti, I. Cornelissen, L. Chan, K. Terayama, S. Naylor, M. Rao, B. Hubbard, and R.V. Farese, Jr. 2010. DGAT1-dependent triacylglycerol storage by macrophages protects mice from diet-induced insulin resistance and inflammation. *J Clin Invest*. 120:756-767.

Kostova, Z., and D.H. Wolf. 2003. For whom the bell tolls: protein quality control of the endoplasmic reticulum and the ubiquitin-proteasome connection. *Embo J*. 22:2309-2317.

Koves, T.R., J.R. Ussher, R.C. Noland, D. Slentz, M. Mosedale, O. Ilkayeva, J. Bain, R. Stevens, J.R. Dyck, C.B. Newgard, G.D. Lopaschuk, and D.M. Muoio. 2008. Mitochondrial overload and incomplete Fatty Acid oxidation contribute to skeletal muscle insulin resistance. *Cell Metab*. 7:45-56.

Krise, J.P., P.M. Sincock, J.G. Orsel, and S.R. Pfeffer. 2000. Quantitative analysis of TIP47-receptor cytoplasmic domain interactions: implications for endosome-to-trans Golgi network trafficking. *J Biol Chem*. 275:25188-25193.

Kuerschner, L., C. Moessinger, and C. Thiele. 2008. Imaging of lipid biosynthesis: how a neutral lipid enters lipid droplets. *Traffic*. 9:338-352.

Kumpula, L.S., J.M. Kumpula, M.R. Taskinen, M. Jauhiainen, K. Kaski, and M. Ala-Korpela. 2008. Reconsideration of hydrophobic lipid distributions in lipoprotein particles. *Chem Phys Lipids*. 155:57-62.

Lass, A., R. Zimmermann, G. Haemmerle, M. Riederer, G. Schoiswohl, M. Schweiger, P. Kienesberger, J.G. Strauss, G. Gorkiewicz, and R. Zechner. 2006. Adipose triglyceride lipase-mediated lipolysis of cellular fat stores is activated by CGI-58 and defective in Chanarin-Dorfman Syndrome. *Cell Metab*. 3:309-319.

Lehner, R., and D.E. Vance. 1999. Cloning and expression of a cDNA encoding a hepatic microsomal lipase that mobilizes stored triacylglycerol. *Biochem J*. 343 Pt 1:1-10.

Lewis, G.F., K.D. Uffelman, L.W. Szeto, and G. Steiner. 1993. Effects of acute hyperinsulinemia on VLDL triglyceride and VLDL apoB production in normal weight and obese individuals. *Diabetes*. 42:833-842.

Li, L., P. Stillemark-Billton, C. Beck, P. Bostrom, L. Andersson, M. Rutberg, J. Ericsson, B. Magnusson, D. Marchesan, A. Ljungberg, J. Boren, and S.O. Olofsson. 2005. Epigallocatechin gallate promotes the formation of cytosolic lipid droplets and causes a subsequent reduction in the assembly and secretion of VLDL-containing apoB-100. *J Lipid Res*.

Liang, J.-S., X. Wu, E.A. Fisher, and H.N. Ginsberg. 2000. The amino-terminal domain of apolipoprotein B does not undergo retrograde translocation from the endoplasmic reticulum to the cytosol. Proteasomal degradation of nascent apolipoprotein B begins at the carboxyl terminus of the protein, while apolipoprotein B is still in its original translocon. *J. Biol. Chem*. 275:32003-32010.

Lippincott-Schwartz, J., T.H. Roberts, and K. Hirschberg. 2000. Secretory protein trafficking and organelle dynamics in living cells. *Annu Rev Cell Dev Biol*. 16:557-589.

Liu, P., Y. Ying, Y. Zhao, D.I. Mundy, M. Zhu, and R.G. Anderson. 2004. Chinese hamster ovary K2 cell lipid droplets appear to be metabolic organelles involved in membrane traffic. *J Biol Chem*. 279:3787-3792.

Londos, C., D.L. Brasaemle, J. Gruia-Gray, D.A. Servetnick, C.J. Schultz, D.M. Levin, and A.R. Kimmel. 1995. Perilipin: unique proteins associated with intracellular neutral lipid droplets in adipocytes and steroidogenic cells. *Biochem Soc Trans*. 23:611-615.

Londos, C., D.L. Brasaemle, C.J. Schultz, J.P. Segrest, and A.R. Kimmel. 1999. Perilipins, ADRP, and other proteins that associate with intracellular neutral lipid droplets in animal cells. *Semin Cell Dev Biol*. 10:51-58.

Londos, C., C. Sztalryd, J.T. Tansey, and A.R. Kimmel. 2005. Role of PAT proteins in lipid metabolism. *Biochimie*. 87:45-49.

Lu, X., J. Gruia-Gray, N.G. Copeland, D.J. Gilbert, N.A. Jenkins, C. Londos, and A.R. Kimmel. 2001. The murine perilipin gene: the lipid droplet-associated perilipins derive from tissue-specific, mRNA splice variants and define a gene family of ancient origin. *Mamm Genome*. 12:741-749.

Magkos, F., and L.S. Sidossis. 2004. Measuring very low density lipoprotein-triglyceride kinetics in man in vivo: how different the various methods really are. *Curr Opin Clin Nutr Metab Care*. 7:547-555.

Magnusson, B., L. Asp, P. Bostrom, M. Ruiz, P. Stillemark-Billton, D. Linden, J. Boren, and S.O. Olofsson. 2006. Adipocyte differentiation-related protein promotes fatty acid storage in cytosolic triglycerides and inhibits secretion of very low-density lipoproteins. *Arterioscler Thromb Vasc Biol*. 26:1566-1571.

Malmstrom, R., C.J. Packard, M. Caslake, D. Bedford, P. Stewart, H. Yki-Jarvinen, J. Shepherd, and M.R. Taskinen. 1997. Defective regulation of triglyceride metabolism by insulin in the liver in NIDDM. *Diabetologia*. 40:454-462.

Malsam, J., S. Kreye, and T.H. Sollner. 2008. Membrane fusion: SNAREs and regulation. *Cell Mol Life Sci*. 65:2814-2832.

Marchesan, D., M. Rutberg, L. Andersson, L. Asp, T. Larsson, J. Boren, B.R. Johansson, and S.O. Olofsson. 2003. A phospholipase D-dependent process forms lipid droplets containing caveolin, adipocyte differentiation-related protein, and vimentin in a cell-free system. *J Biol Chem*. 278:27293-27300.

Martin, S., and R.G. Parton. 2006. Lipid droplets: a unified view of a dynamic organelle. *Nat Rev Mol Cell Biol*. 7:373-378.

Martinez-Botas, J., J.B. Anderson, D. Tessier, A. Lapillonne, B.H. Chang, M.J. Quast, D. Gorenstein, K.H. Chen, and L. Chan. 2000. Absence of perilipin results in leanness and reverses obesity in Lepr(db/db) mice. *Nat Genet*. 26:474-479.

Masuda, Y., H. Itabe, M. Odaki, K. Hama, Y. Fujimoto, M. Mori, N. Sasabe, J. Aoki, H. Arai, and T. Takano. 2006. ADRP/adipophilin is degraded through the proteasome-dependent pathway during regression of lipid-storing cells. *J Lipid Res*. 47:87-98.

Mattsson, L., H. Johansson, M. Ottoson, G. Bondjers, and O. Wiklund. 1993. Expression of lipoprotein lipase mRNA and secretion in macrophages isolated from human atherosclerotic aorta. *J. Clin. Invest*. 92:1759-1765.

McDermott, M., M.J. Wakelam, and A.J. Morris. 2004. Phospholipase D. *Biochem Cell Biol*. 82:225-253.

Mitchell, D.M., M. Zhou, R. Pariyarath, H. Wang, J.D. Aitchison, H.N. Ginsberg, and E.A. Fisher. 1998. Apoprotein B 100 har a prolonged interaction with the translocon during which its lipidation and translocation change from dependence on the microsomal triglyceride transfer protein to independence. *Proc.Natl. Acad. Sci.USA*. 95:14733 - 14738.

Miyoshi, H., J.W. Perfield, 2nd, S.C. Souza, W.J. Shen, H.H. Zhang, Z.S. Stancheva, F.B. Kraemer, M.S. Obin, and A.S. Greenberg. 2007. Control of adipose triglyceride lipase action by serine 517 of perilipin A globally regulates protein kinase A-stimulated lipolysis in adipocytes. *J Biol Chem*. 282:996-1002.

Murphy, D.J., and J. Vance. 1999. Mechanisms of lipid-body formation. *Trends Biochem Sci*. 24:109-115.

Olofsson, S.-O., and L. Asp. 2005. The assembly of Very Low density lipoproteins (VLDL) in the liver. *in Packard CJ and Rader D (eds) Lipid and Atherosclerosis: Advances in translational medicine*. London UK: Taylor and Francis:1-15.

Olofsson, S.-O., L. Asp, and J. Borén. 1999. The assembly and secretion of apolipoprotein B-containing lipoproteins. *Curr. Opin. Lipidol*. 10:341 - 346.

Olofsson, S.-O., G. Bjursell, K. Boström, P. Carlsson, J. Elovson, A.A. Protter, M.A. Reuben, and G. Bondjers. 1987. Apolipoprotein B: Structure, biosynthesis and role in the lipoprotein assembly process. *Atherosclerosis*. 68:1–17.

Olofsson, S.-O., P. Stillemark-Billton, and L. Asp. 2000. The intracellular assembly of VLDL-a process that consists of two major steps that occur in separate cell compartments. *Trends. Cardiovasc. Med*. 10:338 - 345.

Olofsson, S.O., P. Bostrom, L. Andersson, M. Rutberg, M. Levin, J. Perman, and J. Boren. 2008. Triglyceride containing lipid droplets and lipid droplet-associated proteins. *Curr Opin Lipidol*. 19:441-447.

Olofsson, S.O., P. Bostrom, L. Andersson, M. Rutberg, J. Perman, and J. Boren. 2009. Lipid droplets as dynamic organelles connecting storage and efflux of lipids. *Biochim Biophys Acta*. 1791:448-458.

Ost, A., U. Ortegren, J. Gustavsson, F.H. Nystrom, and P. Stralfors. 2005. Triacylglycerol is synthesized in a specific subclass of caveolae in primary adipocytes. *J Biol Chem*. 280:5-8.

Ouguerram, K., T. Magot, Y. Zair, J.S. Marchini, B. Charbonnel, H. Laouenan, and M. Krempf. 2003. Effect of atorvastatin on apolipoprotein B100 containing lipoprotein metabolism in type-2 diabetes. *J Pharmacol Exp Ther*. 306:332-337.

Ozeki, S., J. Cheng, K. Tauchi-Sato, N. Hatano, H. Taniguchi, and T. Fujimoto. 2005. Rab18 localizes to lipid droplets and induces their close apposition to the endoplasmic reticulum-derived membrane. *J Cell Sci*. 118:2601-2611.

Pan, M., V. Maitin, S. Parathath, U. Andreo, S.X. Lin, C. St Germain, Z. Yao, F.R. Maxfield, K.J. Williams, and E.A. Fisher. 2008. Presecretory oxidation, aggregation, and autophagic destruction of apoprotein-B: a pathway for late-stage quality control. *Proc Natl Acad Sci U S A*. 105:5862-5867.

Pariyarath, R., H. Wang, J.D. Aitchison, H.N. Ginsberg, W.J. Welch, A.E. Johnson, and E.A. Fisher. 2001. Co-translational interactions of apoprotein B with the ribosome and translocon during lipoprotein assembly or targeting to the proteasome. *J Biol Chem*. 276:541-550.

Perman, J.C., P. Bostrom, M. Lindbom, U. Lidberg, M. Stahlman, D. Hagg, H. Lindskog, M. Scharin Tang, E. Omerovic, L. Mattsson Hulten, A. Jeppsson, P. Petursson, J. Herlitz, G. Olivecrona, D.K. Strickland, K. Ekroos, S.O. Olofsson, and J. Boren. 2011. The VLDL receptor promotes lipotoxicity and increases mortality in mice following an acute myocardial infarction. *J Clin Invest*. 121:2625-2640.

Powner, D.J., and M.J. Wakelam. 2002. The regulation of phospholipase D by inositol phospholipids and small GTPases. *FEBS Lett*. 531:62-64.

Salter, A.M., D. Wiggins, V.A. Sessions, and G.F. Gibbons. 1998. The intracellular triacylglycerol/fatty acid cycle: a comparison of its activity in hepatocytes which secrete exclusively apolipoprotein (apo) B100 very-low-density lipoprotein (VLDL) and in those which secrete predominantly apoB48 VLDL. *Biochem J*. 332 (Pt 3):667-672.

Samuel, V.T., K.F. Petersen, and G.I. Shulman. 2010. Lipid-induced insulin resistance: unravelling the mechanism. *Lancet*. 375:2267-2277.

Shaw, C.S., D.A. Jones, and A.J. Wagenmakers. 2008. Network distribution of mitochondria and lipid droplets in human muscle fibres. *Histochem Cell Biol*. 129:65-72.

Shelness, G.S., and J.A. Sellers. 2001. Very-low-density lipoprotein assembly and secretion. *Curr Opin Lipidol*. 12:151-157.

Sorensen, L.P., I.R. Andersen, E. Sondergaard, L.C. Gormsen, O. Schmitz, J.S. Christiansen, and S. Nielsen. 2011. Basal and insulin mediated VLDL-triglyceride kinetics in type 2 diabetic men. *Diabetes*. 60:88-96.

Stillemark-Billton, P., C. Beck, J. Boren, and S.O. Olofsson. 2005. Relation of the size and intracellular sorting of apoB to the formation of VLDL 1 and VLDL 2. *J Lipid Res.* 46:104-114.

Stillemark, P., J. Borén, M. Andersson, T. Larsson, S. Rustaeus, K.-A. Karlsson, and S.-O. Olofsson. 2000. The assembly and secretion of apolipoprotein-B48-containing very low density lipoproteins in McA-RH7777 cells. *J.Biol.Chem.* 275:10506 - 10513.

Stone, S.J., M.C. Levin, and R.V. Farese, Jr. 2006. Membrane topology and identification of key functional amino acid residues of murine acyl-CoA:diacylglycerol acyltransferase-2. *J Biol Chem.* 281:40273-40282.

Stone, S.J., M.C. Levin, P. Zhou, J. Han, T.C. Walther, and R.V. Farese, Jr. 2009. The endoplasmic reticulum enzyme DGAT2 is found in mitochondria-associated membranes and has a mitochondrial targeting signal that promotes its association with mitochondria. *J Biol Chem.* 284:5352-5361.

Sudhof, T.C., and J.E. Rothman. 2009. Membrane fusion: grappling with SNARE and SM proteins. *Science.* 323:474-477.

Summers, S.A. 2006. Ceramides in insulin resistance and lipotoxicity. *Prog Lipid Res.* 45:42-72.

Tansey, J.T., C. Sztalryd, J. Gruia-Gray, D.L. Roush, J.V. Zee, O. Gavrilova, M.L. Reitman, C.X. Deng, C. Li, A.R. Kimmel, and C. Londos. 2001. Perilipin ablation results in a lean mouse with aberrant adipocyte lipolysis, enhanced leptin production, and resistance to diet-induced obesity. *Proc Natl Acad Sci U S A.* 98:6494-6499.

Targett-Adams, P., D. Chambers, S. Gledhill, R.G. Hope, J.F. Coy, A. Girod, and J. McLauchlan. 2003. Live cell analysis and targeting of the lipid droplet-binding adipocyte differentiation-related protein. *J Biol Chem.* 278:15998-16007.

Taskinen, M.R. 2003. Diabetic dyslipidaemia: from basic research to clinical practice. *Diabetologia.* 46:733-749.

Taskinen, M.R., W.F. Beltz, I. Harper, R.M. Fields, G. Schonfeld, S.M. Grundy, and B.V. Howard. 1986. Effects of NIDDM on very-low-density lipoprotein triglyceride and apolipoprotein B metabolism. Studies before and after sulfonylurea therapy. *Diabetes.* 35:1268-1277.

Taskinen, M.R., C.J. Packard, and J. Shepherd. 1990. Effect of insulin therapy on metabolic fate of apolipoprotein B-containing lipoproteins in NIDDM. *Diabetes.* 39:1017-1027.

Trayhurn, P., B. Wang, and I.S. Wood. 2008. Hypoxia in adipose tissue: a basis for the dysregulation of tissue function in obesity? *Br J Nutr.* 100:227-235.

Trickett, J.I., D.D. Patel, B.L. Knight, E.D. Saggerson, G.F. Gibbons, and R.J. Pease. 2001. Characterization of the rodent genes for arylacetamide deacetylase, a putative microsomal lipase, and evidence for transcriptional regulation. *J Biol Chem.* 276:39522-39532.

Twisk, J., D.L. Gillian-Daniel, A. Tebon, L. Wang, P.H. Barrett, and A.D. Attie. 2000. The role of the LDL receptor in apolipoprotein B secretion. *J. Clin. Invest.* 105:521 - 532.

van Loon, L.J., and B.H. Goodpaster. 2006. Increased intramuscular lipid storage in the insulin-resistant and endurance-trained state. *Pflugers Arch.* 451:606-616.

Wang, S.M., R.D. Hwang, A.S. Greenberg, and H.L. Yeo. 2003. Temporal and spatial assembly of lipid droplet-associated proteins in 3T3-L1 preadipocytes. *Histochem Cell Biol.* 120:285-292.

Welte, M.A., S.P. Gross, M. Postner, S.M. Block, and E.F. Wieschaus. 1998. Developmental regulation of vesicle transport in Drosophila embryos: forces and kinetics. *Cell*. 92:547-557.

Wiggins, D., and G.F. Gibbons. 1992. The lipolysis/esterification cycle of hepatic triacylglycerol. Its role in the secretion of very-low-density lipoprotein and its response to hormones and sulphonylureas. *Biochem. J.* 284:457–462.

Williams, K.J., R.W. Brocia, and E.A. Fisher. 1990. The unstirred water layer as a site of control of apolipoprotein B secretion. *J. Biol. Chem.* 265:16741-16744.

Wolins, N.E., B.K. Quaynor, J.R. Skinner, A. Tzekov, M.A. Croce, M.C. Gropler, V. Varma, A. Yao-Borengasser, N. Rasouli, P.A. Kern, B.N. Finck, and P.E. Bickel. 2006. OXPAT/PAT-1 is a PPAR-induced lipid droplet protein that promotes fatty acid utilization. *Diabetes*. 55:3418-3428.

Wolins, N.E., B. Rubin, and D.L. Brasaemle. 2001. TIP47 associates with lipid droplets. *J Biol Chem*. 276:5101-5108.

Wolins, N.E., J.R. Skinner, M.J. Schoenfish, A. Tzekov, K.G. Bensch, and P.E. Bickel. 2003. Adipocyte protein S3-12 coats nascent lipid droplets. *J Biol Chem*. 278:37713-37721.

Xu, G., C. Sztalryd, X. Lu, J.T. Tansey, J. Gan, H. Dorward, A.R. Kimmel, and C. Londos. 2005. Post-translational regulation of adipose differentiation-related protein by the ubiquitin/proteasome pathway. *J Biol Chem*. 280:42841-42847.

Yamaguchi, T., S. Matsushita, K. Motojima, F. Hirose, and T. Osumi. 2006. MLDP, a novel PAT family protein localized to lipid droplets and enriched in the heart, is regulated by peroxisome proliferator-activated receptor alpha. *J Biol Chem*. 281:14232-14240.

Ye, J. 2009. Emerging role of adipose tissue hypoxia in obesity and insulin resistance. *Int J Obes (Lond)*. 33:54-66.

3

Role of Triglyceride/Fatty Acid Cycle in Development of Type 2 Diabetes

Chang-Wen Hsieh, David DeSantis and Colleen M Croniger
Case Western Reserve University Cleveland, Ohio
USA

1. Introduction

In United States, the prevalence of obesity has increased from 11.9% to 33.4% in men and from 16.6% to 36.5% in women from 1971 to 2006 (Austin, Spadano-Gasbarro et al. 2011). In general, obesity is caused by energy imbalance where energy intake exceeds energy expenditure for an extended period of time. The excess energy is stored in adipose tissue and results in enlarged fat cells and/or increased number of fat cells. Obesity is of great concern because a subset of the population has co-morbidities that develop as a consequence of obesity. Previous studies have shown that obesity is one of the risk factors linked to metabolic syndrome (Bray 2004). The World Health Organization (WHO) defines metabolic syndrome as a cluster of disorders that require the presence of diabetes, impaired glucose tolerance (IGT), impaired fasting glucose or insulin resistance and any two of the following abnormalities: central obesity, dyslipidemia (high triglycerides or low high-density lipoprotein (HDL) cholesterol concentration), elevated blood pressure, or micro albuminuria (Alberti and Zimmet 1998).

Type 2 diabetes mellitus (T2DM) is well known to be a metabolic disease that is characterized by insulin resistance and impaired insulin secretion. Insulin resistance is a condition in which the peripheral tissues, such as muscle and adipose tissue, lose the ability to uptake plasma glucose efficiently at physiological concentrations of insulin. As a result, the pancreas secretes more insulin to compensate. Therefore, insulin resistance leads to high plasma concentrations of insulin and glucose, and results in T2DM. Moreover, hyperglycemia causes cardiovascular diseases and disease-specific complications such as blindness and kidney failure (Zimmet, Alberti et al. 2001). The increased prevalence of T2DM is strongly associated with obesity (Mokdad, Ford et al. 2003) and is becoming an increasing problem worldwide (King, Abdullaev et al. 1998; Cowie, Rust et al. 2006; Yoon, Lee et al. 2006). In just the United States, 23.6 million people over the age of 20 have diabetes, of which 90% to 95% have T2DM (Cowie, Rust et al. 2006). An overwhelming 25.9% of the US population over 20 years old has early stages of disease by exhibiting impaired fasting glucose levels (Cowie, Rust et al. 2006). Additionally, The International Diabetes Federation predicted that 333 million people will have diabetes by 2025 (King 1998; King, Abdullaev et al. 1998; King, Aubert et al. 1998). Therefore, it is very important to determine the causes of this disease and develop strategies for its prevention.

The correlation between obesity and the prevalence of T2DM has been well established, but how does T2DM develop? In 1963, Randle *et al* proposed that lipids impaired insulin-stimulated glucose uptake in muscle and was caused by inhibition of glycolysis (Randle 1963). Excess circulating free fatty acids (FFA) in obesity is one of the main factors that contribute to development of T2DM (Randle 1963; Randle 1998). Because FFA are elevated in the blood of obese individuals, the muscle has access to more FFA compared to lean individuals and thus obese individuals have increased fatty acid oxidation in their muscles (Boden 1997). This in turn, results in an increased generation of metabolites from FFA β-oxidation such as, nicotinamide adenine dinucleotide (NADH), acetyl-CoA and adenosine triphosphate (ATP). These metabolites inhibit key regulatory enzymes in the glycolytic pathway such as pyruvate dehydrogenase complex (PDC). The increased concentration of ATP also inhibits phosphofructokinase (PFK-1) and pyruvate kinase muscle isoform (PK-M), thus blocking the rate controlling steps in muscle glycolysis and subsequently leads to an accumulation of glucose-6-phosphate (G6P). Increased concentration of G6P inhibit hexokinase and therefore decreases the rate of glucose phosphorylation by muscle which increases the blood glucose concentration (Randle 1963). Randle *et al* also found that FFA oxidation blocks the recycling of the glucose transporter 4 (GLUT4) to the surface of muscle cells, thus decreasing glucose uptake and contributes to the increased blood glucose levels (Randle 1963). In summary, the elevated FFA have been demonstrated to lead to insulin resistance in peripheral tissues by inhibiting insulin-stimulated glucose uptake in the muscle causing elevated blood glucose (Boden 1997).

2. Triglyceride/fatty acid cycle and glyceroneogenesis

What regulates the flux of FFA between tissues? The triglyceride/fatty acid cycle regulates this flux. In the fed state glucose is metabolized to glycerol-3-phosphate via glycolysis and esterifies with three FFA to generate triglycerides (Figure 1). This occurs in both the liver and white adipose tissues (WAT). FFA are derived both from either the diet or *de novo* lipogenesis in the liver. FFA generate energy via β-oxidation as described above in various tissues (muscle, heart) or can be stored as triglycerides in adipose tissue for energy production at a later time.

During fasting however as much as 65% of FFA are re-esterified back to triglycerides in WAT (Jensen, Chandramouli et al. 2001). Since glucose is at a premium during fasting, the synthesis of glycerol-3-phosphate from glucose is minimal. Additionally, in WAT the glycerol released during lipolysis cannot be phosphorylated and used for triglyceride synthesis because the activity of glycerol kinase in this tissue is negligible. Reshef, Ballard and Hanson demonstrated that gluconeogenic precursors such as pyruvate and lactate are converted into glycerol backbone of triglyceride (Reshef, Hanson et al. 1970; Reshef, Meyuhas et al. 1972). This pathway called "glyceroneogenesis" is an abbreviated version of gluconeogenesis. Glyceroneogenesis is defined as the conversion of precursors other than glucose or glycerol into glycerol 3-phosphate for triglyceride synthesis. The pathway is essential for the regulation of the FFA flux between tissues during fasting (Botion, Kettelhut et al. 1995; Botion, Brito et al. 1998; Festuccia, Kawashita et al. 2003).

Glyceroneogenesis, like gluconeogenesis, is regulated by phosphoenolpyruvate carboxykinase (PEPCK-C/*Pck1*), a key enzyme which catalyzes the conversion of oxaloacetate (OAA) to phosphoenolpyruvate (PEP) in both pathways. During fasting, increasing hepatic *Pck1* expression enhances the rates of gluconeogenesis to maintain glucose homeostasis as well as glyceroneogenesis, thus increasing hepatic glucose output and triglycerides synthesis by re-esterification of circulating FFA (Fig. 1). In adipose tissue, glyceroneogenesis controlled by *Pck1* contributes to the regulation of FFA release to the blood. Support for *Pck1* regulation of glyceroneogenesis contributing to the development of disease was shown by Franckhauser et al. They over-expressed of *Pck1* in WAT through a transgene specific for adipose tissue and found increased FFA re-esterification in adipose tissue led to obesity *without* insulin resistance (Franckhauser, Antras-Ferry et al. 1995; Franckhauser, Munoz et al. 2002). The increased glyceroneogenesis reduced the availability of FFA to the muscle and thus prevented impaired glucose tolerance. Therefore the regulation of triglyceride/FFA cycle is important in the development of obesity and T2DM. Figure 1. Triglyceride/FFA cycle regulates the flux of lipids between tissues.

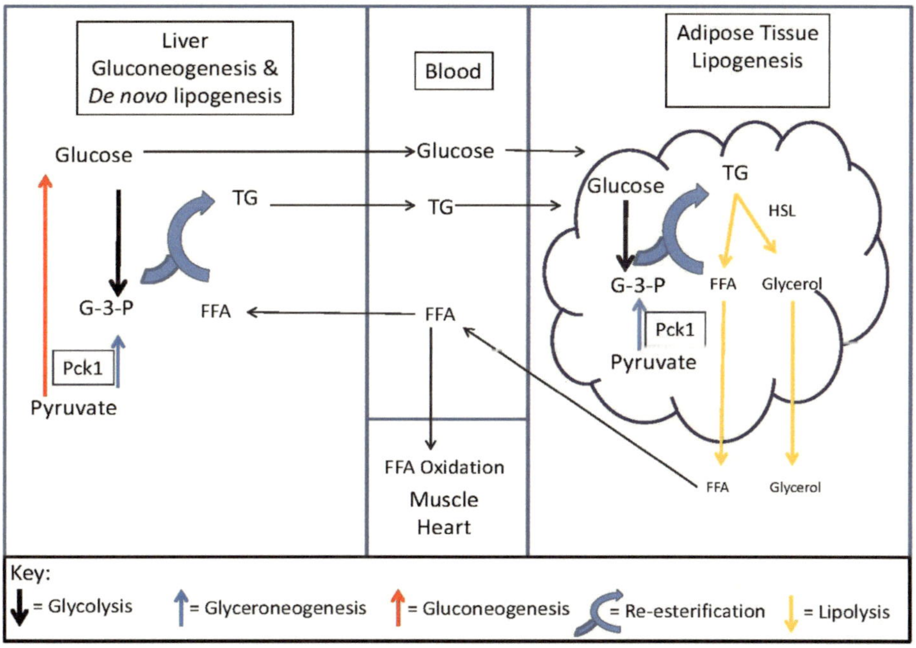

Fig. 1. Triglyceride-fatty acid cycle. During fasting triglycerides are hydrolyzed to glycerol and FFA. However as much as 65% of FFA are re-esterfied back to triglycerides. *Pck1* regulates this process in both adipose tissue and liver.

In order to investigate the disturbance of triglyceride/fatty acid cycle in development of obesity and T2DM, various genetic alterations of the *Pck1* gene have been conducted. Mice with a whole body null mutation of *Pck1* do not survive beyond 3 days after birth (She, Shiota et al. 2000). Therefore, the PPARE$^{-/-}$ mice were generated to circumvent this problem. The binding site for the peroxisome proliferator-activated receptor γ (PPARγ), called the peroxisome proliferator-activated receptor element (PPARE), at -1000 bp of the *Pck1* promoter is essential for adipose tissue expression (Devine, Eubank et al. 1999). The deletion of PPARE region in *Pck1* promoter in mice (PPARE-/-) led to dramatic loss of *Pck1* expression in WAT and mammary gland, and slight reduction in BAT (Hsieh, Millward et al. 2009). Loss of *Pck1* expression in the adipose tissue resulted in reduced adipocyte size and fat content (Olswang, Cohen et al. 2002) due to impaired glyceroneogenesis in adipose tissue. Further research found PPARE$^{-/-}$ mice displayed insulin resistance and altered lipid and glucose homeostasis (Millward, DeSantis et al. 2010). Thus the alteration of the triglyceride/FFA cycle can lead to development of impaired glucose tolerance.

Further evidence for the role of *Pck1* in the regulation of the triglyceride/FFA cycle has been shown in genomic analysis in humans. Beale *et al* have established that two C/T single nucleotide polymorphisms (SNPs) were in complete linkage disequilibrium at position -1097bp and -967bp of the *Pck1* promoter and these SNPs are associated with obesity and T2DM. Patients with T/T polymorphisms have higher HbA1c and higher fasting glucose levels (Beale, Harvey et al. 2007). The region of the identified polymorphisms in these patients is located within the same PPARE site of *Pck1* promoter that has been deleted in PPARE-/- mice (Millward, Desantis et al. 2010). These mice lack *Pck1* expression in WAT and develop insulin resistance with elevated plasma FFA (Millward, DeSantis et al 2010).
In mice that had altered triglyceride/FFA cycle via loss of *Pck1* in mammary gland and WAT, the dams' had 40% reduction of milk triglycerides during lactation. The pups reared by these dams had reduced growth in the perinatal period and developed insulin resistance that persisted into adulthood (Hsieh, Millward et al. 2009). Thus understanding the regulation of lipid metabolism during pregnancy and lactation may provide new insights into the mechanism(s) for development of T2DM.

3. The thrifty hypothesis

How does the alteration of perinatal nutrition program the fetus for T2DM? One theory for the interaction of environment in development of disease is "the thrifty phenotype hypothesis". The thrifty phenotype hypothesis suggested that the metabolic adaption during early life altered "thrifty genes" expression to help people survive when food sources were limited; however, those genes predispose us to diabetes and became detrimental in our modern lifestyle with an abundance of food (Neel 1962). The theory associates poor fetal growth with increased risk for a number of chronic conditions, including diabetes, hypertension, dyslipidemia, coronary artery disease and stroke, in adulthood (Barker 2004; Fernandez-Twinn and Ozanne 2006). Suboptimal nutrition during pregnancy is one of the significant problems that causes infants to suffer from intrauterine growth retardation (IUGR) (Marsal 2002). IUGR has been strongly associated with the development of metabolic disorders, hormone imbalance, organ dysfunction and abnormal development, as well as cardiovascular disorders (Wu, Bazer et al. 2004). Malnutrition and overnutrition during pregnancy as well as alterations in placental function all contribute the development of IUGR and further "program" the fetus to development of a variety of chronic diseases (Wu, Bazer et al. 2004). The "programming" hypothesis suggests that maternal malnutrition can induce permanent changes in the fetal genome through DNA methylation, histone acetylation, or other modifications on transcriptional or translational levels (Meaney and Szyf 2005) and contribute to development of metabolic diseases in the future. Therefore, low birth weight (LBW) is regarded as an independent risk factor for development of T2DM and other adult-onset diseases in adulthood (Hernandez-Valencia and Patti 2006).

4. Animal models for studying programming of the metabolic syndrome during pregnancy/lactation

Several nutritional models have been used to illustrate the mechanism that would explain fetal origins for adult diseases. We summarized some of these models for studying programming of the newborns (Table 1). To investigate the impact of maternal overnutrtion on the fetus, several studies have used the high-fat diet during pregnancy /lactation. They have shown that exposure to the high fat diet during pregnancy results in altered metabolism in the newborn can also lead to the development of metabolic diseases, including insulin resistance and dysfunction of pancreatic β-cells, in the offspring (Elton, Pennington et al. 2002; Buckley, Keseru et al. 2005; Taylor, McConnell et al. 2005). Thus, maternal nutrition directly impacts the developing β-islet cells and can program the fetus for insulin resistance as adults.

Manipulation	Duration	Consequences	Reference
Undernutrition			
Maternal calorie restriction 50% caloric need	3rd week of pregnancy	•Impaired β-cell development	Garofano, Czernichow et al. 1997
	3rd week pregnancy and lactation	•Reduced β-cell mass and number •Fetus has impaired glucose tolerance	Garofano, Czernichow et al. 1998
Maternal caloric restriction 30% Caloric needs	During pregnancy	Fetus develops hypertension, increased fasting insulin concentration and obesity	Vickers, Breier et al. 2000
Maternal protein is reduced to 8% of caloric needs	During pregnancy	•Low birth weight fetus, reduced β-cell islet size •Reduced β-cell islet insulin concentration, adult animals develop insulin rsistance	Snoeck, Remacle et al. 1990 Dahri, Snoeck et al. 1991 Ozanne, Dorling et al. 2001 Ozanne, Olsen et al. 2003
Tubal ligation	During pregnancy	•Reduced β-cell mass	Wigglesworth 1974; De Prins and Van Assche 1982
Maternal diet of conjugated linoleic acid	During pregnancy and lactation Dam's milk had reduced triglycerides	•Impaired fetal growth •Increased pup mortality	Ringseis, Saal et al. 2004
Loss of *Pck1* in mammary gland and WAT	PPARE-/- dams had reduced milk triglycerides during lactation	•Reduced weight gain during lactation •Develop insulin resistance	Hsieh, Millward et al. 2009
Overnutrition			
Reduction of litter size	Reduced from 14 rat pups to 4	•Pups develop obesity and insulin resistance	Plagemann, Heidrich et al 1992
Maternal High fat diet	During pregnancy	•Dysfunction of β-cell •Fetus develops insulin resistance	Elton, Pennington et al. 2002; Buckley, Keseru et al. 2005; Taylor, McConnell et al. 2005
Artificial feeding of pups high carbohydrate diet	Pups fed via intragastric tube high carbohydrate diet for three weeks after birth	•Develop obesity, insulin resistance •Impaired β-cell development	Aalinkeel, Srinivasan et al. 1999; Aalinkeel, Srinivasan et al. 2001; Patel and Srinivasan 2002

Table 1. Imprinting the fetus for T2DM

To investigate the impact of undernutrition on programming the fetus for adult diseases, two different dietary strategies are commonly used, global nutritional restriction and isocaloric low protein manipulation. In rodents, total maternal restriction of 50% of caloric needs in the last week of pregnancy results in impairment of β-cell development (Garofano, Czernichow et al. 1997). If calorie restriction continues during suckling, permanent reduction in β-cell mass and β-cell number occurs resulting in impaired glucose tolerance (Garofano, Czernichow et al. 1998). If rodent dams are more severely restricted to 30% of total caloric intake, the fetus develops systolic hypertension, increased fasting insulin concentrations, increased food intake and obesity (Vickers, Breier et al. 2000). Limiting a single macronutrient in the dams also imprints the fetus. When maternal protein intake during pregnancy is reduced to 8%, the offspring have low birth weight (LBW), reduced β-cell islet size (Snoeck, Remacle et al. 1990) and reduced β- islets insulin content and secretion (Dahri, Snoeck et al. 1991). Peripheral tissues are also affected in the pups from dams fed low protein diet. When the pups were adults (15 months old), insulin stimulated glucose uptake in skeletal and adipose tissues is reduced (Ozanne, Dorling et al. 2001; Ozanne, Olsen et al. 2003). Small birth weight can also be due to impaired nutrient perfusion through the placenta (Haggarty, Allstaff et al. 2002). To mimic placental insufficiency in rodents, unilateral and bilateral uterine artery ligations have been used. These studies established that the fetus develop reduced β-cell mass which persists into adulthood (Wigglesworth 1974; De Prins and Van Assche 1982).

5. Alterations in fetal nutrition

LBW in newborns is a reduction in both lean body mass and fat mass. After birth, these infants have accelerated postnatal growth or catch-up growth (CUG) (Eriksson, Forsen et al. 1999; Bhargava, Sachdev et al. 2004). Several studies have suggested that the fat mass accrues preferentially during CUG and the fat accumulation during childhood is a significant risk factor for T2DM as adults (Crescenzo, Samec et al. 2003; Rasmussen, Malis et al. 2005; Ibanez, Ong et al. 2006; Leunissen, Oosterbeek et al. 2008). Several strategies have been employed to test the consequences of overnutrition on programming the fetus for adult disease. These include reduction of litter size during lactation, high fat diet during pregnancy. Reduction of litter size from 14 to 4 rat pups per litter results in hyperinsulinemia, increased body growth and obesity as adults (Plagemann, Heidrich et al. 1992). Rats fed a high fat diet (20% kcal fat) during pregnancy and lactation had significantly higher milk lipid, protein and lactose concentration compared to the low fat diet group (5%kcal fat). The weights of the pups from the high fat mothers is similar at birth but increases after 6 days and persists into adulthood (Del Prado, Delgado et al. 1997).

During the suckling period, milk lipids provide the major source of both calories and essential fatty acids for the rodent newborn. The neonate uses fatty acids and ketone bodies as their primary energy substrate during lactation and must switch to carbohydrate after weaning (Grigor, Allan et al. 1986; Rolls, Gurr et al. 1986; Del Prado, Delgado et al. 1997; Del Prado, Villalpando et al. 1999).). Patel et al have extensively studied the patterning effect of overnutrtion in the perinatal period by high-carbohydrate feeding during the suckling period (Aalinkeel, Srinivasan et al. 1999; Aalinkeel, Srinivasan et al. 2001; Patel and Srinivasan 2002). They used an artificial rearing technique where newborn rats were raised in styrofoam cups floating in a temperature-controlled water bath called "pup-in-a-cup". At day 4 postpartum, the rats were fed through intragastric cannulas a high carbohydrate formula where 56% of the total calories is carbohydrate compared to 8% normally found in rodent milk. The pups develop hyperinsulinemia within 24 hours which persists into adulthood. Patel et al have investigated both cellular and molecular adaptations in response to the patterning of high carbohydrate diet and insulin secretion. The pancreas has profound changes. The pancreas from the high carbohydrate fed animals has increased number of smaller sized β-islets with an increase of immunopositive staining area for insulin. The islets also has reduced apoptosis (Petrik, Srinivasan et al. 2001). The molecular changes include increases in expression of transcription factors regulating the expression of the preproinsulin mRNA.

Undernutrition during lactation can also impact the fetus. A study using female rats showed that exposure to dietary conjugated linoleic acids resulted in decreased triglyceride concentration in the milk via reduced *de novo* fatty acid synthesis in the mammary gland and an impaired uptake of fatty acids from lipoprotein into mammary gland (Ringseis, Saal et al. 2004). The lower triglyceride concentration of milk led to impaired fetal growth and increased mortality of the suckling pups. As we discussed earlier, alterations in the triglyceride/FFA cycle also reduce triglyceride concentration of milk and lead to programming the fetus to develop insulin resistance (Hsieh, Millward et al 2009). Thus understanding the regulation of lipid metabolism during pregnancy and lactation may provide new insights into the mechanism(s) for development of insulin resistance.

6. Transgenerational programming of fetus

The data described above suggests epigenetic patterning of the fetus for disease due to either genetic or environmental conditions. However there is little evidence for transgenerational effects of the environment in mammals. Most examples of transgenerational environmental effects described in the literature are maternal effects. In Table 2 we have summarized these studies. Aalinkeel et al analyzed pups that were fed a high carbohydrate diet instead of the normal high lipid diet during the first three weeks of life. These pups develop insulin resistance and become obese (Aalinkeel, Srinivasan et al 1999). The F1 generation from these mice also develop obesity and insulin resistance even though the F1 generation had no dietary alterations (Aalinkeel, Srinivasan et al 2001; Patel, Srinivasan 2002). In another study C57BL/6J dams (F0) were fed high fat diet during pregnancy. The pups develop obesity and metabolic syndrome that is transmitted through to the F3 generation (Dunn, Bale et al 2011). Another study showed that caloric restriction of the dam during pregnancy (F0) results in reduced birth weight, impaired glucose tolerance and obesity (Jimenez-Chillaron, Isganaitis et al 2009). The environmental imprinting caused by F0 dam also imprints not only the F1 generation but also the F2 generation (Jimenez-Chillaron, Isganaitis et al 2009). Thus, the original environmental insult to the grandmother or mother imprints not only the fetus but future generations as well.

Recent evidence indicates that it is not just the mother that can imprint the fetus for development of disease. Several studies showed that environmental insults to the grandfather or father imprint the fetus for several generations as well (Table 2). In congenic strains derived from an obesity susceptible strain, C57BL/6J and a resistant strain, A/J, identified a region that protects the fetus from diet-induced obesity on high fat diet. This small region of the A/J chromosome, $Obrq2a^{A/J}$, in an otherwise C57BL/6J background shows that the paternal or grandpaternal allele is sufficient to inhibit diet-induced obesity and reduce food intake in the normally obesity-susceptible C57BL/6J strain (Yazbek, Spiezio et al 2010). In another study when the male C57BL/6J mouse (M) was fed a low-protein diet and then mated to C57BL/6J female mouse (F), the progeny has increased hepatic gene expression for genes in the lipogenic pathway (Carone, Fauquier et al 2010). Finally, when obese male Sprague-Dawley rats were mated to females fed a low-fat diet the F1 generation developed altered β-cell function (Ng, Lin et al 2010). Therefore, environmental insults to the grandfather and father can also imprint the fetus for development of obesity and insulin resistance.

7. Conclusion

The development of obesity and insulin resistance is a complex disease since it is mutlifactorial and both genetics as well as the environment contribute to the development of T2DM. Environmental stresses to either parent can result in imprinting of the fetus for

T2DM. Future studies will define the mechanism(s) responsible for imprinting the fetus for disease and offer new therapeutic strategies for prevention of T2DM.

8. Acknowledgement

This work was supported by the National Institute of Diabetes and Digestive and Kidney Diseases (NIDDK) Grant DK-075040 (CMC). The stable isotope studies were performed at the Case Western Reserve University (Cleveland, Ohio) Mouse Metabolic Phenotyping Center supported by NIDDK Grant DK-76769.

9. References

Aalinkeel, R., M. Srinivasan, et al. (1999). "A dietary intervention (high carbohydrate) during the neonatal period causes islet dysfunction in rats." Am J Physiol 277(6 Pt 1): E1061-9.

Aalinkeel, R., M. Srinivasan, et al. (2001). "Programming into adulthood of islet adaptations induced by early nutritional intervention in the rat." Am J Physiol Endocrinol Metab 281(3): E640-8.

Alberti, K. G. and P. Z. Zimmet (1998). "Definition, diagnosis and classification of diabetes mellitus and its complications. Part 1: diagnosis and classification of diabetes mellitus provisional report of a WHO consultation." Diabet Med 15(7): 539-53.

Austin, S. B., J. Spadano-Gasbarro, et al. (2011). "Disordered weight control behaviors in early adolescent boys and girls of color: an under-recognized factor in the epidemic of childhood overweight." J Adolesc Health 48(1): 109-12.

Barker, D. J. (2004). "The developmental origins of adult disease." J Am Coll Nutr 23(6 Suppl): 588S-595S.

Beale, E. G., B. J. Harvey, et al. (2007). "PCK1 and PCK2 as candidate diabetes and obesity genes." Cell Biochem Biophys 48(2-3): 89-95.

Bhargava, S. K., H. S. Sachdev, et al. (2004). "Relation of serial changes in childhood body-mass index to impaired glucose tolerance in young adulthood." N Engl J Med 350(9): 865-75.

Boden, G. (1997). "Role of fatty acids in the pathogenesis of insulin resistance and NIDDM." Diabetes 46(1): 3-10.

Botion, L. M., M. N. Brito, et al. (1998). "Glucose contribution to in vivo synthesis of glyceride-glycerol and fatty acids in rats adapted to a high-protein, carbohydrate-free diet." Metabolism 47(10): 1217-21.

Botion, L. M., I. C. Kettelhut, et al. (1995). "Increased adipose tissue glyceroneogenesis in rats adapted to a high protein, carbohydrate-free diet." Horm Metab Res 27(7): 310-3.

Bray, G. A. (2004). "Medical Consequences of Obesity." The Journal of Clin. Endo and Metabolism 89(6): 2583-2589.

Buckley, A. J., B. Keseru, et al. (2005). "Altered body composition and metabolism in the male offspring of high fat-fed rats." Metabolism 54(4): 500-7.

Cowie, C. C., K. F. Rust, et al. (2006). "Prevalence of diabetes and impaired fasting glucose in adults in the U.S. population: National Health And Nutrition Examination Survey 1999-2002." Diabetes Care 29(6): 1263-8.

Crescenzo, R., S. Samec, et al. (2003). "A role for suppressed thermogenesis favoring catch-up fat in the pathophysiology of catch-up growth." Diabetes 52(5): 1090-7.

Dahri, S., A. Snoeck, et al. (1991). "Islet function in offspring of mothers on low-protein diet during gestation." Diabetes 40 Suppl 2: 115-20.

De Prins, F. A. and F. A. Van Assche (1982). "Intrauterine growth retardation and development of endocrine pancreas in the experimental rat." Biol Neonate 41(1-2): 16-21.

Del Prado, M., G. Delgado, et al. (1997). "Maternal lipid intake during pregnancy and lactation alters milk composition and production and litter growth in rats." J Nutr 127(3): 458-62.

Del Prado, M., S. Villalpando, et al. (1999). "A high dietary lipid intake during pregnancy and lactation enhances mammary gland lipid uptake and lipoprotein lipase activity in rats." J Nutr 129(8): 1574-8.

Devine, J. H., D. W. Eubank, et al. (1999). "Adipose expression of the phosphoenolpyruvate carboxykinase promoter requires peroxisome proliferator-activated receptor gamma and 9-cis-retinoic acid receptor binding to an adipocyte-specific enhancer in vivo." J Biol Chem 274(19): 13604-12.

Elton, C. W., J. S. Pennington, et al. (2002). "Insulin resistance in adult rat offspring associated with maternal dietary fat and alcohol consumption." J Endocrinol 173(1): 63-71.

Eriksson, J. G., T. Forsen, et al. (1999). "Catch-up growth in childhood and death from coronary heart disease: longitudinal study." Bmj 318(7181): 427-31.

Fernandez-Twinn, D. S. and S. E. Ozanne (2006). "Mechanisms by which poor early growth programs type-2 diabetes, obesity and the metabolic syndrome." Physiol Behav 88(3): 234-43.

Festuccia, W. T., N. H. Kawashita, et al. (2003). "Control of glyceroneogenic activity in rat brown adipose tissue." Am J Physiol Regul Integr Comp Physiol 285(1): R177-82.

Franckhauser, S., J. Antras-Ferry, et al. (1995). "Expression of the phosphoenolpyruvate carboxykinase gene in 3T3-F442A adipose cells: opposite effects of dexamethasone and isoprenaline on transcription." Biochem J 305 (Pt 1): 65-71.

Franckhauser, S., S. Munoz, et al. (2002). "Increased fatty acid re-esterification by PEPCK overexpression in adipose tissue leads to obesity without insulin resistance." Diabetes 51(3): 624-30.

Garofano, A., P. Czernichow, et al. (1997). "In utero undernutrition impairs rat beta-cell development." Diabetologia 40(10): 1231-4.

Garofano, A., P. Czernichow, et al. (1998). "Beta-cell mass and proliferation following late fetal and early postnatal malnutrition in the rat." Diabetologia 41(9): 1114-20.

Grigor, M. R., J. Allan, et al. (1986). "Milk composition of rats feeding restricted litters." Biochem J 233(3): 917-9.

Haggarty, P., S. Allstaff, et al. (2002). "Placental nutrient transfer capacity and fetal growth." Placenta 23(1): 86-92.

Hernandez-Valencia, M. and M. E. Patti (2006). "A thin phenotype is protective for impaired glucose tolerance and related to low birth weight in mice." Arch Med Res 37(7): 813-7.

Hsieh, C. W., C. A. Millward, et al. (2009). "Reduced milk triglycerides in mice lacking phosphoenolpyruvate carboxykinase in mammary gland adipocytes and white adipose tissue contribute to the development of insulin resistance in pups." J Nutr 139(12): 2257-65.

Ibanez, L., K. Ong, et al. (2006). "Early development of adiposity and insulin resistance after catch-up weight gain in small-for-gestational-age children." J Clin Endocrinol Metab 91(6): 2153-8.

Jimenez-Chillaron, J.C., E. Isganaitis et al (2009) " Intergeneratinal transmission of glucose intolerance and obesity by in utero undernutrition in mice."Diabetes 58:460-458.

Jensen, M. D., V. Chandramouli, et al. (2001). "Sources of blood glycerol during fasting." Am J Physiol Endocrinol Metab 281(5): E998-1004.

King, H. (1998). "Epidemiology of glucose intolerance and gestational diabetes in women of childbearing age." Diabetes Care 21 Suppl 2: B9-13.

King, H., B. Abdullaev, et al. (1998). "Glucose intolerance and associated factors in the Fergana Valley, Uzbekistan." Diabet Med 15(12): 1052-62.

King, H., R. E. Aubert, et al. (1998). "Global burden of diabetes, 1995-2025: prevalence, numerical estimates, and projections." Diabetes Care 21(9): 1414-31.

Leunissen, R. W., P. Oosterbeek, et al. (2008). "Fat mass accumulation during childhood determines insulin sensitivity in early adulthood." J Clin Endocrinol Metab 93(2): 445-51.

Marsal, K. (2002). "Intrauterine growth restriction." Curr Opin Obstet Gynecol 14(2): 127-35.

Meaney, M. J. and M. Szyf (2005). "Environmental programming of stress responses through DNA methylation: life at the interface between a dynamic environment and a fixed genome." Dialogues Clin Neurosci 7(2): 103-23.

Millward, C. A., D. Desantis, et al. (2010). "Phosphoenolpyruvate carboxykinase (Pck1) helps regulate the triglyceride/fatty acid cycle and development of insulin resistance in mice." J Lipid Res 51(6): 1452-63.

Mokdad, A. H., E. S. Ford, et al. (2003). "Prevalence of obesity, diabetes, and obesity-related health risk factors, 2001." Jama 289(1): 76-9.

Neel, J. V. (1962). "Diabetes mellitus: a "thrifty" genotype rendered detrimental by "progress"?" Am J Hum Genet 14: 353-62.

Olswang, Y., H. Cohen, et al. (2002). "A mutation in the peroxisome proliferator-activated receptor gamma-binding site in the gene for the cytosolic form of phosphoenolpyruvate carboxykinase reduces adipose tissue size and fat content in mice." Proc Natl Acad Sci U S A 99(2): 625-30.

Ozanne, S. E., M. W. Dorling, et al. (2001). "Impaired PI 3-kinase activation in adipocytes from early growth-restricted male rats." Am J Physiol Endocrinol Metab 280(3): E534-9.

Ozanne, S. E., G. S. Olsen, et al. (2003). "Early growth restriction leads to down regulation of protein kinase C zeta and insulin resistance in skeletal muscle." J Endocrinol 177(2): 235-41.

Patel, M. S. and M. Srinivasan (2002). "Metabolic programming: causes and consequences." J Biol Chem 277(3): 1629-32.

Petrik, J., M. Srinivasan, et al. (2001). "A long-term high-carbohydrate diet causes an altered ontogeny of pancreatic islets of Langerhans in the neonatal rat." Pediatr Res 49(1): 84-92.

Plagemann, A., I. Heidrich, et al. (1992). "Obesity and enhanced diabetes and cardiovascular risk in adult rats due to early postnatal overfeeding." Exp Clin Endocrinol 99(3): 154-8.

Randle, P. J. (1963). "Control of Insulin Secretion in Health and Disease." Isr Med J 22: 408-19.

Randle, P. J. (1998). "Regulatory interactions between lipids and carbohydrates: the glucose fatty acid cycle after 35 years." Diabetes Metab Rev 14(4): 263-83.

Rasmussen, E. L., C. Malis, et al. (2005). "Altered fat tissue distribution in young adult men who had low birth weight." Diabetes Care 28(1): 151-3.

Reshef, L., R. W. Hanson, et al. (1970). "A possible physiological role for glyceroneogenesis in rat adipose tissue." J Biol Chem 245(22): 5979-84.

Reshef, L., O. Meyuhas, et al. (1972). "Physiological role and regulation of glyceroneogenesis in rat adipose tissue." Isr J Med Sci 8(3): 372-81.

Ringseis, R., D. Saal, et al. (2004). "Dietary conjugated linoleic acids lower the triacylglycerol concentration in the milk of lactating rats and impair the growth and increase the mortality of their suckling pups." J Nutr 134(12): 3327-34.

Rolls, B. A., M. I. Gurr, et al. (1986). "Lactation in lean and obese rats: effect of cafeteria feeding and of dietary obesity on milk composition." Physiol Behav 38(2): 185-90.

She, P., M. Shiota, et al. (2000). "Phosphoenolpyruvate carboxykinase is necessary for the integration of hepatic energy metabolism." Mol Cell Biol 20(17): 6508-17.

Snoeck, A., C. Remacle, et al. (1990). "Effect of a low protein diet during pregnancy on the fetal rat endocrine pancreas." Biol Neonate 57(2): 107-18.

Taylor, P. D., J. McConnell, et al. (2005). "Impaired glucose homeostasis and mitochondrial abnormalities in offspring of rats fed a fat-rich diet in pregnancy." Am J Physiol Regul Integr Comp Physiol 288(1): R134-9.

Vickers, M. H., B. H. Breier, et al. (2000). "Fetal origins of hyperphagia, obesity, and hypertension and postnatal amplification by hypercaloric nutrition." Am J Physiol Endocrinol Metab 279(1): E83-7.

Wigglesworth, J. S. (1974). "Fetal growth retardation. Animal model: uterine vessel ligation in the pregnant rat." Am J Pathol 77(2): 347-50.

Wu, G., F. W. Bazer, et al. (2004). "Maternal nutrition and fetal development." J Nutr 134(9): 2169-72.

Yoon, K. H., J. H. Lee, et al. (2006). "Epidemic obesity and type 2 diabetes in Asia." Lancet 368(9548): 1681-8.

Zhou, L. J., H. M. Smith, et al. (1994). "Tissue-specific expression of the human CD19 gene in transgenic mice inhibits antigen-independent B-lymphocyte development." Mol Cell Biol 14(6): 3884-94.

Zimmet, P., K. G. Alberti, et al. (2001). "Global and societal implications of the diabetes epidemic." Nature 414(6865): 782-7.

4

Obesity and Systemic Inflammation: Insights into Epigenetic Mechanisms

Perla Kaliman[1] and Marcelina Párrizas[2]
[1]*Systems Neuroscience Unit, IDIBAPS,*
[2]*Endocrinology and Nutrition Unit, IDIBAPS, CIBERDEM,*
Spain

1. Introduction

The global incidence and prevalence of obesity increase with every passing year, affecting both developed and developing countries. An appalling estimate of 75% of adults are projected to be overweight or obese in the United States by 2015 (Wang and Beydoun, 2007), thus raising serious concerns regarding the social and economic repercussions of obesity. The etiology of obesity is complex, with both genetic and environmental factors influencing its susceptibility and development (Campion et al., 2009; Russo et al., 2010). The detrimental effect of obesity on metabolic, cardiovascular and central nervous system dysfunction is well documented, as is its association with type 2 diabetes and cancer (Andersson et al., 2008; Bruce-Keller et al., 2009; Gallagher and LeRoith, 2010).

The continuing study of the adipose tissue over the past twenty years has transformed the perception that most investigators had of that organ. Despite being considered for decades no more than an uninteresting container for the storage of spare energy endowed with some useful mechanical and thermal insulating characteristics, the white adipose tissue (WAT) is actually an extremely dynamic endocrine organ that secretes a wide variety of hormones and cytokines, some of them in exclusivity, such as adiponectin (Zhang et al., 1994; Scherer et al., 1995; Kershaw and Flier, 2004; Trayhurn and Wood, 2004). Well over fifty adipokines have been described to date, with pleiotropic functions that highlight the involvement of the adipose tissue in the regulation of processes as varied as insulin sensitivity and glucose homeostasis, blood pressure, angiogenesis, fertility, immunity, neuroplasticity or inflammation (Trayhurn and Wood, 2004; Dietrich and Horvarth, 2009; Galic et al., 2010).

Obesity is defined by excess accumulation of white adipose mass, resulting from both an increase in adipocyte cell size (hypertrophy) and the development of new mature cells from undifferentiated precursors (hyperplasia) (Heine et al., 2000; Naaz et al., 2004). Serum levels of most adipokines increase with obesity, whereas others, notably adiponectin, decrease, upsetting the energetic balance of the organism (Trayhurn and Wood, 2004; Smith et al., 2006). Most importantly, the enlarged obese adipose tissue displays enhanced macrophage infiltration and behaves as a chronically inflamed organ (Weisberg et al., 2003; Xu et al., 2003).

The process of inflammation has evolved as a mechanism to repair a tissue after infection or physical damage has taken place. The acute inflammatory response is a controlled process initiated by tissue resident macrophages that after detecting infection or injury secrete a variety of inflammatory mediators that on the one hand attract leukocytes and platelets to the affected site, and on the other hand activate the endothelial cells, increasing their permeability to leukocytes (specifically neutrophils) while avoiding extravasation of erythrocytes (Medzhitov, 2008). The concluding stage of inflammation is resolution, mediated mainly by the tissue resident macrophages that secrete anti-inflammatory mediators to inhibit further recruitment of neutrophils while favoring that of monocytes that remove dead cells and participate in tissue repair and remodeling (Medzhitov, 2008). If resolution is not forthcoming, chronic inflammation ensues, ultimately resulting in tissue damage and metabolic demise of the organism.

Obesity is nowadays being accepted as a state of chronic low-grade inflammation (Xu et al., 2003; Weisberg et al., 2006). This inflammatory state impacts the function of many organs and tissues, from the adipose tissue itself to the endothelium, the central nervous system, the pancreas or the liver, and is being recognized as etiological of the aging process.

2. The proinflammatory features of dysfunctional obese adipose tissue

The white adipose tissue is constituted by a mixture of cell types, amongst which mature adipocytes represent the main fraction. Fat cell number is settled during adolescence or early adulthood in humans, but at least 10% of the total adipose mass is renewed every year (Spalding et al., 2008). In fact, recent reports indicate that 1-5% of total adipocytes may be replaced each day (Rigamonti et al., 2011). Mature adipocytes differentiate from progenitors, i.e. preadipocytes, which are present in the stromal-vascular fraction of the tissue that also contains, together with other minority cell types, a variable number of resident macrophages/monocytes (Rodeheffer et al., 2008). In physiological conditions, macrophages in WAT display an alternatively activated M2 phenotype, characterized by secretion of anti-inflammatory cytokines such as IL-10 (Lumeng et al., 2007; Olefsky and Glass, 2010). However, the cellular composition of WAT is altered in obesity (Figure 1).

On the one hand, the number of committed preadipocytes capable of undergoing adipogenesis is reduced in obese individuals (Tchoukalova et al., 2004; Tchoukalova et al., 2007; Isakson et al., 2009). Conversely, the number of infiltrated macrophages is significantly increased in obesity. Macrophages may represent as much as a 30 % of the total obese adipose tissue cell population, as compared to a 10 % in lean tissue, in both human and rodent models (Weisberg et al., 2003; Xu et al., 2003). Moreover, macrophages infiltrating the obese adipose tissue switch to a classically activated M1 phenotype (Lumeng et al., 2007), resulting in enhanced proinflammatory cytokine production and systemic low-grade inflammation arising from the adipose tissue (Olefsky and Glass, 2010).

Obesity-associated inflammation has been linked to the development of major complications in acute pancreatitis (Evans et al., 2010), non-alcoholic fatty liver disease (Tilg, 2010), vascular inflammation and coronary artery disease (Andersson et al., 2008; Gomes et al., 2010), chronic obstructive pulmonary disease (Tkacova, 2010), risk of cerebral ischemia and brain injury (Denes et al., 2010) and atherosclerotic vascular disease and myocardial infarction (Ohman et al., 2009). Moreover, preclinical data suggest a link between obesity and cancer (Hursting et al., 2008; Roberts et al., 2010). In fact, it has been estimated that overweight and obesity account for approximately 20 % of all cancer cases and scattered evidence indicates beneficial effects of weight loss on susceptibility and prognosis of some types of cancer (Wolin et al., 2010). This inflammatory state also underlies obesity-associated insulin resistance, and genetic inactivation of several inflammatory mediators or their receptors in macrophages improves insulin action and may prevent the development of diabetes in animal models (Arkan et al., 2005; Weisberg et al., 2006; Solinas et al., 2007).

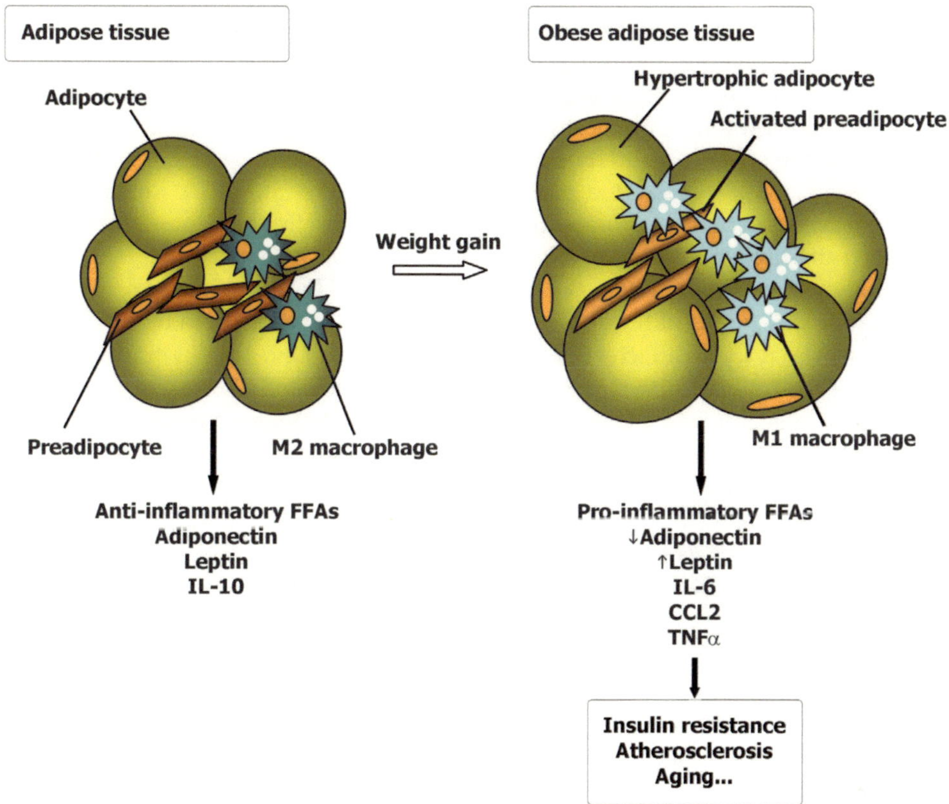

Fig. 1. The cellular composition of the adipose tissue is altered in obesity. Lean adipose tissue is composed of mature adipocytes and the stromal vascular cell fraction characterized by presence of adipose tissue stem cells, committed preadipocytes, endothelial cells and tissue resident macrophages with an alternatively activated M2 phenotype, which secrete anti-inflammatory IL-10. Adipocytes secrete leptin and adiponectin amongst other adipose tissue hormones. The obese adipose tissue is characterized by enlarged adipocytes that secrete increased levels of leptin giving rise to central and peripheral leptin resistance, and decreased levels of anti-inflammatory adiponectin. Macrophages infiltrate the obese adipose tissue in high numbers and polarize to a classically activated M1 phenotype, increasing secretion of proinflammatory cytokines such as TNF-α or IL-6. The inflammatory environment activates the preadipocytes that then acquire macrophage-like characteristics by expressing high levels of inflammatory cytokines and being unable to differentiate.

3. Epigenetics of inflammation

The concept of epigenetics refers to the study of cellular mechanisms that control somatically, and sometimes intergenerationally, inheritable gene expression states that are established in the absence of a change in the DNA sequence itself. Epigenetic mechanisms comprise an array of molecular modifications to both the DNA molecule itself and the histone proteins that associate with it, as well as the regulation by non-coding RNAs (Bernstein et al., 2007). Epigenetic processes drive the response of the cells to environmental cues by selectively activating or repressing transcription of subsets of genes and thus play a crucial role in regulating the transcriptional state and functionality of cells during development or in physiological and pathological conditions. Together with the genetic background (gene variants, polymorphisms) of an individual, the epigenetic modifications accumulated in the course of a lifetime of environmental influences dictate the susceptibility to and development of disease (Fraga et al., 2005; Poulsen et al., 2007). Remarkably, recent findings indicate that inflammation induces epigenetic alterations in tissues that then lay the basis for later disease manifestation (Backdahl et al., 2009).

Two of the most studied epigenetic mechanisms are DNA methylation and the post-translational modifications of histones. DNA methylation is the process by which a cytosine residue present in a CpG dinucleotide is methylated by a DNA methyltransferase (Dnmt) enzyme (Gruenbaum et al., 1981). Methylation of CpGs located close to promoters usually results in gene silencing and plays a crucial role in developmental processes. Recent data have shown that DNA methylation is in some instances dependent on the pattern of histone post-translational modifications in the same gene region and *vice versa* (Fuks, 2005). Histone modifications create new binding sites for regulatory proteins, thus resulting in recruitment of specific activator/repressor complexes (Bartke et al., 2010; Oliver and Denu, 2011). Numerous reports have shown a clear link between the pattern of histone modifications in the chromatin of a given gene and its transcriptional status, and this has been considered indicative of the existence of a histone code, where the pattern of histone modifications at a gene region regulates the transcriptional outcome, as well as other DNA-based processes such as replication or DNA repair, either by modulating access to the DNA or by actively recruiting transcriptional regulators (Strahl and Allis, 2000; Turner, 2000; Jenuwein and Allis, 2001). In this regard, histone lysine acetylation is usually related to gene activation (Pokholok et al., 2005), whereas methylation results in different outcomes, depending on the modified residue (Lachner et al., 2001; Santos-Rosa et al., 2002; Talasz et al., 2005). Histone acetylation is the result of the interplay between histone acetyltransferases (HATs) and deacetylases (HDACs), whereas the enzymes responsible for histone methylation turnover are the histone methytransferases (HMTs) and demethylases (HDMs) (Couture and Trievel, 2006; Smith and Denu, 2009). Interestingly, many components of the basic transcriptional machinery and transcription factors can also undergo acetylation or metylation, which may in turn regulate their activity (Imhof et al., 1997; Egorova et al., 2010).

Non-coding RNAs (ncRNAs), on the other hand, are a large group of RNA molecules that are not translated into protein (Bernstein and Allis, 2005). Recent findings have unravelled a critical role for some of these RNA molecules, such as microRNAs (miRNAs), in the regulation of gene expression and genomic stability. miRNAs are 18-24 nucleotide long, single-stranded RNA molecules that suppress the expression of protein-coding mRNAs, either by directing translational repression or mRNA desestabilization (Bernstein and Allis, 2005).

DNA methylation, histone modifications and miRNAs play key roles in the differentiation of adipocytes and participate in the development of obesity (Esau et al., 2004; Fu et al., 2005; Musri et al., 2006; Noer et al., 2006; Yoo et al., 2006; Musri et al., 2007; Lee et al., 2008; Cho et al., 2009; Horii et al., 2009; Inagaki et al., 2009; Tang et al., 2009; Wakabayashi et al., 2009; Heneghan et al., 2010; Musri et al., 2010; Yang et al., 2010). Epigenetic processes are also implicated in the physiological and pathological inflammatory response (Bayarsaihan, 2011). Increased transcription of proinflammatory cytokine genes by master regulator NF-κB is associated with enhanced histone acetylation at their promoters (Yamamoto et al., 2003), as well as phosphorylation of Ser10 of histone H3 (H3Ser10) (Anest et al., 2003; Yamamoto et al., 2003). NF-κB regulatory kinase IKK-α can in fact phosphorylate H3Ser10 *in vitro* (Anest et al., 2003). On the other hand, expression of NF-κB itself in monocytes or neutrophils is regulated by several miRNAs, such as miR-9, whose expression is in its turn regulated by NF-κB, thus establishing a feedback loop that may control the degree of inflammation (Bazzoni et al., 2009). Dysregulation of any of these processes could generate an anomalous persistence of the inflammatory response in time, resulting in metabolic alterations and tissue damage.

4. Impact of inflammation on the adipose tissue

Several hypotheses have been proposed in an attempt to explain the role of the adipose tissue in the metabolic dysfunction associated with obesity. Thus, the altered pattern of adipokine secretion by the obese adipose tissue (Ukkola and Santaniemi, 2002; Tataranni and Ortega, 2005;), the inflammatory state associated with obesity (Cottam et al., 2004), or the inability of the adipose tissue to expand its mass in response to increased energy intake (Virtue and Vidal-Puig, 2010) have all been signaled as possible culprits. However, all these different hypotheses are not mutually exclusive.

Inflammation of the adipose tissue has been proposed as the critical element that distinguishes metabolically 'healthy' from 'unhealthy' obese subjects (Bluher, 2010), and a recent study has reported that increased inflammation in the adipose tissue precedes the development of obesity and insulin resistance in mice (Mori et al., 2010). Interestingly, preadipocytes display many functional and antigenic features in common with the monocyte/macrophage lineage and can actually be converted into macrophages given the adequate environment (Charriere et al., 2003). In fact, inflammatory cytokines such as tumor necrosis factor (TNF)-α and interleukin 6 (IL-6) block adipogenesis (Gustafson and Smith, 2006) and induce the expression and secretion of molecules that are not usually secreted by preadipocytes, such as IL-1β, IL-6 itself or the monocyte chemoattractant protein MCP-1 (Isakson et al., 2009). Therefore, inflammation has a double-hit effect on adipose tissue dysfunction by on the one hand decreasing adipogenesis and consequently cell turnover and expandability potential, and on the other increasing cytokine production thus establishing a self-sustaining cycle. Epigenetic mechanisms probably underlay this phenotype. In fact, overexpression of DNA methyltransferase Dnmt3a in mouse adipocytes results in enhanced expression of proinflammatory genes by the obese adipose tissue (Kamei et al., 2010). Obesity caused by high-fat diet increases DNA methylation at the leptin promoter in rat adipocytes, and this is associated with decreased circulating leptin levels (Milagro et al., 2009). Inflammatory cytokines such as TNF-α provoke wide transcriptomic changes in adipose tissue *in vivo* and *in vitro* (Ruan et al., 2002b; Isakson et al., 2009). In particular, TNF-α induces expression of the pseudokinase Tribbles 1 (Trb1) in mature adipocytes. Trb1 then binds to NF-κB target promoters and favors transcription of proinflammatory genes (Ostertag et al., 2010), thus creating a vicious circle. On the other hand, incubation of differentiated adipocytes in the presence of TNF-α suppresses expression of mature adipocyte genes, and reactivates the expression of those characteristic of the preadipocyte stage (Ruan et al., 2002a). Obesity produces the same effect, thus suggesting that the changes observed in obese adipose tissue are due to the proinflammatory environment (Xie et al., 2009). Moreover, obesity alters the pattern of adipose tissue-expressed miRNAs in the same fashion, by suppressing expression of mature adipocyte miRNAs, such as miR-103 or mir-143, while reactivating the expression of those highly expressed in preadipocytes, including miR-221 and miR-222, (Xie et al., 2009). Expression of miR-222 is also increased in 3T3-L1 adipocytes maintained under hyperglycemic conditions (Herrera et al., 2010) or in adipose tissue of mice treated with conjugated linoleic acid (Parra et al., 2010), indicating that it is involved in the pathophysiology of diabetes. Interestingly, a number of miRNAs play crucial functions in both the adipose tissue and the immune system. Thus, the miR-17~92 cluster accelerates adipogenesis in 3T3-L1 cells (Wang et al., 2008) and blocks monocytic differentiation of human CD34+ hematopoietic progenitor cells (Fontana et al., 2007), although this later effect is not seen *in vivo* in two different mouse models (Ventura et al., 2008; Xiao et al., 2008). Incidentally, however, no effect of miR-17~92 deficiency on the adipose tissue has been reported to date.

5. Impact of inflammation on the endothelium

Endothelial damage and associated increased cardiovascular risk is a fixture of obesity (Andersson et al., 2008). Endothelial cells incubated in the presence of preadipocytes treated with proinflammatory cytokines as compared with control preadipocytes express high levels of those cytokines themselves and display increased monocyte adhesion to them (Mack et al., 2009).

The regulatory role of epigenetic mechanisms in the pathogenesis of atherosclerosis and risk of coronary artery disease and stroke is increasingly being recognized (Wierda et al., 2010). Recent studies have shown that histone methylation is involved in establishing and maintaining the activated proinflammatory state of vascular smooth muscle cells (VSMC) in diabetic obese *db/db* mice. Histone methyltransferase Suv39h1 is required to maintain high levels of repressive trimethylation of the lysine K9 of the histone H3 (H3K9me3) at the promoters of inflammatory genes in these cells (Villeneuve et al., 2008). In diabetic mice, expression of miR-125b increases in VSMCs and this results in decreased expression of its target Suv39h1 and thus decreased H3K9me3 methylation at the promoters of proinflammatory genes, coupled with increased gene expression (Villeneuve et al., 2010). Similarly, histone demethylase LSD1 is decreased in *db/db* VSMCs, resulting in increased H3K4me2 levels and enhanced expression of inflammatory genes *ccl2* and *il6* (Reddy et al., 2008).

The key proinflammatory transcription factor NF-κB is upregulated in endothelial cells as a response to hyperglycemia in vitro, and this is associated with binding of LSD1 and histone methyltransferase Set7 to its promoter and increased H3K4me1 methylation (Brasacchio et al., 2009). In its turn, NF-κB also associates with Set7 to stimulate transcription of its target genes in monocytes, and Set7 binding to proinflammatory promoters increases in macrophages from diabetic mice (Li et al., 2008). Interestingly, one of the genes whose expression is increased by NF-κB and Set7 in macrophages treated with TNF-α is the histone demethylase JMJD3 (Li et al., 2008), thus suggesting a mechanism by which proinflammatory cytokines induce expression of chromatin-modifying enzymes in target cells to remodel chromatin and amplify the inflammatory response.

The expression of a number of miRNAs is also altered in endothelial cells incubated under inflammatory conditions (Dentelli et al., 2010). Expression of miR-222, for instance, is downregulated in endothelial cells exposed to inflammatory stimuli and its expression is negatively correlated with inflammation-mediated vascular remodeling through regulation of its target Signal Transducer and Activator of transcription 5A (STAT5A) (Dentelli et al., 2010). Treatment with Angiotensin II (Ang II) also has been shown to decrease the expression of miR-221/222 as well as miR-155 in human umbilical vein endothelial cells (HUVEC), and this decrease is associated with increased expression of their target Ets-1, a transcription factor that regulates the expression of adhesion molecules in endothelial cells (Zhu et al., 2011). Overexpression of miR-221/222 and miR-155 in HUVEC effectively decreased the adhesion of Jurkat T cells to Ang II-treated HUVEC (Zhu et al., 2011). Increased expression of adhesion molecules E-selectin and ICAM1 in endothelial cells treated with TNF-α is also mediated through changes in the expression of miRNAs such as miR-31 or miR-17-3p (Suarez et al., 2010).

6. Obesity and aging

Healthy aging and longevity are negatively influenced by inflammatory processes and metabolic alterations. The longevity phenotype seems to arise from a complex network of genetic, epigenetic and environmental factors interacting through still poorly characterized pathways. A negative relationship between adiposity and longevity has been recently proposed in an epidemiological study in healthy centenarians which revealed that low body fat mass, a nonatherogenic lipid profile and a better insulin sensitivity correlate with human longevity (Bluher, 2008). Moreover, telomere length, which is a marker of cellular senescence dependent of intricate epigenetic mechanisms, has recently been found to be decreased in human subjects with higher total and abdominal adiposity, further reinforcing the notion that obesity may accelerate the aging process (Lee et al., 2011).

Most of the longevity gene candidates described so far are related either to inflammatory functions, lipid and glucose metabolism or the stress response. Indeed, aging is characterized by chronic low-grade inflammation termed "inflammaging", in which a two- to fourfold increase in proinflammatory cytokines and acute phase protein production is observed (Jylhävä and Hurme, 2010). Notably, preadipocytes, which as mentioned are closely related to macrophages, dedifferentiate with aging and switch to a proinflammatory, senescent-like state (Tchkonia et al., 2010). However, a senescent-like state also develops in fat cells and preadipocytes from young obese subjects (Villaret et al., 2010).

Changes in DNA methylation levels and histone modification patterns have been detected throughout life although their effect on aging is only just beginning to be revealed (Siegmund et al., 2007; Dang et al., 2009; Greer et al., 2010; Siebold et al., 2010). Whether the age-dependent epigenetic drift is boosted by pathological metabolic situations such as obesity-related inflammation remains an unexplored territory. However, several observations point to a role for epigenetics in the regulation of lipid metabolism, inflammation and longevity. In organisms ranging from yeast to mammals, leanness and caloric restriction have been shown to increase longevity through the class III histone deacetylase sirtuin 1 (SIRT1), which acts in several cell processes by deacetylating both histones and transcription factors. A putative role for sirtuins as metabolic or oxidative sensors that respond to the cellular environment has been proposed (Frye et al, 1999). Interestingly, a potential protective role of SIRT1 against the metabolic consequences of chronic exposure to a high-fat diet has been recently described in a transgenic SIRT1 mouse model (Pfluger et al., 2008). Mice overexpressing SIRT1 and fed a high fat diet showed lower lipid-induced inflammation along with better glucose tolerance, and almost entire protection from hepatic steatosis compared with wild type controls. Such beneficial effects of SIRT1 correlated with increased expression of antioxidant proteins MnSOD and Nrf1 and reduced expression of proinflammatory cytokines, such as TNF-α and IL-6, probably by inhibiting NF-KB activity. Consistent with these observations, the AMP-activated protein kinase AMPK, acting through SIRT1 negatively regulates lipid-induced inflammation, indicating that this protein deacetylase may exert its anti-aging function at least in part through protection against obesity, inflammation, and insulin resistance (Yang et al., 2010). Interestingly, it has been shown that the natural compound resveratrol has anti-inflammatory effects in human adipose tissue through the SIRT1 pathway (Olholm et al., 2010) and several studies have described its capacity to extend lifespan in different species (i.e. *S. cerevisae*, *C. elegans*, and *D. melanogaster*) also through the sirtuin pathway, although other studies did not find an effect of resveratrol on lifespan. (Mouchiroud et al., 2010).

7. Obesity and the central nervous system

In a prospective cohort study conducted from 1997 to 2002 of 3075 subjects aged 70 to 79 years, an increased rate of cognitive decline was detected in those with high levels of serum markers of inflammation (Yaffe et al, 2004). Indeed, subclinical inflammation seems to be involved in the pathogenesis of cognitive impairment. Increased body mass and obesity have been related to cognitive decline, including decreased attentional performance, speed of processing and executive functions (Gunstad et al., 2007; Boeka et al, 2008; Fergenbaum et al, 2009). Moreover, midlife obesity is increasingly being described as a dementia risk factor in later life (Fitzpatrick et al, 2009). Reductions in brain volume in frontal, temporal, parietal, and occipital lobes, gray matter in temporal and frontal regions and white matter have been associated with obesity (Pannacciulli et al., 2006; Gunstad et al., 2008; Taki et al., 2008; Volkow et al., 2009; Ho et al., 2010; Stanek et al, 2011).

Neural oxidative stress, inflammation, and NF-κB activation have been detected in cerebral cortex from rats fed a high fat diet (Zhang et al 2005), suggesting a link between diet-induced obesity and increased risk of dementia. This can be due, at least in part ,to triglyceride breakdown into free saturated fatty acids such as palmitic acid and lauric acid, which have been shown to modulate astrocytic and microglial signaling and to trigger inflammatory signals in macrophages (Patil et al, 2005; Laine et al, 2007). Another mechanism that seems to be involved in the peripheral modulation of CNS function is the impairment by triglycerides of leptin transport through the blood-brain barrier (Banks et al., 2004). Leptin is an afferent fat-to-brain signal entering the brain via a saturable transport mechanism and acting at hypothalamic centers to regulate the feeding behavior. In addition to this well characterized hypothalamic function, leptin receptors are also widely expressed in other regions of the brain, including brain stem, cerebellum, amygdala and hippocampus (Fei et al., 1997; Elmquist et al., 1998) and a role for leptin in cognitive processes has been proposed (Harvey et al., 2005). For example, behavioral performance was improved in rats after intravenous administration of

leptin (Oomura et al., 2006). Notably, leptin has been shown to modulate the inflammatory signaling in microglia (Pinteaux et al, 2007; Tang et al, 2007).
Recently, intergenerational effects of maternal obesity on the CNS have been reported in mouse models, sustained at least in part by epigenetic mechanisms. Indeed, maternal obesity induced by consumption of a high fat diet prior to and during pregnancy and lactation leads to metabolic alterations in the offspring together with behavioral and biochemical alterations within their CNS. For example, effects of prenatal and postnatal exposure to high fat diet (HFD) on the brain were studied by analyzing pups born to HFD-induced obese or control diet (CD) mothers (White et al, 2009). After weaning, male progeny was placed on a CD until 8 weeks old, and then fed either a HFD or a CD themselves. HFD progeny from HFD dams manifested a significantly increased cognitive decline associated with significant increases in 3-nitrotyrosine, iNOS, IL-6, and glial markers Iba-1 and GFAP. These data suggest that brain oxidative and inflammatory signaling is increased by HFD, and that maternal HFD-induced obesity might sensitize offspring. Other studies seem to support some of these observations. Diet-induced maternal obesity has recently been reported to impair hippocampal BDNF production and spatial cognitive function in young offspring, possibly due to metabolic and oxidative changes. (Tozuka et al, 2010). Similarly, in a recent report, rats were fed high-fat diets that created an obese phenotype or were maintained under a low-fat diet for 4 weeks prior to mating, throughout pregnancy and lactation (Bilbo and Tsang, 2010). At birth, pups from obese mothers showed increased serum leptin levels and microglial activation markers in the hippocampus. From weaning to adulthood, in response to a bacterial challenge (LPS), peripheral proinflammatory cytokines were significantly increased in offspring from obese mothers compared to controls. These changes were accompanied by higher anxiety levels in the HFD offspring. Although the cognitive susceptibility of the offspring from obese mothers to inflammatory insults was not evaluated, surprisingly rats born to obese mothers performed better in memory and spatial learning tasks than their low fat diet controls, suggesting that exposure to HFD during development may lead to different cognitive outcomes than during adulthood (Granholm et al., 2008; Murray et al., 2009). On the whole, these data suggest an obesity-induced early life-programming that may be established by epigenetic mechanisms.

8. Obesity and cancer

The connection between obesity and cancer is extensively documented. Obesity has been reported as a cause of approximately 14 % of cancer deaths in men and up to 20 % of cancer deaths in women in a 25-year-prospective study of U.S. adults (Calle et al., 2003). In Europe, a review by the International Agency for Research on Cancer (IARC) in 2002 concluded that obesity was a cause of 39 % of endometrial, 37 % of esophageal, 25 % of kidney, 11 % of colon and 9 % of postmenopausal breast cancer cases (International Agency for Research on Cancer, 2002). By contrast, being overweight or obese during childhood and adolescence appears to be protective against breast cancer (Ahlgren et al., 2004). Body weight has also been inversely associated with breast cancer in premenopausal women (Huang et al, 1997).
Depending of the type of cancer, different mechanisms have been proposed that can be influenced by obesity for example the dysregulation of adipokines. Some of those that regulate the immune and the inflammatory response (i.e. leptin, TNF-α, IL-6, serum amyloid A), seem to contribute to tumorigenesis, tumor progression and metastatic potential. Although evidence is still weak, inflammation is a mechanism gaining interest in

the cancer field mainly because obesity-related inflammatory markers are increasingly associated with worse cancer prognosis (Pierce et al., 2009). Chronic inflammation has been linked to initiation and progression of different cancer types, including gastric (Farinati et al., 2008), hepatocellular (Fernandez-Irigoyen et al., 2008; Lukasiak et al., 2008), and colorectal (Wang & DuBois, 2008) carcinoma. The tumor-associated stroma includes among other cell types adipocytes, inflammatory and immune cells and influences the development and progression of tumors through its interaction with transformed cells *via* soluble mediators, such as growth factors and cytokines (Mantovani et al., 2008; Ono et al., 2008).

Other means through which obesity-related chronic inflammation may influence cancer development is by altering the host antitumor immune response (Nave et al, 2008) and growth factor pathways. Indeed, recent data implicate IGF-I in the obesity-induced increase in tumor cell growth and support a critical role of inflammatory cytokines in the regulation of hepatic metastasis (Wu et al, 2010). Moreover, leptin, a proinflammatory adipokine increased in obesity, can induce eicosanoid production through a PI3K/mTOR-dependent pathway and activate resident macrophages to form adipose differentiation-related protein (ADRP)-enriched lipid droplets (Maya-Monteiro & Bossa, 2008). Notably, human colon adenocarcinoma cell lines and colon cancer biopsies from patients have recently been shown to exhibit a drastic increase in ADRP and COX-2-enriched lipid bodies. The pathological implications of these changes are supported by data showing that inhibition of lipid droplet formation in cancer cells reduces PGE2 production and correlates with diminished cancer cell proliferation (Accioly et al., 2008).

Cells from the white adipose tissue can be recruited by tumors promoting cancer progression in mice. WAT cellular types engrafted in tumors include adipose stromal cells and adipose endothelial cells and their migration has been attributed to obesity-associated inflammation. (Zhang et al., 2009).

Although evidence for specific epigenetic mechanisms linking obesity-related chronic inflammation and cancer is currently lacking, several observations allow a link to be hypothesized. It has been proposed that aberrant epigenetic modifications can be induced by inflammation early in the process of carcinogenesis and that the accumulation of these modifications generates "an epigenetic field for cancerization" (Niwa and Ushijima, 2010). Alterations in cytokine and chemokine signaling seem to be involved in inflammation-induced aberrant DNA methylation. For example, IL-6 promotes the induction of significant global DNA hypomethylation as well as CpG promoter methylation changes in putative tumor suppressor genes such as CHFR, GATA5 and PAX6 in an *in vitro* model of inflammatory stress in squamous cell carcinoma (OSCC) cell lines (Gasche et al., 2011). Disturbances in the activity of DNA methyltransferases are increasingly related to the development of malignant phenotypes and it is interesting to note that the expression of the *de novo* methyltransferase *Dnmt3a* is increased in the adipose tissue and seems to contribute to obesity-related inflammation (Kamei et al., 2010).

Non-coding RNAs are also part of the cellular epigenetic machinery that regulates cell fate and functioning in response to environmental signals. Among them, miRNAs have been implicated in the control of a wide variety of biological processes ranging from proliferation and apoptosis to metabolism (Krol et al., 2010). Notably, several forms of human tumors present a robust upregulation of mir-221 and miR-222, two related miRNAs encoded in cluster on chromosome X (Garofalo et al., 2009; Rao et al., 2010; Pu et al, 2010; Zhang et al., 2010; Pineau et al., 2010; Galardi et al, 2011). Interestingly, miR-221 and miR-222 levels are downregulated during adipogenesis but increased in obese adipocytes. These changes have been attributed to the elevated TNF-α levels and the overall chronic inflammatory environment generated by the obese adipose tissue, as they were mimicked by treatment of differentiated 3T3-L1 adipocytes with TNF-α (Xie et al, 2009).

9. Conclusions

It is becoming increasingly evident that obesity is not only associated with metabolic alterations and decreased general wellbeing but it also represents a risk factor for the development of other chronic diseases such as cardiovascular disease, central nervous system dysfunction, cancer as well as accelerated aging (Figure 2).

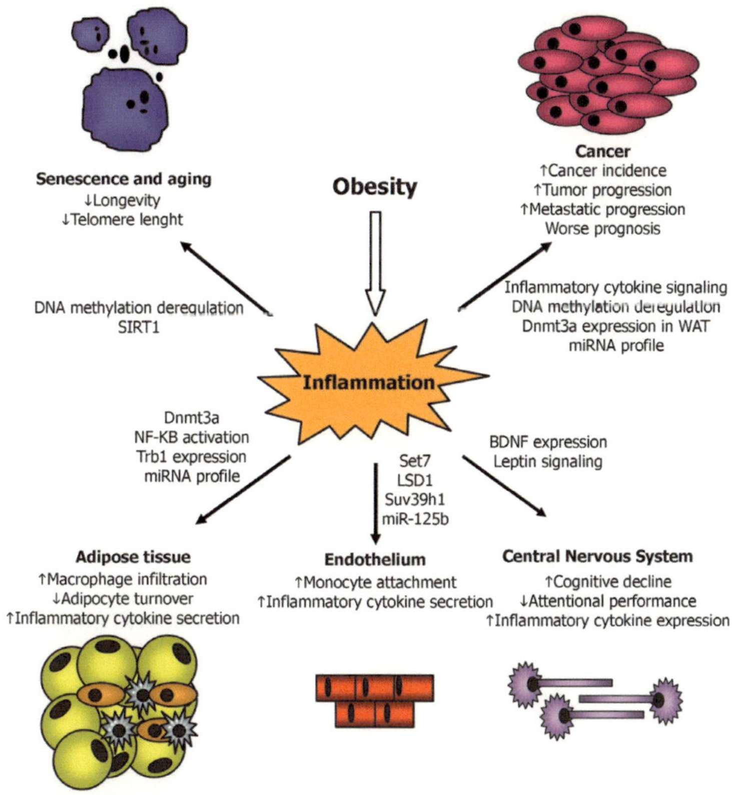

Fig. 2. Inflammation impacts tissue function and organismal aging. Inflammation causes increased macrophage infiltration and decreased adipocyte turnover in the adipose tissue, in part due to increased NF-κB activation, Trb1 expression and alteration of the miRNA profile. Overexpression of DNA methyltransferase Dnmt3a in adipose tissue also results in increased cytokine expression. In the endothelium inflammation increases expression of proiflammatory genes through the regulation of histone demethylases and methyltransferases LSD1, Set7 and Suv39h1, as well as miRNA miR-125b which targets Suv39h1. In the central nervous system, epigenetic effects of inflammation seem to be mediated by decreased BDNF expression and altered leptin signaling. Inflammation also impacts on cell senescence and organismal aging, through deregulation of the pattern of DNA methylation and histone deacetylase Sirt1, and in cancer initiation and progression, by growth-promoting cytokine signaling and deregulation of DNA methylation and the profile of miRNAs.

Obesity is now recognized as an inflammatory disease. Inflammation impacts negatively the function of many organs and tissues through increased macrophage infiltration and decreased adipocyte turnover in the adipose tissue, in part due to increased NF-κB activation and Trb1 expression. Epigenetic mechanisms such as alteration of the miRNA profile and overexpression of DNA methyltransferase Dnmt3a in adipose tissue also result in increased cytokine expression. In the endothelium, inflammation increases expression of proiflammatory genes through the regulation of histone demethylases and methyltransferases LSD1, Set7 and Suv39h1, as well as miRNA miR-125b which targets Suv39h1. In the central nervous system, epigenetic effects of inflammation seem to be mediated by decreased BDNF expression and altered leptin signaling. Inflammation also impacts on cell senescence and organismal aging, through deregulation of the pattern of DNA methylation and histone deacetylase Sirt1. Inflammation may also affect cancer initiation and progression through growth-promoting cytokine signaling and deregulation of DNA methylation and the profile of miRNAs. The emerging picture of potential long lasting systemic alterations induced by obesity-related inflammation, some of which could be transmitted to subsequent generations, raises the urgent need to implement educative, preventive and therapeutic approaches to this serious health concern.

10. Acknowledgments

This work was supported by Ministerio de Ciencia e Innovación grants *SAF2010-15050* to PK and *BFU2009-09988/BMC* to MP

11. References

Accioly, M.T.; Pacheco, P.; Maya-Monteiro, C.M.; Carrossini, N.; Robbs, B.K.; Oliveira, S.S.; Kaufmann C.; Morgado-Diaz, J.A.; Bozza, P.T., & Viola, J.P. (2008) Lipid bodies are reservoirs of cyclooxygenase- 2 and sites of prostaglandin-E2 synthesis in colon cancer cells. *Cancer Res.*, 68, 6, 1732-1740.

Ahlgren, M.; Melbye, M. ; Wohlfahrt, J., & Sorensen, T.I. (2004) Growth patterns and the risk of breast cancer in women. *N. Engl. J. Med.* 351, 16, 1619–1626.

Andersson, C.X.; Gustafson, B.; Hammarstedt, A.; Hedjazifar, S., & Smith, U. (2008) Inflamed adipose tissue, insulin resistance and vascular injury. *Diabetes Metab. Res. Rev.* 24, 595-603.

Anest, V.; Hanson, J.L.; Cogswell, P.C.; Steinbrecher, K.A.; Strahl, B.D., & Baldwin, A.S. (2003) A nucleosomal function for IkappaB kinase-alpha in NF-kappaB-dependent gene expression. *Nature.* 423, 659-663.

Arkan, M.C.; Hevener, A.L.; Greten, F.R.; Maeda, S.; Li, Z.W.; Long, J.M.; Wynshaw-Boris, A.; Poli, G.; Olefsky, J., & Karin, M. (2005) IKK-beta links inflammation to obesity-induced insulin resistance. *Nat. Med.* 11, 191-198.

Backdahl, L.; Bushell, A., & Beck,S. (2009) Inflammatory signalling as mediator of epigenetic modulation in tissue-specific chronic inflammation. *Int. J. Biochem. Cell Biol.* 41, 176-184.

Banks, W.A.; Coon, A.B.; Robinson, S.M.; Moinuddin, A.; Shultz, J.M.; Nakaoke, R., & Morley, J.E. (2004) Triglycerides induce leptin resistance at the blood-brain barrier. *Diabetes*, 53, 5, 1253–1260.

Bartke, T.; Vermeulen, M.; Xhemalce, B.; Robson, S.C.; Mann,M., & Kouzarides, T. (2010) Nucleosome-interacting proteins regulated by DNA and histone methylation. *Cell.* 143, 470-484.

Bayarsaihan, D. (2011) Epigenetic mechanisms in inflammation. *J. Dent. Res.* 90, 9-17.

Bazzoni, F.; Rossato, M.; Fabbri, M.; Gaudiosi, D.; Mirolo, M.; Mori, L.; Tamassia, N.; Mantovani, A.; Cassatella, M.A., & Locati,M. (2009) Induction and regulatory function of miR-9 in human monocytes and neutrophils exposed to proinflammatory signals. *Proc. Natl. Acad. Sci. U.S.A.* 106, 5282-5287.

Bernstein, B.E.; Meissner, A., & Lander, E.S. (2007) The mammalian epigenome. *Cell.* 128, 669-681.

Bernstein, E. & Allis, C.D. (2005) RNA meets chromatin. *Genes Dev.* 19, 1635-1655.

Bilbo, S.D., & Tsang, V. (2010) Enduring consequences of maternal obesity for brain inflammation and behavior of offspring. *FASEB J.* 24, 6, 2104-2115.

Bluher, M. (2008) Fat tissue and long life. *Obes. Facts.*, 1, 4, 176-82.

Bluher, M. (2010) The distinction of metabolically 'healthy' from 'unhealthy' obese individuals. *Curr. Opin. Lipidol.* 21, 38-43.

Boeka, A.G., & Lokken, K.L. (2008) Neuropsychological performance of a clinical sample of extremely obese individuals. *Arch. Clin. Neuropsychol.*, 23, 4, 467–474.

Brasacchio, D.; Okabe, J.; Tikellis, C.; Balcerczyk, A.; George, P.; Baker, E.K.; Calkin, A.C.; Brownlee, M.; Cooper, M.E., & El-Osta, A. (2009) Hyperglycemia induces a dynamic cooperativity of histone methylase and demethylase enzymes associated with gene-activating epigenetic marks that coexist on the lysine tail. *Diabetes.* 58, 1229-1236.

Bruce-Keller, A.J.; Keller, J.N., & Morrison, C.D. (2009) Obesity and vulnerability of the CNS. *Biochim. Biophys. Acta.* 1792, 395-400.

Calle, E.E.; Rodriguez, C.; Walker-Thurmond, K., & Thun, M.J. (2003) Overweight, obesity, and mortality from cancer in a prospectively studied cohort of U.S. adults. *N. Engl. J. Med.* 348, 1625–1163.

Campion, J.; Milagro, F.I., & Martinez, J.A. (2009) Individuality and epigenetics in obesity. *Obes. Rev.* 10, 383-92

Charriere, G.; Cousin, B.; Arnaud, E.; Andre, M.; Bacou, F.; Penicaud, L., & Casteilla, L. (2003) Preadipocyte conversion to macrophage. Evidence of plasticity. *J. Biol. Chem.* 278, 9850-9855.

Cho, Y.W.; Hong, S.; Jin, Q.; Wang, L.; Lee, J.E.; Gavrilova, O., & Ge, K. (2009) Histone methylation regulator PTIP is required for PPARgamma and C/EBPalpha expression and adipogenesis. *Cell Metab.* 10, 27-39.

Cottam, D.R.; Mattar, S.G.; Barinas-Mitchell, E.; Eid, G.; Kuller, L.; Kelley, D.E., & Schauer, P.R. (2004) The chronic inflammatory hypothesis for the morbidity associated with morbid obesity: implications and effects of weight loss. *Obes. Surg.* 14, 589-600.

Couture, J.F. & Trievel, R.C. (2006) Histone-modifying enzymes: encrypting an enigmatic epigenetic code. *Curr. Opin. Struct. Biol.* 16, 753-760.

Dang, W.; Steffen, K.K.; Perry, R.; Dorsey, J.A.; Jonson, F.B.; Shilatifard, A.; Kaeberstein, M.; Kennedy, B.K., & Berger, S.L. (2009) Histone H4 Lysine 16 acetylation regulates cellular lifespan. *Nature*, 459, 7248, 802-807. *Diabetes*. 59, 11, 2755-2763.

Denes, A.; Thornton, P.; Rothwell, N.J., & Allan, S.M. (2010) Inflammation and brain injury: acute cerebral ischaemia, peripheral and central inflammation. *Brain Behav. Immun.* 24, 708-723.

Dentelli, P.; Rosso, A.; Orso, F.; Olgasi, C.; Taverna, D., & Brizzi, M.F. (2010) microRNA-222 controls neovascularization by regulating signal transducer and activator of transcription 5A expression. *Arterioscler. Thromb. Vasc. Biol.* 30, 1562-1568.

Dietrich, M.O., & Horvath, T.L. (2009) Feeding signals and brain circuitry. *Eur. J. Neurosci.* 30, 9, 1688-1696

Egorova, K.S.; Olenkina, O.M., & Olenina,L.V. (2010) Lysine methylation of nonhistone proteins is a way to regulate their stability and function. *Biochemistry (Mosc).* 75, 535-548.

Elmquist, J.K.; Bjorbaek, C.; Ahima, R.S.; Flier, J.S., & Saper, C.B. (1998) Distributions of leptin receptor mRNA isoforms in the rat brain. *J. Comp. Neurol.* 395, 4,535–547.

Esau, C.; Kang, X.; Peralta, E.; Hanson, E.; Marcusson, E.G.; Ravichandran, L.V.; Sun, Y.; Koo, S.; Perera, R.J.; Jain, R.; Dean, N.M.; Freier, S.M.; Bennett, C.F.; Lollo, B., & Griffey, R. (2004) MicroRNA-143 regulates adipocyte differentiation. *J. Biol. Chem.* 279, 52361-52365.

Evans, A.C.; Papachristou, G.I., & Whitcomb, D.C. (2010) Obesity and the risk of severe acute pancreatitis. *Minerva Gastroenterol. Dietol.* 56, 169-179.

Farinati, F.; Cardin, R.; Cassaro, M.; Bortolami, M.; Nitti, D.; Tieppo, C.; Zaninotto, G., & Rugge, M. (2008) Helicobacter pylori, inflammation, oxidative damage and gastric cancer: a morphological, biological and molecular pathway. Eur. J. Cancer Prev., 17, 3, 195–200.

Fei, H.; Okano, H.J.; Li, C.; Lee, G.H.; Zhao, C.; Darnell, R., & Friedman, J.M. (1997) Anatomic localization of alternatively spliced leptin receptors (Ob-R) in mouse brain and other tissues. *Proc. Natl. Acad. Sci. USA.*, 94, 13, 7001–7005.

Fergenbaum, J.H.; Bruce, S.; Lou, W.; Hanley, A.J.; Greenwood, C., & Young, T.K. (2009) Obesity and lowered cognitive performance in a Canadian First Nations population. *Obesity (Silver Spring)* 17, 10, 1957–1963.

Fernandez-Irigoyen J.; Santamaria, M.; Sanchez-Quiles, V.; Latasa, M.U.; Santamaría, E.; Muñoz, J.; Sánchez Del Pino, M.M.; Valero, M.L.; Prieto, J.; Avila, M.A., & Corrales, F.J. (2008) Redox regulation of methylthioadenosine phosphorylase in liver cells: molecular mechanism and functional implications. *Biochem. J.*, 411, 2, 457–465.

Fitzpatrick, A.L.; Kuller, L.H.; Lopez, O.L.; Diehr, P.; O'Meara, E.S.; Longstreth, W.T. Jr., & Luchsinger, J.A. (2009) Midlife and late-life obesity and the risk of dementia: cardiovascular health study. *Arch. Neurol.* 66, 3, 336–342.

Fontana, L.; Pelosi, E.; Greco, P.; Racanicchi, S.; Testa, U.; Liuzzi, F.; Croce, C.M.; Brunetti, E.; Grignani, F., & Peschle, C. (2007) MicroRNAs 17-5p-20a-106a control monocytopoiesis through AML1 targeting and M-CSF receptor upregulation. *Nat. Cell Biol.* 9, 775-787.

Fraga, M.F.; Ballestar, E.; Paz, M.F.; Ropero, S.; Setien, F.; Ballestar, M.L.; Heine-Suner, D.; Cigudosa, J.C.; Urioste, M.; Benitez, J.; Boix-Chornet, M.; Sanchez-Aguilera, A.; Ling, C.; Carlsson, E.; Poulsen, P.; Vaag, A.; Stephan, Z.; Spector, T.D.; Wu, Y.Z.;

Plass,C., & Esteller, M. (2005) Epigenetic differences arise during the lifetime of monozygotic twins. *Proc. Natl. Acad. Sci. U.S.A.* 102, 10604-10609.

Frye, R.A. (1999) Characterization of five human cDNAs with homology to the yeast SIR2 gene: Sir2-like proteins (sirtuins) metabolize NAD and may have protein ADP-ribosyltransferase activity. *Biochem. Biophys. Res. Commun.*, 260, 1, 273-279.

Fu, M.; Rao, M.; Bouras, T.; Wang, C.; Wu, K.; Zhang, X.; Li, Z.; Yao, T.P., & Pestell, R.G. (2005) Cyclin D1 inhibits peroxisome proliferator-activated receptor gamma-mediated adipogenesis through histone deacetylase recruitment. *J. Biol. Chem.* 280, 16934-16941.

Fuks, F. (2005) DNA methylation and histone modifications: teaming up to silence genes. *Curr. Opin. Genet. Dev.* 15, 490-495.

Galardi, S.; Mercatelli, N.; Farace, M.G., & Ciafrè, S.A. (2011) NF-kB and c-Jun induce the expression of the oncogenic miR-221 and miR-222 in prostate carcinoma and glioblastoma cells. *Nucleic. Acids. Res.* (published online January 18 2011).

Galic, S.; Oakhill, J.S., & Steinberg, G.R. (2010) Adipose tissue as an endocrine organ. *Mol. Cell Endocrinol.* 316, 129-139.

Gallagher, E.J. & LeRoith, D. (2010) Insulin, insulin resistance, obesity, and cancer. *Curr. Diab. Rep.* 10, 93-100.

Garofalo, M.; Di Leva, G.; Romano, G.; Nuovo, G.; Suh, S.S.; Ngankeu, A.; Taccioli, C.; Pichiorri, F.; Alder, H.; Secchiero, P.; Gasparini, P.; Gonelli, A.; Costinean, S.; Acunzo, M.; Condorelli, G., & Croce, CM. (2009) miR-221&222 regulate TRAIL resistance and enhance tumorigenicity through PTEN and TIMP3 downregulation. *Cancer Cell.*, 16, 6, 498-509.

Gasche, J.A.; Hoffmann, J.; Boland, C.R., & Goel, A. (2011) Interleukin-6 promotes tumorigenesis by altering DNA methylation in oral cancer cells. *Int. J. Cancer*, (published online 7 January 2011).

Gomes, F.; Telo, D.F.; Souza, H.P.; Nicolau, J.C.; Halpern, A., & Serrano, C.V., Jr. (2010) [Obesity and coronary artery disease: role of vascular inflammation]. *Arq Bras. Cardiol.* 94, 255-260.

Granholm AC.; Bimonte-Nelson HA.; Moore AB.; Nelson ME.; Freeman LR., & Sambamurti K. (2008) Effects of a saturated fat and high cholesterol diet on memory and hippocampal morphology in the middle-aged rat. *J. Alzheimers Dis.*, 14,2, 133-145.

Greer, E.L.; Maures, T.J.; Hauswirth, A.G.; Green, E.M.; Leeman, D.S.; Maro, G.S.; Han, S.; Banko, M.R.; Gozani, O., & Brunet, A. (2010) Members of the H3K4 trimethylation complex regulate lifespan in a germline-dependent manner in *C.elegans*. *Nature*, 7304, 466, 383-387.

Gruenbaum, Y.; Stein, R.; Cedar, H., & Razin,A. (1981) Methylation of CpG sequences in eukaryotic DNA. *FEBS Lett.* 124, 67-71.

Gunstad, J.; Paul, R.H.; Cohen, R.A.; Tate, D.F.; Spitznagel, M.B., & Gordon, E. (2007) Elevated body mass index is associated with executive dysfunction in otherwise healthy adults. *Compr. Psychiatry*, 8, 1, 57–61.

Gunstad, J.; Paul, R.H.; Cohen, R.A.; Tate, D.F.; Spitznagel, M.B.; Grieve, S., & Gordon, E. (2008) Relationship between body mass index and brain volume in healthy adults. *Int. J. Neurosci.*, 118, 11, 1582–1593.

Gustafson, B. & Smith, U. (2006) Cytokines promote Wnt signaling and inflammation and impair the normal differentiation and lipid accumulation in 3T3-L1 preadipocytes. *J. Biol. Chem.* 281, 9507-9516.

Harvey, J.; Shanley, L.J.; O'Malley, D., & Irving, A.J. (2005) Leptin: a potential cognitive enhancer? *Biochem. Soc. Trans.,* 33, 5, 1029–1032.

Heine, P.A.; Taylor, J.A.; Iwamoto, G.A.; Lubahn, D.B., & Cooke, P.S. (2000) Increased adipose tissue in male and female estrogen receptor-alpha knockout mice. *Proc. Natl. Acad. Sci. U.S.A.* 97, 12729-12734.

Heneghan, H.M.; Miller, N., & Kerin, M.J. (2010) Role of microRNAs in obesity and the metabolic syndrome. *Obes. Rev.* 11, 354-361.

Herrera, B.M.; Lockstone, H.E.; Taylor, J.M.; Ria, M.; Barrett, A.; Collins, S.; Kaisaki, P.; Argoud, K.; Fernandez, C.; Travers, M.E.; Grew, J.P.; Randall, J.C.; Gloyn, A.L.; Gauguier, D.; McCarthy, M.I., & Lindgren, C.M. (2010) Global microRNA expression profiles in insulin target tissues in a spontaneous rat model of type 2 diabetes. *Diabetologia.* 53, 1099-1109.

Ho, A.J.; Raji, C.A.; Becker, J.T.; Lopez, O.L.; Kuller, L.H.; Hua, X.; Lee, S.; Hibar, D.; Dinov, I.D.; Stein, J.L.; Jack, C.R. Jr.; Weiner, M.W.; Toga, A.W., & Thompson, P.M. (2010) Obesity is linked with lower brain volume in 700 AD and MCI patients. *Neurobiol. Aging,* 31, 8, 1326-1339.

Horii, T.; Morita, S.; Kimura, M., & Hatada, I. (2009) Epigenetic regulation of adipocyte differentiation by a Rho guanine nucleotide exchange factor, WGEF. *PLoS. ONE. 4,* e5809.

Huang, Z.; Hankinson, S.E.; Colditz, G.A.; Stampfer, M.J.; Hunter, D.J.; Manson, J.E.; Hennekens, C.H.; Rosner, B.; Speizer, F.E., & Willett, W.C. (1997) Dual effects of weight and weight gain on breast cancer risk. *JAMA* 278, 17, 1407–1411.

Hursting, S.D.; Lashinger, L.M.; Wheatley, K.W.; Rogers, C.J.; Colbert, L.H.; Nunez, N.P., & Perkins, S.N. (2008) Reducing the weight of cancer: mechanistic targets for breaking the obesity-carcinogenesis link. *Best. Pract. Res. Clin. Endocrinol. Metab.* 22, 659-669.

Imhof, A.; Yang, X.J.; Ogryzko, V.V.; Nakatani, Y.; Wolffe, A.P., & Ge, H. (1997) Acetylation of general transcription factors by histone acetyltransferases. *Curr. Biol.* 7, 689-692.

Inagaki, T.; Tachibana, M.; Magoori, K.; Kudo, H.; Tanaka, T.; Okamura, M.; Naito, M.; Kodama, T.; Shinkai, Y., & Sakai, J. (2009) Obesity and metabolic syndrome in histone demethylase JHDM2a-deficient mice. *Genes Cells.* 14, 991-1001.

International Agency for Research on Cancer (2002) Weight Control and Physical Activity, Volume 6. *Lyon: International Agency for Research on Cancer,* 1–315.

Isakson, P.; Hammarstedt, A.; Gustafson, B., & Smith, U. (2009) Impaired preadipocyte differentiation in human abdominal obesity: role of Wnt, tumor necrosis factor-alpha, and inflammation. *Diabetes.* 58, 1550-1557.

Jenuwein, T. & Allis, C.D. (2001) Translating the histone code. *Science* 293, 1074-1080.

Jylhävä, J., & Hurme, M. (2010) Gene variants as determinants of longevity: focus on the inflammatory factors. *Pflugers Arch.,* 459, 2, 239-246.

Kamei Y.; Suganami T.; Ehara T.; Kanai S.; Hayashi K.; Yamamoto Y.; Miura S.; Ezaki O.; Okano M., & Ogawa Y. (2010) Increased expression of DNA methyltransferase 3a in obese adipose tissue: studies with transgenic mice. *Obesity (Silver Spring)*, 18, 2, 314-321.

Kershaw, E.E. & Flier, J.S. (2004). Adipose tissue as an endocrine organ. *J. Clin. Endocrinol. Metab.* 89, 2548-2556.

Krol, J.; Loedige, I., & Filipowicz, W. (2010) The widespread regulation of microRNA biogenesis, function and decay. Nat. Rev. Genet., 11, 9, 597-610.

Lachner, M.; O'Carroll, D.; Rea, S.; Mechtler, K., & Jenuwein, T. (2001) Methylation of histone H3 lysine 9 creates a binding site for HP1 proteins. *Nature.* 410, 116-120.

Laine PS.; Schwartz EA.; Wang Y.; Zhang WY.; Karnik SK.; Musi N.; Reaven PD. (2007) Palmitic acid induces IP-10 expression in human macrophages via NF-kappaB activation. *Biochem. Biophys. Res. Commun.*, 358, 1, 150–155.

Lee, M.; Martin, H.; Firpo, M.A., & Demerath, E.W. (2011) Inverse association between adiposity and telomere length: The Fels Longitudinal Study. *Am. J. Hum. Biol.*, 23, 1, 100-106.

Lee, J.; Saha, P.K.; Yang, Q.H.; Lee, S.; Park, J.Y.; Suh, Y.; Lee, S.K.; Chan, L.; Roeder, R.G., & Lee, J.W. (2008) Targeted inactivation of MLL3 histone H3-Lys-4 methyltransferase activity in the mouse reveals vital roles for MLL3 in adipogenesis. *Proc. Natl. Acad. Sci. U.S.A.* 105, 19229-19234.

Li, Y.; Reddy, M.A.; Miao, F.; Shanmugam, N.; Yee, J.K.; Hawkins, D.; Ren, B., & Natarajan, R. (2008) Role of the histone H3 lysine 4 methyltransferase, SET7/9, in the regulation of NF-kappaB-dependent inflammatory genes. Relevance to diabetes and inflammation. *J. Biol. Chem.* 283, 26771-26781.

Lukasiak, S.; Schiller, C.; Oehlschlaeger, P.; Schmidtke, G.; Krause, P.; Legler, D.F.; Autschbach, F.; Schirmacher, P.; Breuhahn, K., & Groettrup, M. (2008) Proinflammatory cytokines cause FAT10 upregulation in cancers of liver and colon. *Oncogene* 27, 46, 6068–6074.

Lumeng, C.N.; Bodzin, J.L., & Saltiel, A.R. (2007) Obesity induces a phenotypic switch in adipose tissue macrophage polarization. *J. Clin. Invest.* 117, 175-184.

Mack, I.; BelAiba, R.S.; Djordjevic, T.; Gorlach, A.; Hauner, H., & Bader, B.L. (2009) Functional analyses reveal the greater potency of preadipocytes compared with adipocytes as endothelial cell activator under normoxia, hypoxia, and TNFalpha exposure. *Am. J. Physiol Endocrinol. Metab.* 297, E735-E748.

Mantovani, A.; Allavena, P.; Sica, A., & Balkwill, F. (2008) Cancer-related inflammation. *Nature*, 454, 7203,436–44.

Maya-Monteiro, C.M., & Bozza, P.T. (2008) Leptin and mTOR: partners in metabolism and inflammation. *Cell Cycle*, 7, 12, 1713-1717.

Medzhitov,R. (2008) Origin and physiological roles of inflammation. *Nature.* 454, 428-435.

Milagro, F.I.; Campion, J.; Garcia-Diaz, D.F.; Goyenechea, E.; Paternain, L., & Martinez, J.A. (2009) High fat diet-induced obesity modifies the methylation pattern of leptin promoter in rats. *J. Physiol Biochem.* 65, 1-9.

Mori, M.A.; Liu, M.; Bezy, O.; Almind, K.; Shapiro, H.; Kasif, S., & Kahn, C.R. (2010) A Systems Biology Approach Identifies Inflammatory Abnormalities between Mouse Strains Prior to Development of Metabolic Disease. *Diabetes.* 59, 2960-71.

Mouchiroud, L.; Molin, L.; Dallière, N., & Solari, F. (2010) Life span extension by resveratrol, rapamycin, and metformin: The promise of dietary restriction mimetics for an healthy aging. *Biofactors*, 36, 5, 377-382.

Murray, A.J.; Knight, N.S.; Cochlin, L.E.; McAleese, S.; Deacon, R.M.; Rawlins, J.N., & Clarke, K. (2009) Deterioration of physical performance and cognitive function in rats with short-term high-fat feeding. *FASEB J.* 23, 12, 4353-4360.

Musri, M.M.; Carmona, M.C.; Hanzu, F.A.; Kaliman, P.; Gomis, R., & Parrizas, M. (2010) Histone demethylase LSD1 regulates adipogenesis. *J. Biol. Chem.* 285, 30034-30041.

Musri, M.M.; Corominola, H.; Casamitjana, R.; Gomis, R., & Parrizas, M. (2006) Histone H3 lysine 4 dimethylation signals the transcriptional competence of the adiponectin promoter in preadipocytes. *J. Biol. Chem.* 281, 17180-17188.

Musri, M.M.; Gomis,R., & Parrizas, M. (2007) Chromatin and chromatin-modifying proteins in adipogenesis. *Biochem. Cell Biol.* 85, 397-410.

Naaz, A.; Holsberger, D.R.; Iwamoto, G.A.; Nelson, A.; Kiyokawa, H., & Cooke, P.S. (2004) Loss of cyclin-dependent kinase inhibitors produces adipocyte hyperplasia and obesity. *FASEB J.* 18, 1925-1927.

Nave, H.; Mueller, G.; Siegmund, B.; Jacobs, R.; Stroh, T.; Schueler, U.; Hopfe, M.; Behrendt, P.; Buchenauer, T.; Pabst, R., & Brabant, G. (2008) Resistance of Janus kinase-2 dependent leptin signaling in natural killer (NK) cells: a novel mechanism of NK cell dysfunction in diet-induced obesity. *Endocrinology*, 149, 7, 3370–3378.

Niwa, T., & Ushijima, T. (2010) Induction of epigenetic alterations by chronic inflammation and its significance on carcinogenesis. *Adv. Genet.*, 71, 41-56

Noer, A.; Sorensen, A.L.; Boquest, A.C., & Collas, P. (2006) Stable CpG hypomethylation of adipogenic promoters in freshly isolated, cultured, and differentiated mesenchymal stem cells from adipose tissue. *Mol. Biol. Cell.* 17, 3543-3556.

Ohman, M.K.; Wright, A.P.; Wickenheiser, K.J.; Luo,W., & Eitzman, D.T. (2009) Visceral adipose tissue and atherosclerosis. *Curr. Vasc. Pharmacol.* 7, 169-179.

Olefsky, J.M. & Glass, C.K. (2010) Macrophages, inflammation, and insulin resistance. *Annu. Rev. Physiol.* 72, 219-246.

Olholm, J.; Paulsen, S.K.; Cullberg, K.B.; Richelsen, B., & Pedersen, S.B. (2010) Anti-inflammatory effect of resveratrol on adipokine expression and secretion in human adipose tissue explants. *Int. J. Obes. (Lond)*, 34, 10, 1546-1553.

Oliver, S.S. & Denu, J.M. (2011) Dynamic interplay between histone H3 modifications and protein interpreters: emerging evidence for a "histone language". *Chembiochem.* 12, 299-307.

Ono M. (2008) Molecular links between tumor angiogenesis and inflammation: inflammatory stimuli of macrophages and cancer cells as targets for therapeutic strategy. *Cancer Sci.*, 99, 8, 1501–1506.

Oomura, Y.; Hori, N.; Shiraishi, T.; Fukunaga, K.; Takeda, H.; Tsuji, M.; Matsumiya, T.; Ishibashi, M.; Aou, S.; Li, X.; Kohno, D.; Uramura, K.; Sougawa, H.; Yada, T.; Wayner, M., & Sasak,i K. (2006) Leptin facilitates learning and memory performance and enhances hippocampal CA1 long-term potentiation and CaMK II phosphorylation in rats. *Peptides*, 27, 11, 2738–2749.

Ostertag, A.; Jones, A.; Rose, A.J.; Liebert, M.; Kleinsorg, S.; Reimann, A.; Vegiopoulos, A.; Berriel, D.M.; Strzoda, D.; Yamamoto, M.; Satoh, T.; Akira, S., & Herzig, S. (2010) Control of adipose tissue inflammation through TRB1. *Diabetes.* 59, 1991-2000.

Pannacciulli, N.; Del Parigi, A.; Chen, K.; Le, D.S.; Reiman, E.M., & Tataranni, P.A. (2006) Brain abnormalities in human obesity: a voxel-based morphometric study. *Neuroimage,* 31, 4, 1419–1425.

Parra, P.; Serra, F., & Palou, A. (2010) Expression of adipose microRNAs is sensitive to dietary conjugated linoleic acid treatment in mice. *PLoS. ONE.* 5, e13005.

Patil, S., & Chan, C. (2005) Palmitic and stearic fatty acids induce Alzheimer-like hyperphosphorylation of tau in primary rat cortical neurons. *Neurosci. Lett.,* 384, 3, 288–293.

Pfluger, P.T.; Herranz, D.; Velasco-Miguel, S.; Serrano, M., & Tschöp, M.H. (2008) SIRT1 protects against high-fat diet-induced metabolic damage. *Proc. Natl. Acad. Sci. U.S.A.* 105, 28, 9793-9798.

Pierce, B.L.; Ballard-Barbash, R.; Bernstein, L.; Baumgartner, R.N.; Neuhouser, M.L.; Wener, M.H.; Baumgartner, K.B.; Gilliland, F.D.; Sorensen, B.E.; McTiernan, A., & Ulrich, C.M. (2009) Elevated biomarkers of inflammation are associated with reduced survival among breast cancer patients. *J. Clin. Oncol.,* 27, 21, 3437–3444.

Pineau, P.; Volinia, S.; McJunkin, K.; Marchio, A.; Battiston, C.; Terris, B.; Mazzaferro, V.; Lowe, S.W.; Croce, C.M., & Dejean, A. (2010) miR-221 overexpression contributes to liver tumorigenesis. *Proc. Natl. Acad. Sc.i U. S. A.* 107, 1, 264-269.

Pinteaux, E.; Inoue, W.; Schmidt, L.; Molina-Holgado, F.; Rothwell, N.J., & Luheshi, G.N. (2007) Leptin induces interleukin-1beta release from rat microglial cells through a caspase 1 independent mechanism. J. Neurochem., 102, 3, 826–833.

Pokholok, D.K.; Harbison, C.T.; Levine, S.; Cole, M.; Hannett, N.M.; Lee, T.I.; Bell, G.W.; Walker, K.; Rolfe, P.A.; Herbolsheimer, E.; Zeitlinger, J.; Lewitter, F.; Gifford, D.K., & Young, R.A. (2005) Genome-wide map of nucleosome acetylation and methylation in yeast. *Cell.* 122, 517-527.

Poulsen, P.; Esteller, M.; Vaag, A., & Fraga, M.F. (2007) The epigenetic basis of twin discordance in age-related diseases. *Pediatr. Res.* 61, 38R-42R.

Pu XX.; Huang GL.; Guo HQ.; Guo CC.; Li H.; Ye S.; Ling S.; Jiang L.; Tian Y., & Lin TY. (2010) Circulating miR-221 directly amplified from plasma is a potential diagnostic and prognostic marker of colorectal cancer and is correlated with p53 expression. *J. Gastroenterol. Hepatol.* 25, 10, 1674-80.

Rao, X.; Di Leva, G.; L,i M.; Fang, F.; Devlin, C.; Hartman-Frey, C.; Burow, ME.; Ivan, M.; Croce, C.M., & Nephew, K.P. (2011) MicroRNA-221/222 confers breast cancer fulvestrant resistance by regulating multiple signaling pathways. *Oncogene,* 30, 9, 1082-1097.

Reddy, M.A.; Villeneuve, L.M.; Wang, M.; Lanting, L., & Natarajan, R. (2008) Role of the lysine-specific demethylase 1 in the proinflammatory phenotype of vascular smooth muscle cells of diabetic mice. *Circ. Res.* 103, 615-623.

Rigamonti, A.; Brennand, K.; Lau, F., & Cowan, C.A. (2011) Rapid cellular turnover in adipose tissue. *PLoS. ONE.* 6, e17637.

Roberts, D.L.; Dive, C., & Renehan, A.G. (2010) Biological mechanisms linking obesity and cancer risk: new perspectives. *Annu. Rev. Med.* 61, 301-316.

Rodeheffer, M.S.; Birsoy, K., & Friedman, J.M. (2008) Identification of white adipocyte progenitor cells in vivo. *Cell.* 135, 240-249.

Ruan, H.; Hacohen, N.; Golub, T.R.; Van, P.L., & Lodish, H.F. (2002a) Tumor necrosis factor-alpha suppresses adipocyte-specific genes and activates expression of preadipocyte genes in 3T3-L1 adipocytes: nuclear factor-kappaB activation by TNF-alpha is obligatory. *Diabetes.* 51, 1319-1336.

Ruan, H.; Miles, P.D.; Ladd, C.M.; Ross, K.; Golub, T.R.; Olefsky, J.M., & Lodish, H.F. (2002b) Profiling gene transcription in vivo reveals adipose tissue as an immediate target of tumor necrosis factor-alpha: implications for insulin resistance. *Diabetes.* 51, 3176-3188.

Russo, P.; Lauria, F., & Siani, A. (2010) Heritability of body weight: Moving beyond genetics. *Nutr. Metab Cardiovasc. Dis.* 20, 691-7

Santos-Rosa, H.; Schneider, R.; Bannister, A.J.; Sherriff, J.; Bernstein, B.E.; Emre, N.C.; Schreiber, S.L.; Mellor, J., & Kouzarides, T. (2002) Active genes are tri-methylated at K4 of histone H3. *Nature* 419, 407-411.

Scherer, P.E.; Williams, S.; Fogliano, M.; Baldini, G., & Lodish, H.F. (1995) A novel serum protein similar to C1q, produced exclusively in adipocytes. *J. Biol. Chem.* 270, 26746-26749.

Siebold, A.P.; Banerjee, R.; Tie, F.; Kiss, D.L.; Moskowitz, J., & Harte, P.J. (2010) Polycomb Repressive Complex 2 and Trithorax modulate *Drosophila* longevity and stress resistance, *Proc. Natl. Acad. Sci. U.S.A.*, 107, 1, 169-179.

Siegmund, K.D.; Connor, C.M.; Campan, M.; Long, T.I.; Weisenberger, D.J.; Biniszkiewicz, D.; Jaenisch, R.; Laird, P.W., & Akbarian, S. (2007) DNA methylation in the human cerebral cortex is dynamically regulated throughout the life span and involves differentiated neurons. *PLoS One,* 2, e895.

Smith, B.C. & Denu, J.M. (2009) Chemical mechanisms of histone lysine and arginine modifications. *Biochim. Biophys. Acta.* 1789, 45-57.

Smith, J.; Al Amri, M.; Dorairaj, P., & Sniderman, A. (2006) The adipocyte life cycle hypothesis. *Clin. Sci. (Lond).* 110, 1-9.

Solinas, G.; Vilcu, C.; Neels, J.G.; Bandyopadhyay, G.K.; Luo, J.L.; Naugler, W.; Grivennikov, S.; Wynshaw-Boris, A.; Scadeng, M.; Olefsky, J.M., & Karin, M. (2007) JNK1 in hematopoietically derived cells contributes to diet-induced inflammation and insulin resistance without affecting obesity. *Cell Metab.* 6, 386-397.

Spalding, K.L.; Arner, E.; Westermark, P.O.; Bernard, S.; Buchholz, B.A.; Bergmann, O.; Blomqvist, L.; Hoffstedt, J.; Naslund, E.; Britton, T.; Concha, H.; Hassan, M.; Ryden, M.; Frisen, J., & Arner, P. (2008) Dynamics of fat cell turnover in humans. *Nature.* 453, 783-787.

Stanek, K.M.; Grieve, S.M.; Brickman, A.M.; Korgaonkar, M.S.; Paul, R.H.; Cohen, R.A., & Gunstad, J.J. (2011) Obesity is associated with reduced white matter integrity in otherwise healthy adults. *Obesity (Silver Spring)*, 19, 3, 500-504.

Strahl, B.D. & Allis, C.D. (2000). The language of covalent histone modifications. *Nature.* 403, 41-45.

Suarez, Y.; Wang, C.; Manes, T.D., & Pober, J.S. (2010) Cutting edge: TNF-induced microRNAs regulate TNF-induced expression of E-selectin and intercellular adhesion molecule-1 on human endothelial cells: feedback control of inflammation. *J. Immunol.* 184, 21-25.

Taki, Y.; Kinomura, S.; Sato, K.; Inoue, K.; Goto, R.; Okada, K.; Uchida, S.; Kawashima, R., & Fukuda, H. (2008) Relationship between body mass index and gray matter volume in 1,428 healthy individuals. *Obesity (Silver Spring),* 16, 1, 119–124.

Talasz, H.; Lindner, H.H.; Sarg, B., & Helliger, W. (2005) Histone H4-lysine 20 monomethylation is increased in promoter and coding regions of active genes and correlates with hyperacetylation. *J. Biol. Chem.* 280, 38814-38822.

Tang, C.H.; Lu, D.Y.; Yang, R.S.; Tsai, H.Y.; Kao, M.C.; Fu, W.M., & Chen, Y.F. (2007) Leptin-induced IL-6 production is mediated by leptin receptor, insulin receptor substrate-1, phosphatidylinositol 3-kinase, Akt, NFkappaB, and p300 pathway in microglia. *J. Immunol.* 179, 2,1292–302.

Tang, Y.F.; Zhang, Y.; Li, X.Y.; Li, C.; Tian, W., & Liu, L. (2009) Expression of miR-31, miR-125b-5p and miR-326 in the Adipogenic Differentiation Process of Adipose-Derived Stem Cells. *OMICS.* 13, 331-336.

Tataranni, P.A. & Ortega, E. (2005) A burning question: does an adipokine-induced activation of the immune system mediate the effect of overnutrition on type 2 diabetes? *Diabetes.* 54, 917-927.

Tchkonia, T.; Morbeck, D.E.; Von Zglinicki, T.;, Van Deursen, J.; Lustgarten, J.; Scrable, H.; Khosla, S.; Jensen, M.D., & Kirkland, J.L.(2010) Fat tissue, aging, and cellular senescence. *Aging Cell,* 9, 5, 667-684.

Tchoukalova, Y.; Koutsari, C., & Jensen, M. (2007) Committed subcutaneous preadipocytes are reduced in human obesity. *Diabetologia.* 50, 151-157.

Tchoukalova, Y.D.; Sarr, M.G., & Jensen, M.D. (2004) Measuring committed preadipocytes in human adipose tissue from severely obese patients by using adipocyte fatty acid binding protein. *Am. J. Physiol Regul. Integr. Comp Physiol.* 287, R1132-R1140.

Tilg, H. (2010) The role of cytokines in non-alcoholic fatty liver disease. *Dig. Dis.* 28, 179-185.

Tkacova, R. (2010) Systemic inflammation in chronic obstructive pulmonary disease: may adipose tissue play a role? Review of the literature and future perspectives. *Mediators. Inflamm.* 585989.

Tozuka, Y.; Kumon, M.; Wada, E.; Onodera, M.; Mochizuki, H., & Wada, K. (2010) Maternal obesity impairs hippocampal BDNF production and spatial learning performance in young mouse offspring. *Neurochem. Int.* 57, 3, 235-247.

Trayhurn, P. & Wood, I.S. (2004) Adipokines: inflammation and the pleiotropic role of white adipose tissue. *Br. J. Nutr.* 92, 347-355.

Turner, B.M. (2000) Histone acetylation and an epigenetic code. *Bioessays.* 22, 836-845.

Ukkola, O. & Santaniemi, M. (2002) Adiponectin: a link between excess adiposity and associated comorbidities? *J. Mol. Med. 80,* 696-702.

Ventura, A.; Young, A.G.; Winslow, M.M.; Lintault, L.; Meissner, A.; Erkeland, S.J.; Newman, J.; Bronson, R.T.; Crowley, D.; Stone, J.R.; Jaenisch, R.; Sharp, P.A., & Jacks, T. (2008) Targeted deletion reveals essential and overlapping functions of the miR-17 through 92 family of miRNA clusters. *Cell.* 132, 875-886.

Villaret, A.; Galitzky, J.; Decaunes, P.; Estève, D.; Marques, M.A.; Sengenès, C.; Chiotasso, P.; Tchkonia, T.; Lafontan, M.; Kirkland, J.L., & Bouloumié, A. (2010) Adipose tissue endothelial cells from obese human subjects: differences among depots in angiogenic, metabolic, and inflammatory gene expression and cellular senescence.

Villeneuve, L.M.; Kato, M.; Reddy, M.A.; Wang, M.; Lanting, L., & Natarajan, R. (2010) Enhanced levels of microRNA-125b in vascular smooth muscle cells of diabetic db/db mice lead to increased inflammatory gene expression by targeting the histone methyltransferase Suv39h1. *Diabetes.* 59, 2904-2915.

Villeneuve, L.M.; Reddy, M.A.; Lanting, L.L.; Wang, M.; Meng, L., & Natarajan, R. (2008) Epigenetic histone H3 lysine 9 methylation in metabolic memory and inflammatory phenotype of vascular smooth muscle cells in diabetes. *Proc. Natl. Acad. Sci. U.S.A.* 105, 9047-9052.

Virtue, S. & Vidal-Puig, A. (2010). Adipose tissue expandability, lipotoxicity and the Metabolic Syndrome--an allostatic perspective. *Biochim. Biophys. Acta.* 1801, 338-349.

Volkow, N.D.; Wang, G.J.; Telang, F.; Fowler, J.S.; Goldstein, R.Z.; Alia-Klein, N.; Logan, J.; Wong, C.; Thanos, P.K.; Ma, Y., & Pradhan, K. (2009) Inverse association between BMI and prefrontal metabolic activity in healthy adults. *Obesity (Silver Spring)* 17, 1, 60–65.

Wakabayashi, K.; Okamura, M.; Tsutsumi, S.; Nishikawa, N.S.,; Tanaka, T.; Sakakibara, I.; Kitakami, J.; Ihara, S.; Hashimoto, Y.; Hamakubo, T.; Kodama, T.; Aburatani, H., & Sakai,J. (2009) The peroxisome proliferator-activated receptor gamma/retinoid X receptor alpha heterodimer targets the histone modification enzyme PR-Set7/Setd8 gene and regulates adipogenesis through a positive feedback loop. *Mol. Cell Biol.* 29, 3544-3555.

Wang, D., & DuBois, R.N. (2008) Pro-inflammatory prostaglandins and progression of colorectal cancer. *Cancer Lett.*, 267, 2,197–203.

Wang, Q.; Li, Y.C.; Wang, J.; Kong, J.; Qi, Y.; Quigg, R.J., & Li, X. (2008) miR-17-92 cluster accelerates adipocyte differentiation by negatively regulating tumor-suppressor Rb2/p130. *Proc. Natl. Acad. Sci. U.S.A.* 105, 2889-2894.

Wang, Y. & Beydoun, M.A. (2007) The obesity epidemic in the United States--gender, age, socioeconomic, racial/ethnic, and geographic characteristics: a *systematic review and meta-regression analysis. Epidemiol. Rev.* 29, 6-28.

Weisberg, S.P.; Hunter, D.; Huber, R.; Lemieux, J.; Slaymaker, S.; Vaddi, K.; Charo, I.; Leibel, R.L., & Ferrante, A.W., Jr. (2006) CCR2 modulates inflammatory and metabolic effects of high-fat feeding. *J. Clin. Invest.* 116, 115-124.

Weisberg, S.P.; McCann, D.; Desai, M.; Rosenbaum, M.; Leibel, R.L., & Ferrante, A.W., Jr. (2003) Obesity is associated with macrophage accumulation in adipose tissue. *J. Clin. Invest.* 112, 1796-1808.

White, C.L.; Pistell, P.J.; Purpera, M.N.; Gupta, S.; Fernandez-Kim, S.O.; Hise, T.L.; Keller, J.N.; Ingram, D.K.; Morrison, C.D., & Bruce-Keller, A.J. (2009) Effects of high fat diet on Morris maze performance, oxidative stress, and inflammation in rats: contributions of maternal diet. *Neurobiol. Dis.*, 35,1, 3-13.

Wierda, R.J.; Geutskens, S.B.; Jukema, J.W.; Quax, P.H., & van den Elsen, P.J. (2010) Epigenetics in atherosclerosis and inflammation. *J. Cell Mol. Med.* 14, 1225-1240.

Wolin, K.Y.; Carson, K., & Colditz, G.A. (2010) Obesity and cancer. *Oncologist.* 15, 556-565.

Wu, Y.; Brodt, P.; Sun, H.; Mejia, W.; Novosyadlyy, R.; Nunez, N.; Chen,, X.; Mendoza, A.; Hong, S.H.; Khanna, C., & Yakar, S. (2010) Insulin-like growth factor-I regulates the liver microenvironment in obese mice and promotes liver metastasis. *Cancer Res.*, 70, 1, 57-67.

Xiao, C.; Srinivasan, L.; Calado, D.P.; Patterson, H.C.; Zhang, B.; Wang, J.; Henderson, J.M.; Kutok, J.L., & Rajewsky, K. (2008) Lymphoproliferative disease and autoimmunity in mice with increased miR-17-92 expression in lymphocytes. *Nat. Immunol.* 9, 405-414.

Xie H.; Lim B., & Lodish HF. (2009) MicroRNAs induced during adipogenesis that accelerate fat cell development are downregulated in obesity. *Diabetes* 58, 5, 1050-1057.

Xu, H.; Barnes, G.T.; Yang, Q.; Tan, G.; Yang, D.; Chou, C.J.; Sole, J.; Nichols, A.; Ross, J.S.; Tartaglia, L.A., & Chen, H. (2003) Chronic inflammation in fat plays a crucial role in the development of obesity-related insulin resistance. *J. Clin. Invest.* 112, 1821-1830.

Yaffe, K.; Kanaya, A.; Lindquist, K.; Simonsick, E.M.; Harris, T.; Shorr, R.I.; Tylavsky, F.A., & Newman, A.B. (2004) The metabolic syndrome, inflammation, and risk of cognitive decline. *JAMA*, 292, 18, 2237-2242.

Yamamoto, Y.; Verma, U.N.; Prajapati, S.; Kwak, Y.T., & Gaynor, R.B. (2003) Histone H3 phosphorylation by IKK-alpha is critical for cytokine-induced gene expression. *Nature.* 423, 655-659.

Yang, Z.; Kahn, B.B.; Shi, H., & Xue, B.Z. (2010) Macrophage alpha1 AMP-activated protein kinase (alpha1AMPK) antagonizes fatty acid-induced inflammation through SIRT1. *J. Biol. Chem.*, 285, 25, 19051-19059.

Yang, Z.; Bian, C.; Zhou, H.; Huang, S.; Wang, S.; Liao, L., & Zhao, R.C. (2010) MicroRNA hsa-miR-138 inhibits adipogenic differentiation of human adipose tissue-derived mesenchymal stem cells through EID-1. *Stem Cells Dev.* 20, 259-67

Yoo, E.J.; Chung, J.J.; Choe, S.S.; Kim, K.H., & Kim, J.B. (2006) Down-regulation of histone deacetylases stimulates adipocyte differentiation. *J. Biol. Chem.* 281, 6608-6615.

Zhang, C.Z.; Zhang, J.X.; Zhang, A.L.; Shi, Z.D.; Han, L.; Jia, Z.F.; Yang, W.D.; Wang, G.X.; Jiang, T.; You, Y.P.; Pu, P.Y.; Cheng, J.Q & Kang, C.S. (2010) MiR-221 and miR-222 target PUMA to induce cell survival in glioblastoma. *Mol. Cancer.* 9, 1, 229-237.

Zhang, X.; Dong, F.; Ren, J.; Driscoll, M.J., & Culver, B. (2005) High dietary fat induces NADPH oxidase-associated oxidative stress and inflammation in rat cerebral cortex. *Exp. Neurol.* 191, 2, 318–325.

Zhang, Y.; Daquinag, A.; Traktue,v D.O.; Amaya-Manzanares, F.; Simmons, P.J.; March, K.L.; Pasqualini, R.; Arap, W., & Kolonin, M.G. (2009) White adipose tissue cells are recruited by experimental tumors and promote cancer progression in mouse models. *Cancer Res.* 69, 12, 5259–5266.

Zhang, Y.; Proenca, R.; Maffei, M.; Barone, M.; Leopold, L., & Friedman, J.M. (1994) Positional cloning of the mouse obese gene and its human homologue. *Nature.* 372, 425-432.

Zhu, N.; Zhang, D.; Chen, S.; Liu, X.; Lin, L.; Huang, X.; Guo, Z.; Liu, J.; Wang, Y.; Yuan, W., & Qin, Y. (2011) Endothelial enriched microRNAs regulate *angiotensin II-induced endothelial inflammation and migration. Atherosclerosis.* 215, 286-93

5

Inflammatory Markers Associated with Chronic Hyperglycemia and Insulin Resistance

Denisa Margina
University of Medicine and Pharmacy, Faculty of Pharmacy, Bucharest, Romania

1. Introduction

Chronic hyperglycemia associated with type 2 diabetes mellitus (T2D) is a result of deficient insulin secretion and/or resistance of target tissues to insulin's action. Chronic hyperglycemia is a major etiological factor causing both micro- and macrovascular lesions associated with diabetes. Numerous biochemical changes initiated by hyperglycemia directly influence cellular function and lead to abnormal vascular remodeling and the development of vascular diabetic complications (Wadham et al., 2007, King et al, 1996, Brownlee, 2001).

Recent literature data states that the innate immune system might be involved in the pathogenesis of type 2 diabetes. It is now commonly accepted that diabetes is associated with low-grade inflammation; there are a lot of human studies that demonstrate an increase for some of the inflammatory markers (hsCRP) including interleukins (IL-6, etc) and several adhesion molecules (intercellular adhesion molecule 1, ICAM-1, E-selectin) in patients with T2D, compared to controls (Garcia et al, 2010). Type 2 diabetes is initiated as a result of both genetic and acquired individual factors associated with triggering stimuli such as overeating, under-activity, increasing age, psychological stress and smoking. All these are also responsible for the activation of innate immunity, leading to insulin resistance (Garcia et al, 2010).

Obesity induces changes in skeletal muscle, adipose tissue and the liver that result in localized inflammation and insulin resistance (IR) through autocrine and paracrine signaling. Excess adiposity is the most important risk factor for the development of insulin resistance, type 2 diabetes and their cardiovascular complications (Tataranni, 2005). Insulin resistance is extensively studied by medical and scientific communities because of its increased prevalence and its association with cardiovascular disease. Even if the precise molecular mechanism(s) linking insulin resistance to the development and/or progression of atherosclerosis remains under debate, it is clear that inflammation is a contributing factor. The exact physiological events leading to the initiation of the inflammatory response in obesity remain incompletely understood. Adipokines such as resistin and leptin, which are secreted by adipocytes, can induce inflammation and the associated insulin resistance. As part of the chronic inflammatory process, chemokines secreted locally, in the adipose tissue, attract pro-inflammatory macrophages that contribute to the acceleration of inflammatory markers' synthesis (Zavaroni I, 2000, De Luca 2008).

Adiponectin is one of the adipocyte-derived proteins that have insulin-sensitizing, antiinflammatory, and antiatherogenic properties. Clinical studies show that decreased plasma levels of adiponectin have been associated with obesity, type 2 diabetes, and hypertension; plasma adiponectin levels are significantly lower in patients with coronary artery disease. Experimental as well as clinical studies strongly suggest that physiologic levels of adiponectin are necessary to maintain the normal, non-inflammatory phenotype of the vascular wall and that the protective role of adiponectin is due to it's capacity to preserve the endothelial cell function (Ouedraogo et al, 2007, Goldstein & Scalia, 2004, Scherer, 2006, Arita et al, 1999, Hotta et al, 2000, Iwashima et al, 2004, Ouchi et al, 2000).
Relative risk of cardiovascular disease is increased 2–3 times in diabetic men and 3–4 times in diabetic women compared to non-diabetic controls; atherosclerosis is the major causal factor for these pathological events (Ray et al, 2009). Blood-borne inflammatory and immune cells constitute an important part of the atheroma lesions; activated immune cells in the atherosclerotic plaque produce inflammatory cytokines (interferonγ, interleukin-1, and tumor necrosis factor), which induce the production of substantial amounts of interleukin-6 (IL6) and other inflammatory factors (Hansson, 2005). Therefore inflammation is an important component in the development of atherosclerosis specifically in the setting of type 2 diabetes and insulin resistance.
In patients at high risk of cardio-vascular disease, the first signs of endothelial dysfunction are observed in morphologically intact vessels, before the onset of clinically manifested vascular disease. There are several lines of evidence indicating especially that endothelial function is compromised in situations associated with reduced sensitivity to endogenous insulin. The adhesion of circulating leukocytes to endothelial cells plays an important role in the initiation of atherosclerosis. Cellular adhesion molecules are poorly expressed by the resting endothelium, but they are up-regulated during atherogenesis; the soluble forms of some cellular adhesion molecules, such as E-selectin, can be found in plasma and it has been suggested that elevated plasma levels of these cellular adhesion molecules may constitute an index of endothelial activation or even a molecular marker of early atherosclerosis (Ceriello, 2004, Stühlinger, 2002). Adhesion molecules (E-selectin, ICAM1, VCAM) as well as cytokines are up-regulated under the effect of hyperglycemia (Zheng et al, 2007, Miyamoto et al, 1999, Joussen et al, 2002).
Nitric-oxide (NO) is synthesized from L-arginine by a family of enzymes, called NO synthases (NOSs) and has antiatherogenic and antithrombotic functions. The constitutively expressed NOS isoforms, endothelial NOS (eNOS) and neuronal NOS (nNOS), are likely to be the major contributors to whole-body NO production. In the last decades, a great effort has been made to understand the role of NO as a modulator of physiological insulin secretion as well as its ability to modulate glucose metabolism and its' involvement in insulin resistance. It has been described that eNOS activation, specifically localized in skeletal muscles, increases muscle blood flow, with increased delivery of glucose to the muscle cell (Monti L.D., 2003). In endothelial cells, insulin stimulates the expression and activity of endothelial NO synthase (eNOS), resulting in increased production of NO. Under normal circumstances, NO is not only critically important in the process of vasodilatation, but it also counteracts the stimulatory effect of VEGF on the expression of adhesion molecules such as E-selectin, intracellular adhesion molecule (ICAM1), and vascular cellular adhesion molecule (VCAM), thereby protecting the endothelial cells from excessive interactions with circulating monocytes (Low Wang, 2004).
Endothelial dysfunction is associated with many pathological conditions, including hyperlipidemia, hypertension, metabolic syndrome, insulin resistance and diabetes.

Endothelial dysfunction is characterized by a loss of nitric oxide bioavailability mainly due to its inactivation under the effect of superoxide excessively produced and is considered a very important cellular event responsible for the adverse effects of high glucose on the blood vesels (Wadham et al, 2007, Brownlee, 2001). Both in vitro and in vivo studies show that exposure to hyperglycemia reduces endothelial NO availability and its bioactivity (Williams et al, 1998, Veves et al, 1998).

The control of blood glucose homeostasis is mainly determined by two closely related physiological mechanisms: the capacity of the pancreas to secrete insulin and the biological action of this hormone on insulin-sensitive tissues, especially liver, muscle and adipose tissue (Foss-Freitas, 2004). It is well known that in type 2 diabetes mellitus and in metabolic syndrome, as well as in various other human pathological states such as glucose intolerance, obesity, polycystic ovary syndrome, essential hypertension, and, more recently, atherosclerosis, insulin resistance is either an associated condition or is considered to be a predictor or pathogenic factor (De Fronzo, 1988, 1991, Guizea, 2008). Insulin resistance is the condition in which normal amounts of insulin are inadequate to produce a normal physiologic response in the main target tissues of the pancreas hormone (fat, muscle, liver).

Insulin resistance reduces the effects of insulin and results in elevated hydrolysis of triglycerides stored in the fat cells, leading to an increase of the free fatty acids' level in plasma. Insulin resistance in muscle cells reduces the glucose uptake, whereas in liver cells results in impaired glycogen synthesis and a failure to suppress glucose production. All these phenomena lead to reduced muscle glucose uptake and increased liver glucose production, thus contributing to the elevation of the blood glucose level, and accelerating the glucose toxicity associated with the insulin resistance (Freitas 2004, De Fronzo 1988, 1991, Guizea 2008).

The medical community agrees that the evaluation of the insulin resistance phenomena might be important for the assessment of hyperglycemia patients. According to literature data, the most efficient and scientifically correct methods for the evaluation of insulin resistance are "clamp" techniques. These procedures require i.v. access, multiple venipunctures, and take a long time, thus being relatively impractical for office assessment and difficult from the patients' point of view. The euglycemic hyperinsulinemic clamp technique is the reference method, the "gold standard" for quantifying insulin sensitivity or resistance in vivo because it directly measures the effects of insulin on glucose use under steady state conditions (Freitas 2004). Besides the euglycemic hyperinsulinemic clamp technique, other clamp techniques have been developed: frequently sampled IV glucose tolerance test (FSIVGTT), insulin tolerance test (ITT), insulin sensitivity test (IST), and continuous infusion of glucose with model assessment (CIGMA). There are also some models available for the evaluation of insulin resistance depending on glucose and insulin levels in oral glucose tolerance tests: Insulin Sensitivity Index (ISI), Matsuda test, Caderholm test, Gut test, etc. Unfortunately, most of these methods share the disadvantages of the euglycemic hyperinsulinemic clamp, requiring i.v. access, multiple blood sampling, glucose/insulin infusion for several hours, being also difficult to use for the patients and for the specialists (McAuley 2001, Matsuda 2010).

Largely because of the fact that the standard methods for assessing beta-cell function and insulin sensitivity, the hyperglycemic and euglycemic glucose clamps, are complex and costly to perform, several studies have been conducted to determine simpler and more applicable assessments (Dansuntornwong 2007).

So the mathematical models for the evaluation of insulin resistance depending on fasting levels of glucose and insulin are presently used. The most popular test of this kind is the Homeostatic model assessment (HOMA) of β-cell function and insulin resistance and it was first described in 1985 (Soonthornpun 2003). This test represents a method for assessing β-cell function and IR from basal glucose and insulin or C peptide concentrations. The model has been widely used since it was first published. (Wallace 2004, Song 2007, Margina 2005).
Recent data mentioned some other models for the evaluation of insulin resistance. Quantitative Insulin Sensitivity Check Index (QUICKI) can be evaluated depending on fasting levels of glucose and insulin. Many investigators believe that QUICKI is superior to HOMA as a way of determining insulin sensitivity (Katz 2000, Mather 2001, Yokoyama 2000).
Since T2D, obesity, insulin resistance, metabolic syndrome, and atherosclerosis, the last one being the main complication of chronic hyperglycemia, share the inflammatory pattern, the aim of this research was to assess the profile of some markers of inflammation (hsCRP, IL6, E-selectin), of the adipocyte function (adiponectin) and of the endothelial status (plasma NO stable end products) in correlation with the insulin resistance indexes, in a Romanian group of patients.
For this purpose 80 patients were selected and their informed consent was obtained. Any past or present insulin treatments, along with hematological, kidney or malignant diseases were exclusion criteria.

2. Materials and methods

2.1 Subjects and study design

We included in our study 80 patients, 40 to 60 years old. Any past or present insulin treatment, along with any hematological or kidney diseases were an exclusion criterion. The protocol was approved by the local ethics committee and the informed consent of the patients was obtained.

2.2 Biochemical evaluation

For the studied patients we assessed, on *à jeun* blood samples, the following parameters: fasting plasma glucose (FPG), fasting plasma insulin, plasma lipids and lipoproteins (total cholesterol - TC, triglycerides –TG, low density lipoproteins - LDL, high density lipoproteins - HDL), plasma insulin level. Fasting plasma glucose and plasma lipids (TC, LDL, and HDL) were determined using automatic devices and commercial kits (Merck and Biorad), on an Olimpus 400 analyzer. Insulin, adiponectin, interleukin 6 and E-selectin were evaluated using ELISA kits (Invitrogen) on a ChemWell 1000 device. The NO stable end products (nitrite and nitrate) were evaluated using enzymatic catalysis coupled with Griess reaction (Gradinaru, 2003, Moshage, 1995, Archer, 2003)
Using the values of fasting plasma glucose and insulin, several insulin sensitivity indexes have been evaluated (Quicki, HOMA-IR, 1/HOMA-IR, log(HOMA-IR), HOMA-B), according to the presented formula (McAuley 2001, Matsuda 2010, Dansuntornwong 2007, Wallace 2004).

2.3 Statistical analysis

Results are reported as means ± standard deviation (SD). Student *t* test was appropriately used for group comparisons. Correlations were assessed by a non-parametric test (Spearman). P values <0.05 were considered statistically significant.

3. Results an discussions

The patients were divided into three groups, according to their BMI:

- control group (n=20), BMI<25 kg/m^2,
- overweight group (n=30), 25 kg/m$^2 \leq$BMI<30 kg/m^2,
- obese group (n=30), BMI$\geq$30 kg/m^2.

Table 1 shows the general biochemical parameters for the three studied groups.

Our results show that the weight increase is associated with a disturbance of the glycemic and lipid homeostasis. The fasting plasma glucose, total cholesterol and the lipoprotein levels increased from the control group to the other two studied groups. The LDL and TG increased significantly at the obese patients compared to controls, but not significantly at overweight patients compared to controls. All the other parameters varied significantly both in the overweight and the obese groups compared to the lean group.

Evaluated parameters	Control group	Overweight group	Obese group
BMI (kg/m^2)	21.46±2.02	27.28±1.61**	35.04±4.74**
Fasting plasma glucose (mg/dL)	85.8±7.25	128.2±74.17**	163.24±73.80**
Total cholesterol (mg/dL)	176.60±34.46	201.05±38.48*	216.8±37.11**
LDL cholesterol (mg/dL)	100.18±39.10	119.48±37.18	133.51±30.72*
HDL cholesterol (mg/dL)	60.20±13.17	48.47±11.34*	48,80±15.52*
Triglycerides (mg/dL)	81.10±55.67	86.75±52.61	173.36±129.21**

*p<0.05, **p<0.01

Table 1. The biochemical parameters for the overweight and obese patients compared to the control group

Analyzing the lipid profile of the selected patients we pointed out that 36% of the overweight and 45.5% of the obese group were hypercholesterolemic (TC>220mg/dL). The HDL level did not meet the cardioprotective (>45mg/dL) level for 29% of the overweight and 54.5% of the obese patients.

So, the analysis of the glucose and lipid markers only shows an increased risk of atherosclerotic events for some of the patients in the obese and overweight groups but does not allow identifying the mechanism involved in the potential endothelial lesions.

Since the discovery of adiponectin, numerous studies have supported the theory that adiponectin has similar action with insulin and increases the pancreatic hormone' metabolic function, as well as its anti-atherogenic properties; animal studies also suggest that adiponectin may exert a protective role in vascular homeostasis. In humans, plasma levels of adiponectin are negatively correlated with adiposity, and decreased plasma adiponectin levels are also observed in patients with diabetes, as well as in subjects with diseases caused by impairment of the endothelial function. Since adiponectin is secreted exclusively from adipose cells, deregulation of adiponectin synthesis and action may provide a link between obesity, insulin resistance, diabetes, vascular complications of diabetes and atherosclerosis (Arita et al, 1999, Hotta et al, 2000, Iwashima et al, 2004, Ouchi et al, 2000). So adiponectin, as well as the endothelial derived relaxing factor (NO), have anti-atherogenic properties. The imbalance of these two markers caused by the weight increase is associated with a general impairment of the vascular function and with a loss of the glycemic, lipid and lipoproteic control.

Statistical analysis of the recorded data revealed that the adiponectin level was significantly lower at overweight (p=0.001) and obese patients (p=0.001) compared to controls (fig 1).

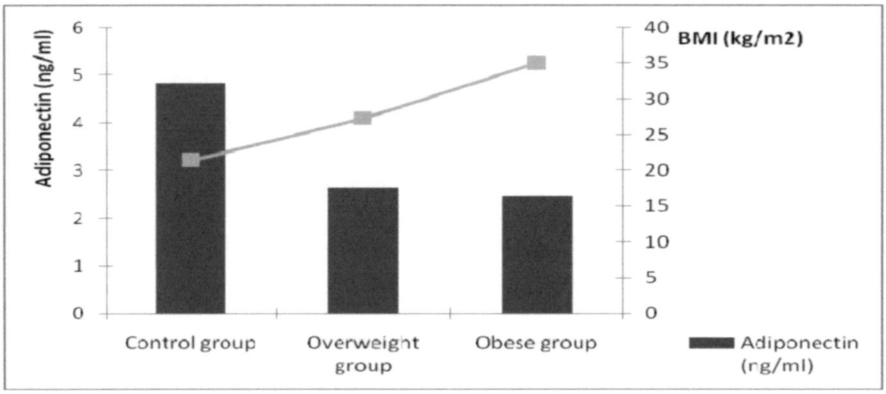

Fig. 1. Dynamics of adiponectin in correlation with the BMI of the studied patients

The nitrite level also decreased inversely correlated with the body mass index of the patients. Our data showing that the synthesis of NO at the endothelial level decreases from lean subjects to the overweight and obese ones might be also explained by the results of Chen et all (2003), which proved that adiponectin stimulates the NO production at the endothelial level (fig 2).

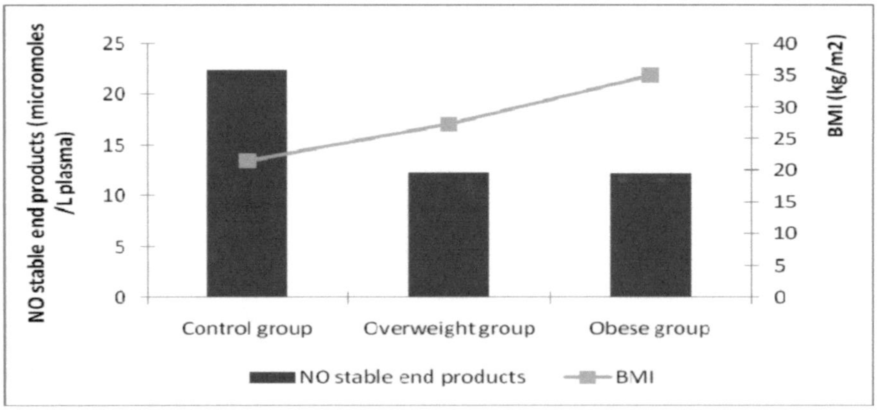

Fig. 2. The NO stable end products level in correlation with the BMI of the studied patients

For all the patients included in the study our results showed a significant, positive correlation between the adiponectin level and the NO stable end products (fig 3). This type of correlation also supports the theory that there is a regulatory mechanism between adiponectin and NO synthesis.

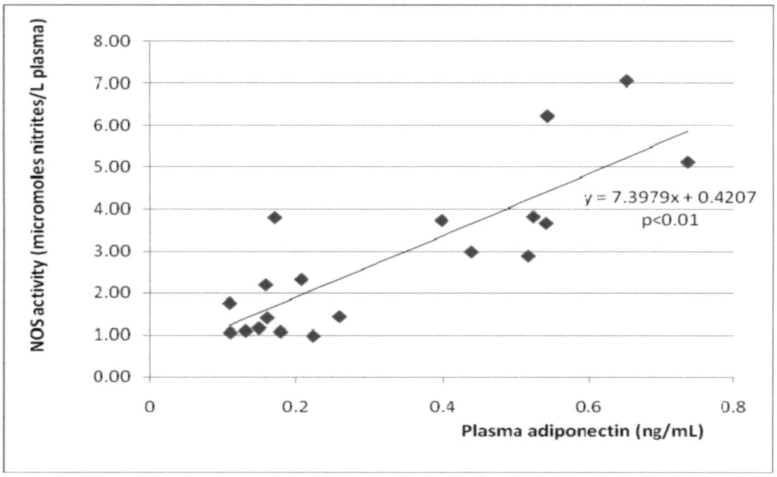

Fig. 3. The correlation between the NO stable end products and the plasma adiponectin level for the study group

The IL6 and hsCRP levels increased significantly at overweight and obese patients, in correlation with the BMI (fig 4). The increase was significant for the obese patients, in the case of both parameters and not significant for both parameters in overweight patients, compared to controls.

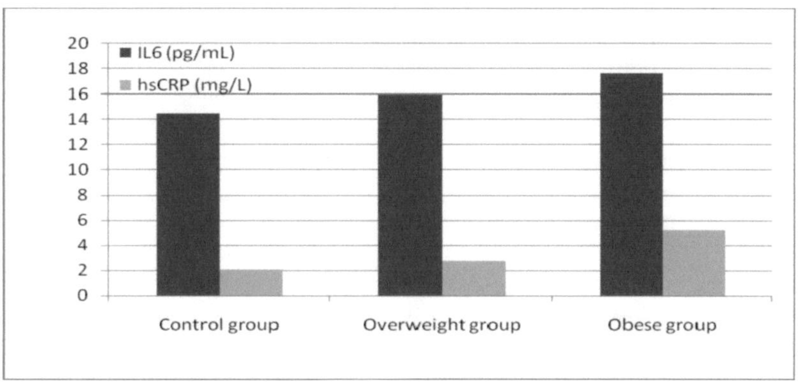

Fig. 4. IL6 and hsCRP levels for the studied groups

The E-selectin level was similar in the overweight and obese groups but was significantly higher ($p<0.001$) compared to lean controls (fig 5). According to literature data, adhesion molecules of the selectin family are poorly expressed by the resting endothelium and are upregulated during atherogenesis, acute infections and granulomatous diseases. Thus, endothelial adhesion molecules are a result of both acute responses against pathogens and chronic inflammatory processes, such as those leading to progressive formation of atherosclerotic plaques (Ferri, 1998, Monaco, 2009). The elevated plasma levels of soluble endothelial adhesins might constitute indexes of increased adhesion molecule expression by the intact vascular endothelium in vivo. The results showing high levels of E-selectin in overweight and obese patients suggest that an early endothelial activation might be present in correlation with the weight increase, favoring the development of overt vascular lesions.

So, the vascular endothelium from obese patients releases endothelium-derived substances that can constitute markers of endothelial damage, such as E-selectin.

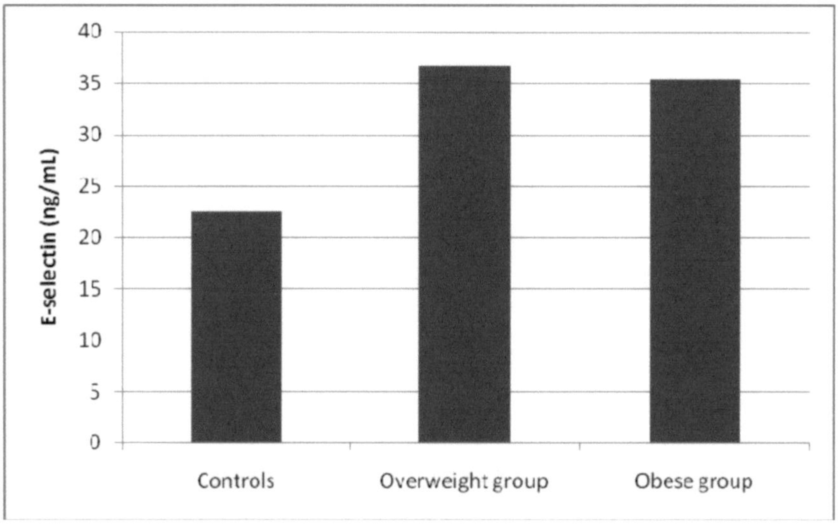

Fig. 5. E-selectin dynamics for the studied groups

The term "insulin resistance" as it is used in clinical and experimental settings refers to the inability of insulin to promote the normal homeostasis of glucose. That means that the reduced insulin action demands the presence of higher-than-normal concentrations of insulin in order to maintain a normal utilization of glucose by insulin target tissues. Thus, the term "insulin resistance" implies the existence of metabolic insulin resistance, which reflects an inadequate effect of insulin on glucose metabolism, but does not address other aspects of insulin action (Low Wang, 2004). Many investigators have studied simple surrogate indices of insulin resistance in comparison with the index assessed by euglycemic-hyperinsulinemic clamp. It has been established that homeostasis model assessment of insulin resistance HOMA-IR is a useful index of insulin resistance in diabetic and nondiabetic subjects and that its logarithmic transformation or its reciprocal value might make it more accurate (Mather et al, 2001, Yokoyama et al, 2003).

The HOMA model allows the evaluation of an insulin resistance index (HOMA-IR) and also of an index for the β-cell function (HOMA-B). These two parameters estimate the deficiency of the pancreatic β-cells based on a mathematical model that takes into account the interrelation (by negative feed-back) between glucose and insulin under normal metabolic control. This interrelation involves both the secretion of the pancreatic hormone and the hypoglycemic insulin action on target tissues. According to this model, the relationship between glucose and insulin, in the basal state, reflects the balance between hepatic glucose output and insulin secretion, which is maintained by a feedback loop between the liver and β-cells (Wallace, 2004, Rutter, 2008). Quicki is also defined as a result of the *in vivo* interaction between glucose and insulin in fasting conditions and, according to some investigators, reflects even better than HOMA, the variations of the insulin sensitivity of target tissues.

The literature data does not define reference values for HOMA and for Quicki parameters; clinical studies show that Quicki and 1/HOMA-IR are significantly lower in obese people compared to healthy subjects (Mather et al, 2001, Yokoyama et al, 2003). For the studied patients we evaluated HOMA-IR and HOMA-B, the reciprocal value of HOMA-IR and Quicki (fig 6 and 7).

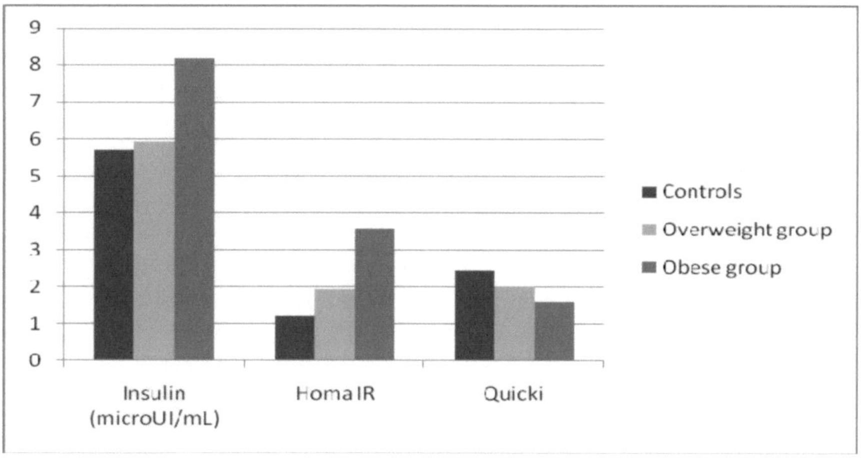

Fig. 6. The insulin as well as HOMA-IR and Quicki parameters for the studied groups

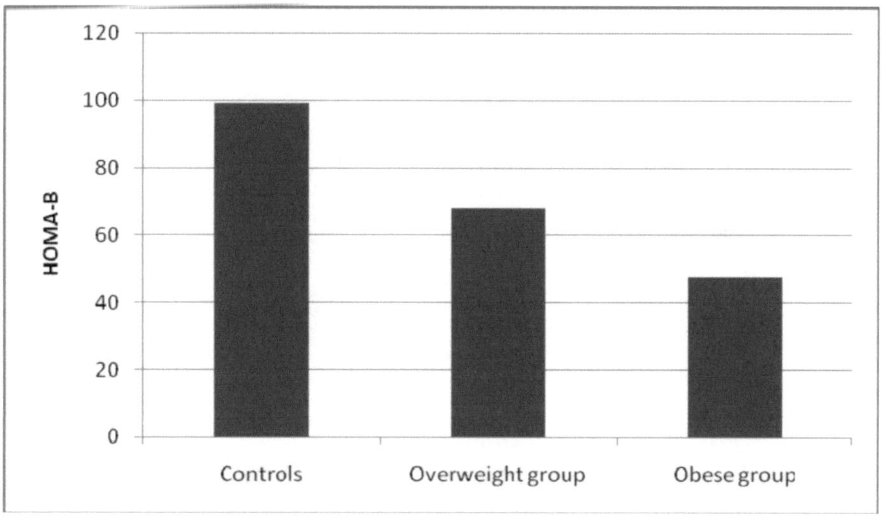

Fig. 7. The HOMA-B parameter for the three study groups

The increase of the insulin level is significant for the obese patients compared to controls. HOMA-IR and Quicki varied significantly in both overweight and obese subjects compared to controls. The insulin level and the insulin resistance index HOMA-IR increase from the control group to the overweight and significantly to the obese patients. So, in obese patients a significantly higher amount of insulin is necessary in order to maintain the normal fasting plasma glucose level; the weight increase might prevent the insulin, even if it's secreted in higher quantity, from exerting its action at the target tissues' level.
In table 2 we present the values obtained for the reciprocal values and the logarithmic values of HOMA-IR, respectively.

Evaluated parameters	Control group	Overweight group	Obese group
Insulin (µUI/mL)	5.73±1.23	5.93±1.65	8.17±4.51**
1/HOMA-IR	0.86±0.17	0.68±0.28*	0.50±0.34**
Log(HOMA-IR)	0.103±0.07	0.24±0.22*	0.46±0.33**

Table 2. The values for 1/HOMA-IR and log (HOMA-IR) for the studied patients

The test used for the evaluation of the insulin resistance/sensitivity phenomena are significantly different both for overweight and obese patients compared to controls. Only the fasting level of insulin does not indicate the degree of insulin resistance. So, the calculated parameters show more precisely than the insulin evaluation the risk of secondary health issues associated with the body mass increase. These changes are revealed starting from the overweight stage and not from the obese stage, as it is the case with insulin.
All the indexes used for the evaluation of insulin resistance/β-cell function are significantly different for both overweight and obese patients compared to controls.
For the studied patients, the decrease of the adiponectin level was correlated with an increase of HOMA-IR. The IL6 and hsCRP levels increased significantly in correlation with HOMA-IR (fig 8).

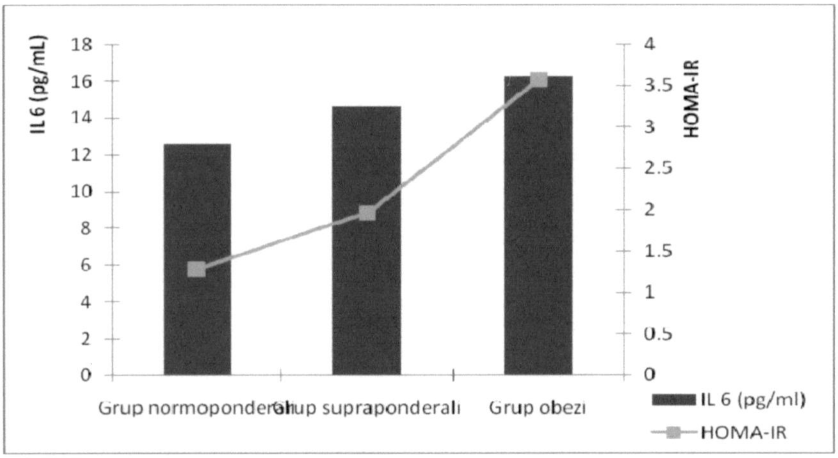

Fig. 8. Correlation of the IL6 level with HOMA-IR

IL6 production is increased in human obesity and the increase is correlated with an increase of the insulin resistance. IL6 can serve as a direct link between adipose tissue and insulin resistance.
The American Diabetes Association defines pre-diabetes by levels of fasting plasma glucose (FPG) between 100 and 125 mg/dL. Analyzing the dynamics of insulin resistance parameters in the group of selected patients in correlation with the fasting plasma glucose level, we obtained the values presented in table 3.
The analysis of the data depending both on the BMI and the fasting plasma glucose, shows that all of the parameters defined for the evaluation of insulin resistance and beta cell function increase significantly in the groups with FPG>125mg/dL, independently of their BMI. The control group and the overweight and obese groups with FPG<100mg/dL had similar values of the evaluated parameters (fig 9).

Evaluated parameters	Overweight group		Obese group	
	FPG<100mg/dL	FPG>125mg/dL	FPG<100mg/dL	FPG>125mg/dL
Insulin (µUI/mL)	5.68±0.81	6.72±2.79	5.53±1.30	10.22±5.29
HOMA-IR	1.22±0.21	3.55±1.63	1.26±0.35	5.58±2.78
1/HOMA-IR	0.85±0.17	0.35±0.18	0.84±0.20	0.22±0.10
Log(HOMA-IR)	0.11±0.05	0.51±0.22	0.12±0.09	0.70±0.21
HOMA-B	96.64±36.39	19.99±13.17	70.51±19.01	25.04±17.92
Quicki	2.42±0.57	1.24±0.36	2.41±0.65	0.99±0.20

Table 3. Parameters for the evaluation of beta cell function and insulin resistance in correlation with the fasting plasma glucose level

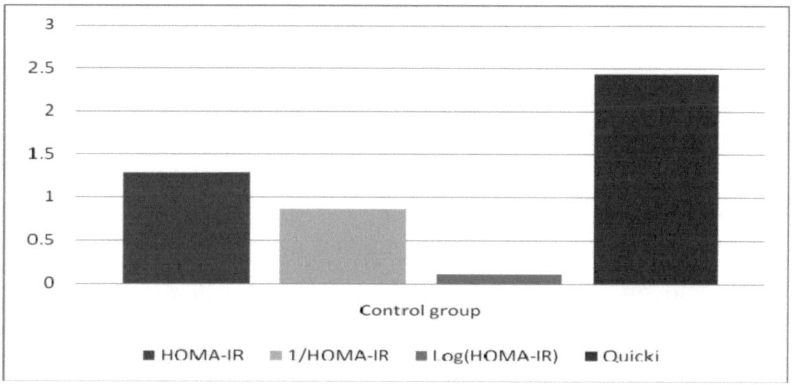

Fig. 9. Parameters for the evaluation of insulin resistance/sensitivity for the control group

The groups with FPG>125mg/dL, either overweight or obese showed significant increases of the parameters for the evaluation of insulin resistance or beta cell function compared to the control group.

The same kind of dynamics was obtained for the IL6 levels, which increased in both overweight and obese groups with FPG>125mg/dL, compared to the FPG<110mg/dl corresponding sub-groups (fig 10). The differences were significant only for the obese subgroups, and not-significant for the overweight ones, compared to controls.

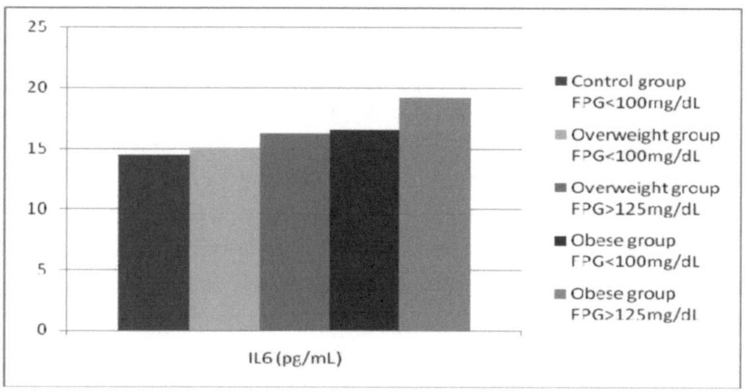

Fig. 10. Interlukin 6 dynamics in the subgroups of patients, defined both according to their BMI and their fasting plasma glucose level

No significant differences were recorded between the sub-groups, regarding the E-selectin levels (fig 11).

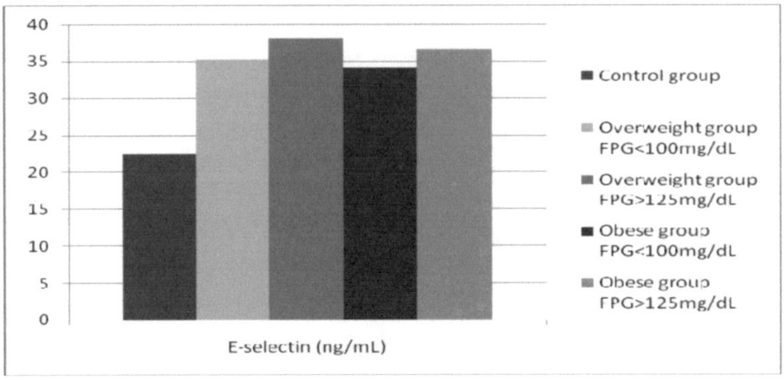

Fig. 11. E-selectin level for the sub-groups of patients, defined according both to their BMI and FPG

4. Conclusions

Our data revealed an impairment of the endothelial function expressed by both the decrease of the NO stable end products' and the adiponectin level, in the overweight and obese groups. These results are in agreement with data from Chen et all (2003), which proved that adiponectin stimulates the NO production at the endothelial level. The synthesis of IL6 as well as the hsCRP plasma level was highly correlated with the body mass index, suggesting the involvement of inflammatory phenomena in the development of endothelial dysfunction associated with the weight gain and the insulin resistance. So, the evaluation of adiponectin as well as of the NOS activity might prove to be useful predictive markers of atherogenic disorders at overweight and obese patients. Interleukin 6 is one of the molecules that contribute to the amplifying of the inflammatory signal in patients with dismetabolic syndrome, taking part into the relationship between the adipose tissue, the liver and the endothelium.

The current study demonstrates elevated plasma soluble adhesion molecule levels in weight increase patients with increased insulin resistance indexes, in spite of the absence of overt vascular damage. On the other hand, the increase of the E-selectin level, associated with the decrease synthesis of NO shows an activation of the endothelium, associated with the insulin resistance. We hypothesized that the early endothelial activation precedes the onset of overt vascular damage in obese patients and might be responsible for the increased release of E-selectin into the bloodstream.

Since insulin resistance is frequently associated as predictor or pathogenic factor in different pathological conditions (type 2 diabetes mellitus, obesity, glucose intolerance, essential hypertension, polycystic ovary syndrome), it is important to have simple, accessible tools for the evaluation of insulin sensitivity of target tissues to the insulin action in humans. The euglycemic hyperinsulinemic clamp technique remains the reference method for quantifying the sensitivity to insulin action but it cannot be applied on a large scale or in the context of routine investigations. For this reason, alternative methods have been developed, including the HOMA model and the Quicki test.

Our results show that the above mentioned parameters vary significantly in correlation with both weight and glucose level in a group of Romanian subjects.

The parameters for the evaluation of insulin resistance and beta cell function might be used in clinical studies in correlation with the level of fasting plasma glucose and not simply as indicators of the degree of insulin resistance in overweight and obese patients.

Since inflammation is an important feature of hyperglycemia and insulin resistance, future therapy for these pathological conditions should focus not only on the reduction of the plasma glucose and/or the glycated hemoglobin levels but also on the decrease of the inflammatory markers, in order to protect the endothelium and to reduce the associated cardio-vascular risk.

5. Acknowledgements

The work was performed under the CNCSIS/UEFISCDI grant PD 132/30.07.2010 (PD 29/2010).

6. References

Archer S. (1999) Measurement of nitric oxide in biological models, 2003, *The FASEB Journal*, Vol 7, No 2, 349-360, ISSN 1530-6860.

Arita Y., Kihara S., Ouchi N., Takahashi M., Maeda K., Miyagawa J., Hotta K., Shimomura I., NakamuraT., Miyaoka K., Kuriyama H., Nishida M., Yamashita S., OkuboK., Matsubara K., Muraguchi M., Ohmoto Y., Funahashi Y. & Matsuzawa Y. (1999) Paradoxical decrease of an adipose-specific protein, adiponectin, in obesity. *Biochem. Biophys. Res. Commun.* Vol 257, No 1, 79–83, ISSN 0006-291X.

Brownlee M (2001) Biochemistry and molecular cell biology of diabetic complications, *Nature*, Vol 414, No 6865, 813-820, 0028-0836.

Ceriello A., Quagliaro L., Piconi L., Assaloni R., Da Ros R., Maier A., Esposito K. & Giugliano D. (2004) Hyperglycemia on Circulating Adhesion Molecules and Oxidative Stress Generation and the Possible Role of Simvastatin Treatment, *Diabetes*, Vol 53, 701–710, ISSN 0012-1797

Chen, H., Montagnani M., Funahashi T., Shimomura I. & Quon M.J. (2003) Adiponectin stimulates production of nitric oxide in vascular endothelial cells, *J Biol Chem*, Vol 45, No 278, 45021-45026, ISSN 1083-351X.

Dansuntornwong B., Chanprasertyothin S., Jongjaroenprasert W., Ngarmukos C., Bunnag P, Puavilai G. & Ongphiphadhanakul B. (2007) The Relation between Parameters from Homeostasis Model Assessment and Glycemic Control in Type 2 Diabetes, *J Med Assoc Thai*, Vol 11, No 90, 2284-2290, ISSN 0007-1323.

De Fronzo R.A. (1988) The triumvirate: beta cell, muscle, liver. A collusion responsible for NIDDM. *Diabetes*, Vol 37, 667-687, ISSN 0012-1797.

De Fronzo RA & Ferrannini E. (1991) Insulin resistance: a multifaceted syndrome responsible for NIDDM, obesity, hypertension, dyslipidemia and atherosclerotic cardiovascular disease, *Diabetes Care*, Vol 14, 173-194, ISSN: 0149-5992.

de Luca C. & Olefsky J.M. (2008) Inflammation and insulin resistance, *FEBS Letters* Vol 1, No 582, 97–105, ISSN: 0014-5793.

Ferri C., Desideri G., Baldoncini R., Bellini C., De Angelis C., Mazzocchi C. & Santucci A. (1998), Early Activation of Vascular Endothelium in Nonobese, Nondiabetic

Essential Hypertensive Patients With Multiple Metabolic Abnormalities, *Diabetes* Vol 47, 660–667, ISSN 0012-1797.

Foss-Freitas M.C. & Foss M.C. (2004) Comparison of the homeostasis model assessment and quantitative insulin sensitivity check index with data from forearm metabolic studies for the *in vivo* assessment of insulin sensitivity, *Brazilian Journal of Medical and Biological Research*, Vol 5, No 37, 663-668, ISSN 1678-4510.

Garcia C. Feve B., Ferré P., Halimi S., Baizri H., Bordier L., Guiu G., Dupuy O., Bauduceau B. & Mayaudon H. (2010) Diabetes and inflammation: Fundamental aspects and clinical implications, *Diabetes & Metabolism*, Vol 5, No 36, 327–338, ISSN: 1262-3636.

Goldstein, B.J. & Scalia R. (2004) Adiponectin: a novel adipokine linking adipocytes and vascular function. *J. Clin. Endocrinol. Metab.* Vol 6, No 89, 2563–2568, ISSN: 1945-7197.

Gradinaru D., Margina D. & Mitrea N., Study Concerning the Influence of Antianginal Therapy on the Activity of Endothelial Nitric Oxide Synthase, Farmacia, Vol 45, Nr. 3, 2003, 42-51, ISSN: 0014-8237.

Guizea L., Panniera B., Thomasa F., Beana K., Jégoa B. & Benetos A. (2008) Recent advances in metabolic syndrome and cardiovascular disease, *Archives of Cardiovascular Disease*, Vol 9, No 101, 577—583, ISSN: 1875-2136.

Hansson G.K. (2005) Inflammation, Atherosclerosis and Coronary Artery Disease, *New England Journal of Medicinel,*Vol 16, No 352, 1685-1695, ISSN 1533-4406.

Hotta K, Funahashi T, Arita Y, Takahashi M, Matsuda M, Okamoto Y, Iwahashi H, Kuriyama H, Ouchi N, Maeda K, Nishida M, Kihara S, Sakai N, Nakajima T, Hasegawa K, Muraguchi M, Ohmoto Y, Nakamura T, Yamashita S. & Hanafusa T, Matsuzawa (2000) Plasma concentrations of a novel, adipose-specific protein, adiponectin, in type 2 diabetic patients. *Arterioscler. Thromb. Vasc. Biol.*, Vol 6, No 20, 1595–1599, ISSN: 1079-5642.

Iwashima Y, Katsuya T, Ishikawa K, Ouchi N, Ohishi M, Sugimoto K, Fu Y, Motone M, Yamamoto K, Matsuo A, Ohashi K, Kihara S, Funahashi T, Rakugi H, Matsuzawa Y. & Ogihara T. (2004) Hypoadiponectinemia is an independent risk factor for hypertension. *Hypertension.*Vol 6, No 43, 1318–1323, ISSN: 02636352.

Joussen AM, Poulaki V, Qin W, Kirchhof B, Mitsiades N, Wiegand SJ, Rudge J, Yancopoulos GD. & Adamis AP (2002) Retinal vascular endothelial growth factor induces intercellular adhesion molecule-1 and endothelial nitric oxide synthase expression and initiates early diabetic retinal leukocyte adhesion in vivo. *Am J Pathol* Vol 2, No 160, 501–509, ISSN 0002-9440.

Katz A, Nambi SS, Mather K, Baron AD, Follmann DA, Sullivan G. & Quon MJ (2000) Quantitative insulin sensitivity check index: a simple, accurate method for assessing insulin sensitivity in humans. *J Clin Endocrinol Metab,*Vol 7, No 85, 2402–2410, ISSN 1945-7197.

King GL, Kunisaki M, Nishio Y, Inoguchi T, Shiba T. & Xia P (1996) Biochemical and molecular mechanisms in the development of diabetic vascular complications. *Diabetes* Vol 45 (Suppl. 3), S105–S108, ISSN 0012-1797.

Low Wang C.C., Goalstone M.L. & Draznin B. (2004) Molecular Mechanisms of Insulin Resistance That Impact Cardiovascular Biology, *Diabetes* Vol 11, No 53, 2735–2740, ISSN 0012-1797.

Margină D, Vlădică M, Grădinaru D, Mitrea N, Dănciulescu R & Radulian G (2005) Clinical study regarding the relationship between the inteleukin 6 level, insulin resistance and endothelial dysfunction, *Farmacia*, No 6, 18-24, ISSN: 0014-8237.

Mather KJ, Hunt AE, Steinberg HO, Paradisi G, Hook G, Katz A, Quon MJ. & Baron AD (2001) Repeatability characteristics of simple indices of insulin resistance: implications for research applications. *J Clin Endocrinol Metab,* Vol 11, No 86, 5457–5464, ISSN 1945-7197.

Matsuda M. (2010) Measuring and estimating insulin resistance in clinical and research settings, *Nutrition, Metabolism & Cardiovascular Diseases* Vol 2, No 20, 79-86, ISSN: 0939-4753.

McAuley KA, Williams SM, Mann JI, Walker RJ, Lewis-Barned NJ, Temple LA. & Duncan AW (2001) Diagnosing insulin resistance in the general population, *Diabetes Care,* Vol 3, No 24, 460-464, ISSN: 0149-5992.

Miyamoto K, Khosrof S, Bursell SE, Rohan R, Murata T, Clermont AC, Aiello LP, Ogura Y. & Adamis AP (1999) Prevention of leukostasis and vascular leakage in streptozotocin-induced diabetic retinopathy via intercellular adhesion molecule-1 inhibition, *Proc Natl Acad Sci U S A* , Vol 19, No 96, 10836 -10841, ISSN 0027-8424.

Monaco C., Gregan S.M., Navin T.J., Foxwell B.M.J., Davies A.H. & Feldmann M (2009) Toll-Like Receptor-2 Mediates Inflammation and Matrix Degradation in Human Atherosclerosis, *Circulation.*, Vol 24, No 120, 2462-2469, ISSN: 0009-7322.

Moshage H., Kok B., Huizenga J.R. & Jansen P.L.M. (1995) Nitrite and nitrate determination in plasma: a critical evaluation, *Clin. Chem.*, Vol 6, No 41, 892-896, ISSN 0009-9147.

Ouchi N., Kihara S., Arita Y., Okamoto Y., Maeda K., Kuriyama H., Hotta K., Nishida M., Takahashi M., Muraguchi M., Ohmoto Y., Nakamura T., Yamashita S., Funahashi T. & Matsuzawa Y. (2000) Adiponectin, an adipocyte derived plasma protein, inhibits endothelial NFkappaB signaling through a cAMP-dependent pathway. *Circulation,* Vol 11, No 102, 1296–1301, ISSN: 0009-7322.

Ouedraogo R., Gong Y., Berzins B., Wu X., Mahadev K., Hough K., Chan L., Goldstein B.J., & Scalia R. (2007) Adiponectin deficiency increases leukocyte-endothelium interactions via upregulation of endothelial cell adhesion molecules in vivo, *J. Clin. Invest.,* Vol 6, No 117, 1718–1726, ISSN: 0021-9738.

Ray A., Huisman M.V., Tamsma J.T.; van Asten J., Bingen B.O., Broeders E.A., Hoogeveen E.S., van Hout F., Kwee V.A., Laman B., Malgo F., Mohammadi M., Nijenhuis M., Rijkée M., van Tellingen M.M., Tromp M., Tummers Q. & de Vries L. (2009) The role of inflammation on atherosclerosis, intermediate and clinical cardiovascular endpoints in type 2 diabetes mellitus, *European Journal of Internal Medicine* Vol 3, No 20, 253–260, ISSN: 0953-6205.

Rutter M.K., Wilson P.W.F, Sullivan L.M., Fox C.S., D'Agostino R.B. & Meigs J.B. (2008) Use of Alternative Thresholds Defining Insulin Resistance to Predict Incident Type 2 Diabetes Mellitus and Cardiovascular Disease, *Circulation.*, Vol 8, No 117, 1003-1009, ISSN: 0009-7322.

Scherer, P.E. (2006) Adipose tissue: from lipid storage compartment to endocrine organ. *Diabetes.* Vol 6, No 55, 1537–1545, ISSN 0012-1797.

Song Y., Manson J.E., Tinker L., Howard B.V., Kuller L.H., Nathan L., Rifai N. & Liu S. (2007) Insulin Sensitivity and Insulin Secretion Determined by the Homeostasis Model Assessment (HOMA) and Risk of Diabetes Mellitus in a Multi-Ethnic Cohort of Women: The Women's Health Initiative Observational Study, *Diabetes Care,* Vol 7, No 30, 1747-52, ISSN: 0149-5992.

Soonthornpun S., Setasuban W., Thamprasit A., Chayanunnukul W., Rattarasarn C. & Geater A. (2003) Novel Insulin Sensitivity Index Derived from Oral Glucose Tolerance Test, *The Journal of Clinical Endocrinology & Metabolism,* Vol 3, No 88 1019–1023, ISSN: 1945-7197.

Stühlinger M.C., Abbasi F., Chu J.W., Lamendola C., McLaughlin T.L., Cooke J.P., Reaven G.M. & Tsao P.S. (2002) Relationship Between Insulin Resistance and an Endogenous Nitric Oxide Synthase Inhibitor, JAMA, Vol 11, No 287, 1420-1426, ISSN 0002-9955.

Wallace T.M., Levy J.C. & Matthews D.R. (2004) Use and Abuse of HOMA Modeling, *Diabetes Care* , Vol 6, No 27, 1487–1495, ISSN: 0149-5992.

Tataranni P.A. & Ortega E. (2005) A Burning Question. Does an Adipokine-Induced Activation of the Immune System Mediate the Effect of Overnutrition on Type 2 Diabetes?, *Diabetes,* Vol 4, No 54, 917–927, ISSN 0012-1797.

Veves A, Akbari CM, Primavera J, Donaghue VM, Zacharoulis D, Chrzan JS, DeGirolami U, LoGerfo FW & Freeman R (1998) Endothelial dysfunction and the expression of endothelial nitric oxide synthetase in diabetic neuropathy, vascular disease, and foot ulceration. *Diabetes* , Vol 3, No 47, 457– 463, ISSN 0012-1797.

Wadham C., Parker A., Wang L. & XiaP. (2007) High Glucose Attenuates Protein *S*-Nitrosylation in Endothelial Cells. Role of Oxidative Stress, *Diabetes,* Vol 11, No 56, 2715–2721, , ISSN 0012-1797.

Williams SB, Goldfine AB, Timimi FK, Ting HH, Roddy MA, Simonson DC & Creager MA: (1998) Acute hyperglycemia attenuates endothelium-dependent vasodilation in humans in vivo. *Circulation* 97:1695–1701, ISSN: 0009-7322.

Yokoyama H., Emoto M., Fujiwara S., Motoyama K., Morioka T., Komatsu M., Tahara H., Shoji T., Okuno Y. & Nishizawa Y. (2003) Quantitative Insulin Sensitivity Check Index and the Reciprocal Index of Homeostasis Model Assessment in Normal Range Weight and Moderately Obese Type 2 Diabetic Patients, *Diabetes Care,*Vol 8, No 26, 2426–2432, ISSN: 0149-5992.

Zavaroni I, Piatti PM, Monti LD, Gasparini P, Barilli LA, Massironi P, Ardigo D, Valsecchi G, Delsignore R& Raven GM (2000): Plasma nitric oxide concentrations are elevated in insulin resistant healthy subjects. *Metabolism,* Vol 8, No 49, 959–961, ISSN: 0026-0495.

Part 2

Oxidative Stress

6

The Regulation of Energy Metabolism Pathways Through L-Carnitine Homeostasis

Edgars Liepinsh, Ivars Kalvinsh and Maija Dambrova
Latvian Institute of Organic Synthesis
Latvia

1. Introduction

Diabetes mellitus is a widespread metabolic disease characterized by hyperglycemia and associated with severe complications, including cardiovascular disease and dyslipidemia. The cardiovascular risk is considerably increased in diabetic patients, and novel cardioprotective strategies are sought that could target both diabetic and cardiovascular outcomes. L-carnitine is a conditionally essential amino acid that plays an important role in cellular energy metabolism. Initial pharmacological studies suggest that preconditioning-like manipulation of substrate metabolism through the regulation of L-carnitine homeostasis could be an effective approach for the prevention of myocardial infarction and the treatment of heart failure, especially for patients with type 2 diabetes. Contradictory data exist concerning the pharmacological outcomes of L-carnitine treatment. It is known that L-carnitine supplementation is beneficial and increases overall glucose utilisation in animals and humans.

Interestingly, a state of limited L-carnitine availability also induces compensatory mechanisms that alter the pathways of energy metabolism. In some experimental studies, a decrease in L-carnitine concentration was achieved by the administration of 3-(2,2,2-trimethylhydrazinium)-propionate (mildronate). In addition to its cardioprotective and anti-atherosclerotic effects, it was shown recently that mildronate, by decreasing L-carnitine concentration, decreases fed and fasted blood glucose concentrations and prevents diabetic complications in an experimental model of type 2 diabetes, Goto-Kakizaki (GK) rats, and an obesity model using Zucker rats. Recently presented mildronate-induced gene expression profiles suggest the peroxisome proliferator-activated receptors (PPARs) as possible nuclear factors underlying the effects of mildronate and decreased L-carnitine availability on FA metabolism. The effects of mildronate might depend on dosing and the length of treatment, which could differentially compensate for the decreased L-carnitine availability and thereby inhibit FA metabolism by activating glucose utilisation. Thus, it is possible that a limited availability of tissue L-carnitine might improve the metabolic flexibility of muscle tissues and enhance the preconditioning-like adaptive responses.

2. Effects of L-carnitine

L-carnitine is a conditionally essential amino acid that plays an important role in cellular energy metabolism. In heart and skeletal muscle, L-carnitine aids the translocation of long-chain FA into the mitochondria for subsequent beta-oxidation, which is a major energy source in muscle cells. L-carnitine is absorbed from dietary products and biosynthesised from lysine and methionine; its excretion is efficiently regulated by renal re-absorption. The physiological range of L-carnitine concentrations in various tissues is maintained by complex transporter systems.

2.1 L-carnitine in pathways of energy metabolism

The homeostasis of cellular energy metabolism relies on the availability of two major sources of substrates: FA and carbohydrates. Through catabolic processes, both substrates provide a metabolite, acetyl coenzyme A (acetyl-CoA), which further undergoes oxidation in the mitochondrial machinery to provide cellular metabolism with adenosine-5'-triphosphate (ATP) molecules, the "molecular unit of currency" of intracellular energy transfer (Koves et al., 2008a). The role of L-carnitine in regulating cellular energy metabolism is schematically summarised in Fig. 1. First, L-carnitine is a substrate of the enzyme L-carnitine palmitoyltransferase-1 (CPT I), which catalyses the rate-limiting reaction in the transfer of FA into the mitochondria (Kuhajda et al., 2007). The key mechanism for regulation of CPT I activity is allosteric inhibition by malonyl CoA (Cuthbert et al., 2005).

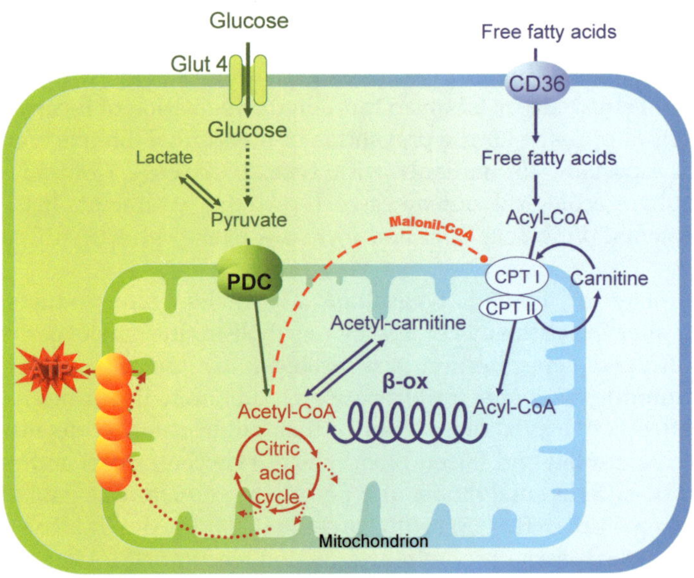

Fig. 1. The cellular pathways of energy metabolism

In the CPT I-catalysed reaction, L-carnitine and acyl-CoA-activated long-chain FA interact to form long-chain acyl-L-carnitine esters that are then shuttled across the mitochondrial membranes by L-carnitine/acyl-L-carnitine translocase (CACT) (Bremer, 1983). Inside the mitochondrial matrix, acyl-L-carnitine is converted back to L-carnitine and long-chain FA by the enzyme CPT II. Thus, L-carnitine aids the import of long-chain FA to the mitochondria for β-oxidation, which is the major provider of energy for muscle cells.

In addition to its role in FA transport pathways, L-carnitine is also involved in the export of acetyl groups out of the mitochondria (Stephens et al., 2007). In the mitochondrial matrix, lumen of the endoplasmic reticulum and peroxisomes, L-carnitine acetyltransferase (CrAT;

EC 2.3.1.7) catalyses the reversible transfer of acetyl groups between acetyl-CoA and L-carnitine (Ramsay et al., 2001). By catalysing its reaction in a reversible manner, CrAT regulates the cellular pool of CoA, which serves as a carrier of activated acetyl groups in the oxidation of energy metabolism substrates and in the synthesis of FA and lipids (Ramsay et al., 2001). Glucose metabolism pathways are also regulated through the homeostasis of the ratio of acetyl-CoA/CoA. An increase in this ratio is sensed by pyruvate dehydrogenase kinase, which phosphorylates and thereby leads to the inhibition of the pyruvate dehydrogenase complex (PDC), the key rate-limiting step in carbohydrate oxidation (Lopaschuk, 2001; Rebouche, 2004), with L-carnitine being a pivotal regulator of these pathways. For example, during high-intensity exercise, L-carnitine enters the CrAT-catalysed reaction and buffers the excess acetyl groups formed. As a result, a pool of free CoA is maintained for the continuation of the PDC and citric acid cycle reactions (Stephens et al., 2007). It can be concluded that L-carnitine is important for the regulation of both long-chain FA and carbohydrate metabolism. L-carnitine-dependent pathways are strongly involved in the regulation of the adaptive responses related to the overall homeostasis of cellular energy metabolism.

2.2 The bioavailability of L-carnitine

The homeostasis of L-carnitine (Fig. 2) is maintained through biosynthesis, efficient reabsorption in the kidneys and food intake, particularly from meat and dairy products (Rebouche, 2004). The physiological range of different L-carnitine concentrations in various tissues is maintained by complex transporter systems (Ramsay et al., 2001). The biosynthesis of L-carnitine from the amino acids lysine and methionine proceeds in the liver, kidney and testis, with γ-butyrobetaine (GBB) being an intermediate precursor (Bieber, 1988). It has been estimated that in the case of a non-vegetarian diet, only about 25% of the necessary L-carnitine is biosynthesised, and 75% is ingested from food (Longo et al., 2006). Interestingly, the blood plasma concentration in women is about 20% lower than in men (Cederblad, 1976). Additionally, in vegetarians, the L-carnitine concentration in the blood serum is 20-30% lower than that in the reference population (Delanghe et al., 1989).

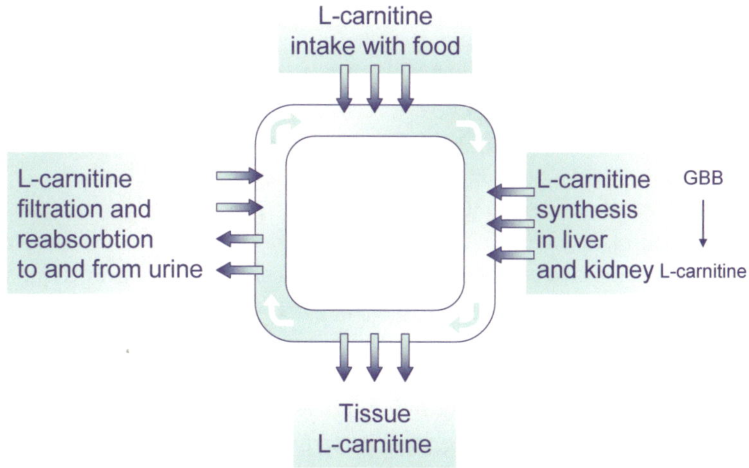

Fig. 2. The body L-carnitine pools and turnover.

After oral intake, the absorption of L-carnitine proceeds by active transport and passive diffusion (Ramsay et al., 2001). It has been shown experimentally that the absolute bioavailability of L-carnitine after a peroral dose of 1-6 g was only 5-18%, while the intake of L-carnitine by food resulted in an absorption of up to 75% (Evans et al., 2003). When the peroral dose was higher than 6 g, a specific smell was noted, possibly due to an increased concentration of trimethylamine in sweat (Hathcock et al., 2006).
Interestingly, the L-carnitine concentration that is required to support long-chain FA oxidation spans a wide range among different tissues of the same species and in the same tissue across species (Long et al., 1982; McGarry et al., 1983) because different tissues express different isoforms of CPT I, which are, in turn, differentially sensitive to L-carnitine. For example, the rat isoforms of CPT I in the liver (CPT IA) and muscle (CPT IB) have Km values for L-carnitine of 30 and 500 μM, respectively (McGarry et al., 1983). In the heart, both CPT I isoforms, CPT IA and CPT IB, are present, and as a result, the average Km for L-carnitine in the heart is 200 μM (McGarry et al., 1983). Therefore, the liver is much less sensitive to lower L-carnitine concentrations than the muscles and the heart. Additionally, in cases of a reduced L-carnitine concentration, a compensatory increase in CPT I is observed (Uenaka et al., 1996). In a recent publication, it was demonstrated that systemic L-carnitine deficiency causes severe hypoglycaemia in mice (Kuwajima et al., 2007). Similarly, after treatment with sodium pivalate, glucose oxidation was increased in L-carnitine-deficient hearts (Broderick, 2006). Thus, the bioavailability of L-carnitine changes along with the amounts of its dietary intake, and its requirements could be different in different tissues, reflecting the energy needs under certain conditions.

2.3 Effects of L-carnitine supplementation

During the last decades, the intake of L-carnitine as a food supplement has become very popular even though scientific evidence of its efficacy is not always available. Undoubtedly, L-carnitine is effective for the treatment of inherited disorders related to functional anomalies in a specific organic cation/carnitine transporter (OCTN2), in drug-induced L-carnitine deficiency and in cases of excessive excretion of L-carnitine because of renal tubular disorders and in patients on haemodialysis (Angelini et al., 2006; Fornasini et al., 2007; Lheureux et al., 2005). The safety profile of L-carnitine allows its frequent use in cocktails of food additives that are aimed to increase the oxidation of FA to eliminate body fat and thus produce cosmetic effects. However, thus far, the body weight-reducing effect of L-carnitine supplementation has not been proven clinically (Saper et al., 2004). A similar situation is characteristic for the use of L-carnitine for improved physical activity. The ineffectiveness of L-carnitine might be related to its low bioavailability during normal homeostasis (Hathcock et al., 2006). As a result, additional L-carnitine does not reach the cellular mitochondria where it could bring about the desired effects and drive the processes of FA metabolism. Recent developments in the use of L-carnitine to stimulate the oxidation of FA are linked to novel approaches to increase the bioavailability of L-carnitine (Stephens et al., 2007).
In addition to being an important cofactor for the L-carnitine mediated transport of long-chain FA into the mitochondrial matrix, as a pharmacological agent, L-carnitine enhances the glycolytic processing of carbohydrates (Foster, 2004; Mingrone, 2004; Stephens et al., 2007). The suggested mechanisms of pharmacological action of L-carnitine are increased

PDC activity, regulation of acetyl- and acyl-cellular trafficking and changes in the acetyl CoA/CoA ratio and expression of key glycolytic and gluconeogenic enzymes (Mingrone, 2004; Uziel et al., 1988). L-carnitine also stimulates glucose oxidation in intact fatty acid-perfused rat heart (Broderick, 2006). The beneficial effects of L-carnitine supplementation in animal models of diabetes also have been demonstrated (Malone et al., 1999; Malone et al., 2006; Sena et al., 2008). L-carnitine supplementation is believed to be beneficial for diabetic patients (Mingrone, 2004). In type 2 diabetic patients, L-carnitine increases the amount of whole-body glucose utilisation and glucose oxidation (Capaldo et al., 1991; De et al., 1999). However, for use in the management of diabetic complications, L-carnitine is listed between antioxidants for which no established benefit has been found (Golbidi et al., 2011), and the effects of L-carnitine in healthy subjects or in type 2 diabetic patients are still controversial (Gonzalez-Ortiz et al., 2008). Nevertheless, additional intake of L-carnitine is recommended for diabetic patients with late complications (Poorabbas et al., 2007; Power et al., 2007).
Because FA metabolism is the main source of energy for muscle cells, including cardiomyocytes, the effects of L-carnitine have been evaluated for the treatment of different cardiovascular diseases (Ferrari et al., 2004). The evidence for the cardioprotective effectiveness of L-carnitine is also not unambiguous. Treatment with L-carnitine was protective against ischemia-reperfusion injury (Cui et al., 2003), but another experimental study provided evidence that L-carnitine worsens ischemic injury under conditions where L-carnitine does not facilitate glucose metabolism (Diaz et al., 2008). For example, in the CEDIM 2 trial, L-carnitine therapy led to a reduction in early mortality without affecting the risk of death and heart failure at 6 months in patients with anterior acute myocardial infarction, resulting in a non-significant finding with respect to the primary end-point (Tarantini et al., 2006).
Even though the clinical and experimental evidence for the effects of supplementary L-carnitine intake are not always convincing, it is a very popular food additive due its safety profile, antioxidant-type activity and suggested effects on energy metabolism pathways.

3. Metabolic consequences of pharmacologically decreased availability of L-carnitine

Mildronate (3-(2,2,2-trimethylhydrazinium)propionate dihydrate) (Fig. 3) represents the only pharmacological agent that effectively reduces L-carnitine concentration and in turn induces protective effects against diabetes and cardiovascular diseases. The mechanism of action of mildronate is believed to involve a decreased tissue concentration of L-carnitine (Dambrova et al., 2002), even though other possible interactions between mildronate and pathways of energy metabolism signalling cannot be excluded.

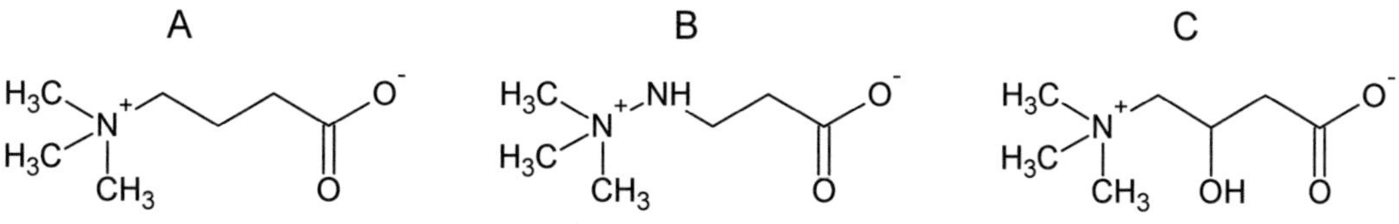

Fig. 3. Structural formulas or GBB (A), mildronate (B) and carnitine (C).

3.1 Inhibitory effect of mildronate on L-carnitine content

Mildronate is known to be an inhibitor of L-carnitine biosynthesis (Simkhovich et al., 1988), its transport into tissues and its reabsorption in the kidney (Kuwajima et al., 1999). The K_i for GBB hydroxylase enzyme inhibition by mildronate has been determined to be 19 μM (enzyme prepared as described by (Tars et al., 2010)). The EC50 for OCTN2 inhibition by mildronate was calculated to be 21 μM (Grube et al., 2006). At a dose of 100 mg/kg, the mildronate concentration in rat blood plasma reached 20 μM after a single administration; however, after 3 days of repeated administration, the mildronate concentration remained at 20 μM even 24 h after the last administration (Liepinsh 2006). Mildronate is actively transported into tissues by OCTN2 (Grigat et al., 2009), and the mildronate concentration in liver and heart reaches 500-1000 μM (Liepinsh et al., 2009a). Thus, mildronate concentrations are able to completely inhibit L-carnitine biosynthesis and substantially decrease L-carnitine transport into tissues and reabsorption in the kidneys. As a result, mildronate (100 mg/kg) induces a significant reduction of the L-carnitine concentration in blood plasma and different tissues by 60-70% (Liepinsh et al., 2009a). In our recent human study, it was shown that mildronate also decreases L-carnitine concentrations by 20% in healthy human non-vegetarian volunteers (Liepinsh et al., 2011a). A less-pronounced effect of mildronate on L-carnitine content in humans could be explained by meat consumption, which is the most important source of L-carnitine (Rebouche, 2004). Compared to a human non-vegetarian diet, in standard laboratory animal feed, the content of L-carnitine is very low (unpublished data). Overall, after long-term treatment, the plasma concentration of mildronate reaches a level that is able to induce changes in the homeostasis of L-carnitine. However, it must be noted that to our knowledge, an acute mildronate treatment does not induce any metabolic or gene expression changes, and therefore, long-term treatment (at least 10-14 days) is necessary to achieve regulatory effects. In addition, all changes induced by mildronate are highly related to the decrease in the L-carnitine concentration in tissues. The modulation of L-carnitine pathways by mildronate then changes the activity of cellular enzymes and receptor systems in a manner that could maintain sufficient energy metabolism and induce adaptive-like changes.

By inhibiting the biosynthesis of L-carnitine, mildronate increases the concentration of its substrate, γ-butyrobetaine (GBB, Fig. 3.), which is mostly known as a bio-precursor of L-carnitine (Bremer, 1983). We have investigated the effects of mildronate administration (4-12 weeks, 100 mg/kg) on both L-carnitine and GBB contents in rat plasma and tissues and have shown that in concert with a decrease in L-carnitine concentration, the administration of mildronate causes a significant increase in GBB concentration (Liepinsh et al., 2009a). There have been speculations regarding the cholinergic activity of GBB; however, only the methyl-ester of GBB produces this activity (Dambrova et al., 2004). The physiological and pharmacological consequences of increased GBB concentration remain to be discovered.

3.2 Metabolic changes in fatty acid metabolism

3.2.1 The effects on CPT I and mitochondrial fatty acid metabolism

Mildronate-decreased tissue L-carnitine concentrations induce changes in the energy metabolism pathways, especially in mitochondrial long-chain FA oxidation (Fig. 4). These changes are exclusively related to CPT I activity and FA transport into the mitochondria. If the L-carnitine content is lowered by mildronate treatment, a subsequent decrease in CPT I activity and a decreased CPT I-driven FA oxidation rate is observed (Kuka et al., 2011;

Simkhovich et al., 1988). Interestingly, due to the differences in L-carnitine content and the K_m values of CPT I for L-carnitine, at least a 60-70% reduction in L-carnitine content in the heart is necessary to reduce CPT I-dependent long-chain FA transport and oxidation.

Additionally, if the L-carnitine content is lowered significantly below the K_m value of CPT I, a compensatory increase in CPT I expression is observed (Uenaka R 1996). After long-term mildronate treatment, a 2 to 2.5-fold increase in the expression of CPT IA and CPT IB was found in the heart and liver (Degrace et al., 2007; Liepinsh et al., 2008). However, the increase in CPT I protein expression cannot compensate for significantly reduced L-carnitine availability, and therefore, subsequent changes in metabolic pathways occur. Although the expression of CPT I after mildronate treatment is increased, the overall FA oxidation rate in mitochondria is decreased (Kuka, et al. 2011; Simkhovich et al., 1988).

In a recent study, the effects of mildronate, L-carnitine and a combination of both substances on myocardial infarction were compared (Kuka et al., 2011). Mildronate treatment markedly decreased the L-carnitine concentration of the heart tissue and significantly decreased the infarct size. Administration of mildronate together with L-carnitine restored the L-carnitine concentration, and therefore, CPT I activity was similar to that in control samples; as a consequence, the infarct size was not reduced. Therefore, we conclude that the decrease of L-carnitine concentration is the main mechanism of action of mildronate, and this decrease is necessary to induce changes in cellular energy metabolism.

3.2.2 The modulation of PPARs and fatty acid metabolism-related gene expression

Peroxisome proliferator-activated receptors (PPARs) are central regulators of energy metabolism that mediate adaptive metabolic responses to increased systemic lipid availability following activation by the binding of endogenous or dietary lipids or lipid derivatives (Grimaldi, 2007; Sugden et al., 2009). Several genes that are induced by mildronate treatment, particularly CPT I (Degrace et al., 2007; Liepinsh et al., 2008), suggest PPARs as possible nuclear factors involved in the mildronate-induced effects on glucose and FA metabolism (Fig. 4). In a very recent study to elucidate the molecular mechanism of mildronate, PPAR-α and PPAR-γ nuclear content and the expression of glucose and FA metabolism genes were determined in obese Zucker rats (Liepinsh et al., 2011b). The hearts of obese Zucker rats had a significant impairment in the PPAR-α system, and the response to increased FA and triglyceride (TG) was disrupted. Thus, the expression of PPAR-α and its target genes in obese Zucker rat heart tissue was reduced compared to their expression in lean animals. Mildronate treatment restored the sensitivity of PPAR-α, which is manifested as significantly increased nuclear expression of PPAR-α in heart tissue and the expression of genes involved in FA metabolism. In cell culture, we found that mildronate and L-carnitine did not change PPAR activity *in vitro*. Thus, PPAR activation is instead induced as a result of a reduced FA oxidation rate and some FA accumulation.

Interestingly, increased expression of FA metabolic genes, particularly CPT-I, did not compensate for a reduction in the L-carnitine content, and therefore, the CPT I-dependent FA oxidation rate in heart tissue was significantly reduced. However, PPAR-α activation also induces genes that are involved in intra-mitochondrial FA β-oxidation. Thus, mildronate treatment could stimulate mitochondrial β-oxidation of FA transported into the mitochondria by CPT I (mildronate induces partial reduction in CPT I activity) and carnitine-acylcarnitine transport system. This could be another mechanism to protect the mitochondria from lipid overload and the accumulation of FA in mitochondria. To test this hypothesis, mitochondrial respiration measurements were performed on energy substrates like palmitoyl-CoA and palmitoyl-L-carnitine. CPT I-dependent mitochondrial oxidation of palmitoyl-CoA was reduced in mildronate-treated rat hearts, while palmitoyl-L-carnitine oxidation in mildronate-treated heart mitochondria was even faster than in the control group (unpublished data). In contrast, the expression of PPAR-α and target genes in the liver of obese Zucker rats was not significantly affected by treatment. The effects of mildronate on PPAR-γ and PPAR-δ and the expression of their target genes are rather unclear and should be clarified in future studies. In conclusion, mildronate-dependent gene expression is, to some extent, dependent on the activation of PPAR-α in heart tissue but not in liver tissue.

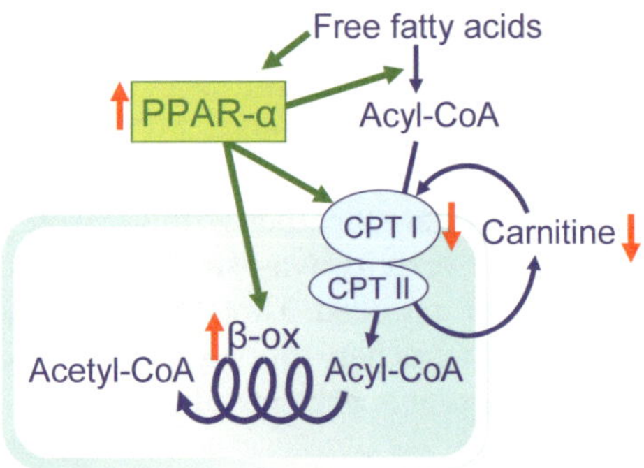

Fig. 4. The effects of pharmacologically decreased availability of L-carnitine on PPAR-α activity and fatty acid metabolism pathways. The red arrows indicate mildronate-induced changes; green arrows indicate stimulating effects of PPAR-α.

3.2.3 Metabolic flexibility and protection against lipid overload

Healthy subjects, depending on the availability of glucose or FA, are able to switch appropriately between the available energy substrates (Fig. 5A). At a postprandial state, the glucose and insulin concentrations are increased, and glucose oxidation dominates over FA oxidation. In contrast, in a fasted state, the glucose concentration is significantly lower, and energy metabolism is switched to FA. As shown in Fig. 5B, in obese subjects, lipid overload induces a metabolic inflexibility that is characterised by the reduced ability of cells to appropriately move between energy metabolism substrates (Larsen et al., 2008). Thus, an increase in circulating lipids stimulates FA influx into the mitochondria (Koves et al., 2008b; Petersen et al., 2004). Then, the increased concentration of long-chain FA and intermediates of FA metabolism, in particular acetyl-CoA, mediates the inhibition of the PDC and CPT I activity and induces the impairment of the citric acid cycle and respiratory chain functions (Koves et al., 2008b; Wang et al., 2007). These changes result in a pathologically decreased oxidation rate of both glucose and FA and deteriorate the mitochondrial capacity to produce ATP (Kelley et al., 2002). Therefore, lipid overload-induced metabolic inflexibility and lipotoxicity is primarily associated with FA accumulation in the mitochondria.

Mildronate treatment prevents lipid overload by decreasing the L-carnitine content in tissues and subsequently decreasing CPT I-mediated long-chain FA transport and pathological accumulation in the mitochondria (Asaka et al., 1998; Kirimoto et al., 1996). In obese Zucker rats, mildronate induced a moderate increase in the FA and TG concentrations, and it significantly improved insulin sensitivity and reduced blood glucose and insulin concentrations (Fig. 5C) (Liepinsh et al., 2011b). Thus, mildronate treatment, by decreasing L-carnitine content, improves metabolic flexibility and adaptive responses to hyperglycaemia- and hyperlipidaemia-induced metabolic disturbances.

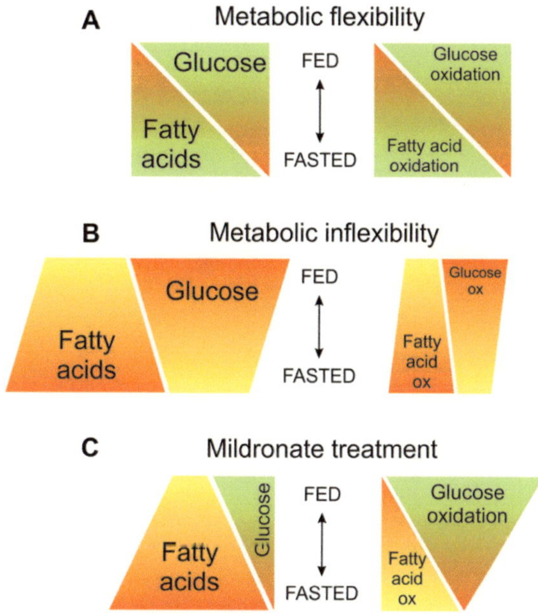

Fig. 5. Metabolic flexibility, inflexibility and mildronate treatment induced protection against lipid overload.

3.2.4 Comparison of mildronate to other inhibitors of fatty acid oxidation

Different approaches are used to inhibit FA oxidation and to switch energy metabolism from FA to glucose oxidation (Table 1). The most similar to the mildronate mechanism of action is the direct inhibition of CPT I or targeting malonyl-CoA, which is a potent endogenous inhibitor of CPT I (Anderson et al., 1995; Cuthbert et al., 2005). Because CPT I is the rate-limiting enzyme in FA oxidation, the inhibition of CPT I is an effective way to achieve a decrease in the long-chain FA oxidation rate. Several irreversible and reversible inhibitors of CPT I, such as etmoxir and teglicar, were synthesised and tested experimentally (Table 1). A significant myocardial infarction-lowering effect for etmoxir was demonstrated; however, its toxicity strongly limits its usage in clinic. Teglicar, both *in vitro* and in animal models, reduces gluconeogenesis and improves glucose homeostasis (Table 1) (Conti et al., 2011). Another approach is to inhibit malonyl-CoA decarboxylase, an enzyme that degrades malonyl-CoA to acetyl-CoA. The inhibition of this reaction by selective inhibitors leads to the accumulation of malonyl-CoA which inhibits CPT I and related FA oxidation. The inhibitors of CPT II have also been considered to be potentially useful for the treatment of type 2 diabetes (Rufer et al., 2009). Overall, the direct inhibition of CPT I or CPT II as well as an increase in malonyl-CoA and reduction in L-carnitine concentrations are similarly effective ways to target CPT I-dependent FA oxidation As a result, cardiac metabolism is switched from FA to glucose oxidation.

In contrast, trimetazidine and ranolazine inhibit 3-ketoacyl coenzyme-A thiolase, which catalyses the last step in mitochondrial FA β-oxidation. A potential benefit offered by trimetazidine and ranolazine in myocardial dysfunction is the ability to increase the utilisation of glucose and lactate, improving oxygen consumption of the myocardium. Overall, free FA inhibitors effectively act as metabolic modulators in the protection of ischemic myocardium both in non-diabetic and diabetic subjects.

Name	Mechanism of action	Effect on myocardial infarction	Effect on blood glucose metabolism	Benefit against diabetes complications	Literature
Mildronate	Lowered L-carnitine conc. and CPT I dependent FA oxidation	↓	↑	+	(Liepinsh et al., 2009b; Sesti et al., 2006)
Trimetazidine	Inhibition of 3-KAT in mitochondrial FA β-oxidation	↓	↑	+	(Monti et al., 2006; Mouquet et al., 2010)
Ranolazine	Inhibition of 3-KAT in mitochondrial FA β-oxidation	↓	↑	+	(Hale et al., 2008; Morrow et al., 2009)
Etmoxir	Inhibition of CPT I and dependent FA oxidation	↓	↑	?	(Gunther et al., 2000; Wolf et al., 1988)
Teglicar	Inhibition of liver CPT IA and dependent FA oxidation	?	↑	?	(Conti et al., 2011)

3-KAT – 3-ketoacyl coenzyme-A thiolase, FA – fatty acids, CPT I – L-carnitine palmitoyl transferase, ↑ – stimulate, ↓ – decrease, + – beneficial effect, ? – under investigation.

Table 1. Comparison of mildronate to other inhibitors of fatty acid oxidation.

3.3 Metabolic changes in glucose metabolism

3.3.1 Switch to glucose metabolism

It is generally accepted that better survival of ischemic myocardium cells can be achieved by stimulating glucose oxidation, either directly or secondarily, to partially inhibited FA oxidation (Lopaschuk, 2001). The beneficial effects of metabolic modulators in cardiac tissue are based on the increased efficiency of the obtained ATP per mole of oxygen for glucose oxidation compared to FA oxidation and, more importantly, the increased coupling of glycolysis to glucose oxidation resulting in a net reduction of the proton burden in the ischemic tissue (Schofield et al., 2001; Taegtmeyer et al., 1998). Moreover, insulin resistance and lowered glucose uptake and oxidation have been associated with the progression of cardiovascular pathologies such as coronary heart disease and heart failure (Kamalesh, 2007;

Taegtmeyer et al., 1998). A shift of the energy substrate preference from FA oxidation to glucose oxidation was suggested as a basis for the cardioprotective effects of mildronate long before it was demonstrated experimentally (Asaka et al., 1998; Dambrova et al., 2002). Indeed, the reduction of L-carnitine content by mildronate treatment leads to a decrease in the CPT I-dependent FA oxidation rate in mitochondria, and in turn, due to a Randle cycle, a substantial increase is expected in the rate of glucose uptake, as was found in mouse hearts after mildronate treatment (Liepinsh et al., 2008). Thus, in cases of partially decreased FA oxidation, changes in glucose metabolism could play a compensatory role. In contrast to mouse and diabetic rat models, where a significant blood glucose-lowering effect was observed, the glucose concentration was not significantly decreased in rats treated with mildronate at doses up to 400 mg/kg (Liepinsh et al., 2009a). These results suggest that mildronate treatment does not directly stimulate but rather facilitates glucose metabolism and that the effect of mildronate strongly depends on substrate availability and energy requirements.

3.3.2 Effects on insulin signalling

Insulin is the major regulator of glucose homeostasis in the body. The insulin signalling pathway is responsible for controlling substrate preference in the heart, muscles and adipose tissues. Insulin stimulates myocardial glucose uptake and accelerates glucose oxidation (Benecke et al., 1993). Both in non-diabetic and diabetic animals, mildronate treatment significantly facilitates insulin-dependent glucose uptake and metabolism (Fig. 6). At the same time, mildronate, which decreases the blood glucose concentration in mice and diabetic rats, usually does not affect plasma insulin and C-peptide levels (Liepinsh et al., 2008; Liepinsh et al., 2009b). In addition, in study in Zucker rats mildronate along with decrease in glucose concentration also decreased pathologically elevated insulin concentration in fed Zucker rats (Liepinsh et al., 2011b). Moreover, mildronate induces a statistically significant 35% increase in insulin-stimulated glucose uptake in isolated mouse hearts (Liepinsh et al., 2008). Mildronate action could be explained by specific insulin pathway-related gene expression. During insulin-stimulated conditions, glucose transport by GLUT 4 is the rate-limiting step for glucose uptake in muscles and the heart. In genetically manipulated mice overexpressing GLUT 4, improvement in both glucose tolerance and insulin action were noted (Hansen et al., 1995). Mildronate treatment induces an increase in GLUT 4 protein expression in heart tissues, which explains the increase in insulin-stimulated glucose uptake.

The important intracellular regulators of aerobic oxidation of glucose are the enzymes of the PDC, which links the glycolysis metabolic pathway to the mitochondrial citric acid cycle (Fig. 6). A significant 2-fold increase in the expression of both PDC enzymes, E1/E2, in mildronate-treated mouse hearts compared with non-treated controls was observed. In addition, in several studies, a decrease in lactate concentration in ischemic hearts of mildronate-treated animals has been noted, which indicates that long-term mildronate treatment not only facilitates glucose uptake but also enhances the aerobic oxidation of glucose (Asaka et al., 1998; Hayashi et al., 2000b; Liepinsh et al., 2011b). Besides the direct effects of insulin on glucose homeostasis, stimulation of the insulin receptor leads to the activation of signalling pathways such as the phosphatidylinositol-3-kinase and the mitogen-activated protein kinase cascades, which are involved in cardioprotection from reperfusion injury (Jonassen et al., 2001; Youngren, 2007). Overall, the observed increase of insulin receptor sensitivity could be important for the manifestation of the cardioprotective and antidiabetic effects of the mildronate treatment.

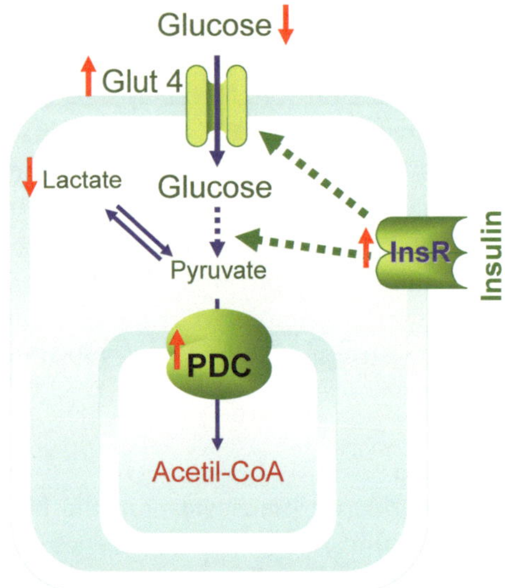

Fig. 6. The effects of pharmacologically decreased availability of L-carnitine on glucose metabolism. The red arrows indicate mildronate-induced changes; green arrows indicate stimulating effects of insulin.

4. Pharmacological effects of decreased availability of L-carnitine

4.1 Effects on myocardial infarction

Mildronate is primarily known as a cardioprotective drug, the mechanism of action of which is based on a decrease of L-carnitine concentration, regulation of energy metabolism and enhancement of preconditioning-like adaptive responses (Dambrova et al., 2002). In the past 10 years, cardioprotective effects of mildronate have been extensively studied in different models of heart infarction and heart failure (Hayashi et al., 2000b; Liepinsh et al., 2006; Sesti et al., 2006; Vilskersts et al., 2009a). It was shown that long-term treatment with mildronate preserved ATP production by optimisation of energy metabolism. Then, a significant reduction of infarct size was shown in an isolated heart infarction model both in vitro (Liepinsh et al., 2006) and in vivo (Sesti et al., 2006). In addition, mildronate was recently demonstrated to be cardioprotective in diabetic Goto-Kakizaki (G-K) rats, where besides the glucose-lowering effect, mildronate treatment at doses of 100 and 200 mg/kg decreased the infarct size by 30% (Liepinsh et al., 2009b). Overall, mildronate treatment effectively reduces myocardial infarction in diabetic GK and non-diabetic Wistar rats.

Treatment with mildronate did not have a significant effect on haemodynamic parameters either before or during ischemia-reperfusion, indicating that the observed effects on infarct size are not related to changes in the cardiac workload. This result gives evidence that mildronate primarily acts as metabolic regulator and provides opportunities to effectively combine mildronate with agents affecting haemodynamic parameters. In animal studies, mildronate is combined with orotic acid, which is also known as an energy metabolism-influencing metabolite (Vilskersts et al., 2009a). Mildronate possesses additive pharmacological effects with orotic acid, and mildronate orotate might be considered a powerful therapeutic agent facilitating recovery from ischemia-reperfusion injury. In the same study, we found that the administration of mildronate and its orotate salt decreased the duration and incidence of arrhythmias in experimental arrhythmia models.

4.2 Heart failure

The effects of mildronate on haemodynamics, cardiac hypertrophy and metabolic consequences in rats after coronary artery ligation were also studied. Mildronate induces significant attenuation of the development of left ventricular (LV) hypertrophy and of increased LVEDP. These results suggest that mildronate improved LV hypertrophy and LV dysfunction in rats with heart failure induced by myocardial ischemia (Nakano et al., 1999). In a similar study performed by Hayashi et al., the effects of mildronate were examined in rats with congestive heart failure following myocardial infarction (Hayashi et al., 2000b). A survival study was conducted for 6 months, and ventricular remodelling, cardiac function, and myocardial high-energy phosphate levels after treatment for 20 days were measured. Mildronate prolonged survival, prevented expansion of the left ventricular cavity (ventricular remodelling), attenuated the rise in right atrial pressure and augmented cardiac functional adaptability against an increased load. Additionally, an improved myocardial energy state in mildronate-treated rats was observed. A different study by the same authors demonstrated that the mechanisms of mildronate action in heart failure are based on the amelioration of [Ca2+]i transients through an increase in SR Ca2+ uptake activity (Hayashi et al., 2000a).

Several clinical studies evaluated the efficacy of mildronate in the complex therapy of chronic heart failure (CHF). Statsenko, ME et al. evaluated the clinical efficacy of mildronate in addition to basic therapy in patients with CHF and type 2 diabetes mellitus (DM2) during the postinfarction period (Statsenko et al., 2007). The subjects were 60 II to III NYHA CHF patients aged 43 to 70 years who were also suffering from DM2. The patients were observed during the early postinfarction period (weeks 3 to 4 from the onset of myocardial infarction). The use of mildronate in addition to basic therapy was associated with a more evident decrease in CHF functional class, an increase in 6-min walking test distance, a tendency towards normalisation of diastolic heart function and an increase in LVEF. Also, in a recent study, the advantage of treatment with mildronate (1 g/day) as a corrector of metabolism in combination with standard therapy for the exercise tolerance of patients with CHD over treatment with a placebo in combination with standard therapy was noted (Dzerve et al., 2010). The overall conclusion from clinical studies is that the use of mildronate in basic therapy favours the normalisation of vegetative homeostasis and improves the quality of life.

4.3 Metabolic syndrome and diabetes

The effects of mildronate on glucose metabolism and its benefits in the treatment of diabetes have been proven experimentally only during the last decade, even though they had been suggested previously (Dambrova et al., 2002). This delay could be because mildronate at doses up to 400 mg/kg did not affect the blood glucose concentration in non-diabetic rats. Mildronate reduced blood glucose in Wistar rats only at a dose of 800 mg (Degrace et al., 2007). The possible anti-diabetic effects of mildronate were then examined in an experimental model of type 2 diabetes in GK rats (Liepinsh et al., 2009b).

The main finding of this study was that decreased L-carnitine availability leads to fed and fasted blood glucose concentration-lowering effects without increasing the insulin concentration in diabetic GK rats. As mentioned before, mildronate also induced cardioprotective effects in GK rat hearts. At the end of an 8-week treatment, the necrosis zone in mildronate-treated diabetic rat hearts was significantly decreased by 30%. Overall, these findings directly indicate that mildronate treatment could be beneficial in diabetes patients with cardiovascular diseases. Furthermore, mildronate effectiveness was tested in rats with streptozotocin-induced diabetes mellitus (Sokolovska et al., 2011). As expected, long-term mildronate treatment caused a significant decrease in the mean blood glucose and glycated haemoglobin (HbA1c) concentrations in streptozotocin-treated rats. Thus, the glucose-lowering effects were shown experimentally both in type 1 and type 2 diabetes mellitus.

In a recent study, the effects of mildronate treatment were compared to the effects of metformin treatment in obese Zucker rats (Liepinsh et al., 2011). In this study, mildronate treatment, to the same extent as metformin, significantly reduced the blood glucose concentration in the fed and fasted states and increased the insulin concentration in obese Zucker rats. In addition, several effects caused by the combination of mildronate and metformin treatment were additive or even synergistic. An additive effect in an oral glucose tolerance test and in the reduction of insulin concentration was observed. Moreover, treatment with the combination of both drugs increased liver glycogen content, suggesting a significant improvement in liver insulin sensitivity. Thus, the additional increase in body insulin sensitivity is a benefit of treatment with this combination. These changes may be explained by an increase in the expression of glucose metabolism genes, such as Glut-1, HK-2 and, in particular, GLUT 4. Furthermore, treatment with mildronate or metformin alone did not significantly change the weight gain of obese Zucker rats. In contrast to monotherapy, treatment with the combination of mildronate and metformin induced a significant reduction in weight gain and especially fat mass, which was decreased by 47% in combination-treated rats. Thus, the combination therapy of mildronate with metformin could have a potential therapeutic value in the treatment of obese patients with type 2 diabetes. Additionally, one of the well-known side effects of metformin is related to an increased lactate level. In this study, mildronate treatment separately or in combination with metformin reduced the lactate concentration in obese Zucker rat plasma, and therefore, mildronate used in combination could reduce the risk of metformin-induced lactate acidosis.

4.4 Diabetes complications

Mildronate treatment induces protective effects not only in the heart but also in other tissues. Vilskersts et al. demonstrated that chronic treatment with mildronate at a dose of 100 mg/kg significantly reduced the size of atherosclerotic plaques in the aortic roots and in the whole aorta in apoE/LDLR(-/-) mice (Vilskersts et al., 2009b). The effect of long-term treatment with mildronate on the functional manifestation of metabolic disturbances and diabetes-induced complications in diabetic animals was also studied (Liepinsh et al., 2009b). The contractile responsiveness to phenylephrine was significantly enhanced in the aortas of GK rats, and this hypersensitivity was normalised by mildronate at a dose of 200 mg/kg. The functional impairment of coronary arteries characterised by significantly lower coronary flow was observed in isolated GK rat hearts compared to those of Wistar rats.

After treatment by mildronate, coronary flow was significantly increased, indicating that long-term treatment with mildronate prevents endothelial dysfunction in animals with type 2 diabetes.

Peripheral neuropathy characterised by abnormality in the thermal pain threshold of diabetic GK rats was associated with the development of diabetes (Ueta et al., 2005). The loss of thermal response is dependent on the severity and duration of hyperglycaemia and is also a characteristic diabetic complication in the clinic. Long-term mildronate administration both controlled hyperglycaemia and prevented diabetic neuropathy. It is very likely that by influencing energy metabolism, mildronate reduces neuropathy in type 2 diabetes animals.

An open randomised trial in diabetic patients investigated 70 matched patients with type 2 diabetes mellitus and sensomotor neuropathy; the effectiveness of mildronate was evaluated for 3 months in addition to basic therapy (Statsenko et al., 2008). Mildronate administration did not influence glucose and Hb1Ac concentration, but it significantly improved the clinical condition of the study group patients vs. the controls by neuropathy and symptoms count scales, electrophysiological properties of the nerve fibres and optimisation of oxygen tissue balance. Overall, mildronate is suggested for the treatment of diabetes at a dose of 1 g/day as an addition to standard therapy.

5. Conclusion

In conclusion, a mildronate-induced decrease in L-carnitine concentration leads to a partial reduction in FA oxidation and shifts energy metabolism from free FA towards predominantly glucose utilisation by the myocardium to increase the effectiveness of ATP generation. Long-term pharmacologically decreased availability of L-carnitine induces adaptive effects by causing changes in FA and glucose metabolism-related gene expression, which are beneficial in the treatment of heart diseases and diabetes. The L-carnitine homeostasis is a valuable target for the regulation of energy metabolism pathways and treatment of metabolic diseases.

6. Acknowledgment

This work was supported by the EFSD grant program New Horizons Collaborative Research Initiative and the ERDF grant Nr. 2DP/2.1.1.1.0/10/APIA/VIAA/063.

7. References

Anderson, R.C., Balestra, M., Bell, P.A., Deems, R.O., Fillers, W.S., Foley, J.E., Fraser, J.D., Mann, W.R., Rudin, M., & Villhauer, E.B. (1995). Antidiabetic agents: a new class of reversible carnitine palmitoyltransferase I inhibitors. *J Med Chem,* Vol.38, No.18, pp. 3448-3450

Angelini, C., Federico, A., Reichmann, H., Lombes, A., Chinnery, P., & Turnbull, D. (2006). Task force guidelines handbook: EFNS guidelines on diagnosis and management of fatty acid mitochondrial disorders. *Eur J Neurol,* Vol.13, No.9, pp. 923-929

Asaka, N., Muranaka, Y., Kirimoto, T., & Miyake, H. (1998). Cardioprotective profile of MET-88, an inhibitor of carnitine synthesis, and insulin during hypoxia in isolated perfused rat hearts. *Fundam Clin Pharmacol,* Vol.12, No.2, pp. 158-63

Benecke, H., Flier, J.S., Rosenthal, N., Siddle, K., Klein, H.H., & Moller, D.E. (1993). Muscle-specific expression of human insulin receptor in transgenic mice. *Diabetes,* Vol.42, No.1, pp. 206-212

Bieber, L.L. (1988). Carnitine. *Annu Rev Biochem,* Vol.57, pp. 261-83

Bremer, J. (1983). Carnitine--metabolism and functions. *Physiol Rev,* Vol.63, No.4, pp. 1420-1480

Broderick, T.L. (2006). Hypocarnitinaemia induced by sodium pivalate in the rat is associated with left ventricular dysfunction and impaired energy metabolism. *Drugs R D,* Vol.7, No.3, pp. 153-161

Capaldo, B., Napoli, R., Di, B.P., Albano, G., & Sacca, L. (1991). Carnitine improves peripheral glucose disposal in non-insulin-dependent diabetic patients. *Diabetes Res Clin Pract,* Vol.14, No.3, pp. 191-195

Cederblad, G. (1976). Plasma carnitine and body composition. *Clin Chim Acta,* Vol.67, No.2, pp. 207-212

Conti, R., Mannucci, E., Pessotto, P., Tassoni, E., Carminati, P., Giannessi, F., & Arduini, A. (2011). Selective reversible inhibition of liver carnitine palmitoyl-transferase 1 by teglicar reduces gluconeogenesis and improves glucose homeostasis. *Diabetes,* Vol.60, No.2, pp. 644-651

Cui, J., Das, D.K., Bertelli, A., & Tosaki, A. (2003). Effects of L-carnitine and its derivatives on postischemic cardiac function, ventricular fibrillation and necrotic and apoptotic cardiomyocyte death in isolated rat hearts. *Mol Cell Biochem,* Vol.254, No.1-2, pp. 227-234

Cuthbert, K.D. & Dyck, J.R. (2005). Malonyl-CoA decarboxylase is a major regulator of myocardial fatty acid oxidation. *Curr Hypertens Rep,* Vol.7, No.6, pp. 407-411

Dambrova, M., Chlopicki, S., Liepinsh, E., Kirjanova, O., Gorshkova, O., Kozlovski, V.I., Uhlen, S., Liepina, I., Petrovska, R., & Kalvinsh, I. (2004). The methylester of gamma-butyrobetaine, but not gamma-butyrobetaine itself, induces muscarinic receptor-dependent vasodilatation. *Naunyn Schmiedebergs Arch Pharmacol,* Vol.369, No.5, pp. 533-539

Dambrova, M., Liepinsh, E., & Kalvinsh, I. (2002). Mildronate: cardioprotective action through carnitine-lowering effect. *Trends Cardiovasc Med,* Vol.12, No.6, pp. 275-279

De, G.A., Mingrone, G., Castagneto, M., & Calvani, M. (1999). Carnitine increases glucose disposal in humans. *J Am Coll Nutr,* Vol.18, No.4, pp. 289-295

Degrace, P., Demizieux, L., Du, Z.Y., Gresti, J., Caverot, L., Djaouti, L., Jourdan, T., Moindrot, B., Guilland, J.C., Hocquette, J.F., & Clouet, P. (2007). Regulation of lipid flux between liver and adipose tissue during transient hepatic steatosis in carnitine-depleted rats. *J Biol Chem,* Vol.282, No.29, pp. 20816-20826

Delanghe, J., De Slypere, J.P., De, B.M., Robbrecht, J., Wieme, R., & Vermeulen, A. (1989). Normal reference values for creatine, creatinine, and carnitine are lower in vegetarians. *Clin Chem,* Vol.35, No.8, pp. 1802-1803

Diaz, R., Lorita, J., Soley, M., & Ramirez, I. (2008). Carnitine worsens both injury and recovery of contractile function after transient ischemia in perfused rat heart. *J Physiol Biochem,* Vol.64, No.1, pp. 1-8

Dzerve, V., Matisone, D., Pozdnyakov, Y., & Oganov, R. (2010). Mildronate improves the exercise tolerance in patients with stable angina: results of a long term clinical trial. *Seminars in Cardiovascular Medicine,* Vol.16, No.3, pp. 1-8

Evans, A.M. & Fornasini, G. (2003). Pharmacokinetics of L-carnitine. *Clin Pharmacokinet,* Vol.42, No.11, pp. 941-967

Ferrari, R., Merli, E., Cicchitelli, G., Mele, D., Fucili, A., & Ceconi, C. (2004). Therapeutic effects of L-carnitine and propionyl-L-carnitine on cardiovascular diseases: a review. *Ann N Y Acad Sci,* Vol.1033, pp. 79-91

Fornasini, G., Upton, R.N., & Evans, A.M. (2007). A pharmacokinetic model for L-carnitine in patients receiving haemodialysis. *Br J Clin Pharmacol,* Vol.64, No.3, pp. 335-345

Foster, D.W. (2004). The role of the carnitine system in human metabolism. *Ann N Y Acad Sci,* Vol.1033, pp. 1-16

Golbidi, S., Ebadi, S.A., & Laher, I. (2011). Antioxidants in the treatment of diabetes. *Curr Diabetes Rev,* Vol.7, No.2, pp. 106-125

Gonzalez-Ortiz, M., Hernandez-Gonzalez, S.O., Hernandez-Salazar, E., & Martinez-Abundis, E. (2008). Effect of Oral L-Carnitine Administration on Insulin Sensitivity and Lipid Profile in Type 2 Diabetes Mellitus Patients. *Ann Nutr Metab,* Vol.52, No.4, pp. 335-338

Grigat, S., Fork, C., Bach, M., Golz, S., Geerts, A., Schomig, E., & Grundemann, D. (2009). The carnitine transporter SLC22A5 is not a general drug transporter, but it efficiently translocates mildronate. *Drug Metab Dispos,* Vol.37, No.2, pp. 330-337

Grimaldi, P.A. (2007). Peroxisome proliferator-activated receptors as sensors of fatty acids and derivatives. *Cell Mol Life Sci,* Vol.64, No.19-20, pp. 2459-2464

Grube, M., Meyer zu Schwabedissen, H.E., Prager, D., Haney, J., Moritz, K.U., Meissner, K., Rosskopf, D., Eckel, L., Bohm, M., Jedlitschky, G., & Kroemer, H.K. (2006). Uptake of cardiovascular drugs into the human heart: expression, regulation, and function of the carnitine transporter OCTN2 (SLC22A5). *Circulation,* Vol.113, No.8, pp. 1114-1122

Gunther, J., Wagner, K., Theres, H., Schimke, I., Born, A., Scholz, H., & Vetter, R. (2000). Myocardial contractility after infarction and carnitine palmitoyltransferase I inhibition in rats. *Eur J Pharmacol,* Vol.406, No.1, pp. 123-126

Hale, S.L. & Kloner, R.A. (2008). The antianginal agent, ranolazine, reduces myocardial infarct size but does not alter anatomic no-reflow or regional myocardial blood flow in ischemia/reperfusion in the rabbit. *J Cardiovasc Pharmacol Ther,* Vol.13, No.3, pp. 226-232

Hansen, P.A., Gulve, E.A., Marshall, B.A., Gao, J., Pessin, J.E., Holloszy, J.O., & Mueckler, M. (1995). Skeletal muscle glucose transport and metabolism are enhanced in transgenic mice overexpressing the Glut4 glucose transporter. *J Biol Chem,* Vol.270, No.4, pp. 1679-1684

Hathcock, J.N. & Shao, A. (2006). Risk assessment for carnitine. *Regul Toxicol Pharmacol,* Vol.46, No.1, pp. 23-28

Hayashi, Y., Ishida, H., Hoshiai, M., Hoshiai, K., Kirimoto, T., Kanno, T., Nakano, M., Tajima, K., Miyake, H., Matsuura, N., & Nakazawa, H. (2000a). MET-88, a gamma-butyrobetaine hydroxylase inhibitor, improves cardiac SR Ca2+ uptake activity in rats with congestive heart failure following myocardial infarction. *Mol Cell Biochem,* Vol.209, No.1-2, pp. 39-46

Hayashi, Y., Kirimoto, T., Asaka, N., Nakano, M., Tajima, K., Miyake, H., & Matsuura, N. (2000b). Beneficial effects of MET-88, a gamma-butyrobetaine hydroxylase inhibitor in rats with heart failure following myocardial infarction. *Eur J Pharmacol,* Vol.395, No.3, pp. 217-224

Jonassen, A.K., Sack, M.N., Mjos, O.D., & Yellon, D.M. (2001). Myocardial protection by insulin at reperfusion requires early administration and is mediated via Akt and p70s6 kinase cell-survival signaling. *Circ Res,* Vol.89, No.12, pp. 1191-1198

Kamalesh, M. (2007). Heart failure in diabetes and related conditions. *J Card Fail,* Vol.13, No.10, pp. 861-873

Kelley, D.E., He, J., Menshikova, E.V., & Ritov, V.B. (2002). Dysfunction of mitochondria in human skeletal muscle in type 2 diabetes. *Diabetes,* Vol.51, No.10, pp. 2944-2950

Kirimoto, T., Nobori, K., Asaka, N., Muranaka, Y., Tajima, K., & Miyake, H. (1996). Beneficial effect of MET-88, a gamma-butyrobetaine hydroxylase inhibitor, on energy metabolism in ischemic dog hearts. *Arch Int Pharmacodyn Ther,* Vol.331, No.2, pp. 163-178

Koves, T.R., Ussher, J.R., Noland, R.C., Slentz, D., Mosedale, M., Ilkayeva, O., Bain, J., Stevens, R., Dyck, J.R., Newgard, C.B., Lopaschuk, G.D., & Muoio, D.M. (2008a). Mitochondrial overload and incomplete fatty acid oxidation contribute to skeletal muscle insulin resistance. *Cell Metab,* Vol.7, No.1, pp. 45-56

Kuhajda, F.P. & Ronnett, G.V. (2007). Modulation of carnitine palmitoyltransferase-1 for the treatment of obesity. *Curr Opin Investig Drugs,* Vol.8, No.4, pp. 312-317

Kuka, J. Vilskersts, R., Cirule, H., Makrecka, M,. Pugovics, O., Kalvinsh, I., Dambrova, M,. Liepinsh, E. (2011). The cardioprotective effect of mildronate is diminished after co-treatment with L-carnitine. *J Cardiovasc Pharmacol Ther,* in press.

Kuwajima, M., Fujihara, H., Sei, H., Umehara, A., Sei, M., Tsuda, T.T., Sukeno, A., Okamoto, T., Inubushi, A., Ueta, Y., Doi, T., & Kido, H. (2007). Reduced carnitine level causes death from hypoglycemia: possible involvement of suppression of hypothalamic orexin expression during weaning period. *Endocr J,* Vol.54, No.6, pp. 911-925

Kuwajima, M., Harashima, H., Hayashi, M., Ise, S., Sei, M., Lu, K., Kiwada, H., Sugiyama, Y., & Shima, K. (1999). Pharmacokinetic analysis of the cardioprotective effect of 3-(2,2, 2-trimethylhydrazinium) propionate in mice: inhibition of carnitine transport in kidney. *J Pharmacol Exp Ther,* Vol.289, No.1, pp. 93-102

Larsen, T.S. & Aasum, E. (2008). Metabolic (in)flexibility of the diabetic heart. *Cardiovasc Drugs Ther,* Vol.22, No.2, pp. 91-95

Lheureux, P.E., Penaloza, A., Zahir, S., & Gris, M. (2005). Science review: carnitine in the treatment of valproic acid-induced toxicity - what is the evidence? *Crit Care,* Vol.9, No.5, pp. 431-440

Liepinsh, E., Konrade, I., Skapare, E., Pugovics, O., Grinberga, S., Kuka, J., Kalvinsh, I., Dambrova, M. (2011a). Mildronate treatment alters γ-butyrobetaine and l-carnitine concentrations in healthy volunteers. *J Pharm and Pharmacol,* in press.

Liepinsh, E., Kuka, J., Svalbe, B., Vilskersts, R., Skapare, E., Cirule, H., Pugovics, O., Kalvinsh, I., & Dambrova, M. (2009a). Effects of long-term mildronate treatment on cardiac and liver functions in rats. *Basic Clin Pharmacol Toxicol,* Vol.105, No.6, pp. 387-394

Liepinsh, E., Skapare, E., Svalbe, B., Makrecka, M., Cirule, H., & Dambrova, M. (2011b). Anti-diabetic effects of mildronate alone or in combination with metformin in obese Zucker rats. *Eur J Pharmacol,* Vol.658, No.2-3, pp. 277-283

Liepinsh, E., Vilskersts, R., Loca, D., Kirjanova, O., Pugovichs, O., Kalvinsh, I., & Dambrova, M. (2006). Mildronate, an inhibitor of carnitine biosynthesis, induces an increase in gamma-butyrobetaine contents and cardioprotection in isolated rat heart infarction. *J Cardiovasc Pharmacol,* Vol.48, No.6, pp. 314-319

Liepinsh, E., Vilskersts, R., Skapare, E., Svalbe, B., Kuka, J., Cirule, H., Pugovics, O., Kalvinsh, I., & Dambrova, M. (2008). Mildronate decreases carnitine availability and up-regulates glucose uptake and related gene expression in the mouse heart. *Life Sci,* Vol.83, No.17-18, pp. 613-619

Liepinsh, E., Vilskersts, R., Zvejniece, L., Svalbe, B., Skapare, E., Kuka, J., Cirule, H., Grinberga, S., Kalvinsh, I., & Dambrova, M. (2009b). Protective effects of mildronate in an experimental model of type 2 diabetes in Goto-Kakizaki rats. *Br J Pharmacol,* Vol.157, No.8, pp. 1549-1556

Long, C.S., Haller, R.G., Foster, D.W., & McGarry, J.D. (1982). Kinetics of carnitine-dependent fatty acid oxidation: implications for human carnitine deficiency. *Neurology,* Vol.32, No.6, pp. 663-666

Longo, N., Amat di San Filippo, C., & Pasquali, M. (2006). Disorders of carnitine transport and the carnitine cycle. *Am J Med Genet C Semin Med Genet,* Vol.142C, No.2, pp. 77-85

Lopaschuk, G.D. (2001). Optimizing cardiac energy metabolism: how can fatty acid and carbohydrate metabolism be manipulated? *Coron Artery Dis,* Vol.12 Suppl 1, pp. S8-11

Malone, J.I., Cuthbertson, D.D., Malone, M.A., & Schocken, D.D. (2006). Cardio-protective effects of carnitine in streptozotocin-induced diabetic rats. *Cardiovasc Diabetol,* Vol.5, pp. 2-

Malone, J.I., Schocken, D.D., Morrison, A.D., & Gilbert-Barness, E. (1999). Diabetic cardiomyopathy and carnitine deficiency. *J Diabetes Complications,* Vol.13, No.2, pp. 86-90

McGarry, J.D., Mills, S.E., Long, C.S., & Foster, D.W. (1983). Observations on the affinity for carnitine, and malonyl-CoA sensitivity, of carnitine palmitoyltransferase I in animal and human tissues. Demonstration of the presence of malonyl-CoA in non-hepatic tissues of the rat. *Biochem J,* Vol.214, No.1, pp. 21-28

Mingrone, G. (2004). Carnitine in type 2 diabetes. *Ann N Y Acad Sci,* Vol.1033, pp. 99-107

Monti, L.D., Setola, E., Fragasso, G., Camisasca, R.P., Lucotti, P., Galluccio, E., Origgi, A., Margonato, A., & Piatti, P. (2006). Metabolic and endothelial effects of trimetazidine on forearm skeletal muscle in patients with type 2 diabetes and ischemic cardiomyopathy. *Am J Physiol Endocrinol Metab,* Vol.290, No.1, pp. E54-E59

Morrow, D.A., Scirica, B.M., Chaitman, B.R., McGuire, D.K., Murphy, S.A., Karwatowska-Prokopczuk, E., McCabe, C.H., & Braunwald, E. (2009). Evaluation of the glycometabolic effects of ranolazine in patients with and without diabetes mellitus in the MERLIN-TIMI 36 randomized controlled trial. *Circulation,* Vol.119, No.15, pp. 2032-2039

Mouquet, F., Rousseau, D., Domergue-Dupont, V., Grynberg, A., & Liao, R. (2010). Effects of trimetazidine, a partial inhibitor of fatty acid oxidation, on ventricular function and survival after myocardial infarction and reperfusion in the rat. *Fundam Clin Pharmacol,* Vol.24, No.4, pp. 469-476

Nakano, M., Kirimoto, T., Asaka, N., Hayashi, Y., Kanno, T., Miyake, H., & Matsuura, N. (1999). Beneficial effects of MET-88 on left ventricular dysfunction and hypertrophy with volume overload in rats. *Fundam Clin Pharmacol,* Vol.13, No.5, pp. 521-526

Petersen, K.F., Dufour, S., Befroy, D., Garcia, R., & Shulman, G.I. (2004). Impaired mitochondrial activity in the insulin-resistant offspring of patients with type 2 diabetes. *N Engl J Med,* Vol.350, No.7, pp. 664-671

Poorabbas, A., Fallah, F., Bagdadchi, J., Mahdavi, R., Aliasgarzadeh, A., Asadi, Y., Koushavar, H., & Vahed, J.M. (2007). Determination of free L-carnitine levels in type II diabetic women with and without complications. *Eur J Clin Nutr,* Vol.61, No.7, pp. 892-895

Power, R.A., Hulver, M.W., Zhang, J.Y., Dubois, J., Marchand, R.M., Ilkayeva, O., Muoio, D.M., & Mynatt, R.L. (2007). Carnitine revisited: potential use as adjunctive treatment in diabetes. *Diabetologia,* Vol.50, No.4, pp. 824-832

Ramsay, R.R., Gandour, R.D., & van der Leij, F.R. (2001). Molecular enzymology of carnitine transfer and transport. *Biochim Biophys Acta,* Vol.1546, No.1, pp. 21-43

Rebouche, C.J. (2004). Kinetics, pharmacokinetics, and regulation of L-carnitine and acetyl-L-carnitine metabolism. *Ann N Y Acad Sci,* Vol.1033, pp. 30-41

Rufer, A.C., Thoma, R., & Hennig, M. (2009). Structural insight into function and regulation of carnitine palmitoyltransferase. *Cell Mol Life Sci,* Vol.66, No.15, pp. 2489-2501

Saper, R.B., Eisenberg, D.M., & Phillips, R.S. (2004). Common dietary supplements for weight loss. *Am Fam Physician,* Vol.70, No.9, pp. 1731-1738

Schofield, R.S. & Hill, J.A. (2001). Role of metabolically active drugs in the management of ischemic heart disease. *Am J Cardiovasc Drugs,* Vol.1, No.1, pp. 23-35

Sena, C.M., Nunes, E., Louro, T., Proenca, T., Fernandes, R., Boarder, M.R., & Seica, R.M. (2008). Effects of alpha-lipoic acid on endothelial function in aged diabetic and high-fat fed rats. *Br J Pharmacol,* Vol.153, No.5, pp. 894-906

Sesti, C., Simkhovich, B.Z., Kalvinsh, I., & Kloner, R.A. (2006). Mildronate, a novel fatty acid oxidation inhibitor and antianginal agent, reduces myocardial infarct size without affecting hemodynamics. *J Cardiovasc Pharmacol,* Vol.47, No.3, pp. 493-499

Simkhovich, B.Z., Shutenko, Z.V., Meirena, D.V., Khagi, K.B., Mezapuke, R.J., Molodchina, T.N., Kalvins, I.J., & Lukevics, E. (1988). 3-(2,2,2-Trimethylhydrazinium)propionate (THP)--a novel gamma-butyrobetaine hydroxylase inhibitor with cardioprotective properties. *Biochem Pharmacol,* Vol.37, No.2, pp. 195-202

Sokolovska, J., Isajevs, S., Sugoka, O., Sharipova, J., Lauberte, L., Svirina, D., Rostoka, E., Sjakste, T., Kalvinsh, I., & Sjakste, N. (2011). Correction of glycaemia and GLUT1 level by mildronate in rat streptozotocin diabetes mellitus model. *Cell Biochem Funct,* Vol.29, No.1, pp. 55-63

Statsenko, M.E., Belenkova, S.V., Sporova, O.E., & Shilina, N.N. (2007). [The use of mildronate in combined therapy of postinfarction chronic heart failure in patients with type 2 diabetes mellitus]. *Klin Med (Mosk),* Vol.85, No.7, pp. 39-42

Statsenko, M.E., Poletaeva, L.V., Turkina, S.V., Inozemtseva, M.A., & Apukhtin, A.F. (2008). [Clinical efficiency of milrdonate in combined treatment of peripheral diabetic (sensory-motor) neuropathy]. *Klin Med (Mosk),* Vol.86, No.9, pp. 67-71

Stephens, F.B., Constantin-Teodosiu, D., & Greenhaff, P.L. (2007). New insights concerning the role of carnitine in the regulation of fuel metabolism in skeletal muscle. *J Physiol,* Vol.581, No.Pt 2, pp. 431-444

Sugden, M.C., Zariwala, M.G., & Holness, M.J. (2009). PPARs and the orchestration of metabolic fuel selection. *Pharmacol Res,* Vol.60, No.3, pp. 141-150

Taegtmeyer, H., King, L.M., & Jones, B.E. (1998). Energy substrate metabolism, myocardial ischemia, and targets for pharmacotherapy. *Am J Cardiol,* Vol.82, No.5A, pp. 54K-60K

Tarantini, G., Scrutinio, D., Bruzzi, P., Boni, L., Rizzon, P., & Iliceto, S. (2006). Metabolic treatment with L-carnitine in acute anterior ST segment elevation myocardial infarction. A randomized controlled trial. *Cardiology,* Vol.106, No.4, pp. 215-223

Tars, K., Rumnieks, J., Zeltins, A., Kazaks, A., Kotelovica, S., Leonciks, A., Sharipo, J., Viksna, A., Kuka, J., Liepinsh, E., & Dambrova, M. (2010). Crystal structure of human gamma-butyrobetaine hydroxylase *Biochem Biophys Res Commun,* Vol.398, No.4, pp. 634-639

Uenaka, R., Kuwajima, M., Ono, A., Matsuzawa, Y., Hayakawa, J., Inohara, N., Kagawa, Y., & Ohta, S. (1996). Increased expression of carnitine palmitoyltransferase I gene is repressed by administering L-carnitine in the hearts of carnitine-deficient juvenile visceral steatosis mice. *J Biochem,* Vol.119, No.3, pp. 533-540

Ueta, K., Ishihara, T., Matsumoto, Y., Oku, A., Nawano, M., Fujita, T., Saito, A., & Arakawa, K. (2005). Long-term treatment with the Na+-glucose cotransporter inhibitor T-1095 causes sustained improvement in hyperglycemia and prevents diabetic neuropathy in Goto-Kakizaki Rats. *Life Sci,* Vol.76, No.23, pp. 2655-2668

Uziel, G., Garavaglia, B., & Di, D.S. (1988). Carnitine stimulation of pyruvate dehydrogenase complex (PDHC) in isolated human skeletal muscle mitochondria. *Muscle Nerve,* Vol.11, No.7, pp. 720-724

Vilskersts, R., Liepinsh, E., Kuka, J., Cirule, H., Veveris, M., Kalvinsh, I., & Dambrova, M. (2009a). Myocardial infarct size-limiting and anti-arrhythmic effects of mildronate orotate in the rat heart. *Cardiovasc Drugs Ther,* Vol.23, No.4, pp. 281-288

Vilskersts, R., Liepinsh, E., Mateuszuk, L., Grinberga, S., Kalvinsh, I., Chlopicki, S., & Dambrova, M. (2009b). Mildronate, a regulator of energy metabolism, reduces atherosclerosis in apoE/LDLR-/- mice. *Pharmacology,* Vol.83, No.5, pp. 287-293

Wang, W. & Lopaschuk, G.D. (2007). Metabolic therapy for the treatment of ischemic heart disease: reality and expectations. *Expert Rev Cardiovasc Ther,* Vol.5, No.6, pp. 1123-1134

Wolf, H.P. & Brenner, K.V. (1988). The effect of etomoxir on glucose turnover and recycling with [1-14C], [3-3H]-glucose tracer in pigs. *Horm Metab Res,* Vol.20, No.4, pp. 204-207

Youngren, J.F. (2007). Regulation of insulin receptor function. *Cell Mol Life Sci,* Vol.64, No.7-8, pp. 873-891

7

Oxidative Stress in Type II Diabetes Mellitus and the Role of the Endogenous Antioxidant Glutathione

Stephney Whillier[1], Philip William Kuchel[2] and Julia Elizabeth Raftos[1]
[1]*Macquarie University,*
[2]*University of Sydney, Sydney,*
Australia

1. Introduction

Oxidative stress appears to be involved in aging and a great many diseases, including diabetes mellitus (Lang, Naryshin et al. 1992; Fletcher and Fletcher 1994; Julius, Lang et al. 1994; Richie, Skowronski et al. 1996; Nuttall, Martin et al. 1998; Lang, Mills et al. 2000; Erden-Inal, Sunal et al. 2002; Junqueira, Barros et al. 2004; Gil, Siems et al. 2006). 'Oxidative stress' is a term that was introduced by Sies in 1985 and refers to any situation where there is a serious imbalance between the production of free radicals (FR) or reactive oxygen species (ROS), called the oxidative load, and the antioxidant defense system. The oxidative load is described as "a measure of the steady-state level of reactive oxygen or oxygen radicals in a biological system" (Baynes 1991). Oxidative stress has been defined as "a disturbance in the pro-oxidant-antioxidant balance in favour of the former, leading to potential damage" (Sies 1985). Because it is hard to measure oxidative stress directly, it is inferred from the accumulation of oxidation products, such as plasma $O_2^{\bullet-}$ radicals or high levels of peroxidation products such as thiobarbituric acid-reactive substances (TBARS) in plasma (Dominguez, Ruiz et al. 1998).

Cells can tolerate moderate oxidative loads by increasing gene expression to up-regulate their reductive defense systems and restore the oxidant/antioxidant balance. But when this increased synthesis cannot be achieved due to damage to enzymes, or substrate limitations, or when the oxidative load is overwhelming, an imbalance persists and the result is oxidative stress. Persisting imbalance leads to damage to DNA, proteins and lipids, and cell death. Oxidative stress has been implicated in over 100 diseases, more as a consequence of the pathology than as the causative factor (Halliwell 2005).

Glutathione, the tripeptide γ-L-glutamyl-L-cysteinyl-glycine (GSH), is an antioxidant molecule synthesised in almost all living cells from prokaryote organisms to the eukaryote kingdoms (Griffith and Mulcahy 1999). Glutathione is able to protect cells from oxidation by virtue of the reducing power of the thiol group on the cysteine portion of the molecule. Normally ~98% of the total GSH in healthy human cells exists in the reduced form (Griffith 1981; Kennett, Bubb et al. 2005). When GSH is oxidised to glutathione disulphide (GSSG), the enzyme GSH reductase (GR; EC 1.6.4.2) rapidly reduces it back to GSH using NADPH as an electron donor, thus ensuring that the cycling of ROS does not alter the GSH to GSSG concentration ratio of ≥ 100 (Griffith 1999; Griffith and Mulcahy 1999). It is only when the oxidative load on the cell reaches the high levels usually associated with a variety of disease states, that a shift in this redox buffer can occur, and can result in oxidative damage to cellular constituents and the especially vulnerable plasma membrane (Kennett and Kuchel 2006).

The red blood cell (RBC) is susceptible to oxidative damage through its role as the main oxygen transporting cell, and is protected from a constant flux of reactive oxygen metabolites. Glutathione is the main source of RBC antioxidant protection and its redox status is often used as a measure of oxidative stress (Kennett and Kuchel 2006). In addition, RBC GSH has far reaching effects in being the largest mobile antioxidant pool, detoxifier and chemokine scavenger in the body (Keenoy, Vertommen et al. 2001; Sailaja, Baskar et al. 2003). Its membrane is permeable to $O_2^{\bullet-}$ and H_2O_2 (via the band 3 transporter, also called capnophorin) and so the RBC scavenges these ROS and protects cells and tissues of the body (Aoshiba, Nakajima et al. 1999).

A consistent finding in type II diabetes mellitus (non-insulin dependent diabetes mellitus, NIDDM) is a high FR load, which is associated with the hyperglycemia. The elevated glucose binds to proteins, glycating them, and leads to the formation of advanced glycation end products (AGEs) and many FRs (Keenoy, Vertommen et al. 2001). Advanced glycation end products are associated with tissue damage and aging (Sullivan 1996; Wautier and Schmidt 2004). The glycation of proteins in diabetes increases the rate of FR production by nearly 50-fold, and the generated FRs were found to increase peroxidation of polyunsaturated fatty acids (PUFAs) in the cell membrane nearly 2-fold over control levels (Mullarkey, Edelstein et al. 1990).

The less well the diabetes is controlled, i.e., the higher the blood glucose concentration, the more likely is the formation of glycated proteins. Glycated haemoglobin (HbA_{1c}), an Amadori product, is routinely measured in NIDDM, because once formed, it remains for the lifetime of the RBC (120 days), and therefore acts as a reliable monitor of blood glucose control over 4 months. Glycation of haemoglobin of under 6% is normal, but in NIDDM it can be measured in the teens. HbA_{1c} is more negatively charged than haemoglobin and has a higher oxygen affinity, therefore reducing gaseous exchange at the tissues (Arese and Schwarzer 2003).

A decrease in GSH concentration in the RBCs of NIDDM patients is widely reported, and this depletion of GSH is considered to be indicative of increased oxidative stress (Bono, Caimi.G et al. 1986; Tho, Candlish et al. 1988; Murakami, K. et al. 1989; Jain and McVie 1994; Yoshida, Hirokawa et al. 1995; Vijayalingam, Parthiban et al. 1996; Lang, Mills et al. 2000; Dincer, Akcay et al. 2002; Arese and Schwarzer 2003; Beard, Shangari et al. 2003; Martin-Gallan, Carrascosa et al. 2003; Sailaja, Baskar et al. 2003; Darmaun, Smith et al. 2005; Sampathkumar, Balasubramanyam et al. 2005). However, many authors report unchanged or elevated GSH concentrations in the RBCs of NIDDM patients (Caren and Carne 1951; Matsubara, Ferreira et al. 1992; Sinclair, Girling et al. 1992; Di Simplicio, De Giorgio et al. 1995; Laaksonen, Atalay et al. 1996; Thornalley, McLellan et al. 1996; Atalay, Laaksonen et al. 1997; Straface, Rivabene et al. 2002; Nwose, Jelinek et al. 2006; Ozkilic, Cengiz et al. 2006). Reported concentrations depend upon the form of glutathione measured (oxidised, reduced, total free, protein-bound), the analytic methods used, whether the subjects have been receiving treatment, and the particular drugs used in treating the disease (Yoshida, Hirokawa et al. 1995; Bravi, Armiento et al. 2006). Compounding this is the wide range of GSH concentrations in the healthy population, and subjects who vary in age and extent of pathology (Richie, Skowronski et al. 1996; Lang, Mills et al. 2000).

In this chapter we explored the nature of the FR, what GSH is and how it works to neutralise FRs, and how FR and AGE induced damage is implicated in the pathogenesis and complications of NIDDM. We explore the literature on the purported levels of GSH in patients with NIDDM, and finally we discuss the research done by the authors on the concentration of GSH and the rate of synthesis of GSH in a group of patients with NIDDM, compared to a group of healthy controls.

2. The nature of Free Radicals (FRs)

A FR is any species that is capable of an independent existence and is reactive because it contains at least one unpaired electron in its outer atomic orbital. The lone hydrogen atom is reactive because it has one unpaired electron. When the unpaired electron (denoted by •) resides on an oxygen atom it is called an oxygen-centred radical, and examples are the superoxide ($O_2{\bullet}^-$) and hydroxyl (OH•) radicals (Halliwell 2005). ROS are both oxygen-centred FRs as well as nonradical derivatives (e.g. H_2O_2). Radicals can react with each other to form nonradical derivatives that are often more damaging than the parent radicals (Halliwell 2005). For example $O_2{\bullet}^-$ and nitric oxide (NO•) can form the nonradical derivative peroxynitrite ($ONOO^-$). When FRs react with nonradicals, a chain reaction of FR formation can develop. One example is the reaction between OH• and a fatty acid that produces a chain reaction of lipid peroxidation. Some FRs are beneficial to a cell; e.g. $O_2{\bullet}^-$ produced by phagocytes kills bacteria and endothelial derived NO• has a vasodilatory function and is also produced by macrophages to kill invading microbes.

When a FR or ROS reacts with another atom or molecule, it captures one or more electrons. The FR or ROS is the electron acceptor because it will pair up its own unpaired electrons as a result of this reaction. The removal of an electron from an atom is a process called 'oxidation', thus FRs or ROS act as oxidising agents. In its broadest sense, oxidation occurs in an atom or molecule when it is involved in a reaction that increases its oxidation number; this can result from the loss of an electron or a hydrogen atom, or the addition of an oxygen atom, or it can be viewed as the relative increase in the proportion of oxygen in a molecule due to the loss of other atoms. The FR or ROS, having gained an electron is said to be reduced, and its oxidation number is decreased as a result of this reaction. Oxidation of one molecule is always accompanied by the reduction of another molecule, and so these interactions are called reduction-oxidation (redox) reactions (Hill and Kolb 2001) .

The activity of cellular antioxidants should be in balance with the oxidative load. The body has a number of antioxidant defenses that prevent the damaging effects of oxidation caused by FRs or ROS. An antioxidant is any substance, present usually in low concentrations compared to the oxidising agent, that significantly delays or prevents oxidation of other molecules by acting as a reducing agent. The most important antioxidants found in the cell are superoxide dismutase (SOD) (EC 1.15.1.1); catalase (EC 1.11.1.6); thioredoxin reductase (EC 1.8.1.9); vitamins C; vitamin E; glutathione (GSH), glutathione -*S*-transferase (GST; EC 2.5.1.18) and glutathione peroxidase (GPx; EC 1.11.1.9) (Halliwell 2005).

3. What is GSH and how does it neutralise FRs?

As noted above, GSH is synthesised in almost all living cells from prokaryote organisms to the eukaryote kingdoms (Griffith and Mulcahy 1999), which emphasises both its ancient origin and its persistent cell-protective function (see Figure 1). GSH plays a major role in defending the cell against oxidative and nitrosative damage by reacting with ROS; and the GSH in red blood cells (RBCs) has even been proposed as an indicator of health status although concentrations have been shown to vary almost two fold even among healthy individuals (Richie, Abraham et al. 1996).

The highest concentrations of GSH in mammals are found in the liver, spleen, kidneys, pancreas, and the lens of the eye. The liver is the main site of GSH production in the body where it remains largely localised, and has the highest concentration (~10 mM) (Burk and Hill 1995), while in plasma the concentration is only ~0.90 μM (Chawla, Lewis et al. 1984; Beutler and Gelbart 1985; Yang, Chou et al. 1995). Glutathione is a major metabolite of the human RBC (Lunn, Dale et al. 1979), and has a steady-state concentration of ~2 mmol (L RBC) $^{-1}$ (~3 mM in the free water space) (Raftos, Dwarte et al. 2006). Recent evidence indicates that the RBC can export GSH at a rate of up to ~0.35 μmol (L RBC)$^{-1}$ min^{-1} and thus contribute to the extracellular GSH pool (Giustarini, Dalle-Donne et al. 2008). It is hypothesised that the rate of *de novo* synthesis of GSH in healthy RBCs balances the rate of efflux of GSH, oxidised glutathione (GSSG) and GSH-conjugates (Srivastava and Beutler 1969; Srivastava, Awasthi et al. 1976; Lunn, Dale et al. 1979; Griffith 1999), and has a turnover of 4 - 6 days (Lunn, Dale et al. 1979; Griffith 1981). There is no known mechanism for the breakdown of GSH inside the RBC, as the enzyme γ-glutamyl transpeptidase (GGTP; EC 2.3.2.2), which cleaves the γ bond in GSH in many cells of the body, is absent in the RBC (Board and Smith 1977).

Glutathione is synthesised from three amino acids: glutamate, cysteine and glycine. The synthesis of GSH was first demonstrated in extracts of pigeon liver and yeast, by Snoke and Bloch (1954) and was shown to be a process requiring two enzymes (see Figure 2) (Snoke, Yanari et al. 1953; Snoke and Bloch 1954; Snoke 1955).The condensation of glutamate and cysteine requires γ-L-glutamyl-L- cysteine synthetase now more commonly called γ-L-glutamate-L-cysteine ligase (GCL;). Addition of glycine is by glutathione synthetase (GS). γ -L-Glutamate-L-cysteine ligase is the main flux controlling enzyme, and is inhibited by GSH with a K_i of 2.3 mM in the free water of the cell (1.6 mmol (L RBC) $^{-1}$) which is within the normal range of the GSH concentration in RBCs (Richman and Meister 1975). However, 5 and 10 mM GSH, greatly in excess of normal physiological concentrations, has been shown to inhibit the activity of the enzyme by only 22 and 31% respectively (Richman and Meister 1975), suggesting that the inhibitory effect of GSH under normal conditions is not the only factor controlling GSH synthesis in RBCs. The GSH inhibition appeared to be reduced by glutamate, indicating that GSH was binding to the glutamate receptor on the enzyme (Richman and Meister 1975).

Glutamate-L-cysteine ligase is a heterodimer, composed of a heavy catalytic subunit (GCLC), and a lighter modifier subunit (GCLM). The catalytic unit can support GSH production alone, but the modifier unit increases the rate of GSH production in the RBC by increasing the K_i for GSH inhibition and decreasing the K_m for glutamate utilisation. These subunits are encoded by separate genes on different chromosomes (Griffith 1999; Yang, Dieter et al. 2002; Chen, Shertzer et al. 2005), and it may be the inherited ratio of GCLC:GCLM that determines the steady state GSH concentration of an individual. In addition, polymorphisms in both the GCLC and GCLM gene promoters have been shown to be associated with variations in the expression of these subunits, their inducibility and consequent GSH concentrations, and a number of studies have identified specific polymorphisms that increase the risk of diseases including cystic fibrosis, cardiovascular disease, schizophrenia, diabetes mellitus and asthma (Franklin, Backos et al. 2008). The modifier subunit is not essential for viability, even though *gclm*(-/-) knockout mice have decreased levels of GSH that vary between different tissues, and their GSH concentration is substantially reduced in RBCs (Yang, Dieter et al. 2002). Both subunits can be up-regulated at the transcriptional level by oxidative stress, and especially by H_2O_2 and TNF-α (Yang, Dieter et al. 2002).

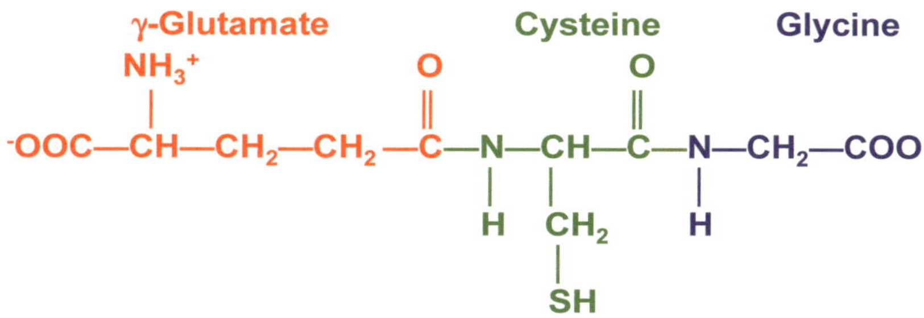

Fig. 1. **Chemical structure of GSH.** The tripeptide is composed of glutamate, cysteine and glycine residues with a γ-peptide bond between the glutamate and cysteine residues. The cysteine residue has a thiol functional group that imparts the reducing potential to the molecule.

As noted above, normally ~98% of the total GSH in healthy human cells exists in the reduced form (Griffith 1981; Kennett, Bubb et al. 2005). When GSH is oxidised to GSSG, the GR rapidly catalyses its reduction back to GSH using NADPH as an electron donor, thus ensuring that the cycling of ROS does not alter the GSH to GSSG concentration ratio of ≥ 100 (Griffith 1999; Griffith and Mulcahy 1999). It is only when the oxidative load on the cell reaches the high levels usually associated with a variety of disease states, that a shift in this redox buffer can occur, and can result in oxidative damage to cellular constituents including the especially vulnerable plasma membrane (Kennett and Kuchel 2006). A marked fall in the GSH to GSSG ratio can also act as a signal that leads to decreased cell proliferation and increased apoptosis (Schafer and Buettner 2001; Wu, Fang et al. 2004).

3.1 Free radicals and GSH in the RBC

Mammalian reticulocytes are formed in the marrow and mature into RBCs that are enucleated biconcave discs that survive for ~120 days in the circulation carrying O_2 and CO_2. Haemoglobin occupies ~33% of the RBC volume. Thus the RBC is susceptible to oxidative damage through its role as the O_2 transporter, and is protected from a constant flux of reactive O_2 metabolites. When O_2 binds to haemoglobin, iron remains in its ferrous (Fe^{2+}) form, but occasionally water or a small anion causes the transfer of an electron from the Fe^{2+} to oxygen to form methaemoglobin. Such autoxidation of haemoglobin occurs at a rate of up to 3% a day and results in the release of $O_2^{\bullet-}$ radicals (Rice-Evans and Baysal 1987; Low, Hampton et al. 2008). The release of ferric iron (Fe^{3+}) from haemoglobin leads to free radical damage by the Fenton reaction in which Fe^{3+} binding to H_2O_2 results in the formation of highly reactive $OH^{\bullet-}$ radicals. Release of Fe^{3+} can lead to oxidative changes in membrane proteins and rapid RBC aging (Burak Cimen 2008). Glutathione is the main source of RBC antioxidant protection and its redox status is often used as a measure of oxidative stress (Kennett and Kuchel 2006).

Methaemoglobin is converted back to haemoglobin by the methaemoglobin reductase system (NADH:cytochrome b_5 reductase E.C. 1.6.2.2 and cytochrome b_5: methaemoglobin reductase).

The RBC has high concentrations of SOD for the dismutation of $O_2^{\bullet-}$ to H_2O_2, making autoxidation the major source of H_2O_2 in the RBC, although H_2O_2 from extracellular sources is able to permeate RBCs, and oxidants are also generated by the interaction of xenobiotics with haemoglobin. The H_2O_2 is reduced by catalase to O_2 and H_2O, especially when concentrations of the ROS are high, and GPx, a selenium-containing enzyme, converts H_2O_2 to H_2O at lower concentrations and is the flux controlling step of GSH recycling (Low, Hampton et al. 2008). The schemes for these reactions are shown in Figure 3. Peroxide metabolism in RBCs cannot be explained by these two enzymes (catalase and GPx) alone, and kinetic modeling has shown that peroxiredoxins (Prxs), especially Prx2, which use thioredoxin as the reductant, are also important in the RBC for reducing the daily H_2O_2 load (Low, Hampton et al. 2008).

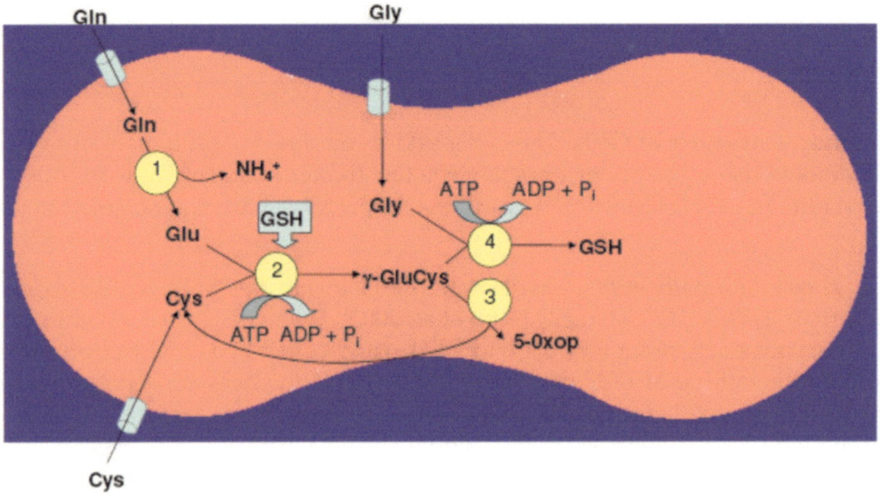

Fig. 2. **GSH synthesis in the human RBC.** The metabolite labels denote: Cys, cysteine; Gln, glutamine; Glu, glutamate; Gly, glycine; GSH, glutathione; NH_4^+, ammonium; γ-GluCys, γ-glutamylcysteine; 5-Oxop, 5-oxoproline. The enzymes are numbered as follows: (1) glutaminase (2) γ-L-glutamate-L-cysteine ligase or γ-glutamylcysteine synthetase (3) γ-glutamyl cyclotransferase (4) glutathione synthetase. (Adapted from Raftos, Whillier et al. 2007.)

Glutathione-disulphide is reduced back to GSH using GR and NADPH. The oxidative pentose phosphate pathway generates NADPH when glucose 6-phosphate is converted to 6-Phospho-glucolactone via glucose-6-phosphate dehydrogenase (G6PDH; E.C. 1.1.1.49) (Mulquiney and Kuchel 2003), and this appears to be the main role of this pathway in the RBC, as the formation of ribose 5-phosphate and the other end products of the pentose phosphate pathway are of no direct synthetic use in an enucleated cell.

The reductive activity of NADPH also competes against the oxidation of PUFAs in the membrane and retains the iron in haemoglobin (Hb) in the Fe^{2+} form (Lehninger 1984). In G6PDH deficiency, there is an increased sensitivity to H_2O_2, mainly due to low NADPH concentrations. Loss of both NADPH and GSH in this inherited condition may account for enhanced methaemoglobin formation and lipid peroxidation in the propositi (Burak Cimen 2008).

Young healthy subjects have been shown to have higher GSH and lower H_2O_2 concentrations in their RBCs than healthy elderly subjects; and both have higher GSH concentrations than elderly patients with a variety of chronic diseases (Nuttall, Martin et al. 1998). In addition, 36% of newly admitted typical hospital patients with a wide variety of chronic diseases have markedly reduced RBC total GSH concentrations compared to age-matched controls (Lang, Mills et al. 2000), which suggests that adverse changes in the redox status accompanies many chronic pathologies. There is evidence that a decrease in RBC GSH occurs in HIV, diabetes mellitus, kwashiorkor, malnutrition, magnesium-ion deficiency, alcoholic liver disease, progeria, rheumatoid arthritis, muscular dystrophy, amyotrophic lateral sclerosis, atherosclerosis, Alzheimer disease, cataractogenesis, sickle cell trait, thalassemia, and malaria (Murakami, K. et al. 1989; Sorensen, Rubin et al. 1990; Jain and McVie 1994; Becker, Leichsenring et al. 1995; Grinberg, Rachmilewitz et al. 1995; Sullivan 1996; Erden-Inal, Sunal et al. 2002; Rossi, Milzani et al. 2002).

4. How is FR and AGE damage implicated in the pathogenesis and complications of NIDDM?

Diabetes mellitus in its primary presentation is either the result of decreased pancreatic β-islet insulin production (type I or IDDM), or a resistance of cells to insulin (type II or NIDDM). The incidence of NIDDM has increased rapidly in recent years. It is estimated that the morbidities due to this illness will more than double within 15 years. Once a disease of slow-onset, appearing in middle-aged adults, it is now appearing in children (Ceriello and Motz 2004). Pathognomonic of the disease is hyperglycaemia, and this is associated with many systemic complications associated with the disease, that include pathology in the cardiovascular, neural, renal, visual and other organ systems.

A consistent finding in NIDDM is a high FR load, which is associated with hyperglycaemia. The elevated amounts of glucose lead to binding of glucose to proteins, and leads to the formation of AGEs and many FRs.

4.1 Glycation as a cause of oxidation in NIDDM

Glycation of proteins is initiated when a reducing sugar such as glucose, which in its acyclic form has an exposed aldehyde functional group, forms a double bond with the amine group of an amino acid residue (commonly lysine) in a protein (Figure 4). This is called the Maillard reaction (also called browning). The result is the formation of an imine called a Schiff base, in which the covalent bonds are rearranged to yield a ketoamine called an Amadori product. These reactions are reversible in the presence of reducing agents. Further oxidation over months results in the formation of irreversibly damaged proteins; these are the AGEs that are associated with tissue damage and aging (Sullivan 1996; Wautier and Schmidt 2004) as well as the liberation of many FRs (Keenoy, Vertommen et al. 2001). The glycation of proteins in diabetes increases the rate of FR production by nearly 50-fold; and the generated FRs increase peroxidation of PUFAs in the cell membrane nearly 2-fold over control levels (Mullarkey, Edelstein et al. 1990).

Monosaccharides become autoxidised in the presence of metal-catalysts and oxygen to yield ketoaldehydes (Wolff and Dean 1987) that then catalyse autoxidative glycosylation, in which the more reactive dicarbonyl sugars such as glucosone react with proteins to form ketoimine adducts. In turn these are more reactive than Amadori adducts and can initiate further Maillard reactions. Superoxide and H_2O_2 are formed in these autoxidation reactions (Wolff and Dean 1987). Autoxidative glycosylation therefore produces FRs, leading to damaged proteins and peroxidation of associated lipids during glycation reactions.

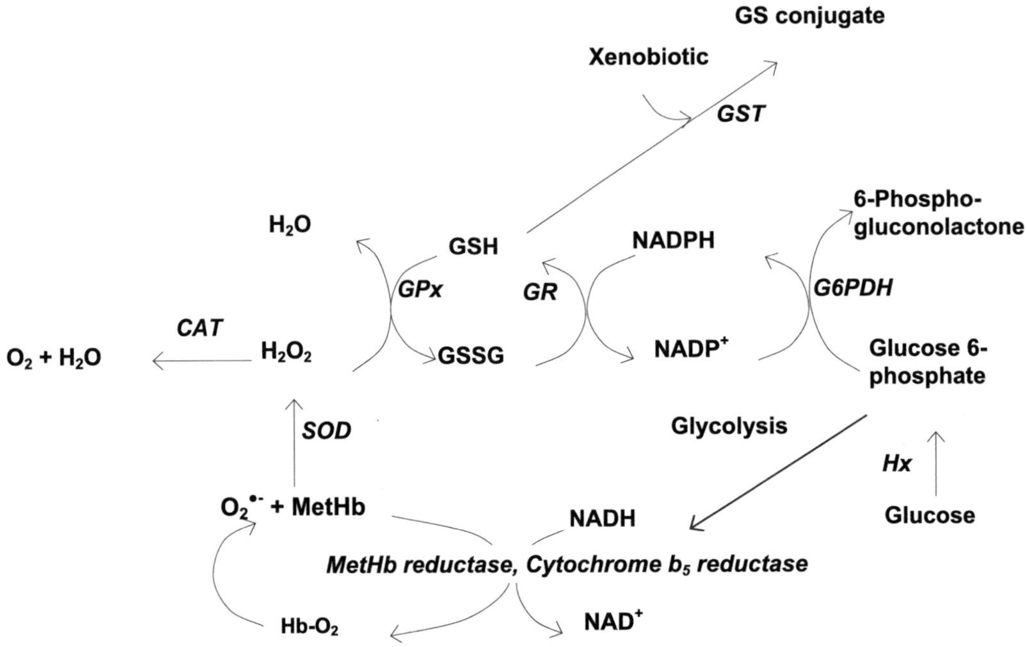

Fig. 3. **Antioxidants in the RBC.** A daily 3% formation of methaemoglobin (metHb) from oxyhaemoglobin (Hb-O_2) results in the formation $O_2^{\bullet-}$. The metHb is reduced to Hb via metHb reductase, cytochrome b_5 reductase and NADH. The $O_2^{\bullet-}$ is converted to H_2O_2 by SOD. The H_2O_2 is converted via either catalase (CAT) to $O_2 + H_2O$, or via GPx to H_2O, resulting in the formation of GSSG, which is reduced back to GSH using GSH-reductase (GR) and NADPH. The electron donors NADPH and NADH are derived from glycolysis and the oxidative pentose phosphate shunt respectively. The $NADP^+$ is reduced to NADPH via glucose-6-phosphate dehydrogenase (G6PDH) and glucose 6-phosphate formed via the phosphorylation of glucose using hexokinase (Hx). GSH conjugates xenobiotics which are pumped out of the RBC via ATP-dependent glutathione transferase transporters (Board 1981; Board 1993)

There are many molecules with a reactive aldehyde group that generate AGEs (Figure 5). They include acyclic fructose, formed from glucose via the sorbitol or polyol pathway; triose intermediates, such as glyceraldehyde 3-phosphate, formed in glycolysis; oxoaldehydes such as glyoxal and methylglyoxal formed from the autoxidation of these triose intermediates, the latter in a side reaction of triose phosphate isomerase (E.C. 5.3.1.1); and aldehydes such as hydroxynonenal (HNE) and malondialdehyde (MDA) formed from peroxidation of PUFAs (Dominguez, Ruiz et al. 1998; Dincer, Akcay et al. 2002; Arese and Schwarzer 2003; Beard, Shangari et al. 2003; Memisogullari, Taysi et al. 2003).

The increased polyol pathway flux only becomes significant in hyperglycaemia because the K_m for glucose is high (Brownlee 2001). In this pathway, aldose reductase (E.C. 1.1.1.21) converts carbonyl compounds like glucose to sorbitol by oxidising NADPH (Figure 5). Sorbitol can be oxidised to fructose, and NADH is generated in the process. An increase in the NADH: NAD ratio inhibits glyceraldehydes-3-phosphate dehydrogenase (GAPDH; 1.2.1.12), which requires NAD as a co-substrate. The enzyme has a thiol group at its active

site, so it is also inhibited by oxoaldehydes, glycating agents and oxidative radicals (Beisswenger, Howell et al. 2003). The consumption of NADPH decreases the ability of cells to regenerate GSH from GSSG, which elevates oxidative stress. Aldose reductase inhibition reduces diabetic neuropathy (Brownlee 2001).
The oxoaldehydes such as methylglyoxal, formed from glyceraldehyde 3-phosphate (see above), react spontaneously with GSH to form hemithioacetal. The glyoxylase pathway of two enzymes converts hemithioacetal to S-D-lactoylglutathione via glyoxylase I (E.C. 4.4.1.5), and then glyoxylase II (E.C. 3.1.2.6) converts this to D-lactate and thus regenerates GSH (Thornalley 1988; Rae, Berners-Price et al. 1990; Beard, Shangari et al. 2003). But if GSH concentrations are decreased, the tendency to form hemithioacetal, and flux via the glyoxylase pathway is diminished, and methylglyoxal will accumulate.
Methylglyoxal is increased threefold in NIDDM patients, despite significantly increased activity of the glyoxalase I enzyme and this was found to be associated with complications of the disease (Thornalley, McLellan et al. 1996). The oxoaldehyde glyoxal can also be produced from a slow non-enzymatic autoxidation of glucose (Abordo, Minhas et al. 1999).

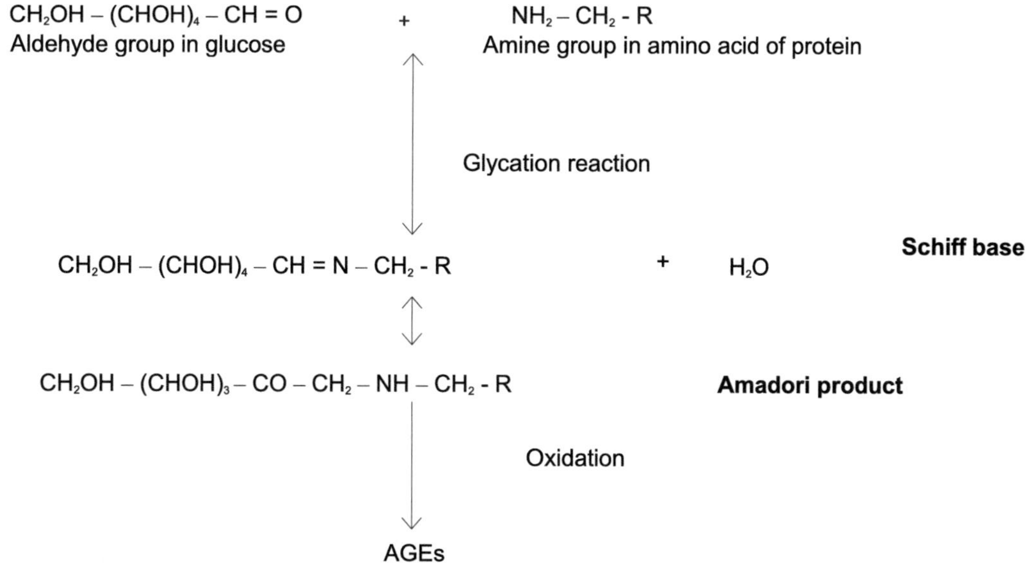

Fig. 4. **Formation of AGEs.** In the Maillard or glycation reaction, glucose forms a covalent bond with the amine group of an amino acid residue such as lysyl in a protein, resulting in the formation of an imine called a Schiff base, which has its covalent bonds rearranged into an Amadori product. Further oxidation over a time scale of months results in the formation of irreversibly damaged proteins called AGEs.

Oxidative damage to the lipids of the RBC membrane and alterations in the protein cytoskeleton result in RBC adhesion and aggregation, decreased deformability, accelerated senescence, and a reduced lifespan with increased macrophage removal (Thornalley 1988; Laaksonen, Atalay et al. 1996; Straface, Rivabene et al. 2002; Arese and Schwarzer 2003). AGEs have been identified on the RBC surface, and AGE receptors (RAGE) exist on a variety of cells, including the vascular endothelium. Binding of AGE to RAGEs on these cells leads to vascular damage and complications of cardiovascular disease (Arese and

Schwarzer 2003). This outcome is supposedly due to an inflammatory response and the generation of FRs in these cells have a disruptive effect on NO-mediated vasodilation. Superoxide in particular can directly cause vasoconstriction and decrease NO. Acute hyperglycaemia impairs endothelial cell function within 15 minutes of onset, and produces an increase in catecholamine concentrations, hence elevated mean arterial blood pressure and heart rate (Marfella, Verrazzo et al. 1995).

4.2 Oxidation in the aetiology of NIDDM

Major contributing factors to the development of NIDDM are weight gain and the deposition of excessive amounts of visceral fat (waist circumference > 94 cm in men or > 80 cm in women) (Caterson and Broom 2001). Accumulation of visceral fat is due to a reduced capacity to store excess energy subcutaneously, and is seen as a marker of 'dysfunctional adipose tissue' (Rosen and Spiegelman 2006). This fat is more lipolytic (rapidly turned over) than subcutaneous fat and less sensitive to the anti-lipolytic effect of insulin. As abdominal fat develops, the adipocytes release non-esterified fatty acids (NEFAs), many inflammatory products, and FRs (Rosen and Spiegelman 2006). Both the weight gain and inflammation are correlated with oxidative stress, which gives them an integral role in the pathogenesis as well as the complications of NIDDM.

Obesity and NIDDM are considered to be inflammatory states, and the concentration of plasma C-reactive protein, an inflammatory marker, is elevated in both conditions (Rosen and Spiegelman 2006) while macrophages are recruited to the fat deposits (Rosen and Spiegelman 2006). The potential for fat deposits to be involved in the inflammatory response may be explained by the common ontological and phylogical origin of the liver, haemopoietic and immune systems in the fat body, a structure considered to be the equivalent of mammal fat tissue. In drosophila, the fat body coordinates pathogen response with metabolic status. Specialisation occurred in the mammal, but hepatocytes are still found in close association with Kupffer cells (macrophages that are part of the immune system) with close access to blood vessels. This suggests overlapping pathways in mammals allowing for nutritionally induced inflammation (Hotamisligil 2006).

The normal physiological response to postprandial hyperglycemia is the secretion of insulin from the pancreas into the bloodstream. The hormone binds to its receptor on the cell membrane, which via its tyrosine-kinase activity initiates the phosphorylation of a tyrosine residue on an insulin receptor substrate (IRS-1). The phosphorylation stimulates a second messenger system that alters the metabolic environment in the cell, and causes the intracytoplasmic migration of vesicles that contain GLUT4 protein and their fusion into the cell's plasma membrane. GLUT4 mediates the exchange of glucose into the cell, thus rapidly lowering blood glucose concentrations to normal values within 2 h (Silverthorn 2007).

When NEFAs accumulate in cells they undergo β-oxidation, forming acetyl-CoA that enters the Krebs cycle. The excessive amount of NADH formed passes electrons into the electron transport chain, and creates a proton gradient that favours the transfer of the electrons freed from a hydrogen atom onto an oxygen molecule, forming many $O_2^{\bullet -}$ FRs. Entry of glucose into the cell increases amounts of acetyl-CoA even more; thus inhibiting the phosphorylation of tyrosine in IRS-1 as a 'protective mechanism' that down-regulates insulin sensitivity, reduces glucose entry into the cell, and thus reduces the amount of $O_2^{\bullet -}$ formed (Ceriello and Motz 2004). The NEFAs increase the concentrations of metabolites such as diacylglycerol, fatty acyl-CoA and ceramides, and these down-regulate the number of expressed insulin receptors (Frayn 2003). Inflammatory chemicals like TNF-α also disrupt insulin action in the cell by promoting serine phosphorylation of the IRS-1, which also down-regulates the cell's sensitivity to insulin (Hotamisligil 2006).

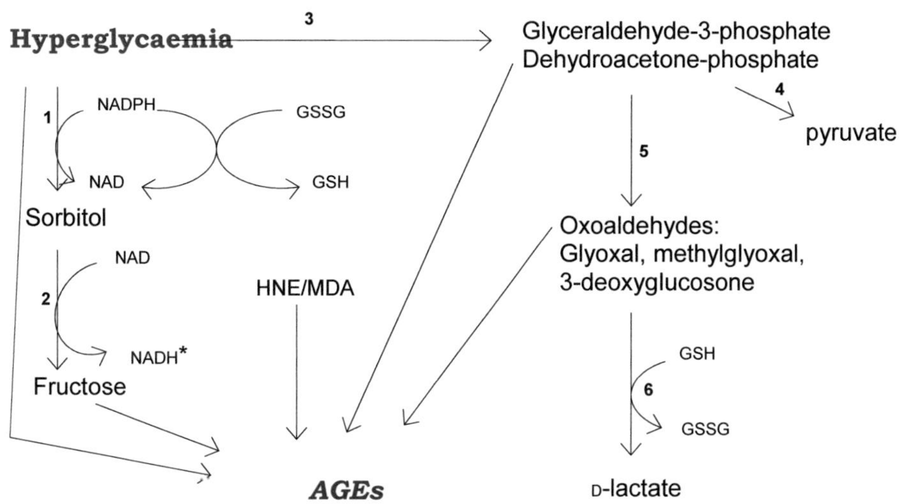

Fig. 5. **Formation of AGEs in NIDDM.** Glucose, a reducing sugar with an exposed aldehyde group in its acyclic form can directly and non-enzymatically glycate proteins and result in AGEs. It can also enter glycolysis and the triose intermediates glyceraldehydes 3-phosphate and dehydroacetone phosphate can be converted to oxoaldehydes by non-enzymatic autoxidation, particularly if GAPDH is inhibited by high levels of NADH. These oxoaldehydes can glycate proteins and result in AGE formation. Oxoaldehydes can be converted to D-lactate using 2 GSH molecules and re-releasing GSH via the glyoxylase pathway. Glucose can also enter the sorbitol, or polyol, pathway with the formation of another reducing sugar, fructose, which is more reactive than glucose in glycating proteins, and causing AGEs. The polyol pathway also depletes NADPH that is required to reduce GSSG to GSH. It results in the formation of NADH that inhibits pyruvate production and creates a favourable circumstance for more oxoaldehyde formation. Finally, aldehydes such as HNE and MDA formed from the peroxidation of PUFAs, can glycate proteins and cause AGE formation. The numbers are as follows: (1) aldose reductase (2) sorbitol dehydrogenase (3) glycolysis (4) GAPDH (5) non-enzymatic autoxidation (6) glycoxalase I and II. *NADH inhibits (4).

Randle *et al.* first showed this reciprocal interaction between the two major fuel sources (glucose and NEFAs) in 1963. It is referred to as the glucose-fatty acid cycle: high fatty acid oxidation in muscle reduces glucose uptake and oxidation i.e. insulin resistance develops (Frayn 2003). Chronically high concentrations of NEFAs released from visceral fat travel to the liver and promote hepatic insulin resistance, resulting in an impaired glucose tolerance test. Insulin resistance also results in an inability to suppress gluconeogenesis in the liver; so glucose production is increased, making the hyperglycaemia worse (Van Gaal, Mertens et al. 2006). There is also a change in activity of lipoprotein lipase (E.C. 3.1.1.34) and triglyceride lipase (E.C. 3.1.1.3) activity in the liver, resulting in dyslipidaemias of raised total triglycerides and lowered HDL concentrations (Caterson and Broom 2001).

A vital component of the development of NIDDM is diminished pancreatic β-cell function. Many obese, insulin-resistant patients do not develop hyperglycaemia. The β-cells can increase insulin release up to fivefold, and cell volume by 50%. If blood glucose is raised artificially in healthy subjects, insulin sensitivity increases and β-cell function is enhanced within 20 h. For NIDDM to develop, the pancreas must be unable to increase insulin secretion to compensate for this insulin-resistance. By the stage that the disease is diagnosed, the β-cells are operating at 25% or less of their original capacity. The disease is progressive, and the functionality of the β-cells progressively declines (Rosen and Spiegelman 2006). Once the disease is established, hyperglycaemia has a further glucotoxic effect on the β-cells and on insulin sensitivity (Kahn, Hull et al. 2006). Non-esterified fatty acids have been shown to act directly on β-cells to regulate glucose-stimulated insulin secretion. At first they potentiate the effects of glucose, but prolonged high NEFAs inhibit insulin release (Frayn 2003).

5. Glutathione concentrations and synthesis in NIDDM; A study

Animal studies show that antioxidants such as GSH improve insulin sensitivity, and clinical trials with vitamins C and E and GSH in insulin-resistant non-diabetic subjects improves insulin sensitivity (Ceriello and Motz 2004). It has also been shown that pancreatic β-cells have few antioxidants, and therefore oxidative stress can damage mitochondria and depress insulin secretion in these cells (Ceriello and Motz 2004). However, whether the GSH concentration is altered or not in NIDDM is not clear. Quite a few authors report unchanged or elevated GSH concentrations in RBCs in diabetes (Matsubara, Ferreira et al. 1992; Sinclair, Girling et al. 1992; Di Simplicio, De Giorgio et al. 1995; Laaksonen, Atalay et al. 1996).

Glutathione is protective in oxidative stress as it forms conjugates with reactive products of lipid peroxidation such as HNE, and it participates in the conversion of methyglyoxal to D-lactate, and scavenges $O_2^{\bullet -}$ and H_2O_2 generated by AGEs (Yoshida, Hirokawa et al. 1995; Thornalley, McLellan et al. 1996; Griffith and Mulcahy 1999; Beard, Shangari et al. 2003; Beisswenger, Howell et al. 2003; Robertson, Harmon et al. 2003; Constantin, Constantinescu et al. 2005; Iles and Liu 2005; Gil, Siems et al. 2006). When loss of GSH occurs, due to an increased rate of these reactions, it is important that the metabolic machinery in RBCs react with an increased rate of GSH synthesis.

As mentioned above some authors report unchanged or elevated GSH concentrations in the RBCs of NIDDM patients (Caren and Carne 1951; Matsubara, Ferreira et al. 1992; Sinclair, Girling et al. 1992; Di Simplicio, De Giorgio et al. 1995; Laaksonen, Atalay et al. 1996; Thornalley, McLellan et al. 1996; Atalay, Laaksonen et al. 1997; Straface, Rivabene et al. 2002; Nwose, Jelinek et al. 2006; Ozkilic, Cengiz et al. 2006). A second group of authors report decreased GSH concentrations in NIDDM (Bono, Caimi.G et al. 1986; Murakami, K. et al. 1989; Yoshida, Hirokawa et al. 1995; Vijayalingam, Parthiban et al. 1996; Seghrouchni, Drai et al. 2002; Memisogullari, Taysi et al. 2003; Sailaja, Baskar et al. 2003; Constantin, Constantinescu et al. 2005; Sampathkumar, Balasubramanyam et al. 2005). It has been suggested that the GSH synthetic enzymes are glycated when glucose levels are raised, and this affects their function (Dincer, Akcay et al. 2002).

Where a decrease in GSH concentration is reported it is considered to be indicative of increased oxidative stress (Bono, Caimi.G et al. 1986; Tho, Candlish et al. 1988; Murakami, K. et al. 1989; Jain and McVie 1994; Yoshida, Hirokawa et al. 1995; Vijayalingam, Parthiban et al. 1996; Lang, Mills et al. 2000; Dincer, Akcay et al. 2002; Arese and Schwarzer 2003; Beard, Shangari et al. 2003; Martin-Gallan, Carrascosa et al. 2003; Sailaja, Baskar et al. 2003; Darmaun, Smith et al. 2005; Sampathkumar, Balasubramanyam et al. 2005).

In order to clarify this, a study was conducted to measure the GSH concentrations and rates of synthesis in the intact RBCs of 20 NIDDM patients (58.3 ± 2.5 y) with a mean HbA_{1c} of 8.34 ± 0.2%, and 20 healthy controls (ND group) (46.6 ± 3.3 y) with a mean HbA_{1c} of 5.7 ± 0.1%. Ten NIDDM subjects were being treated with both insulin and oral hypoglycemics, four were receiving insulin alone and six were receiving oral hypoglycemics alone (Whillier, Raftos et al. 2008). Ethics approval was obtained from Sydney South West Area Health Service, and the Macquarie University Human Ethics Committee.

Subjects were not fasted prior to sampling their blood. Twelve to 18 mL of blood was drawn into 6 mL lithium heparin vacutainers using a 23-gauge needle/butterfly needle and barrel. The blood was separated by centrifugation (20 min at 4°C and 3000 × g). The plasma buffy coat (white cell layer) was aspirated and the packed cells were resuspended in 45 mL of washing solution and washed three times. A small sample of blood was used to measure the HbA_{1c} using the Micromat TM II HbA_{1c} analyser (280-0016EX) from BioRad Laboratories Pty Ltd (Regents Park, NSW, Australia). The RBCs were then resuspended to a haematocrit (Hct) of 10% in incubation solution. Samples of an Hct = 10% suspension were retained to measure the original GSH concentration of the donor's RBCs.

The Hct = 10% suspensions of intact RBCs were GSH-depleted using 1-chloro-2,4-dinitrobenzene (CDNB) (Raftos, Dwarte et al. 2006), and then incubated in a solution containing substrates for GSH synthesis (alanine, α-ketoglutarate, glycine and *N*-acetyl cysteine) and sampled for total free GSH (TFG) using a DTNB/enzymatic recycling micro-method developed by Raftos *et al* (Raftos, Dwarte et al. 2006), based on the earlier procedures of 5,5′-γ-dithiobis-(2-nitrobenzoic acid) (DTNB)/enzymatic recycling by Tietze (Tietze 1969), Owens and Belcher (Owens and Belcher 1965) and Richie *et al.* (Richie, Skowronski et al. 1996). The rate of GSH synthesis directly correlates with the rate of increase in TFG. Total RBC thiols were measured by Beutler's DTNB-based method (Beutler 1975). Plates were read on a multiskan spectrophotometer (Labsystems Original Multiscan from Pathtech Pty Ltd, Chatswood, NSW 2067).

The comparative statistics of the ND and NIDDM subjects are shown in Table 1 below. When the RBCs from control and NIDDM subjects were compared, no differences were found in their TFG concentration and in the uninhibited rate of *de novo* TFG synthesis after GSH depletion ($P > 0.05$). The NIDDM and ND control groups were also analysed for differences in TFG concentration between males and females, both between and within the groups. No differences were found ($P > 0.05$).

In subjects with NIDDM, there was a significant increase in TFG concentration with increasing age ($P = 0.0001$ for slope, ANCOVA for TFG, $F_{(1,38)} = 7.5624$, $P = 0.0093$), and a trend towards an increasing rate of TFG synthesis with age ($P = 0.09$ for slope, ANCOVA for the rate of synthesis, $F_{(1,38)} = 1.4826$, $P = 0.2313$). Neither TFG nor TFG synthesis appeared to be correlated with age in the ND controls ($P = 0.41$ for GSH concentration; $P = 0.94$ for TFG synthesis) (Figure 6).

Variable	ND subjects	NIDDM subjects	Comparison (P value)
Age (y)	46.6 ± 3.32	58.3 ± 2.49	P < 0.01
Duration of illness (y)		15.1 ± 2.5	
HbA_{1c} (%)	5.68 ± 0.08	8.34 ± 0.22	P < 0.005
TFG concentration [mmol (LRBC) $^{-1}$]	1.91 ± 0.09	1.89 ± 0.10	P > 0.05
Maximal rate of TFG synthesis [μmol (LRBC) $^{-1}$ min $^{-1}$]	1.06 ± 0.07	1.14 ± 0.06	P > 0.05

* All values mean ± SEM

Table 1. Comparison of ND and NIDDM subjects

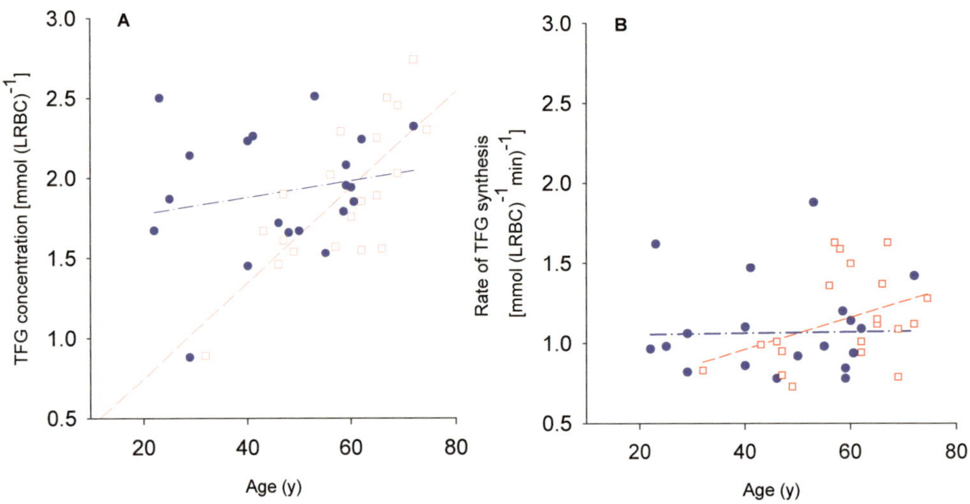

Fig. 6. **RBC GSH concentration and synthesis rate in ND and NIDDM RBCs.** A. Effect of age on TFG concentration. For ND controls blue (•), linear regression gave $r = 0.20$, $P = 0.41$; NIDDM subjects red (□), linear regression gave $r = 0.76$, $P = 0.0001$. B. Effect of age on the rate of TFG synthesis. For ND controls blue (•), linear regression gave $r = 0.02$, $P = 0.94$; NIDDM subjects red (□), linear regression gave $r = 0.39$, $P = 0.09$.

Non-diabetic subjects showed a significant correlation between the rate at which the TFG was synthesised in their RBCs, and the initial TFG concentration prior to CDNB-dependent depletion of TFG ($r = 0.71$, $P = 0.0005$). This was not the case for NIDDM subjects ($r = 0.05$, $P = 0.731$) (see Figure 7). The r and P values in Figure 7 are for the relationship between the initial TFG concentration and the rates of TFG synthesis after both variables had been corrected for the age of the subject.

In NIDDM, there was a downward trend in HbA_{1c} with age (-0.017 ± 0.02 % HbA_{1c} y^{-1}) (Figure 8) but the statistical analysis indicated that this was non-significant with the sample size that was used. Therefore this was investigated in data from a further 6775 NIDDM patients where it was found to be significant with a slope of - 0.019 ± 0.002 % HbA_{1c} y^{-1} (r = 0.126, P < 0.0001). When TFG concentration and rate of TFG synthesis were corrected for age in the NIDDM group, there was no correlation between these two variables and the extent of glycation (% HbA_{1c}).

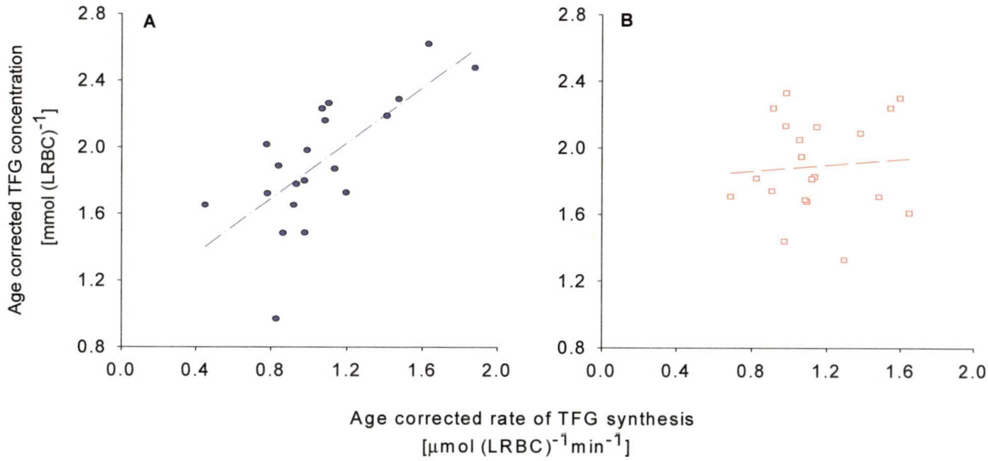

Fig. 7. **TFG synthesis rate versus concentration in ND and NIDDM A.** For ND controls (age-corrected) blue (•), linear regression gave r = 0.71 (0.69)*, P = 0.0005 (0.0006)*. B. For NIDDM subjects (age-corrected) red (□), linear regression gave r = 0.05 (0.35)*, P = 0.73 (0.14)*. (**non-age-corrected values).*

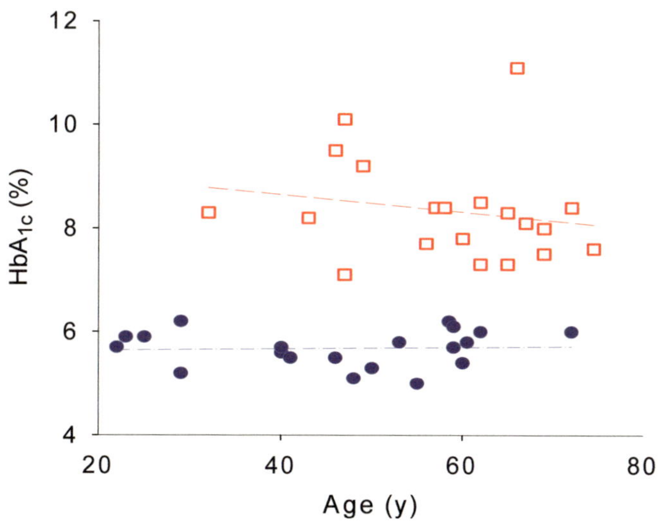

Fig. 8. **Relationship between age and Hb_{A1c}.** For ND controls blue (•), linear regression gave r = 0.06, P = 0.80. For NIDDM subjects red (□), linear regression gave r = - 0.19, P = 0.43. Additional data from 6775 NIDDM patients showed that the decline in HbA_{1c} with age was significant (slope of the linear regression -0.02 ± 0.002 % HbA_{1c} y^{-1}, r = 0.13, P < 0.0001).

5.1 Discussion of the results

Researchers are conflicted with regard to the activity of individual enzymes in the GSH synthetic pathway in RBCs in diabetic patients. Studies of purified isolated enzymes have shown decreased activity of GCL (Murakami, K. et al. 1989; Yoshida, Hirokawa et al. 1995) , GR (Murakami, K. et al. 1989; Sailaja, Baskar et al. 2003), GPx (Dincer, Akcay et al. 2002; Martin-Gallan, Carrascosa et al. 2003; Memisogullari, Taysi et al. 2003; Sailaja, Baskar et al. 2003) and GST in NIDDM (Sailaja, Baskar et al. 2003). But these findings are not supported by others (Bono, Caimi.G et al. 1986; Matsubara, Ferreira et al. 1992; Vijayalingam, Parthiban et al. 1996; Atalay, Laaksonen et al. 1997). More importantly, results obtained from individual enzyme concentrates do not necessarily reflect the overall state of GSH synthesis and utilisation in intact RBCs. The results of the present study using intact RBCs suggested that the enzymes that synthesise GSH are not damaged by glycoxidation.

When GSH-depleted RBCs are supplied with glucose and the amino acid substrates for GSH synthesis, the rate of TFG synthesis increases almost five fold compared to RBCs with normal GSH concentration (Raftos, Dwarte et al. 2006). Under these experimental conditions, the mean rate of GSH synthesis in RBCs from both NIDDM subjects and ND is the same, indicating that enzyme function had not been compromised in the NIDDM RBCs. In addition, the pre-depletion mean-TFG concentrations in RBCs in the NIDDM patients were the same as the ND subjects; this implies that the circulating RBCs of NIDDM patients are capable of increasing their rate of TFG synthesis to compensate for increased oxidative loads thought to occur in this disease.

There is evidence for increased oxidative loads in NIDDM in the present study. In the ND group there was a correlation between the rate of GSH synthesis and total GSH concentration. If the rate of oxidation were similar in healthy individuals, then the rate of synthesis in these individuals would be reflected in the GSH concentration. This was not the case in the RBCs from the NIDDM patients, and indicated that the larger variable oxidative load in NIDDM interferes with the relationship between the rate of GSH synthesis and the GSH concentration achieved in the RBC.

A novel finding in the present study was an increase in TFG concentration and to a lesser extent rate of GSH synthesis with increasing age in the RBCs from the NIDDM group but not the ND group. In addition, there was a decrease in HbA_{1c} with increasing age in the NIDDM group. This differs from reports on healthy subjects, in which GSH declined with age, and GSSG and various markers of oxidative stress, including HNE, increased (Lang, Naryshin et al. 1992; Matsubara, Ferreira et al. 1992; Gil, Siems et al. 2006). However, an increase in GSH with age in NIDDM has been shown by a few authors and has been explained variously as an up-regulation, compensation or stimulation of the GSH biosynthetic pathway by either the condition itself and/or the medication used (Matsubara, Ferreira et al. 1992; Atalay, Laaksonen et al. 1997; Nwose, Jelinek et al. 2006). In this context, the work of Matsubara *et al* is of particular interest, in showing that although the GSH concentration, GR and GPx activities do decrease with age in healthy individuals, in older NIDDM patients these values are similar to young healthy subjects. They proposed that the GSH redox system of aged subjects with diabetes is stimulated by the condition itself and/or its treatment with oral hypoglycaemics and insulin (Matsubara, Ferreira et al. 1992). Indeed, a study using *in vivo* euglycaemic hyperinsulinaemic clamping, found that administered insulin reduces RBC oxidative stress and results in a higher GSH/GSSG ratio in NIDDM patients to almost normal levels after 2 h (Bravi, Armiento et al. 2006). The decline in HbA_{1c} seen in the NIDDM group in the present study suggests good management of the condition, and/or a decline in the oxidative load; and it may be that the treatment and management of the NIDDM patients stimulated the GSH biosynthetic pathway.

An adaptive response has been described to account for normal GSH concentrations in the RBCs of NIDDM patients. Cellular stresses such as hydrogen peroxide, TNF-α, oxidised LDL, nitric oxide and particularly HNE, are known to up-regulate GCL. Initially, GST mediates the binding of HNE with GSH to form a Michael adduct that is pumped from the cell. This results in an initial decline in GSH. But HNE and other stressors themselves increase the activity of GCL, and result in an increase in GSH. Increased GCL gene expression maintains GSH homeostasis when oxidative stress is increased (Iles and Liu 2005). GCL consists of a catalytic (GCLC) and a modulator (GCLM) subunit. It is the GCLM subunit that increases the rate of GSH synthesis by increasing the K_i for GSH inhibition and decreasing the K_m for glutamate utilisation (Yang, Dieter et al. 2002); and it has been shown that increased circulating concentrations of ROS can up-regulate the production of GCLM in certain cell types (Yang, Dieter et al. 2002).

Another possibility for the observed increase in GSH with age in the NIDDM group is that, because this was not a longitudinal study, we may have been witnessing "the survivors" in the population age-group who have genetically higher levels of GSH that actually protect them from oxidative damage. Some studies suggest this to be the case (Lang, Naryshin et al. 1992; Julius, Lang et al. 1994). Lang *et al* (1992) showed that while ~50% of healthy subjects between the ages of 60 – 79 y have low GSH concentrations, only ~25% did in the 80 – 99 y age group; so they suggested that individuals with low GSH concentrations die before reaching 80 y (Lang, Naryshin et al. 1992), and this accounts for their observed mean GSH concentrations increasing with age (Julius, Lang et al. 1994). Another study reported normal concentrations of three indicators of oxidative stress (GSH, thiobarbituric acid and diene conjugates) in elderly (>60 y) NIDDM patients (Sinclair, Girling et al. 1992). Longitudinal studies on healthy individuals and subjects with NIDDM are needed to determine whether we are observing a true maintenance in GSH concentration in NIDDM patients with age, or simply the survival of those with inherently high GSH concentrations.

6. Conclusion

Oxidative stress refers to an imbalance between oxidative load and antioxidant defenses. Type II diabetes mellitus is considered an inflammatory state with a high oxidative load. The accumulation of visceral fat results in the release of NEFAs and FR, and these are implicated in the down regulation of the insulin sensitivity of plasma membranes and in the inhibition of the release of insulin from the pancreas. The resulting hyperglycaemia causes the formation of AGEs and FR that damage endothelial linings, the kidney, nervous tissue, and the eye; and this manifests as the many complications of the disease.

Glutathione is an endogenously produced antioxidant that protects cells by virtue of the reducing power of its thiol group located on the cysteine moiety of the tripeptide. Red blood cell GSH constitutes a large mobile antioxidant pool that is able to scavenge ROS and protect tissues in the body. Glutathione is beneficial in oxidative stress in conjugating reactive products and scavenging FRs. It is important that the metabolic machinery of the RBC reacts to increase the rate of GSH synthesis when oxidative loads are high.

There is controversy in the literature on the role of GSH in NIDDM, with various authors reporting increased, unchanged, or decreased concentrations of RBC GSH. The results of the study presented here are unique in showing that the intact RBC maintains its ability to synthesise GSH at the same rate as found in healthy controls when given glucose and the amino acid substrates. This suggests that the enzymes involved in the metabolic pathway function normally. A surprising finding was an increase in TFG concentration and rate of synthesis with increasing age in NIDDM subjects but not in ND subjects; and a decrease in HbA_{1c} levels with increasing age in NIDDM subjects. It is proposed that the treatment of the condition in the form of insulin and/or oral hypoglycaemics causes an upregulation in the GSH pathway. It is also proposed that older subjects who were seen in this study are "the survivors" with genetically higher concentrations of GSH, which suggests an overall protective function of this antioxidant in this disease.

7. Acknowledgements

Many thanks to Prof. Dennis Yue, Lynda Molyneaux, Belinda Brooks and the Metabolic Unit at Royal Prince Alfred Hospital's Diabetes Centre, the doctors at the University Health Services at Macquarie University and the volunteer blood donors. BioRad Labs Pty Ltd (NSW Australia) supplied the Micromat II Alc analyser.

8. References

Abordo, E., H. Minhas, et al. (1999). Accumulation of α-oxoaldehydes during oxidative stress: a role in cytotoxicity. *Biochemical Pharmacology* 58: 641-648.

Aoshiba, K., Y. Nakajima, et al. (1999). Red blood cells inhibit apoptosis of human neutrophils. *Blood* 93(11): 4006-4010.

Arese, P. and E. Schwarzer (2003). *Metabolic Disorders: Red Cell Alterations in Diabetes Mellitus*. Berlin, Springer-Verlag.

Atalay, M., D. Laaksonen, et al. (1997). Altered antioxidant enzyme defences in insulin-dependent diabetic men with increased resting and exercise-induced oxidative stress. *Acta Physiologica Scandinavica* 161(2): 195-201.

Baynes, J. (1991). Perspectives in diabetes: Role of oxidative stress in development of complications in diabetes. *Diabetes* 40: 405-412.

Beard, K., N. Shangari, et al. (2003). Metabolism, not auto-oxidation, plays a role in α-oxoaldehyde and reducing sugar-induced erythrocyte GSH depletion: Relevance for diabetes mellitus. *Molecular and Cellular Biochemistry* 252: 331-338.

Becker, K., M. Leichsenring, et al. (1995). Glutathione and association antioxidant systems in protein energy malnutrition: results of a study in Nigeria. *Free Radical Biology and Medicine* 18(2): 257-263.

Beisswenger, P. J., S. Howell, et al. (2003). Glyceraldehyde-3-phosphate dehydrogenase activity as an independent modifier of methylglyoxal levels in diabetes. *Biochimica et Biophysica Acta* 1637: 98-106.

Beutler, E. (1975). *Red cell metabolism: a manual of biochemical methods*. New York, Grune & Stratton.

Beutler, E. and T. Gelbart (1985). Plasma glutathione in health and in patients with malignant disease. *Journal of laboratory & clinical medicine* 105(5): 581-584.

Board, P. (1981). Transport of glutathione S-conjugate from human erythrocytes. *FEBS Letters* 124(2): 163-165.

Board, P. (1993). Inhibition of erythrocyte glutathione conjugate transport by polyethoxylated surfactants. *FEBS* 315(3): 298-300.

Board, P. G. and J. Smith (1977). Erythrocyte γ-glutamyl transpeptidase. *Blood* 49: 667-668.

Bono, A., Caimi.G, et al. (1986). Red cell peroxide metabolism in diabetes mellitus. *Hormone and metabolic Research* 19: 264-266.

Bravi, M. C., A. Armiento, et al. (2006). Insulin decreases intracellular oxidative stress in patients with type 2 diabetes mellitus. *Metabolism: Clinical and Experimental* 55: 691-695.

Brownlee, M. (2001). Biochemistry and molecular cell biology of diabetic complications. *Nature* 414: 813-319.

Burak Cimen, M. (2008). Free radical metabolism in human erythrocytes. *Clinica Chimica Acta* 390: 1 - 11.

Burk, R. and K. Hill (1995). Reduced glutathione release into rat plasma by extrahepatic tissue. *American Journal of Physiology* 269(3 pt 1): G396-399.

Caren, R. and H. O. Carne (1951). The blood glutathione level and its response to insulin in diabetic and non-diabetic patients and a case of insulin resistance. *The American Journal of Medical Sciences* 221: 307-313.

Caterson, I. D. and J. Broom (2001). *Obesity*. London, Harcourt Health Com.

Ceriello, A. and E. Motz (2004). Is oxidative stress the pathogenic mechanism underlying insulin resistance, diabetes, and cardiovascular disease? The common soil hypothesis revisited *Arteriosclerosis, Thrombosis, and Vascular Biology* 24: 816-823.

Chawla, R., F. Lewis, et al. (1984). Plasma cysteine, cystine, and glutathione in cirrhosis. *Gastroenterology* 87(4): 770-776.

Chen, Y., H. G. Shertzer, et al. (2005). Glutamate cysteine ligase catalysis; dependence on ATP and modifier subunit for regulation of tissue glutathione levels. *The Journal of Biological Chemistry* 280(40): 33766 - 33774.

Constantin, A., E. Constantinescu, et al. (2005). Effects of ageing on carbonyl stress and antioxidant defense in red blood cells of obese Type 2 diabetic patients. *Journal of Cellular and Molecular Medicine* 9(3): 683-691.

Darmaun, D., S. D. Smith, et al. (2005). Evidence for accelerated rates of glutathione utilization and glutathione depletion in adolescents with poorly controlled type I diabetes. *Diabetes* 54: 190-196.

Di Simplicio, P., L. A. De Giorgio, et al. (1995). Glutathione, glutathione utilizing enzymes and thioltransferase in platelets of insulin-dependent diabetic patients: relation with platelet aggregation and with microangiopathic complications. *European Journal of Clinical Investigation* 25(9): 665-669.

Dincer, Y., T. Akcay, et al. (2002). Effect of oxidative stress on glutathione pathway in red blood cells from patients with insulin-dependent diabetes mellitus. *Metabolism* 51(10): 1360-1362.

Dominguez, C., E. Ruiz, et al. (1998). Oxidative stress at onset and in early stages of type I diabetes in children and adolescents. *Diabetes Care* 21: 1736-1742.

Erden-Inal, M., E. Sunal, et al. (2002). Age-related changes in the glutathione redox system. *Cell Biochemistry and Function* 20: 61 - 66.

Fletcher, R. H. and S. W. Fletcher (1994). Glutathione and ageing: ideas and evidence. *Lancet* 344(8934): 1379 - 1380.

Franklin, C. C., D. S. Backos, et al. (2009). Structure, function, and post-translational regulation of the catalytic and modifier subunits of glutamate cysteine ligase. *Molecular Aspects of Medicine* 30(1-2): 86-98.

Frayn, K. N. (2003). *The glucose-fatty acid cycle: a physiological perspective.* Biochemical Society, Essex, Colchester.

Gil, J., W. Siems, et al. (2006). Age-associated analysis of oxidative stress parameters in human plasma and erythrocytes. *Free Radical Research* 40(5): 495-505.

Giustarini, D., I. Dalle-Donne, et al. (2008). Red blood cells as a physiological source of glutathione for extracellular fluids. *Blood Cells, Molecules and Diseases* 40(2): 174-179.

Griffith, O. W. (1981). Glutathione turnover in human erythrocytes. *Journal of Biological Chemistry* 256(10): 4900-4904.

Griffith, O. W. (1999). Biologic and pharmacologic regulation of mammalian glutathione synthesis. *Free Radical Biology and Medicine* 27(9-10): 922-935.

Griffith, O. W. and R. T. Mulcahy (1999). The enzymes of glutathione synthesis: gamma-glutamylcysteine synthetase. *Advances in Enzymology*. New York, John Wiley & sons Inc. 73: 60-80.

Grinberg, L., E. Rachmilewitz, et al. (1995). Hydroxyl radical generation in B-thalassemia. *Free Radical Biology and Medicine* 18: 611-615.

Halliwell, B. (2005). *Free Radicals and Other Reactive Species in Disease*. John Wiley & Sons.

Hill, J. W. and D. K. Kolb (2001). *Chemistry for Changing Times*. New Jersey, Prentice Hall.

Hotamisligil, G. S. (2006). Inflammation and metabolic disorders. *Nature* 444: 860-867.

Iles, K. E. and R. M. Liu (2005). Mechanisms of glutamate cysteine ligase (GCL) induction by 4-hydroxynonenal. *Free Radical Biology and Medicine* 38: 547-556.

Jain, S. and R. McVie (1994). Effect of glycemic control, race (white versus black), and duration of diabetes on reduced glutathione content in erythrocytes of diabetic patients. *Metabolism* 43: 306-309.

Julius, M., C. Lang, et al. (1994). Glutathione and morbidity in a community-based sample of elderly. *Journal of Clinical Epidemiology* 47(9): 1021-1026.

Junqueira, V. B. C., S. B. M. Barros, et al. (2004). Aging and oxidative stress. *Molecular Aspects of Medicine* 25: 5-16.

Kahn, S. E., R. L. Hull, et al. (2006). Mechanisms linking obesity to insulin resistance and type 2 diabetes. *Nature* 444: 840-846.

Keenoy, B. M., J. Vertommen, et al. (2001). Divergent effects of different oxidants on glutathione homeostasis and protein damage in erythrocytes from diabetic patients: effects of high glucose. *Molecular and Cellular Biochemistry* 225: 59-73.

Kennett, E., W. Bubb, et al. (2005). NMR studies of exchange between intra- and extracellular glutathione in human erythrocytes. *Redox Report* 10(2): 83-90.

Kennett, E. C. and P. W. Kuchel (2006). Plasma membrane oxidoreductases: effects on erythrocyte metabolism and redox homeostasis. *Antioxidants & Redox Signaling* 8(7 & 8): 1241 - 1247.

Laaksonen, D. E., M. Atalay, et al. (1996). Increased resting and exercise-induced oxidative stress in young IDDM men. *Diabetes Care* 19(6): 569-574.

Lang, C., S. Naryshin, et al. (1992). Low blood glutathione levels in healthy aging adults. *Journal of Laboratory and Clinincal Medicine* 120(5): 720-725.

Lang, C. A., B. J. Mills, et al. (2000). Blood glutathione decreases in chronic diseases. *Journal of Laboratory and Clinical Medicine* 135: 402-405.

Lang, C. A., S. Naryshin, et al. (1992). Low blood glutathione levels in healthy aging adults. *Journal of Laboratory and Clinical Medicine* 120(5): 720-725.

Lehninger, A. L. (1984). *Lehninger, Principles of biochemistry.* New York, Worth Publishers, Inc.

Low, F. M., M. B. Hampton, et al. (2008). Peroxiredoxin 2 and peroxide metabolism in the erythrocyte. *Antioxidants & Redox Signaling* 10(8): 1621-1629.

Lunn, G., G. L. Dale, et al. (1979). Transport accounts for glutathione turnover in human erythrocytes. *Blood* 54(1): 238-244.

Marfella, R., G. Verrazzo, et al. (1995). Glutathione reverses systemic hemodynamic changes induced by acute hyperglycemia in healthy subjects. *American Journal of Physiology* 268(31): E1167-1175.

Martin-Gallan, P., A. Carrascosa, et al. (2003). Biomarkers of diabetes-associated oxidative stress and antioxidant status in young diabetic patients with or without subclinical complications. *Free Radical Biology and Medicine* 34(12): 1563-1574.

Matsubara, L., A. Ferreira, et al. (1992). Influence of diabetes mellitus on the glutathione redox system of human red blood cells. *Brazilian Journal of Medical and Biological Research* 25: 331-335.

Memisogullari, R., S. Taysi, et al. (2003). Antioxidant status and lipid peroxidation in type II diabetes mellitus. *Cell biochemistry and function* 21: 291-296.

Mullarkey, C. J., D. Edelstein, et al. (1990). Free radical generation by early glycation products: a mechanism for accelerated atherogenesis in diabetes. *Biochemical and Biophysical Research Communications* 173(3): 932-939.

Mulquiney, P. J. and P. W. Kuchel (2003). *Modelling Metabolism with Mathematica.* Boca Raton, Florida, CRC Press.

Murakami, K., T. K., et al. (1989). Impairment of glutathione metabolism in erythrocytes from patients with diabetes mellitus. *Metabolism* 38(8): 753-758.

Nuttall, S. L., U. Martin, et al. (1998). Glutathione: in sickness and in health. *Lancet* 351(9103): 645.

Nwose, E. U., H. F. Jelinek, et al. (2006). Changes in the erythrocyte glutathione concentration in the course of diabetes mellitus. *Redox Report* 11(3): 99-104.

Owens, C. and R. Belcher (1965). A colorimetric micro-method for the determination of glutathione. *Journal of Biological Chemistry* 94: 705-711.

Ozkilic, A. C., M. Cengiz, et al. (2006). The role of N-acetylcysteine treatment on anti-oxidative status in patients with type II diabetes mellitus. *Journal of Basic & Clinical Physiology & Pharmacology* 17(4): 245-254.

Rae, C., S. Berners-Price, et al. (1990). Kinetic analysis of the human erythrocyte glyoxalase system using H NMR and a computer model. *European Journal of Biochemistry* 193: 83-90.

Raftos, J., S. Whillier, et al. (2007). Kinetics of uptake and deacetylation of N-acetylcysteine by human erythrocytes. *The International Journal of Biochemistry and Cell Biology* 39(9): 1698-1706.

Raftos, J. E., T. M. Dwarte, et al. (2006). Direct measurement of the rate of glutathione synthesis in 1-chloro-2,4-dinitrobenzene treated human erythrocytes. *Redox Report* 11(1): 9-14.

Rice-Evans, C. and E. Baysal (1987). Iron-mediated oxidative stress in erythrocytes *The Biochemical Journal* 244: 191 - 196.

Richie, J. J., P. Abraham, et al. (1996). Long-term stability of blood glutathione and cysteine in humans. *Clinical Chemistry* 42(7): 1100-1105.

Richie, J. J., L. Skowronski, et al. (1996). Blood glutathione concentrations in a large-scale human study. *Clinical Chemistry* 42: 71-75.

Richman, P. and A. Meister (1975). Regulation of gamma-glutamyl-cysteine synthetase by nonallosteric feedback inhibition by glutathione. *Journal of Biological Chemistry* 250(4): 1422-1426.

Robertson, R. P., J. Harmon, et al. (2003). Glucose toxicity in b-cells: Type 2 diabetes, good radicals gone bad, and the glutathione connection. *Diabetes* 52: 581-587.

Rosen, E. D. and B. M. Spiegelman (2006). Adipocytes as regulators of energy balance and glucose homeostasis. *Nature* 444: 847-853.

Rossi, R., A. Milzani, et al. (2002). Blood glutathione disulfide: in vivo factor or in vitro artifact? *Endocrinology and Metabolism* 48(5): 742-753.

Sailaja, Y. R., R. Baskar, et al. (2003). The antioxidant status during maturation of reticulocytes to erythrocytes in type 2 diabetes. *Free Radical Biology and Medicine* 35(2): 133-139.

Sampathkumar, R., M. Balasubramanyam, et al. (2005). Increased glutathionylated hemoglobin (HbSSG) in type 2 diabetes subjects with microangiopathy. *Clinical Biochemistry* 38(10): 892-899.

Schafer, F. Q. and G. R. Buettner (2001). Redox environment of the cell as viewed through the REDOX state of the GSSG/GSH couple. *Free Radical Biology and Medicine* 30(11): 1191-1212.

Seghrouchni, I., J. Drai, et al. (2002). Oxidative stress parameters in type I, type II and insulin-treated type 2 diabetes mellitus; insulin treatment efficiency. *Clinica Chimica Acta* 321: 89-96.

Sies, H. (1985). *Oxidative stress: oxidants and antioxidants*. New York, Academic Press.

Silverthorn, D. U. (2007). *Human Physiology*. San Francisco, Pearson Benjamin Cummings.

Sinclair, A. J., A. J. Girling, et al. (1992). An investigation of the relationship between free radical activity and vitamin C metabolism in elderly diabetic subjects with retinopathy. *Gerontology* 38: 268-274.

Snoke, J. (1955). Isolation and properties of yeast glutathione synthetase. *The Journal of Biological Chemistry* 213: 813.

Snoke, J. and K. Bloch (1954). *Glutathione-A Symposium*. NY, Academic Press.

Snoke, J., S. Yanari, et al. (1953). Synthesis of glutathione from γ-glutamylcysteine. *the Journal of Biological Chemistry* 201: 573.

Sorensen, S., E. Rubin, et al. (1990). The role of membrane skeletal-associated α-globin in the pathophysiology of β-thalassemia. *Blood* 75: 1333-1336.

Srivastava, A. K., Y. Awasthi, et al. (1976). Studies on γ-glutamyl transpeptidase in human and rabbit erythrocytes. *Blood* 47(4): 645-650.

Srivastava, S. and E. Beutler (1969). The Transport of Oxidised Glutathione from human Erythrocytes. *Journal of Biological Chemistry* 244(1): 9-16.

Straface, E., R. Rivabene, et al. (2002). Structural changes of the erythrocyte as a marker of non-insulin-dependent diabetes: protective effects of N-acetylcysteine. *Biochemical and Biophysical Research Communications* 290: 1393-1398.

Sullivan, R. (1996). Contributions to senescence: non-enzymatic glycosylation of proteins. *Archives of Physiology and Biochemistry* 104(7): 797-806.

Tho, L., J. Candlish, et al. (1988). Correlates of diabetes markers with erythrocytic enzymes decomposing reactive oxygen species. *Annals of Clinical Biochemistry* 25: 426-431.

Thornalley, P. (1988). Modification of the glyoxalase system in human red blood cells by glucose *in vitro*. *Journal of Biochemistry* 254: 751-755.

Thornalley, P., A. McLellan, et al. (1996). Negative association between erythrocyte reduced glutathione concentration and diabetic complications. *Clinical Science* 91(5): 575-582.

Tietze, F. (1969). Enzymatic method for quantitative determination of nanogram amounts of total and oxidised glutathione applications to mammalian blood and other tissues. *Analytical Biochemistry* 27: 502-522.

Van Gaal, L. F., I. L. Mertens, et al. (2006). Mechanisms linking obesity with cardiovascular disease. *Nature* 444: 875-880.

Vijayalingam, S., A. Parthiban, et al. (1996). Abnormal antioxidant status in impaired glucose tolerance and non-insulin-dependent diabetes mellitus. *Diabetic Medicine* 13: 715-719.

Wautier, J. L. and A. M. Schmidt (2004). Protein glycation: a firm link to endothelial cell dysfunction. *Circulation Research* 95: 233-238.

Whillier, S., J. Raftos, et al. (2008). Glutathione synthesis by red blood cells in type 2 diabetes mellitus. *Redox Report* 13(6): 277-282.

Wolff, S. P. and R. T. Dean (1987). Glucose autoxidation and protein modification. *The Biochemical Journal* 245: 243-250.

Wu, G., Y. Fang, et al. (2004). Glutathione metabolism and its implications for health. *Journal of Nutrition* 134(3): 489-492.

Yang, C., S. Chou, et al. (1995). Effect of ageing on human plasma glutathione concentrations as determined by high-performance liquid chromatography with fluorimetric detection. *Journal of Chromatography: Biomedical Sciences and Applications* 674(1): 23-30.

Yang, Y., M. Z. Dieter, et al. (2002). Initial characterization of the glutamate-cysteine ligase modifier subunit Gclm(-/-) knockout mouse - Novel model system for a severely compromised oxidative stress response. *Journal of Biological Chemistry* 277(51): 49446-49452.

Yoshida, K., J. Hirokawa, et al. (1995). Weakened cellular scavenging activity against oxidative stress in diabetes mellitus: regulation of glutathione synthesis and efflux. *Diabetologia* 38: 201-210.

8

The Role of Oxidative Stress in Pathogenesis of Diabetic Neuropathy: Erythrocyte Superoxide Dismutase, Catalase and Glutathione Peroxidase Level in Relation to Peripheral Nerve Conduction in Diabetic Neuropathy Patients

Gordana M. Djordjević[1], Stojanka S.Djurić[1], Vidosava B. Djordjević[1], Slobodan Apostolski[2] and Miroslava Živković[1]
[1]University of Niš, Medical Faculty,
[2] University of Belgrade, Medical Faculty,
Serbia

1. Introduction

Distal symmetrical polyneuropathy is the most common form of neurological complications in diabetes mellitus (DM). It is sensory-motor polyneuropathy dominated by sensitive symptoms and signs, primarily decrease or loss of sensibility in distal parts of extremities, or positive symptoms of prickling, burning pain and tingling. These symptoms can be extremely unpleasant for patients but at the same time they are a huge therapeutic problem as well. Motor symptoms and signs in early phase of DSP are often absent, although by neurophysiologic tests motor fibers damaging signs can be detected and this damage often leads to loss of functions in patients in advanced phase of the disease. The most significant clinical consequence of sensitive and autonomic fibers damage is feet ulceration, what is a leading cause for hospitalization and for lower extremities amputations, if trauma factors are excluded. Thus, diabetic DSP is important not only for clinical reasons but for economic ones as well, especially regarding the fact that DM prevalence is rapidly growing. For many years scientists have done numerous researches for therapeutic solutions to prevent, delay or slow the progression of the disease, aiming to better understanding of ethiopathogenesis of this disease. Special attention has been paid to oxidative stress (OS) role in pathogenesis of DM and diabetic neuropathy. Despite numerous experimental confirmations of OS in diabetic patients, there is still controversy about whether oxidative stress is just a side effect or it is a possible cause of diabetic neuropathy. More than thousand studies about this problem have already been reported and since this problem is not completely solved, further investigations are required. Therefore, a good knowledge of biochemistry of oxidative stress, cell signal transduction and antioxidative protection is necessary.

2. Biochemistry of oxidative stress

Oxidative stress is a consequence of the imbalance between reactive oxygen species (ROS) production and antioxidant capacity. This can occur as a result of either increased ROS generation, impaired antioxidant system, or a combination of both. Free radicals are defined as an atoms or molecules that contain one or more unpaired electrons, making them unstable and highly reactive (Halliwell , 1999). The most important free radicals are reactive oxygen species (ROS) and reactive nitrogen species (RNS). ROS include free radicals such as superoxide (O_2^-), hydroxyl (OH), peroxyl (RO_2), hydroperoxyl (HRO_2^-) as well as nonradical species such as hydrogen peroxide (H_2O_2) and hydrochlorous acid (HOCl) (Turko et al., 2001; Evans et al., 2002; Ziegler, 1994; Soliman & Gellido,2004.). Other non-oxygen species existing as reactive nitrogen species (RNS) include free radicals like nitric oxide (NO) and nitrogen dioxide (NO_2^-), as well as nonradicals such as peroxynitrite ($ONOO^-$), nitrous oxide (HNO_2) and alkyl peroxynitrates (RONOO) (Ziegler, 1994; Soliman and Gellido,2004).

In aerobic cells, free radicals are constantly produced mostly as reactive oxygen species. Once produced, free radicals are removed by antioxidants defenses including enzyme superoxide dismutase, catalase and gluthation peroxidise. Reactive oxygen species, including nitric oxide and related species, commonly exert a series of useful physiological effects. However, imbalance between prooxidant and antioxidant defenses in favour of prooxidants results in oxidative stress associated with the oxidative modification of biomolecules such as lipids, proteins and nucleic acids.

Hyperglycemia is the main cause of increased concentration of free radicals in the plasma of diabetic patients.

Chronic hyperglycemia causes oxidative stress (OS) in a number of ways including enzymatic, non-enzymatic and mitochondrial pathways, thus disrupting the prooxidative/antioxidative balance in cellular systems.

Nonenzymatic sources of oxidative stress originate from the oxidative biochemistry of glucose. Hperglycemia can directly cause increased ROS generation. Glucose can undergo autoxidation and generate OH radicals. A second consequence of hyperglycemia is nonenzymatic glycation of proteins.

Nonenzymatic glycation of proteins implies the ability of glucose to react in a nonenzymatic process with proteins, reducing molecular oxygen to highly reactive products (superoxide radical, hydrogen peroxide, and hydroxyl radical). The glycation process occurs in two phases: early – reversible, and late – irreversible phase. The early phase is characterized by the development of Amadori products followed by formation of stable adducts - advanced glycation end products (AGEs) in the later phase. The production of intracellular AGE precursors damages target cells via three pathways. First, intracellular proteins, modified by AGE, alter their own function. Second, extracellular matrix components modified by AGEP precursors interact abnormally with other matrix components and with matrix protein receptors on the cells. Third, plasma proteins modified by AGE precursors bind to the AGE receptors on endothelial cells, mesangial cells, and macrophages, causing receptor-mediated production of reactive oxygen species (ROS).

Enzymatic sources of augmented generation of reactive species in diabetes include NOS, NAD(P)H oxidase and xanthine oxidase (Guzik et al.,2000; Guzik et al., 2002; Aliciguzel et al.,2003) , where it is considered that the NAD(P)H oxidase is the major source of O_2^-productionf (Guzik, 2000; Ergul et al., 2004).

The mitochondrial respiratory chain is another source of nonenzymatic generation of reactive species. Hyperglycemia-induced generation of $\cdot O_2^-$ at the mitochondrial level is the initial trigger of vicious cycle of oxidative stress in diabetes (Schultz et al., 2005, Nishikawa et al., 2000, Brownlee, 2001). Iincreased generation of ROS, especially O_2^- precedes the activation of four major pathways involved in the development of diabetic complications.

In hyperglicemia there is enhanced metabolism of glucose through the polyol (sorbitol) pathway, which also results in inhanced productions of $O_2^{-\cdot}$ Glucose is a poor substrate for aldose reductase, but at high concentrations this enzyme converts glucose to sorbitole, initiating the polyol pathway of glucose conversion to fructose.

This pathway of glucose metabolism implies the participation of aldosoreductase enzyme, which using the NADPH cofactor, catalyzes the reduction of glucose into sorbitol, which can be further transformed into fructose. Aldosoreductase is widespread in the mammalian tissues such as peripheral nerves, retina, renal glomeruli, eye lenses. Stimulation of this pathway in hyperglycemic conditions is one of the pathogenetic mechanisms responsible for the development of diabetic neuropathy, nephropathy, and cataract. Activation of this pathway leads to structural changes in the tissues via several mechanisms, out of which most significant are increased osmotic pressure in the cell, depletion of myoinositol, and disordered redox potential of the cell due to reduced NADPH concentration, on the account of which the activity of NADPH dependent enzymes (including glutathione reductase and NO synthase) is diminished. Reduced production of NO leads to vasoconstriction, and impossibility of reduced glutathione regeneration in the so called glutathione redox cycle leads to depletion of reduced glutathione, since it is regenerated by the action of NADPH-dependent glutathione reductase (Garlberg & Mannervik, 1975), ultimately producing a permanent oxidative stress. Change of redox status of the cell, as determined by the cellular content of thiol compounds, glutathione above all, is a significant factor in the regulation of signal transduction to appropriate genes. This signal transduction pathway is effectuated via so called redox sensors which react to any change of concentration of intracellular thiols responsible for upkeeping of the cellular redox status. Numerous regulatory transcription factors supress transcription if bound in reduced state to regulatory sequences of certain genes. In the absence of GSH in the cell and in the state of intensified polyol metabolic pathway, the oxidized form of regulatory nuclear transcription factors loses the affinity for regulatory gene sequence, which results in increased transcription and synthesis of appropriate functional and structural proteins responsible for complications in diabetes and dysregulation of glucose metabolism homeostasis. Disturbed redox potential initiates the activation of stress-signaling cascade, resulting in direct activation of other kinases and transcription factors and/or indirect modulation (oxidation) of cysteine-rich redox-sensitive proteins, such as thioredoxin and glutathione S-transferase (Adler et al., 1999).

2.1 Modulation of cell signal transduction

Results of recent clinical and experimental *in vivo* and *in vitro* studies unequivocally suggest that DM is a disease followed by intensified oxidative stress which modulates numerous cell transduction pathways (Pavlović et al.,2002;Tomlinson & Gardiner,2008). This eventually results in tissue damage and the emergence of numerous diabetic complications, including peripheral neuropathy.

Hyperglycemia leading to oxidative stress induces diabetic complications via two signaling pathways: activation of protein kinase C (PKC) (Tomkin, 2001), and activation of mitogen-activated protein kinases (MAPK) (Tomlinson, 1999). PKC represents a family of multifunctional enzymes synthesized on at least three separate genes. They play a fundamental role in signal transduction in various tissues via phosphorylation (up and down regulation) of enzymes, receptors, transcription factors, and other kinases. PKC family consists of at least 11 isoforms, out of which 9 are activated by way of lipid secondary messenger diacylglycerol (DAG). High glucose concentration increases the level of DAG stimulating de novo synthesis of DAG, which activates PKC. Hyperglycemia can also activate PKC isoforms via AGE receptors (Portilla et al., 2000) and by increased activity of the polyol pathway (Keogh, Dunlop & Larkins,1997.), probably by incresing reactive oxygen species (ROS). Intensified DAG-PKC signaling pathway is responsible for the disorders which represent the basic mechanisms in the development of vascular complications in diabetes mellitus.

In the complex process of signal transduction there are interactions of numerous receptor proteins and impulses are being amplified, so that joint, cascade pathways of signal transduction may be talked about. One of these pathways is the PKC-MAPK signal transduction pathway (Tomlinson & Gardiner,2008). Specific isoforms of PKC can activate MAPK, which via phosphorylation of transcription factors lead to altered expression of certain genes, making conditions for the change of cellular phenotype, apoptosis, or survival with a resultant disbalance producing complications in particular organs and systems. Thus MAPK activation represents a key event in the development of diabetic complications, especially diabetic neuropathy. Activation of this signaling pathway induces changes at the level of ion channels or disturbed gene expression, directly leading to nerve conduction disorders and development of axonopathy.

MAP kinases are group of serin/threonine specific kinases which are activated in response to extracellular stimuli through dual phosphorylation at conserved threonine and tyrosine residues. There are three main groups of MAP kinases: extracellular signal-regulated protein kinases (ERK), p38 and c-Jun N-terminal kinases (JNK). Results of recent clinical and experimental *in vivo* and *in vitro* studies show that all three groups of MAP kinases are activated in sensory neurons in hyperglicemia conditions in both diabetic rats and patients. (Purves at al, 2001) . In general the JNK and p38 group mediate responses to osmotic stress and is likely to be involved in the regulation of aldose reductase expression . Activation of p38 MAPK results in generating reduced nerve conduction velocity (NCV). These changes in NCV results from phosphorilation of the sodium channel Na 1.6 (Wittmack et al., 2005), which is the main voltage-activated channel at the node of Ranvier in myelinated fibres. In later stages of DM, other factors prevail: neurofilaments perturbation occurs, as a result of JNK activation and hyperphosphorylation of neurofilament proteins.

2.2 Antioxidant protection

The biological oxidative effects of free radicals on macromolecules are controlled by a spectrum of enzymatic and nonenzymatic antioxidants. Intracellular antioxidative defense is primarily enabled by the antioxidative enzymes, most significant of which are SOD, CAT and GSH-Px (Andrea et al.,2004; Maritim et al., 2003; Szaleczky et al., 1999; Djordjević, 2004). These three antioxidant enzymes differ in their structure, tissue distribution and cofactors required for functioning. SOD works as the first line of enzymatic protection against superoxide radicals. This enzyme catalyses the dismutation of superoxide anion radicals into hydrogen peroxide and oxygen. Hydrogen peroxide is further metabolized by CAT and GSH-Px, and due to lower Km values, GSH-Px is active in lower concentrations of hydrogen peroxide, while CAT activity increases with increased hydrogen peroxide concentration (Djordjević, 2004; Djordjević et al.,2000). Glutathione, together with its related enzymes, comprises a system that maintains the intracellular reducing environment and acts as primary defense against excessive generation of harmful ROS.

During reduced antioxidative protection and/or increased production of free radicals, OS occurs, playing an important role as a mediator of the apoptosis of both neurons and supportive glial cells, which has been confirmed in studies using animal models and tissue cultures (Schmeichel et al.,2003; Russel et al., 1999;Russel et al., 2002; Polydefkis et al., 2003; Person et al., 2003; Chiarelli et al., 2000; Sakaue et al., 2003).

2.2.1 Superoxide dismutase (SOD)

SOD catalyzes the conversion of superoxide anion into hydrogen peroxide and oxygen.

$$O_2^{-} + O_2^{-} + 2H+ \rightarrow H_2O_2 + O_2$$

SOD activity was originally described by McCord and Fridovich in 1969 (Szaleczky et al., 1999); they subsequently established that this enzyme is essential in sustaining life in aerobic conditions (McCord et al.,1971). There are several forms of SOD. These are metalloproteins, each containing a metal ion in its center (CuZn SOD, Mn SOD, Fe SOD, and Ni SOD) (Fridovich,1998). Fe SOD can be found in procaryotes and plants, while in humans intra- and extracellular CuZn SOD as well as mitochondrial Mn SOD were identified.
Intracellular CuZn is composed of two identical subunits (Tainer et al.,1982), each containing Cu (II) and Zn (II). Cu (II) is responsible for catalytic activity of SOD, while Zn (II) has a role in the stabilization of enzyme conformation (Djordjević, 2004). Cytosolic CuZn SOD can be inactivated by hydrogen peroxide, leading to the formation of either Cu (II) - OH or the ionized form Cu (II) -O-. This enzyme can further catalyze peroxidation of various substances. The gene coding for CuZn SOD is located on chromosome 21. In connection with that, the results of some studies have demonstrated a significantly elevated activity of this enzyme in the patients with Down syndrome (*Kurobe et al.,1990*).
Extracellular SOD (ECSOD) is structurally similar to intracellular SOD, but it is present in the extracellular space. The gene for ECSOD is located on the chromosome 4. ECSOD is a tetrameric glycoprotein, each subunit of which contains a Cu and Zn atom and has a high affinity for heparin sulphate, enabling its existence in relatively high concentrations in specific regions of extracellular space or on the cell surface. ECSOD expression is principally regulated by cytokines, such as IFNγ, which stimulates the enzyme expression, while TNFα and TGFβ reduce its expression (Marklund,1992). Reduced ECSOD expression lead to reduced mitochondrial GSH and increased oxidative stress (Lebovitz RM et al.,1996). ECSOD is also significant in modulating NO activity. The superoxide can react with NO and form peroxynitrite, which by way of dissociation can form both hydroxil radical and nitric dioxyde, potent oxydants (Fukai T et all, 2000; Oury TD et al., 1996).
Mitochondrial SOD (MnSOD) is located in the mitochondrial matrix. There are two isoforms of MnSOD, dimeric MnSOD and tetrameric MnSOD, each subunit of which contains one Mn (III) ion. It is produced in a constitutive manner, but can also be induced by IL-1, TNF, or an endotoxin (Tang et al.,1994). In addition to cytokines, numerous oxygen metabolites can also induce MnSOD expression in particular cell types, which can be of critical importance in the occurrence of tissue damage in the situation of oxidative stress (Djordjević, 2004; Yoshioka T et al.,1994). It is believed that transcriptional regulation of MnSOD is mediated by the activation of nuclear transcription factor κB (NF- κB), supported by oxidants. Congenital complete inactivity of MnSOD lead to lethal outcome within few days after birth due to renal dysfunction (Lebovitz RM et al.,1996).

2.2.2 Catalase (CAT)

Catalase is a homotetrameric enzyme found in the tissues of almost all mammals, and demonstrating the highest activity in the liver and erythrocytes. Within the cell, catalase is localized primarily in the peroxisomes and mitochondria. The principal role of catalase lies in the degradation of H_2O_2, produced with support of peroxisomal oxidases. In the erythrocytes, catalase constitues the first line of defense against H_2O_2 (Mueller et al., 1997). In the situations of normal H_2O_2 concentration, the reaction goes towards H_2O_2 conversion into water and oxygen:

$$\text{Catalaza} + 2\,H_2O_2 \rightarrow \text{Compaund I} + H_2O$$

$$\text{Compaund I} + H_2O_2 \rightarrow \text{Katalaza} + H_2O + O_2$$

The second H_2O_2 molecule serves as the donor of hydrogen ion.

In the situations of low H_2O_2 concentration and in the presence of small molecular electron donors, catalase may act as peroxydase as well (Ghadermarzi & Moosavi-Movahedi,1996). Catalase forms a firm bond with NADPH, which can prevent the accumulation of inactive forms of the enzyme slowly created when catalase is exposed to hydrogen peroxide. These effects of NADPH are evident in low concentrations in the cell as well (<0.1 μM) (Kirkman et al., 1987).

Numerous diseases can be accompanied with altered catalase activity. Reduced catalase activity has been documented in diabetes mellitus (DM), malignant diseases, Down syndrome, as well as in regenerating tissues and in experimental conditions of nephrotoxicity (Djordjević et al., 2000). Since catalase has a predominant role in the control of H_2O_2 concentration (Mueller et al., 1997; Gaetani et al., 1996), which has been shown to damage pancreatic β cells and inhibits insulin activity (Murata et al.,1998; Tiedge et al., 1998; Jorns et al., 1999), it is believed that catalase in that manner protects β cells from the harmful action of H_2O_2 (Murata et al.,1998).

In the literature, two categories of genetic deficiency of erythrocyte catalase have been described (Eaton and Ma, 1995): acatalasemia (<10% of normal activity) and hypocatalasemia (about 50% of normal activity). In Hungary, a family with acatalasemia and 12 families with hypocatalasemia have been reported (Góth & Eaton, 2000; Góth, 1992; Vitai & Góth, 1997). These families comprised 2 acatalasemic individuals, 61 individuals had hypocatalasemia, while 66 individuals had normal values of catalase. In the group with hereditary catalase deficiency, the incidence of diabetes was 12.7%. DM was diagnosed in 8 persons, in both acatalasemic and 6 persons with hypocatalasemia; all of them had DM type 2. None of those with normal catalase values had DM. These data can indicate the significance of catalase in the pathogenesis of DM.

2.2.3 Glutathione peroxidase (GSH-Px)

GSH-Px is a selenium-dependent enzyme naturally occurring in three isoforms. The so called „classical" GSH-Px is a homotetramer with a molecular mass of 80 kDa, containing four atoms of selenium. GSH-Px demonstrates a special affinity for hydrogen peroxide and glutathione (Djordjević, 2004). It reduces H_2O_2 and organic alkaline hydroperoxides into water and appropriate alcohols, and oxidizes GSH into an appropriate disulfide (GSSG).

$$2GSH + H_2O_2\ (ROOH) \rightarrow GSSG + ROH + H2O$$

GSSG is converted back into GSH by glutathione reductase, which utilizes NADPH for its activity. It is thought that NAD(P)H, by itself, as an antioxidant, can act as a scavenger of toxic free radicals, as well as the radicals originating from repaired biomolecules (Kirsch and De Groot, 2001). The classical, selenium-dependent GSH-Pxs, isolated from various organs (erythrocytes, liver, lungs), demonstrate similar features and catalytic properties regardless of their origin. The maximum rate of reaction of GSH-Px depends on the concentrations of GSH and H_2O_2. In contrast to catalase, GSH-Px demonstrates a higher affinity for the substrate (H_2O_2) at low H_2O_2 concentrations, since the Michaelis constant (K_M) of peroxidase is lower than that of catalase. That is why GSH-Px plays a key role in the tissue detoxication from H_2O_2 at low H_2O_2 concentrations and normal GSH concentrations, while catalase is actively involved at higher H_2O_2 concentrations in the cell. The role of GSH-Px in erythrocytes is predominantly associated with detoxification from organic hydroperoxides and with keeping in reduced state the SH groups of structural and functional erythrocyte proteins, while its role in H_2O_2 degradation is of a lesser significance compared to catalase. The activity of erythrocyte selenium-dependent GSH-Px correlates with the erythrocyte content of selenium, so that the activity of this enzyme can be used as a functional index to assess selenium deficiency.

The second type of peroxidase is extracellular GSH-Px, with a molecular mass of 21.5 kDa. It is a tetramer too, the subunits of which contain an atom of selenium each. It is thought that extracellular GSH-Px is most important regarding the reduction of H_2O_2 in the plasma. GSH-Px in the plasma is a glycoprotein, believed to be most probably a secretory enzyme released from organ cells into the plasma. This enzyme demonstrates significant kinetic differences compared to erythrocyte GSH-Px. In contrast to erythrocyte GSH-Px, GSH-Px in the plasma demonstrates saturation kinetics compared to GSH (Đorđević et all, 2000). The activity of this enzyme declines with increased glutathione via the value of saturation concentration for GSH of 5 mmol. Moreover, GSH-Px in the plasma demonstrates higher affinity for organic hydroperoxides and H_2O_2. It is thought that selenium-dependent plasma GSH-Px is responsible for the process of detoxication from H_2O_2 and organic hydroperoxides created in the process of synthesis of eicosanoids in entothelial cells (Đorđević et all, 2000). Although the concentration of reduced glutathione in the plasma is very low, it is conceivable that the change in glutathione concentration (interorgan distribution, release from the liver into the plasma) can modulate the enzyme activity.

The third type of peroxidase is phospholipid hydroperoxide GSH-Px (PHGpx). It is too a selenium-dependent enzyme which differs from the first two types in view of the substrate and localization. PHGpx is a monomer, with the molecular mass of 23 kDa. This enzyme has a special characteristic – it directly reduces lipid hydroperoxides in the membranes.

Reduced GSH-Px activity can be found in numerous pathologic conditions and diseases, such as in chronic etilism, chronic renal insufficiency, hypertension, endemic nephropathy (Djordjević et all 1998). Altered GSH-Px activity can also be detected in DM (Kaji et al., 1985; Cser et al., 1993; Matkovics et al., 1982).

GSH-Px activity in the nervous system is low (in both peripheral nerves and in the central nervous system). Low values of GSH-Px compared to catalase activity in the peripheral nerves could lead to the conclusion that this enzyme has a minor role in H_2O_2 inactivation. However, GSH-Px function is prominent in the mitochondria, where the enzyme is necessary for the inactivation of H_2O_2 generated during the electron transport (McClain and Crook , 1996) where the catalase activity is insufficient.

2.2.4 Glutathione (GSH)

Glutathione is one of the most important nonenzymatic antioxidant in mammal cells. This ubiquitous tripeptide (γ-Glu-Cys-Gly) accounts for 90% of total non-protein sulphydril compounds in the cell. In the cell, it is most commonly found as a thiol – in a reduced form – and less as a disulfide – in an oxidized form (Toyokuni, 1996; Hann et al., 1990; Natarajan, 1995).

GSH concentration in the cell is determined by the control of enzymes involved in its synthesis, availability of synthesis precursors, intensity of GSH depletion for cellular detoxification processes, interorgan GSH distribution, as well as GSH regeneration in the so called glutathione redox cycle.

Erythrocytes represent a unique transport system for glutathione and its conjugates. In contrast to other cells, GSH appears in erythrocytes in several intermediary metabolic forms. In physiologic conditions, reduced GSH form appears in the highest percentage. The other GSH form is oxidized glutathione (GSSG), occurring in the process of nonenzymatic oxidation or oxidation mediated by GSH-peroxidase. The third erythrocyte form is the disulphide form of glutathione bound to proteins and non-protein sulphydril compounds. Glutathione S-conjugates (occurring via the action of glutathione S-transferase) are the fourth potential intracellular-intermediary form of GSH in the erythrocytes. Erythrocytes take up toxic molecules from the plasma, to be excreted back into plasma after conjugation with GSH. Further detoxification of S-conjugates continues in the liver and kidneys; non-toxic compounds are then excreted from the organism via the bile or urine.

GSH is involved in many cellular functions. Many cells synthesize GSH *de novo* by γ-glutamyl transferase, forming firstly a γ-peptide bond between one cystein and one glutamate residue. The next phase is the addition of glycine, assisted by GSH synthetase. Neurons do not contain γ-glutamyl-cystein synthetase; instead, GSH is synthesized in the glial cells controlling this synthesis via the mechanisms of transcription regulation (Iwata-Ichikawa et al., 1999; Keelan et al., 2001). It is thought that during the evolution, depending on the cellular metabolic needs, glutathione is engaged in the regulation of different processes. Though the role of glutathion has been commonly associated with the protection of the cell from active free radicals, glutathione is involved in many other processes such as detoxification from xenobiotics, synthesis of eicosanoids, synthesis of nucleic acids and proteins, cell signaling, proliferation, and differentiation (Djordjević,2000). However, its essential role lies in the protective antioxidant system. GSH, GSH-Px, GSH-transferase, GSH-reductase, and NAD(P)H constitute an antioxidant system of glutathione, in which GSH-reductase and NAD(P)H are required for the reduction of oxidized glutathione and consequential glutathione recycling in the so called glutathione redox cycle. Depletion of GSH in the cell increases its sensitivity to oxidative damage (Rizzardini et al., 2003). In contrast, accumulation of GSH in the cell, especially in the mitochondria, can prevent neural apoptosis caused by ischemia (Li et al., 2002) and excitotoxicity (Kobayashi et al., 2000). The involvement of GSH in the limitation of prooxidative cell status, has as the ultimate consequence deceleration of aging, atherogenesis, mutagenesis, and cancerogenesis (Anghileri and Thouvenot ,1997; Vostreis et al., 1988)

3. Aim of study

Research in patients with diabetic neuropathy (DN) is mainly based on studying the influence of antioxidative substances on certain biomarkers of oxidative stress and on the function of peripheral nerves (Ziegler et al., 1995; Reljanović et al., 1999; Ziegler et al., 1999; Ametov et al., 2003; Ziegler and Gries, 1997; Ziegler et al., 1997). However, there are no enough studies, testing the direct correlation between prooxidative/antioxidative parameters and the development of DN, especially in humans. Additional difficulties occur when different kinds of reactive oxygen are directly determined in biological systems due to their short life. For this reason, the measurement of oxidative stress is mainly based on indirect and non-specific measurement of products of their activity.

Considering that antioxidant enzymes are important biomarkers of oxidative stress, the aim of this study was to determine the activities of antioxidant enzymes (SOD, CAT, GSH-Px) and glutathione in the erythrocytes of patients with type 2 diabetes mellitus (DM) in relation to presence or absence of distal symmetrical polyneuropathy (DSP), as well as to analyze the possible connection between the activity of these antioxidant parameters and the function of peripheral nerves. In this way we tried to determine the level of antioxidant defense in erythrocytes of diabetic patients and to establish the potential role of oxidative stress in the development of diabetic neuropathy.

4. Materials and methods

The research took the form of a prospective study, which included 100 patients suffering from type 2 DM and diabetic distal symmetric polyneuropathy (DDSP). Patients suffering from another acute or chronic illness, patients previously subjected to cytotoxic therapy or radiotherapy, and patients who had been treated with antioxidative substances were excluded from the experimental group. The control group gathered 50 healthy individuals who denied ailments and diseases and whose clinical observations and laboratory tests showed no abnormalities. The DDSP was diagnosed after clinical and electrophysiological testing.

The electrophysiological testing checked the conductivity of sensory and motor fibers of upper and lower extremity peripheral nerves. Due to the symmetric nature of the disease, the protocol included the unilateral (right) testing of sural, peroneal, tibial, ulnar and median nerves. We analyzed the latency, amplitude, and conduction velocity of the tested nerves. The minimal criterion for the electrophysiological validation of diabetic neuropathy (DN) was the abnormality of any electroneurographic (ENG) conduction parameter in at least two nerves, one of which had to be sural nerve (England et al., 2005). The values of tested electroneurographic parameters were expressed as the score from 1 to 4, where 1 corresponded to a normal result, while 4 meant that the motor or sensory evoked potential was absent. The ENG testing was carried out on the ENG device (Schwartzer, Mios 2+). During the testing, the surface electrodes were used: the stimulation electrode - for the electrical stimulation of the peripheral nerve and the registration electrode - for the registration of the motor evoked potential (MEP). In order to increase the diagnostic sensitivity of the electrophysiological tests, in addition to the standard ENG, we also tested the conduction sensitivity of the median plantar nerve. Since the sensory evoked potential (SEP) amplitude of medial plantar nerve is distinctly low, a separate technique was used to test this on an evoked potential device (Medelec Sapphire 2). A large number (236) of stimuli were used and the values were subsequently averaged by the computer. The following parameters were analyzed: the peak latency of the sensory neurogram, expressed in milliseconds, and the amplitude of the sensory neurogram, expressed in μV. The stimulation was carried out with a surface electrode positioned on the plantar part of the thumb. The response was registered via a surface electrode located behind the internal malleolus, proximal to the retinaculum flexorum.

Laboratory analysis determined the level of morning glycemia and glycosylated hemoglobin (HbA1c) by the standard laboratory tests from the venous blood of patients and halthy persons. Erythrocyte SOD activity was determined by a commercial test Ransod provided by Randox (Randox Laboratories, Crumlin, UK), based on the McCord and Fridovich method (Mccord and Fridovich, 1969). Erythrocyte CAT activity was determined by the method of Beutler (*Beutler, 1982*). Erythrocyte GSH-Px activity was determined by commercial test Ransel (Randox Laboratories, Crumlin, UK). Glutathione was measured as total glutathione in the erythrocytes as described by Tietze (1969). Caiman's GSH Assay kit utilizes a carefully optimized enzymatic recycling method, using glutathione reductase for quantification of GSH.

Statistical method: To process results we used widely accepted statistical techniques: means and standard deviation, statistical significance calculation tests, correlation tests. We utilized standard statistics software tools (Origin Pro and MATLAB Statistics Toolbox). The results are presented as mean ± SD.

5. Results

The study encompassed 100 type 2 DM patients who showed signs of distal symmetrical polyneuropathy, whose average age was 58.62±11.62 years. The average duration of the disease was 11.32±7.05 years. The control group included 50 healthy individuals, whose average age was 51.64±12.25 years (Tab. 1). There was significant increase in glycemia and HbA1c values in the patients compared with the control group (*p<0. 0001).

	Number	Sex(M/F)	Age (years) mean ±SD	Duration of DM (years)	Glycemia (mmol/L) mean ±SD	HbA1C (%) mean ±SD
Control	50	22 / 28	51.64±12.25	0	4.81 ±0.63	5.73 ± 0.56
Patients without DSP	40	24 / 16	57.73±11.08	11.23±7.94	8.99±3.11*	9.26 ± 3.33*
Patients with DSP	100	55 / 45	58.62±11.62	11.32±7.05	9.50 ±4.13*	9.09 ±2.13*

Table 1. Demographic and biochemical characteristics of diabetic neuropathy patients and the control group.

There was a statistically significant decrease SOD and GSH-Px activity and GSH level in erythrocyte of diabetic neuropatrhy patients compared with the control group and patients without DN. The values of erythrocyte CAT were lower in patients compared to the control ones, but this difference did not reach statistical significance (Tab. 2).

	SOD (U/gr Hb) mean ±SD	CAT (U/gr Hb) mean ±SD	GSH-Px(U/gr Hb) mean ±SD	GSH (μmol/grHb) mean ±SD
Control	1238.36 ± 136.86	7.34 ± 1.62	67.35 ± 11.39	0.24 ± 0.05
Patients without DSP	1144.26 ± 103.92**	7.22 ± 2.01	55.63 ±13.07**	0.22 ± 0.05**
Patients with DSP	1101.00 ± 64.36**,*	6.68 ± 1.26	50.25 ± 10.42**,*	0.21 ± 0.04**

Table 2. SOD and CAT in the diabetic neuropathy patients and in the control group. ** p<0,001 vs. control, * p<0,05 vs. patients without DN

Values of antioxidant parameters were variable at different stages of the disease in patients with DDSP (Fig. 1-4).

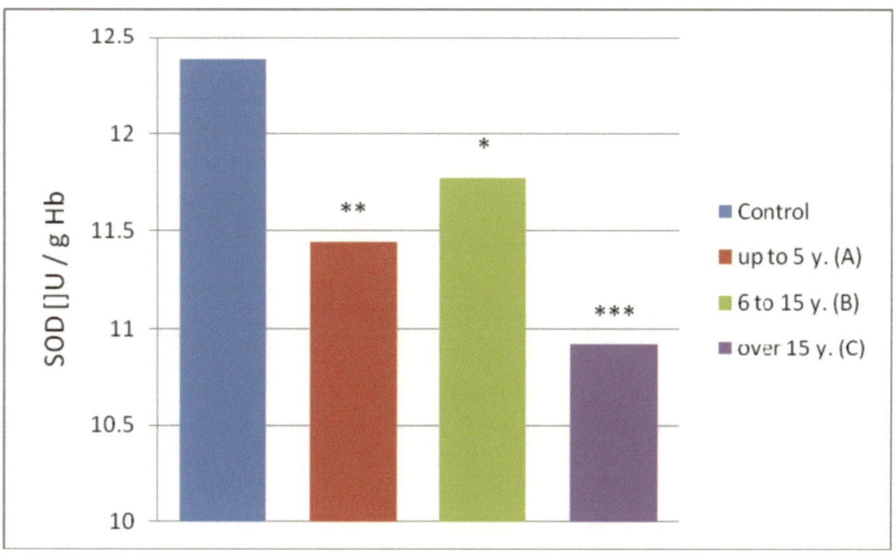

* p<0.05 vs. control; **p<0.01 vs. control; *** p<0.001 vs. control; A:B p=0.202; A:C p<0.05; B:C p<0.001, y. =year

Fig. 1. SOD values in different periods of illness in patients with DDSP as compared to the control group

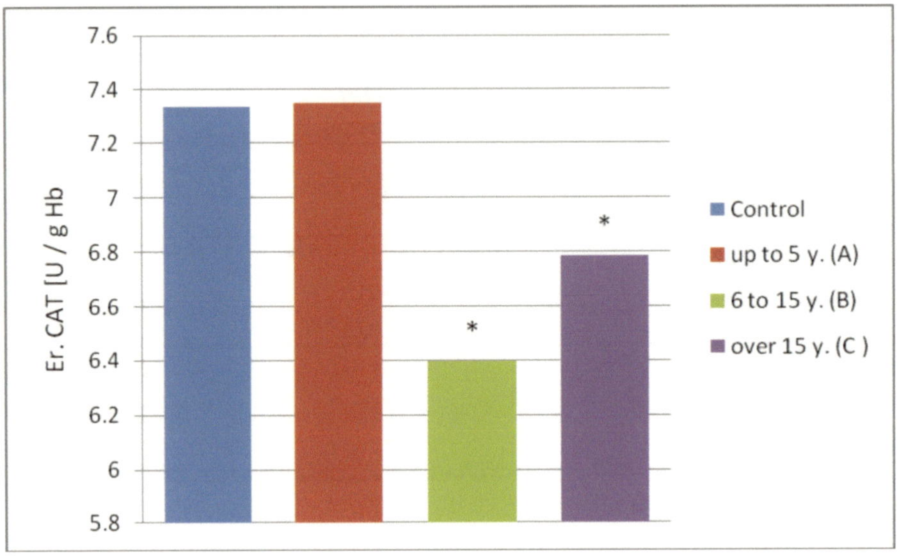

Fig. 2. Erythrocite CAT values in different periods of illness in patients with DDSP as compared to the control group * $p<0.05$ vs. control, A:B $p<0.01$; A:C $p=0.15$; B:C $p=0.24$, y.= year

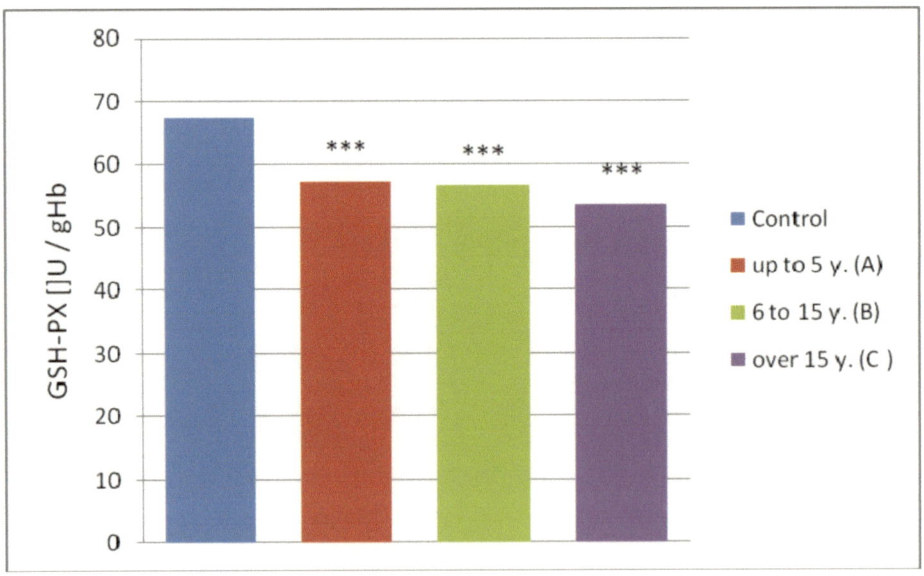

*** $p<0.001$ vs. control A:B $p=0.97$; A:C $p=0.38$; B:C $p=0.28$, y= year

Fig. 3. GSH-PX values in different periods of illness in patients with DDSP as compared to the control group

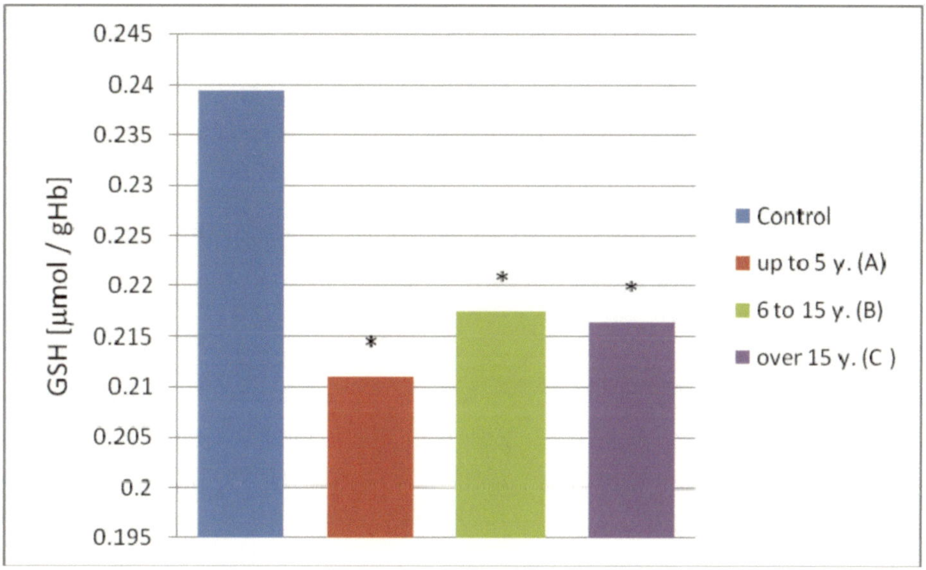

Fig. 4. GSH values in erythrocytes in different periods of illness in patients with DDSP as compared to the control group * $p<0.05$ vs. control A:B $p=0.4$; A:C $p=0.5$; B:C $p=0.9$, y= year

There was statistically significant difference between the latency and amplitude of sensory evoked potentials (SEP) of *medial plantar nerve* in the patients and the controls (Tab. 3).

SEP n.plantaris medialis	Patients mean± SD	Controls mean ± SD	t	p
Latency [ms]	7.50 ± 1.36	5.56 ± 0.89	-8.90	<0. 0001
Amplitude [µV]	0.381± 0.358	0.849 ± 0.606	5.37	<0. 0001

Table 3. Latency and amplitude of the SEP of medial plantar nerve in the diabetic neuropathy patients and in the control

All electrophysiological parameters related to the conduction of motor and sensory fibers of the tested upper and lower extremity nerves showed that there was a statistically significant difference between diabetic neuropathy patients and controls (Tab. 4).

ENG parameters		Controls mean±SD	Patients mean±SD	t	p
CMAP peroneal nerve	Latency (ms)	3.54±0.56	4.66±1.13	-6.64	<0. 0001
	Amplitude (mV)	5.77±2.47	3.46±2.13	5.88	<0. 0001
	NCV (m/s)	51.65±5.79	41.24±6.77	9.20	<0. 0001
CMAP tibial nerve	Latency (ms)	3.56±0.51	4.94±1.32	-7.13	<0. 0001
	Amplitude (mV)	11.19±4.73	4.62±2.98	10.28	<0. 0001
	NCV (m/s)	43.37±3.07	35.72±7.30	7.083	<0. 0001
CMAP median nerve	Latency (ms)	3.45±0.55	4.88±2.24	-4.47	<0. 0001
	Amplitude (mV)	7.00±2.51	4.90±2.35	5.23	<0. 0001
	NCV (m/s)	56.57±7.01	49.52±6.22	6.27	<0. 0001
CMAP ulnar nerve	Latency (ms)	2.90±0.63	3.17±0.78	-2.12	0. 0359
	Amplitude (mV)	7.87±3.35	4.93±7.27	6.36	0. 0025
	NCV (m/s)	57.54±8.57	48.59±8.00	6.30	<0. 001
SEP sural nerve	Latency (ms)	2.93±0.50	4.14±0.90	-8.60	<0. 0001
	Amplitude (mV)	15.61±6.16	8.79±5.77	6.31	<0. 0001
	NCV (m/s)	36.37±4.48	29.49±6.35	6.63	<0. 0001
SEP median nerve	Latency (ms)	3.96±0.49	4.70±0.82	-5.83	<0. 0001
	Amplitude (mV)	43.07±9.33	15.75±9.70	16.47	<0. 0001
	NCV (m/s)	47.36±5.63	38.77±7.85	6.86	<0. 0001
SEP ulnar nerve	Latency (ms)	3.28±0.68	4.12±0.82	-6.23	<0. 0001
	Amplitude (mV)	36.46±11.63	17.28±12.22	9.16	<0. 0001
	NCV (m/s)	46.32±6.10	38.20±7.37	6.69	<0. 0001

Table 4. ENG parameters in the diabetic neuropathy patients and in the control group. CMAP - compound muscle action potential, SEP - sensory evoked potentials, NCV-nerve conduction velocity

A number of scored ENG parameters correlated significantly with erythrocyte SOD and CAT level in the patients studied (Tab. 5 and Tab. 6).

SEP of medial plantar nerve	SOD		CAT		GSH-px		GSH	
	r	p	r	p	r	p	r	p
Latency	-0.1621	0.1071	-0.0488	0.6295	-0.1149	0.2550	-0.0492	0.6265
Amplitude	0.0995	0.3248	0.2059	**0.0399**	0.0580	0.5564	-0.0570	0.5734

Table 5. Correlation between SEP parameters of medial plantar nerve and parameters of OS (SOD and CAT) in diabetic neuropathy patients. Marked values point out a statistically significant correlation.

Nerve	ENG parameters	SOD		CAT		GPx		GSH	
		r	p	r	p	r	p	r	p
CMAP Peroneal nerve	Latency	-0.1096	0.2777	-0.1597	0.1126	-0.0577	0.5683	-0.0605	0.5497
	Amplitude	-0.2526	**0.0112**	-0.2859	**0.0039**	-0.1096	0.2777	-0.0662	0.5129
	MEP NCV	-0.2633	**0.0081**	0.0199	0.8442	-0.1417	0.1598	0.0097	0.9238
CMAP Tibial nerve	Latency	-0.1866	0, 0630	0.0406	0.6883	0.0130	0.8977	-0.0476	0.6383
	Amplitude	-0.1575	0.1175	-0.0568	0.5747	-0.0233	0.8184	0.0148	0.8837
	NCV	-0.2524	**0.0113**	0.0254	0.8016	-0.0910	0.3681	0.0618	0.5416
CMAP Median nerve	Latency	-0.2326	**0.0199**	-0.0959	0.3425	-0.0694	0.4929	0.0140	0.8901
	Amplitude	-0.0663	0.5123	0.0188	0.8529	-0.1198	0.2352	0.1366	0.1753
	NCV	-0.2171	**0.0301**	0.0462	0.6483	-0.0469	0.6431	0.1887	0.0601
CMAP Ulnar nerve	Latency	-0.0442	0.6627	-0.0043	0.9659	-0.1294	0.1996	-0.0209	0.8366
	Amplitude	-0.1531	0.1282	0.0174	0.8639	0.0327	0.7466	0.0224	0.8252
	NCV	-0.1387	0.1687	-0.0629	0.5339	-0.0694	0.4927	-0.0655	0.5174
SEP Median nerve	Latency	-0.2183	**0.0291**	-0.0501	0.6205	-0.0771	0.4456	-0.1923	0.0552
	Amplitude	-0.0881	0.3836	-0.0057	0.9549	0.0904	0.3710	-0.1230	0.2227
	NCV	-0.2079	**0.0379**	-0.0569	0.5741	-0.1253	0.2143	-0.2805	**0.0047**
SEP Ulnar nerve	Latency	-0.1679	0.0949	-0.1659	0.0991	-0.0095	0.9252	-0.1094	0.2786
	Amplitude	-0.0213	0.8336	-0.0997	0.3239	-0.0866	0.3914	-0.1710	0.0889
	NCV	-0.1202	0.2336	-0.0627	0.5357	-0.1009	0.3178	-0.1344	0.1826
SEP Sural nerve	Latency	-0.1129	0.2636	-0.3837	**0.0001**	-0.0245	0.8088	0.0443	0.6613
	Amplitude	-0.2896	**0.0035**	-0.1449	0.1505	-0.0275	0.7861	-0.0194	0.8481
	NCV	-0.1122	0.2662	-0.3840	**0.0001**	0.0035	0.9723	0.0798	0.4298

Table 6. Correlation between ENG parameters and parameters of OS (SOD and CAT) in diabetic neuropathy patients. MEP- Motor Evoked Potential, SEP- Sensory Evoked Potentials, NCV – Nerve Conduction Velocity. Marked values point out a statistically significant correlation.

6. Discussion

Results of experimental studies, conducted both *in vivo* and *in vitro*, suggest that the peripheral nervous system is sensitive to oxidative damage (Schmeichel et al.,2003; Russel et al., 1999;Russel et al., 2002). Neurons take over glucose from the blood by the concentration dependent transport, so that hyperglycemia is always associated with increased glucose values in the neurons, which results in oxidative stress (Tomlinson and Gardiner,2008; Andrea et al.,2004). On the other hand, antioxidative defense in peripheral nerves is thought to be limited due to primary lower values of glutathione and glutathione-dependent enzymes (GSH-Px and GSH-r) (Romero et al., 1991; Schmeichel et al.,2003), which further increases the sensitivity of nerves to oxidative damage. SOD could provide efficient antioxidative protection, since, contrary to glutathione-dependent enzymes, it is relatively more active in the peripheral nerves. However, in spite of such a theoretical position, studies carried out on experimental models have not shown any significant changes of the endoneural antioxidative status in the experimentally induced DN, except an increased CAT levels which could not be able to correct by insulin therapy (Van Dam et al., 1996). On the other side, positive effects of antioxidants on the antioxidative capacity of blood, and also on the disturbed function of peripheral nerves in the very same experimental models, lead one to conclude that systemic OS can have a more significant role compared to endoneural OS in the development of neuropathic changes.

The determination of OS biomarkers is an important step in the understanding of DN pathogenesis. Recent research suggests that there are tissue- and time-dependent changes in the activity of various antioxidative enzymes. The results of our study show that there is a statistically significant reduction of erythrocyte SOD levels in patients with type 2 DM and DDSP in comparison with healthy controls, which corresponds to the data from the literature (Arai et al., 1987; Kawamura et al., 1992; Vijaylingam et al., 1996). Eerythrocyte SOD level was significantly lower in patients with diabetic neuropathy compared with patients without diabetic neuropathy, suggesting the importance of antioxidant protection in the prevention of nerve injury. The main reason for the reduced SOD activity is the glycolization of Cu, Zn-SOD, which has been documented in both *in vitro* and *in vivo* experiments (Arai et al., 1987; Kawamura et al., 1992). However, there are also studies which show no changes in erythrocyte SOD activity (Peuchant et al.,1997; Walter et al.,1991; Faure et al.,1995), or which, quite the contrary, suggest an increased activity of this enzyme (Yaqoob et al., 1994).

In most cases, CAT activity in erythrocytes was not changed in either experimental animals or type 1 and type 2 DM patients (Wohaieb & Godi, 1987; Godin et al., 1988; Matkovich et al., 1982). However, some studies have noted changes in CAT activity, in particular its reduction (Vijaylingam et al., 1996; Alphonsus et al., 2007). In this study, erythrocyte CAT values were reduced in patients as compared with the controls, but this reduction did not reach statistically significant levels, which correlates with the literature data listed above. Catalase values were reduced in patients with DSP, compared with patients without DSP, although these deviations were not statistically significant. Reduced CAT activity could be explained by the accumulation of H_2O_2 in the cells, as a result of glucose autooxidation. As the principal enzymatic role of CAT is to control H_2O_2 concentration, H_2O_2 accumulation in the cells is believed to lead to the exhaustion of this enzyme, which primarily reflects erythrocytes, where CAT is otherwise most active. Studies have shown that in other tissues H_2O_2 accumulation may stimulate CAT synthesis, thus increasing its activity. However, erythrocytes lack the genetic apparatus for such a synthesis, which is a reason that the increased H_2O_2 concentration results in the exhaustion and inactivation of catalase (Alphonsus et al., 2007).

Changes in the activity of glutathione-dependent enzymes were different in experimental models. Most studies have shown tissue and time dependent changes of enzyme activity. However, even if we acknowledge these factors, we cannot precisely match the results of various studies of the association of DM and activity of glutathione-dependent enzymes. The studies dealing with the GSH-Px activity in the erythrocytes have demonstrated variable results. A large number of studies demonstrated that GSH-Px activity in the blood, erythrocytes, and leukocytes was similar in DM patients (types 1 and 2) and in healthy controls (Walter RM et al., 1991; Leonard M.B. et al., 1995; Akkus I et al., 1996). On the other hand, there are studies clearly confirming altered activity of glutathione-dependent enzymes in DM, above all in the form of reduced activity of GSH-Px and increased activity of GSH reductase (Godin et al., 1988; Dohi et al.,1988; Tagami et al., 1992; Langenstroer & Pieper, 1992; Blakytny and Harding,1992). Murakami (1991), studying the erythrocytes in DM, concluded that reduced erythrocyte GSH was caused by reduced activity of gamma glutamyl-cystein synthetase in connection with its glycation, reduced activity of GSH-reductase and defective glutathione transport. Yoshida (1995) confirmed that in the erythrocytes of diabetics with poorly controlled disease the synthesis of GSH and thiol transport were damaged, rendering the cells more sensitive to oxidative damage. In diabetics with permanently higher values of glucose Uzel et al. (1987) established reduced GSH-Px activity and lower erythrocyte GSH values, with increased products of lipid peroxidation, with changes more apparent in patients with retinopathy. GSH reduction in the erythrocytes in DM was confirmed by Bono et al. (*1987*) as well. Stahlberg and Hietanen (1991) observed a reduced activity of GSH reductase in children with DM but Walter et al. (1991) were not able to demonstrate any difference in GSH-Px and GSH reductase activities in diabetics and nondiabetics. Kaji et al. (1985) failed to find a difference in activity of erythrocyte GSH-Px, but established increased GSH-Px activity in the plasma in women with DM. Osterod et al. (1996) found in their studies a reduced erythrocyte GSH-Px activity in DM type 1. Authors of some studies also described an increased erythrocyte GSH-Px activity in DM (Matkovics et al., 1982). Literature data mostly indicated an unaltered or reduced activity of erythrocyte GSH-Px. The results obtained in this study indicate a statistically significant reduction of GSH-Px activity both in patients with DSP and in patients without DSP, compared to controls. Erythrocyte GSH-Px values were significantly lower in patients with diabetic neuropathy compared with patients without diabetic neuropathy. Reduced GSH-Px could be directly explained by reduced GSH content in studied patients, representing otherwise a substrate and cofactor for GSH-Px enzyme.

The studies of glutathione homeostasis in DM have so far shown tissue differences in the levels of GSH, although in most of the cases reduced GSH contents have been found. The studies of glutathione level in the blood of diabetics demonstrated that those with DM type 2 had reduced erythrocyte level of GSH and increased level of GSSG (De Mattia at all, 1994; Jain & McVie, 1994). The blood level of GSH was significantly reduced in various phases of the type 2 DM, such as glucose intolerance, early hyperglycemia (Vijayalingam et al., 1996) in the first two years and before complications developed (Sundaram et al., 1996), as well as in poorly controlled glycemia (Peuchant et al., 1997). Yoshida et al. (1995) observed reduced GSH in the erythrocytes of type 2 diabetics, with disturbed activity of gamma glutamyl transferase and thiol transport. In contrast to a clear reduction of blood GSH in type 2 DM, in type 1 disease the results were not entirely convincing. The role of GSH in the occurrence of diabetes complications has not been elucidated. Thornalley et al. (1996) found an inverse correlation between the level of erythrocyte GSH and presence of diabetes complications (neuropathy, retinopathy, and nephropathy) in patients with DM type 1 and 2, leaving unanswered the question whether GSH levels were reduced in those without complications, ot these patients have an even more significant reduction GSH levels.

The results of our investigation showed a statistically significant reduction of erythrocite GSH level both in patients with DSP and in patients without DSP compared to controls, which was in accordance with the literature data. In the group of patiens without DSP, erythrocite GSH-Px value did not show larger deviations compared to patients with DSP.

Some studies of the antioxidative protection system in DM, principally in experimental animal models, were related to the study of impact of disease duration on the activity of antioxidative enzymes. Time-dependent changes of the activity of antioxidative enzymes and prooxidative-antioxidative balance were thus observed in DM in various tissues. (Majythija & Jayesh, 2005; Sasvári and Nyakas, 2003**)**. Kishi et al.(2005) based on their own study, came to the conclusion that changes in the activity of antioxidative enzymes in peripheral nerves were not the result of reduced gene expression, but can be linked to the duration of DM or posttranslational modifications.

Bearing these information in mind, this study analyzed the activity of antioxidative enzymes and glutathione in the blood of patients which disease had lasted up to 5 years, 5-15 years, and over 15 years. The activity of SOD enzyme was generally lower in patients in each phase of the disease, though the reduction was variable. The smallest reduction was observed in the first 5 years of DM, while the reduction was most evident in advanced disease phases - in those affected for more than 15 years. More intense inactivation of SOD in more advanced DM could be explained by increased production of H_2O_2 in the processes of non-enzymatic glycation predominating with time, which can further inhibit SOD. In the group of those affected for 5-15 years, a slight increase of SOD activity can be observed related to other two groups, which can be explained by an adaptive increase of antioxidative protection pathways. Increased H_2O_2 production inhibited SOD activity, but, on the other hand, formation of superoxide radicals presents a signal for increased gene expression of SOD (Matsuyama et al. 1993). Available amount and activity of SOD should represent a balance between the enzyme production and its degradation. As shown here, the balance demonstrated time-dependent modulation in different disease phases.

The activity of erythrocyte catalase also demonstrated a declining tendency, with the smallest decline in the first 5 years of DM. The decline of catalase activity was greatest in those affected for 5-15 years. In this group, the values of erythrocyte catalase were significantly different from control ones.

In all groups, a statistically significant reduction of erythrocyte GSH level was observed compared to controls. Among the groups of different disease phases, there was no statistically significant difference in the erythrocyte GSH level.

Changes were observed also with the enzyme associated with glutathione metabolism – GSH-Px. This enzyme demonstrated a statistically significant decline of activity in all disease phases compared to controls. The decline was most evident in advanced DM (>15 years), though there were no statistically significant deviations among the individual groups of patients in different disease phases. Reduced GSH-Px activity can be directly explained by low GSH content in diabetics, in view of the fact that GSH is the substrate and cofactor of GSH-Px. Reduced GSH-Px activity can be caused by the enzyme inactivation as the consequence of increased glycation in the situation of hyperglycemia. Increased glycation and consequential protein reactions can affect amino acids in active enzyme domain or disturb stereochemical configuration and cause structural and functional molecular changes (Bonnefont-Rousselot et al., 2000). Reduced GSH-Px activity causes H_2O_2 accumulation, which also contributes to progressive reduction of activity of SOD in advanced DM.

These changes in the activity of antioxidative enzymes in DM confirm the notion that disturbed carbohydrate metabolism have an impact on the function of antioxidative protection which by itself can affect the development of late complications of DM. In recent years, it has been definitely confirmed that the frequency of late diabetic complications is higher with poorer metabolic control. If oxidative stress has a role in the development of diabetic complications, we should expect adaptive changes in the system of antioxidative protection. These changes would be more or less evident in different situations of metabolic control and largely depend on the duration of unfavorable metabolic status.

Similarly to the literature data, our results suggest that blood of type 2 DM patients has decreased antioxidative protection. However, in spite of strong evidence in the literature that OS is increased in DM, there is still no definite connection between OS levels and the development of late diabetic complications. Accordingly, in this study, we have looked into the interrelation between the tested antioxidative enzyme levels and the functional damage of peripheral nerves. Our previous study did not show any correlation between plasma total antioxidant capacity (TAC) and the degree of damage of peripheral nerves in type 2 DM and DDSP patients (Djordjević et al., 2008). Having in mind that TAC is not a mere sum of various antioxidant activity, but a dynamical system of interdependent individual serum antioxidant parameters (Koraćević et al., 2001), we have designed this study in such a way as to observe and analyze the influence of individual TAC constituents on the development of peripheral nerve dysfunction in type 2 DM patients.

All electroneurographic parameters of peripheral nerve conduction have showed deviation in the patients as compared with the control group and these deviations have been statistically significant. In the studied patients, we have found a significant negative linear correlation between erythrocyte SOD levels and a number of scored ENG parameters - indicators of DDSP (the lower the SOD values, the higher the ENG score, i.e. the more pronounced the functional damage). The correlation that was found between SOD and ENG indicators of the degree of neuronal damage indicates that there was an important role of toxic effects of superoxide anion radicals in the development of neuronal damage. In vivo, superoxide anion radicals are mostly removed enzymatically, by SOD. When superoxide anion radicals are excessively produced, they react with nitric oxide and form a peroxynitrite, which has numerous cytotoxic effects. A tenfold increase in superoxide anion radicals and nitric oxide has been found to increase peroxynitrite production one hundred times (Djordjević et al.,2000). Excessive production of superoxide anion radicals, nitric oxide and peroxynitrite may, thus, be a significant pathogenetic factor for neuronal damage.

As for catalase, even though the reduced activity of this enzyme did not reach statistical significance in this study, the correlation analysis between CAT blood levels and the electrophysiological conduction parameters of the peroneal, sural, median, and plantar nerves (MEP-amplitude of peroneal nerve, the latency and NCV of the sural nerve, the SEP amplitude of medial plantar nerve) has revealed a statistically significant value. Such results suggest that CAT has a pathogenetic importance, i.e. that hydrogen peroxide has toxic effects on the degree of neuronal damage.

There was no correlation between erythrocite GSH-Px and ENG parameters which could be explained by lower Km and lower GSH-Px activity in erythrocytes, compared to CAT activity. Erythrocite GSH-Px value correlated with censory nerve condaction of median nerve only. This results could be explained by limited activity of GSH and GSH-dependent enzymes in periferal nerves. It should also bear in mind that the values of GSH and GSH-px in our group of patients showed small variation over the course of DM, which could also be the explanation for the lack of correlation with the ENG parameters, given the progressive course of diabetic neuropathy.

7. Conclusion

DM is closely linked to an imbalance in pro/antioxidant status of cells and changes in redox potential. Oxidative stress, as a common denominator, is the biochemical mechanism by which disturbed glucose metabolism and deregulation of cell signaling leads to the development of diabetic complications. Results of our study pointed out a reduced systemic antioxidative defense in the patients with type 2 DM and diabetic distal symmetrical polyneuropathy and indicate that systemic oxidative stress plays a potential role in the development of diabetic neuropathy. For better understanding of the role of oxidative stress and antioxidative mechanisms, further investigations with standardized methodology, molecular biological technique and better defined experimental models and subjects are required, aiming to prevent, delay or slow the progression of the disease.

8. References

Adler, V.; Yin Z.; Tew K.D.; Ronai Z.(1999). Role of redox potential and reactive oxygen species in stress signalling. *Oncogene*, 18:6104-6111.

Akkus, I.; Kalak, S.; Vural, H.; Caglayan, O.; Menekse, E.; Can, G.; Durmus, B. (1996). Leukocyte lipid peroxidation, superoxide dismutase, glutathione peroxidase and serum and leukocyte vitamin C levels of patients with type II diabetes mellitus. *Clinica Chimica Acta*, 244, 221-227.

Aliciguzel, Y.; Ozen, I.; Aslan, M.; Karayalcin, U. (2003). Activities of xanthine oxidoreductase and antioxidant enzymes in different tissues of diabetic rats. *J Lab Clin Med* , 142(3):172-177

Alphonsus, E.U.; Iya, N.; Okon, E.; Mary, N. (2007). Red cell catalase activity in diabetics. *Pakistan Journal of nutrition* 6 (5): 511-515.

Ametov, A.S;, Barinov, A.; Dyck, P.J.; Hermann, R.; Kozlova, N.; Litchy, W.J.; et al (2003). The sensory symptoms of diabetic polyneuropathy are improved with alpha-lipoic acid: the SYDNEY trial. *Diabetes Care* 26 (3): 770–6.

Anghileri, L.J.; Thouvenot, P. (1997). Non-transferrin-bound iron and tumor cells. Anticancer research, 17(4A):2529-33.

Arai, K.; Iizuka, S.; Tada, Y.; Oikawa, K.; Taniguchi, N. (1987). Increase in the glucosylated form of erythrocyte Cu-Zn-superoxide dismutase in diabetes and close association of the nonenzymatic glucosylation with the enzyme activity. *Biochimica et Biophysica Acta* 924: 292-296.

Beutler, E. (1982). CatalaseIn: Beutler E (ed). Red cell metabolism, a manual and biochemical method. 3rd ed. *Grune and Stratton, New York*, pp 105–6.

Blakytny, R.; Harding, J.J. (1992). Glycation (non-enzymatic glycosylation) inactivates glutathione reductase. *Biochem J*, 288:303-307.

Bonnefont-Rousselot, D.; Bastard, J.P.; Jaudon, M.C.; Delattre, J. (2000). Consequences of the diabetic status on the oxidant/antioxidant balance. *Diabetes & Metabolism*,26,:163-176

Bono, A.; Caimi, G.; Catania, A.; Sarno, A.; Pandolfo, L.(1987). Red cell peroxide metabolism in diabetes mellitus. Horm Metab Res, 19:264-266

Brownlee, M. (2001). Biochemistry and molecular cell biology of diabetic complications. *Nature* , 414(6865):813-820.

Chiarelli, F.; Santilli, F.; Mohn, A. (2000). Role of growth factors in the development of diabetic complications. *Horm Res* 53:53–67.

Cser, A.; Sziklai, L.I.; Menzel H.; Lombeck, I. (1993). Selenium status and lipoproteins in healthy and diabetic children. *Trace Elem Electroly*, 7:205-210.

De Mattia, G.; Laurenti, O.; Bravi, C.; Ghiselli, A.; Iuliano, L.; and Balsano, F. (1994). Effect of aldose reductase inhibition on glutathione redox status in erythrocytes of diabetic patients. *Metabolism*, 43, 965-968.

Djordjević, B. V.; Ćosić, V.; Pavlović, D.; Vlahović, P.; Jevtović T.; Kocić G.; Savić, V. (2000). Does captopril change oxidative stress in puromycin aminonucleoside nepropathy? *Renal. Fail.*, 22, 535-544.

Djordjević, B. V. (2004). Free Radicals in Cell Biology. *International Review of Cytology*, Vol.237: 57-89.

Djordjević B.V.; Grubor-Lajšić,G.; Jovanović-Galović, A.; Pavlović, D.; Cvetković, T.; Pejović, M.; Lečić, N. (1998). Selenium-dependent GSH-Px in erythrocites of patients with hypertension treated with ACE inhibitors. *J. Environ. Pathol. Toxicol. Oncol.*, 17, 277-280.

Djordjević, G.; Đurić, S.; Apostolski, S.; Djordjević, V.B.; Živković, M. (2008). Total antioxidant blood capacity in patients with type 2 diabetes mellitus and distal symmetrical polyneuropathy. *VSP*, 65 (9):1-7.

Djordjević, V.B.; (2004). Free radicals in cell biology. *International review of cytology* 237:57-89.

Djordjević, V.B.; Pavlović, D.D.; Kocić, G.M. (2000). Biochemistry of free radicals. Medical Faculty Niš.

Dohi T, Kawamura K, Morita K, Okamoto H, Tsujimoto A. (1988). Alterations of plasma selenium concentrations and the activities of tissue peroxide metabolism enzymes in streptozotocin induced diabetic rats. *Horm Metab Res*, 20:671-675.

Đorđević, V.B.; Pavlović, D.D.; Kocić, G.M.(2000). Biohemija slobodnih radikala, *Medicinski fakultet, Niš.* (Byochemistry of free radicals, *Medical faculty, Nis, Serbia)*

Eaton, J.W., Ma, M. (1995). Acatalasemia. In The Metabolic Bases of Inherited Disease. 7th ed. Scriver C, Beudet A, Sly W, Valle DL, Eds. New York, McGraw-Hill, , p. 2371–2383.

England, J.D.; Gronseth G.S.; Franklin, G.; Miller, R.G.; Asbury, A.K.; Carter, G.T.; Cohen,J.A.; Fisher, M.A.; Howard, J.F.; Kinsella, L.J.; Latov,N.; Lewis, A.; Low, P.A.; Sumner, A.J. (2005). Distal symmetric polyneuropathy: A definition for clinical research. *Neurology* 64:199-207.

Ergul, A.; Schultz Johansen J.; Stromhaug C.; Harris, A.K.; Hutchinson J.; Tawfik,A.; Rahimi, A.; Rhim, E.; Wells, B.; Caldwell, R.W., et al. (2004). Vascular dysfunction of venous bypass conduits is mediated by reactive oxygen species in diabetes: Role of endothelin-1. *J Pharmacol Exp Ther*, 313:70–77.

Evans, J.L.; Goldfine, I.D.; Maddux, B.A.; Grodsky, G.M. (2002). Oxidative stress and stress-activated signaling pathways: a unifying hypothesis of type 2 diabetes. *Endocr Rev*, 23(5):599-622.

Faure,P.; Benhamou, P.Y.; Perard,A.; Halimi, S.; Roussel, A.M- (1995). Lipid peroxidation in insulindependent diabetic patients with early retina degenerative lesions: effects of an oral zinc supplementation. *Eur. J. Clin. Nutr.* 49: 282-288.

Faure, P.; Benhamou, P.Y.; Perard, A.; Halimi, S.; Roussel, A.M. (1995). Lipid peroxidation in insulindependent diabetic patients with early retina degenerative lesions: effects of an oral zinc supplementation. *Eur. J. Clin. Nutr.* 49: 282-288.

Fridovich, I. (1998). Oxygen toxicity: A radical explanation. *J. Exp. Biol.* 201, 1203-1209.

Gaetani, G.F;, Ferraris, A.M.; Rolfo, M.; Mangerini, R.; Arena, S.; Kirkman, H.N. (1996). Predominant role of catalase in the disposal of hydrogen peroxide within human erythrocytes. *Blood*, 87:1569–1599.

Garlberg, I.; Mannervik, B. (1975). Purification and characterization of the flavoenzime glutathione reductase from rat liver. *J Biol Chem*, 250:5475-5480

Ghadermarzi, M.; Moosavi-Movahedi A.A.(1996). Determination of the kinetic parameters for the suicide substrate inactivation of bovine liver catalase by hidrogen peroxide. *J. Enzime Inhibition*, 10, 167-175.

Godin, D.V.; Wohaieb, S.A.; Garnett, M.E.; Goumeniouk, A.D. (1988). Antioxidant enzyme alterations in experimental and clinical diabetes. *Mol Cell Biochem* 84:223-231

Góth, L.; Eaton, J. (2000). Hereditary catalase deficiencies and increased risk of diabetes. *Lancet*, 356:1820–1821.

Góth, L. (1992). Two cases of acatalasemia in Hungary. *Clin Chim Acta*,207:155–158.

Guzik, T.J.; Mussa, S.; Gastaldi, D.; Sadowski, J.; Ratnatunga, C.; Pillai, R.; Channon, K.M. (2002). Mechanisms of increased vascular superoxide production in human diabetes mellitus: role of NAD(P)H oxidase and endothelial nitric oxide synthase. *Circulation*, 105(14):1656-1662.

Guzik, T.J.; West, N.E.; Black, E.; McDonald, D.; Ratnatunga, C.; Pillai, R.; Channon, K.M. (2000). Vascular superoxide production by NAD(P)H oxidase: association with endothelial dysfunction and clinical risk factors. Circ Res, 86(9):E85-90.

Halliwell, B. (1999). Antioxidant defense mechanisms:from the beginning to the end (of the beginning). *Free Rradic. Res.*, 31:261-272

Hann, H.L.; Stahlhut, M.W.; Hann, C.L. (1990). Effect of iron and deferoxamine on cell growth and in vitro ferritin synthesis in human hepatoma cell lines. *Hepatology*, 11:566-569.

Iwata-Ichikawa, E.; Kondo, Y.; Miyazaki, I.; Asanuma, M.; Ogawa, N. (1999). Glial cells protect neurons against oxidative stress via transcriptional up-regulation of the glutathione synthesis. *J Neurochem*, 72:2334–2344.

Jain, S.K. and McVie, R. (1994). Effect of glycemic control, race (white versus black), and duration of diabetes on reduced glutathione content in erythrocytes of diabetic patients. *Metabolism* 43, 306-309.

Jörns, A.; Munday, R.; Tiedge, M., Lenzen, S. (1999). Effect of superoxide dismutase, catalase, chelating agents, and free radical scavengers on the toxicity of alloxan to isolated pancreatic islets in vitro. *Free Rad Biol Med*, 26:1300–1304.

Kaji, H.; Kurasaki, M.; Ito, K. et al. (1985). Increased lipoperoxide value and glutathione peroxidase activity in blood plasma of type Í diabetic women. *Klin Wochenschr*, 63:76576-76578.

Kaneto, H.; Fujii, J.; Myint, T.; Miyazawa, N.; Islam,K.N.; Kawasaki, Y.; Suzuki, K.; Nakamura, M.; Tatsumi, H.; Yamasaki, Y.; Taniguchi, N. (1996). Reducing sugars trigger oxidative modification and apoptosis in pancreatic beta-cells by provoking oxidative stress through the glycation reaction. *Biochemical Journal* 320: 855-863

Kawamura, N.; Okawara, T.; Suzuki, K.; Konishi, K.; Mino, M.; Taniguchi, N. (1992). Increased glycated cu, Zn.SOD levels in erythrocites of patients with IDDM. *J. Clin. Endocrinol. Metab.* 74: 1352-1354.

Keelan, J.; Allen, N.J.; Antcliffe, D.; Pal, S.; Duchen, M.R. (2001). Quantitative imaging of glutathione in hippocampal neurons and glia in culture using monochlorobimane. *J Neurosci Res*; 66:873–884.

Keogh, R.J.; Dunlop, M.E. & Larkins R.G. (1997). Effect of inhibition of aldose reductase on glucose flux, diacylglycerol formation, protein kinase C, and phospholipase A2 activation. *Metabolism*; 46, 41–47.

Kirkman, H.N.; Galiano, S.; Gaetani, G.F. (1987). The function of catalase-bound NADPH. *J. Biol. Chem.*, Vol. 262, Issue 2, 660-666.

Kirsch, M. & De Groot,, H. (2001). NAD (P) H, a directly operating antioxidant? *The FASEB Journal.*, 15:1569-1574.

Kishi, Y.; Nickander, K.K.; Schmelzer, J.D.; Low, P.A. (2000). Gene expression of antioxidant enzymes in experimental diabetic neuropathy. *Journal of the Peripheral Nervous System*, Volume 5, Issue 1: 11-18,

Kobayashi, M.S.; Han, D.; Packer, L. (2000). Antioxidants and herbal extracts protect HT-4 neuronal cells against glutamate-induced cytotoxicity. *Free Radic Res* , 32:115–124.

Koraćević, D;, Koraćević, G.; Djordjević, V.; Andrejević, S.; Ćosić, V. (2001). Method for the measurement of antioxidant activity in human fluids. *J Clin Pathol.* 54 (5): 356–61.

Kurobe, N.; Suzuki, F.; Okajima, K.; Kato, K. (1990). Sensitive enzyme immunoassay for human Cu/Zn superoxide dismutase. *Clin Chim Acta.* 31;187 (1):11-20.

Langenstroer, P., Pieper, G.M. (1992). Regulation of spontaneous EDRF release in diabetic rat aorta by oxygen free radicals. *Am J Physiol*, 63:H257-H265.

Lebovitz, R.M.; Zhang, H.; Vogel, H.; Cartwright, J.; Dionne, L.; Lu, N.; Huang, S.; Matzuk, M.M. (1996). Neurodegeneration, myocardial injury, and perinatal death in mitochondrial superoxide dismutase-deficient mice. *Proc Natl Acad Sci*, 93:9782–9787.

Leonard, M.B.; Lawton, K.; Watson, I.D.; Patrick, A.; Walker, A.; MacFarlane I. (1995). Cigarette smoking and free radical activity in young adults with insulin- dependent diabetes. *Diabetic Medicine*, 12, 46-50.

Li, L.; Shen, Y.M.; Yang, X.S.; Wu, W.L.; Wang, B.G.; Chen, Z.H.; Hao, X.J. (2002). Effects of spiramine T on antioxidant enzymatic activities and nitric oxide production in cerebral ischemia-reperfusion gerbils. Brain Res, 944:205–209.

Majythija, J.B.; Balaraman, R.(2005). Time depemdent changes in antioxidant enzyme and vascular reactivity of aorta in streptozotocin-induced diabetic rats treated with Curcumin. *Journal of Cardiovascular farmacology Novembar*, 46(5):697-705.

Maritim, A.C.; Sanders, R.A.; Watkins, III J.B. (2003). Diabetes, oxidative stress and antioxidants: A Review. *J.Biochem Molecular Toxicology* 17(1): 24-38.

Matkovics, B.; Varga, S.I.; Szabo, L.; Witas, H. (1982). The effect of diabetes on the activities of the peroxide metabolism enzymes. *Horm Metab* Res14:77-79.

Matsuyama, T., Michishita, H., Nakamure, H., Tsuchiyama, M., Shimizu, S., Watanabe, K., Sugita, M. (1993). Induction of copper-zinc superoxide dismutase in gerbil hippocampus after ischemia. J Cereb Blood Flow Metab, 13:135-144.

McCord, J.M., Fridovich, I. (1969). Superoxide dismutase. An enzymic function for erythrocuprein (hemocuprein). *J Biol Chem* 244: 6049–6055

McCord, J.M.; Keele, B.; Fridovich, I. (1971). An enzyme based theory of obligate anaerobiosis: the physiological function of SOD. *Proc Natl Acad Sci*, 68:1024–7.

McClain, D.A. & Crook, E.D. (1996). Perspectives in diabetes. Hexosamines in insulin resistance. *Diabetes*, 45: 1003–1009.

Mueller, S.; Riedel, H.D.; Stremmel, W. (1997). Direct evidence for catalase as the predominant H2 O2– removing enzyme in human erythrocites. *Blood* 90, 4973-4978.

Mukherjee, B., Mukherjee, J.R., Chatterjee, M. (1994). Lipid peroxidation, glutathione levels and changes in glutathione related enzyme activities in streptozotocin induced diabetic rats. *Immun Cell Biol*, 72:109-114

Murakami, K. (1991). Glutathione metabolism in erythrocytes from patients with diabetes mellitus. *Hokkaido-Igaku-Zasshi*, 66:29-40.

Murata, M.; Imada, M.; Inoue, S.; Kawanishi, S. (1998). Metal mediated DNA damage by diabetogenic alloxan in the presence of NADH. *Free Radic Biol Med*, 25:586–595.

Natarajan, V. (1995). Oxidants and signal transduction in vascular endothelium [Review]. *J Lab Clin Med*, 125: 26-37.

Nishikawa, T.; Edelstein, D.; Du, X.L.; Yamagishi, S.; Matsumura, T.; Kaneda, Y.; Yorek, M.A.; Beebe, D.; Oates, P.J. Hammes HP, *et al.* (2000). Normalizing mitochondrial superoxide production blocks three pathways of hyperglycaemic damage. *Nature*, 404(6779):787-790.

Osterode, W.; Holler, C.; Ulberth, F. (1996). Nutritional antioxidants, red cell membrane fluidity and blood viscosity in type 1 (insulin dependent) diabetes mellitus, *Diabet Med.*, 13, 1044–1050.

Oury, T.D.; Day, B.J.; Crapo, J.D. (1996). Extracellular superoxide dismutase: a regulator of nitric oxide bioavailability. *Lab. Invest.*, 75:617-636.

Pavlović, D.; Djordjević, V.; Kocić, G., (2002). Ćelijska signalna transdukcija-modulacija slobodnim radikalima, *Jugoslov. Med. Biohem.* 21:69-84

Peuchant, E.; Delmas Beauvieux, M.C.; Couchouron, A.; Dubourg, L.; Thomas, M.J.; Perromat, A.; Clerc, M.; Gin, H. (1997). Short-term insulin therapy and normoglycemia. Effects on erythrocyte lipid peroxidation in NIDDM patients. *Diabetes Care* 20: 202-207.

Pierson, C.R.; Zhang, W.; Sima, A.A. (2003). Proinsulin C-peptide replacement in type 1 diabetic BB/Wor-rats prevents deficits in nerve fiber regeneration. *J Neuropathol Exp Neurol* 62:765–779.

Polydefkis, M.; Griffin, J.W.; McArthur, J. (2003). New insights into diabetic polyneuropathy. JAMA 290:1371–1376.

Portilla, D. et al. Etomoxir -induced PPARalpha-modulated enzymes protect during acute renal failure. *Am. J. Physiol. Renal Physiol.* 2000; 278, F667–F675 .

Purves, T.; Middlemas, A.; Agthong, S.; Jude, E.B.; Boulton, A.J.; Fernyhough, P.;Tomlinson, D.R. (2001). A role for mitogen-activated protein kinases in the etiology of diabetic neuropathy. *Fed Am Soc Exp Biol J*, 15:2508–14.

Reljanović, M.; Reichel, G.; Rett, K.; Lobisch, M.; Schuette, K.; Möller, W.; et al. (1999). Treatment of diabetic polyneuropathy with the antioxidant thioctic acid (alpha-lipoic acid): a two year multicenter randomized double-blind placebo-controlled trial (ALADIN II). Alpha Lipoic Acid in Diabetic Neuropathy. *Free Radic Res* 31 (3): 171–9.

Rizzardini, M., Lupi, M.; Bernasconi, S.; Mangolini, A.; Cantoni, L. (2003). Mitochondrial dysfunction and death in motor neurons exposed to the glutathione-depleting agent ethacrynic acid. *J Neurol Sci*, 207:51–58.

Romero, F.J.; Monsalve, E.; Hermenegildo, C.; Puertas, F.J.; Higueras, V., Nies, E.; Segura-Aguilar, J.; Roma, J. (1991). Oxygen toxicity in the nervous tissue: comparison of the antioxidant defense of rat brain and sciatic nerve. *Neurochem Res*, 16:157–161.

Russell, J.W.; Golovoy, D.; Vincent, A.M.; Mahendru, P.; Olzmann, J.A.; Mentzer, A.; Feldman, E.L. (2002). High glucose induced oxidative stress and mitochondrial dysfunction in neurons. *FASEB J* 16:1738–1748.

Russell, J.W.; Sullivan, K.A.; Windebank, A.J.; Herrmann, D.N.; Feldman, E.L. (1999). Neurons undergo apoptosis in animal and cell culture models of diabetes. *Neurobiol Dis* 6:347–363

Sakaue, Y.; Sanada, M.; Sasaki, T.; Kashiwagi, A.; Yasuda, H. (2003). Amelioration of retarded neurite Zutgrowth of dorsal root ganglion neurons by overexpression of PKC in diabetic rats. *Neuroreport* 14:431–436.

Sasvári, M.; Nyakas, C.(2003). Time dependent changes in oxidative metabolism during chronic diabetes in rats. *Acta Biologica Szegediensis,* Volume 47(1-4):153-158.

Schmeichel, A.M.; Schmelzer, J.D.; Low, P.A. (2003). Oxidative injury and apoptosis of dorsal root ganglion neurons in chronic experimental diabetic neuropathy. *Diabetes* 52:165–171.

Soliman, E.; Gellido, C. Diabetic Neuropathy. *In eMedicine Septembar, 2004. Available from URL: http://www.emedicine.com/NEURO.*

Schultz, J.J.; Harris A.K.; Richly, D.J.; Ergul,A. (2005). Oxidative stress and the use of antioxidants in diabetes: Linking basic science to clinical practice. *Cardiovascular diabetology*.4:5.

Stahlberg, M.R.; Hietanen, E. (1991). Glutathione and glutathione metabolizing enzymes in the erythrocytes of healthy children and children with insulin dependent diabetes mellitus, juvenile rheumatoid arthritis, coeliac disease and acute lymphoblastic leukemia. *Scand J Clin Lab Invest*, 51:125-130

Sundaram, R.K.; Bhaskar, A.; Vijayalingam, S.; Viswanathan, M.; Mohan, R.; and Shanmugasundaram, K.R. (1996). Antioxidant status and lipid peroxidation in type II diabetes mellitus with and without complications. *Clinical Science*,90, 255-260.

Szaleczky, E.; Prechl, J.; Feher, J.; Somogyi, A. (1999). Alterations in enzymatic antioxidant defense in diabetes mellitus – a rational approach. *Postgrad Med J*, 75 (879): 13–17.

Tagami, S.; Kondo, T.; Yoshida, K.; Hirokawa, J.; Ohtsuka, Y.; Kawakami, Y. (1992). Effect of insulin on impaired antioxidant activities in aortic endothelial cells from diabetic rabbits. Metabolism, 41:1053-1058

Tainer, J.A., Getzoff, E.D., Beem, K.M., Richardson, J.S., Richardson, D.C. (1982). Determination and analysis of the 2 Å structure of copper, zinc superoxide dismutase. *J Mol Biol*, 160: 181–217.

Tang, L.; Ou, X.; Henkle-Dührsen, K.; Selkirk, M. E. (1994). Extracellular and cytoplasmic CuZn superoxide dismutases from Brugia lymphatic filarial nematode parasites. *Infect Immun*, 62 (3): 961–967.

Thornalley, P.J.; McLellan, A.C.; Lo, T.W., Benn, J.; Sonksen, P.H. (1996). Negative association between erythrocyte reduced glutathione concentration and diabetic complications. *Clinical Science*, 91, 575-582.

Tiedge, M.; Lortz, S.; Drinkgern, J.; Lenzen, S. (1997). Relation between antioxidant enzymes gene expression and antioxidative defense status of insulin producing cells. *Diabetes*, 46:1733–1742.

Tiedge, M.; Lortz, S.; Munday, R.; Lenzen, S. (1998). Complementary action of anti-oxidant enzymes in the protection of bioengineered insulin-producing RINm5F cells against toxicity of reactive oxygen species. *Diabetes*, 47:1578–1585.

Tietze, F. (1969). Enzymic method for quantitative determination of nanogram amounts of total and oxidized glutathione: Applications to mammalian blood and other tissues. *Anal Biochem*, 27: 502-522.

Tomkin, G.H. (2001). Diabetic vascular disease and the rising star of protein kinase C. Diabetologia, 44:657-658.

Tomlinson, D,R.; Gardiner, N.J. (2008). Diabetic neuropathies: components of etiology; *Journal of the peripheral Nervous* System 13:112-121.

Tomlinson, D.R. (1999). Mitogen-activated protein kinases as glucose trasducers. *Diabetologia*, 42:1271-1281.

Toyokuni, S. (1996). Iron-induced carcinogenesis: the role of redox regulation. *Free Radic Biol Med*, 20:553-566

Turko, I,V.; Marcondes, S.; Murad, F.(2001). Diabetes-associated nitration of tyrosine and inactivation of succinyl-CoA:3-oxoacid CoA-transferase. *Am J Physiol Heart Circ Physiol*, 281(6):H2289-2294.

Uzel, N.; Sivas, A.; Uysal, M.; Oz, H. (1987). Erythrocyte lipid peroxidation and glutathione peroxidase activities in patients with diabetes mellitus. *Horm Metab Res*, 19:89-90

Van Dam, P.S.; Bravenboer, B.; Van Asbeck, B.S.; Van Oirschot, J.F.L.M.; Marx, j. J,M.; Gispen, W.H. (1996). Effects of insulin treatment on endoneurial and systemic oxidative stress in relation to nerve conduction in streptozotocin-diabetic rats. *European Journal of Clinical Investigation* 26 (12): 1143-1149 (7).

Vijayalingam, S.; Parthiban, A.; Shanmugasundaram, K.R.; Mohan, V. (1996). Abnormal antioxidant status in impaired glucose tolerance and non-insulindependent diabetes mellitus. *Diabetic Medicine*, 13, 715-719.

Vincent, A.M.; Russell, J.W.; Low, P.; Feldman, E.L. (2004). Oxidative Stress in the Pathogenesis of Diabetic Neuropathy. *Endocrine Reviews* 25 (4): 612-628.

Vitai, M.; Góth, L.(1997). Reference ranges of normal blood catalase activity and levels in familial hypocatalasemia in Hungary. *Clin Chim Acta*, 261:35–42.

Vostreis, M.; Moran, P.L.; Seligman, P.A. (1988). Transferrin synthesis by small cell lung cancer cells acts as an autocrine regulator of cellular proliferation.; *J Clin Invest* 82:331.

Walter, R.M. Jr.; Uriu Hare J.Y.; Olin, K.L.; Oster, M.H.; Anawalt, B.D.; Critchfield, J.W.; Keen, C.L. (1991). Copper, zinc, manganese, and magnesium status and complications of diabetes mellitus. *Diabetes Care* 14: 1050-1056.

Wittmack, E.K.; Rush, A.M.; Hudmon, A.; Waxman, S.G.; Dib-Hajj, S.D. (2005). Voltage-Gated Sodium Channel Nav1.6 Is Modulated by p38 Mitogen-Activated Protein Kinase *J. Neurosci.*, 13, 25 (28): 6621-6630.

Wohaieb, S.A., Godin, D.V. (1987). Alterations in free radical tissue defense mechanisms in streptozotocin induced diabetes in rat. *Diabetes* 36:1014-1018.

Yaqoob, M.; McClelland, P.; Patrick, A.W.; Stevenson, A.; Mason, H.; White, M.C.; Bell, G.M. (1994). Evidence of oxidant injury and tubular damage in early diabetic nephropathy. *Q. J. Med.* 87: 601-607.

Yoshida, K.; Hirokawa, J.; Tagami, S.; Kawakami, Y.; Urata, Y.; Kondo, T. (1995). Weakened cellular scavenging activity against oxidative stress in diabetes mellitus: regulation of glutathione synthesis and efflux. *Diabetologia*, 38, 201-210.

Yoshioka, T.; Homma, T.; Meyrick, B.; Takeda, M.; Moore-Jarrett, T.; Kon, V.; Ichikawa, I. (1994). Oxidants induce transcriptional activation of manganese superoxide dismutase in glomerular cells. Kidney Int., 46 (2):405-13.

Ziegler, D.; Gries, F.A. (1997). Alpha-lipoic acid in the treatment of diabetic peripheral and cardiac autonomic neuropathy. *Diabetes* 46 (Suppl 2): 62–6.

Ziegler, D.; Hanefeld, M.; Ruhnau, K.J.; Hasche, H.; Lobisch, M.; Schütte, K., et al. (1999). Treatment of symptomatic diabetic polyneuropathy with the antioxidant alpha-lipoic acid: a 7-month multicenter randomized controlled trial (ALADIN III Study). ALADIN III Study Group. Alpha-Lipoic Acid in Diabetic Neuropathy. *Diabetes Care* 22 (8): 1296–301.

Ziegler, D.; Hanefeld, M.; Ruhnau, K.J.; Meissner, H.P.; Lobisch, M.; Schütte, K., et al. (1995). Treatment of symptomatic diabetic peripheral neuropathy with the anti-oxidant alpha-lipoic acid. A 3-week multicentre randomized controlled trial (ALADIN Study). *Diabetologia* 38 (12): 1425–33.

Ziegler, D.; Schatz, H.; Conrad, F.; Gries, F.A.; Ulrich, H.; Reichel, G. (1997). Effects of treatment with the antioxidant alpha-lipoic acid on cardiac autonomic neuropathy in NIDDM patients. A 4-month randomized controlled multicenter trial (DEKAN Study). Deutsche Kardiale Autonome Neuropathie. *Diabetes Care* 20 (3): 369–73.

Ziegler, D. (1994). Diagnosis, staging and epidemiology of diabetic peripheral neuropathy. *Diabetes Nutrition and Metabolism*, 7:342-348.

9

Interactions Between Total Plasma Homocysteine, Oxidized LDL Levels, Thiolactonase Activities and Dietary Habits in Tunisian Diabetic Patients

Nadia Koubaa et al.*
Bichemistry laboratory, UR"Human Nutrition & Metabolic Disorders" Faculty of Medicine Monastir, Tunisia

1. Introduction

Cardiovascular disease (CVD) is the predominant cause for morbidity and mortality in diabetes mellitus (DM). Patients with diabetes mellitus have two to three times the incidence of atherosclerotic disease compared to the general population (Kannel & McGee, 1979). Several etiologic factors increase susceptibility to CVD in DM including insulin resistance, dyslipidemia, endothelial dysfunction, prothrombosis, and increased protein glycation (Baynes & Thorpe, 1999).

Plasma homocysteine levels are elevated in patients with diabetes, particularly in patients with type 2 diabetes as well as in individuals in prediabetic states who exhibit insulin resistance. Homocysteine (Hcy) is a non-essential amino acid that is produced from demethylation of methionine. Hcy can be remethylated into methionine by means of vitamin B12-dependent methionine synthase and 5-methyltetrahydrofolate as a methyl donor. Hcy can be also catabolized into cysteine (the transsulfuration pathway) via cystathionine beta synthase and cystathioninase, both enzymes being vitamin B6-dependent. A third way to remove Hcy is conversion to S-adenosylhomocysteine (SAH). The last reaction is mediated by SAH-hydrolase and favors the SAH formation in case of increased Hcy concentrations. S-Adenosyl methionine (SAM) is a universal methyl donor that is formed from methionine and converted into SAH after donating its methyl group. SAH is a potent inhibitor of most known methyltransferases (Kloor & Osswald, 2004).

Among the main determinants of tHcy levels in non-diabetic subjects are age, sex, renal function, several diseases, drugs, coffee and chronic alcohol consumption, smoking and physical inactivity (Refsum et al., 2006). Genetic factors and nutritional deficiencies of folate

---

* Maha Smaoui[1], Sounira Mehri[1], Amel Nakbi[1], Sonia Hammami[2], Raja Chaaba[1], Khaldoun Ben Hamda[3], Fethi Betbout[3], Mohamed Ameur Frih[2] and Mohamed Hammami[1].
1 Bichemistry laboratory, UR"Human Nutrition & Metabolic Disorders" Faculty of Medicine Monastir, Tunisia
2 Department of Internal Medicine, CHU F.Bourguiba, Monastir, Tunisia
3 Department of cardiology, CHU F.Bourguiba, Monastir, Tunisia

or of the vitamin cofactors (vitaminsB12, B6 and B2) involved in Hcy metabolism may also promote hyperhomocysteinemia. Besides other genetic defects, a thermolabile variant of Methylene Tetrahydrofolate Reductase (MTHFR), a key enzyme of the remethylation pathway, has been described (Frosst et al., 1995). It has been shown that this gene variation was associated with increased levels of homocysteine; Heterozygotes carrying MTHFR thermolabile variant have a reduced enzyme activity (down to 65% of normal levels), while homozygotes have only 30% of normal activity (Frosst et al., 1995). In type 2 diabetic patients, levels of homocysteine are influenced by their insulin concentrations, therapy with insulin, and medications such as metformin and glitazones that can either raise or lower homocysteine levels.

Epidemiological studies have identified elevated homocysteine (hyperhomocysteinaemia) as an independent risk factor for cardiovascular disease. Elevated levels of homocysteine (Hcy) above 12.1μmol/L have been shown to double the risk of pathophysiological conditions such as atherosclerosis, myocardial infarction, cerebral or peripheral vascular diseases (Castro et al., 2006). Mean plasma total Hcy (tHcy) was found to be significantly higher both in male and female patients with CAD compared to controls with angiographically normal coronary arteries (Kang et al., 1992). An increase in plasma Hcy of only 12% greater than the upper limit of normal was shown to be associated with an increase by 3.4- fold in the risk of myocardial infarction (Stampfer et al., 1992). After adjusting for possible confounders, Arnsen et al. (Arnsen et al., 1995) found a relative risk for coronary heart disease of 1.32 for an increase in serum Hcy of 4 μmol/l. A meta-analysis of 27 studies relating Hcy to coronary, cerebro vascular and peripheral arterial vascular diseases showed a very strong relationship between these diseases and tHcy (Boushey et al., 1995).

Elevated Hcy may also contribute to progressive atherosclerosis by several mechanisms, including arterial endothelial function impairment, oxidative stress induction, and the promotion of inflammation and thrombosis (Castro et al., 2006; Wald et al., 2002; 2004; Jakubowski, 2006). A unifying hypothesis for the mechanism of Hcy-mediated vascular injury has not yet been established. One frequently described mechanism involves oxidative damage, as Hcy can undergo autoxidation in the plasma or intracellularly, to form various reactive oxygen species (Welch & Loscalzo, 1998). The potent reactive superoxide and hydrogen peroxides, which are produced during this process, are mainly responsible for the vascular toxicity of homocysteine via the formation of oxidized low density lipoprotein (ox-LDL). The oxidation of LDL in the artery wall is believed to be the primary event leading to the initiation and progression of atherosclerosis (Steinberg & Witztum, 2002; Parthasarathy et al., 1998). Hcy has also been shown to decrease the activity (Nishio & Watanabe, 1997) as well as the expression of the antioxidant enzyme glutathione peroxidase (Upchurch et al., 1997). Creation of a prothrombotic environment by the action of Hcy on various factors involved in coagulation has also been proposed (Ratnoff, 1968; Fryer et al., 1993; Nishinaga et al., 1993). The reaction of Hcy with nitric oxide (NO) acts to prevent oxidative damage caused by Hcy but at the same time reduces the bioavailability of NO by trapping it intracellularly as a nitrosothiol (Jacobsen, 2001). Hcy is also a potent mitogen for vascular smooth-muscle cells (Harker et al., 1983; Tsai et al., 1994). Aggregates formed by the combination of Hcy thiolactone, a cyclical product of Hcy, with LDL (low-density lipoprotein) were shown to be taken up by intimal macrophages and be incorporated into atheromatous plaques (Naruszewicz et al., 1994). Hcy thiolactone is also incorporated into cellular and secretory proteins through lysine homocysteinylation, leading to the dysfunction of the proteins (Jakubowski, 1997). The high density lipoprotein (HDL) particle(s) is known to prevent the

formation of ox-LDL by means of the HDL-associated enzyme paraoxonase (PON); its antioxidant properties prevent the accumulation of lipid peroxides on LDL (Shih et al., 1998). Paraoxonase is a multifunctional antioxidant enzyme that not only can destroy Ox-LDL but also can detoxify the homocysteine metabolite, homocysteine thiolactone (Jakubowski H, 1997). In fact, human paraoxonase possesses a thiolactonase (HTase) activity, hydrolyzing Hcy thiolactone to Hcy (Jakubowski, 1999). Hcy thiolactone is likely a natural substrate of HTase/paraoxonase (Jakubowski, 2004) a product of the PON1 gene (Furlong et al., 1988).
The effect of diet on human health has already been underlined in many studies. During the past years population-based surveys and large-scale clinical trials have provided scientific evidence that diets, and especially those rich in fruits, vegetables, legumes, whole grains, fish and low-fat dairy products, are associated with lower incidence of various chronic diseases, including diabetes, cardiovascular disease and cancer (Ascherio et al., 1992; appel et al., 1997; Price & Fowkes, 1997; koubaa et al., 2007). Diet has also an important role among the factors affecting homocysteine levels. Mediterranean diet, with a high proportion of bioactive compounds (vitamins, polyphenols and flavonoids) proved its efficiency in lowering plasma homocysteine levels and reducing the incidence of cardiovascular disease.
The aim of the current study was to investigate whether elevated Hcy levels are associated with oxidation of LDL, and thiolactonase activity in type 2 diabetic patients, and further explore the contribution of various dietary components to prevent diabetes vascular complications and atherosclerosis progression.

2. Patients and methods

2.1 Study population

110 diabetic patients (54.2 ± 10.7 years) and 120 non diabetic healthy controls (44 ± 12.3 years) with available metabolic and life style informations were involved in this study. These patients did not receive any antioxidant drugs and none used hormonal replacement therapy. The following data were obtained: age, sex, weight. Height hip and waist circumference were measured using a standard scale. The study was approved by our hospital ethical committee, and informed consent was obtained from all patients before their enrolment. Major requirements for enrolment in all the groups were: absence of infectious or acute/chronic inflammatory diseases, known malignancy, absence of acute/chronic renal failure, or hepatic failure.

2.2 Laboratory procedures

Validated laboratory procedures were used as described previously (Koubaa et al., 2008). Plasmatic total homocysteine (free and protein bound) was determined by a validated highly sensitive and accurate capillary gas chromatography mass spectrometry method (GC-MS) using a stable isotope as internal standard. Thiolactonase (HTLase) activity was estimated by a commercially available kit assay (Alfresa Auto HTLase; Alfresa Pharma Corporation, Japan). This method utilizes gamma-thiobutyrolactone as substrate and Ellman's procedure to monitor the accumulation of free sulfhydryl groups via coupling with 5,5-dithiobis(2-nitrobenzoicacid). Lipids and lipoproteins (Triglycerides: TG; total cholesterol: TC mmol/l, High density lipoproteins- cholesterol HDL mmol/l, Low density lipoproteins cholesterol: LDL mmol/l, triglycerides: TG mmol/l) concentrations were determined by enzymatic way. Apolipoproteins Apo A1 and Apo B were determined by an immunoturbidimetric method (Randox, Antrim, UK). Oxidized LDL levels (ox-LDL) were measured by a sandwich ELISA method using a commercial kit (ox-LDL ELISA Kit; immunodiagnostic Bensheim,Germany). The dietary habits of the diabetic patients were evaluated. Food intakes were estimated by two dieticians using one-week diet recalls. Subjects were asked about their daily diet over a week period: they were asked about amounts, frequencies and variations in consumption. Nutrient intakes were calculated using the software Nutritionist IV computer analysis (Nutritionist IV Computer Analysis Program, 1994, Version 3.1, N2 Computing, Hearst Corp. Salem, OR).

2.3 Statistical analysis

Statistical analyses were assessed using the Statistical Package for Social Sciences (SPSS Inc., Chicago). Data are presented as median (25th to 75th interquartile range I.R) for several variables that were not normally distributed and comparison between the 2 groups was performed with the Mann-Whitney *U* test. The normally distributed values were expressed as means with standard deviations and group differences analyzed using the Student's t test. To test the association between the variables, either Pearson's correlations or Spearman's correlation rank (R) were used. Values of $p<0.05$ were considered to be statistically significant.

3. Results

3.1 Participants characteristics

The clinical and biochemical features of the healthy and diabetic patients are listed in table 1. Diabetic patients exhibited significantly higher mean values of systolic and diastolic blood

	Healthy controls (n=120)	Diabetics (n=110)	p
Age (years)	44 ± 12.3	54.2 ± 10.7	0.00
BMI (kg/m^2)	26.7 ± 4.0	28.9 ± 5.7	0.00
WHR	0.91 ± 0.08	0.96 ± 0.07	0.01
SBP (mm Hg)	12.1 ± 1.2	14.6 ± 9	0.033
DBP (mm Hg)	7.06 ± 0.9	7.8 ± 1.2	0.00
Glucose (mmol/L)	5.23 ± 1	10.98 ± 4.2	0.00
Creatinine (µmol/L)	88.2 ± 19.3	85.8 ± 39.2	0.58
Urea (mmol/L)	4.9 ± 1.6	6.8 ± 2.7	0.00
Cholesterol (mmol/L)	4.4 ± 1.2	4.9 ± 1.4	0.00
Triglycerides (mmol/L)	1.3 ± 0.8	2.1 ± 1.2	0.00
HDL-C (mmol/L)	1.01 ± 0.28	1.01 ± 0.28	0.97
LDL-C (mmol/L)	2.7 ± 1.1	3 ± 1.5	0.08
ApoA1 (g/L)	1.29 ± 0.27	1.39 ± 0.43	0.1
ApoB (g/L)	0.83 ± 0.28	1.39 ± 0.43	0.03
tHcy (µmol/L) [£]	11.76 (10.7 - 12.81)	12.87 (9.7 - 17.5)	0.01
ox-LDL (ng/mL)	78.4 ± 23.7	139.6 ± 52.2	0.00
HTase (U/L)	569.9 ± 254	442.8 ± 211.8	0.01

SBP, DBP: systolic and diastolic blood pressure
Values are expressed as mean ± SD
*: $p<0.05$; **: $p<0.001$
£: expressed as median (I.R) and tested with the Mann Whitney's U test

Table 1. Clinical and biochemical features of the healthy Tunisians and diabetic patients

pressure (SBP and DBP), Waist to hip Ratio (WHR) and body mass index (BMI). As far as the biochemical features of the patients and healthy groups were examined, the diabetics exhibited significantly elevated urea levels as compared to healthy subjects (4.9 ± 1.6 vs. 6.8 ± 2.7, p= 0.00). Serum triglycerides and total cholesterol levels were also significantly higher in these patients (p = 0.00 and p=0.003 respectively) associated to significantly higher Apo B levels. In addition we found a significant increase in plasma homocysteine levels (11.76 (10.7 - 12.81) vs. 12.87 (9.7 - 17.5) µmol/l; P=0.01) associated with lower Thiolactonase activities (442.8 ± 211.8 vs. 569.9 ± 254 U/ml, P=0.01) and higher oxidized LDL levels (139.6 ± 52.2 vs. 78.4 ± 23.7 ng/ml p = 0.00) as compared to healthy subjects (table 1).

3.2 Correlations analysis

The correlations between plasma homocysteine levels, thiolactonase activities and oxidized LDL levels were then evaluated with some clinical and biochemical features in the diabetic patient's group. As expected, thiolactonase activities were associated negatively with tHcy levels (r= -0.554, p= 0.00), total cholesterol (r= -0.345, p< 0.05), LDL levels (r= -0.358, p< 0.05). Oxidized LDL levels were in opposite positively correlated with total cholesterol (r= 0.313, p< 0.05), creatinine levels (r= 0.353, p< 0.05) and BMI (r= 0.315, p< 0.05).

	tHcy	HTase	ox-LDL	BMI	TC	LDL-C	creatinine
tHcy	1.00	**-.554****	-.060	.080	.068	.036	.039
HTase	**-.554****	1.000	-.198	-.115	**-.345***	**-.358***	-.013
ox-LDL	-.060	-.198	1.00	**.315 ***	**.313***	.260	**.353***

*: p<0.05; **: p<0.001
£: tested with the Spearman's test of correlation

Table 2. Correlations between thiolactonase activity, plasma total homocysteine and oxidized LDL levels, with some clinical and biochemical features in the diabetic patients

3.3 Dietary surveys

As far as the dietary habits were considered we established that in the diabetic patients, the relative percentages of protein intakes per total calories were higher (12.4 ± 1.9 vs. 13.7 ± 3.8 %, p< 0.05) but the relative percentages of carbohydrate intakes per total calories were lower (50.7 ± 7.7 vs. 56.8 ± 5.4 %, p<0.001). The diabetic patient's diet was significantly richer in fats (30.8 ± 5.9 vs. 35.9 ± 7.5 %, p<0.00). They were consuming higher polyunsaturated fatty acids (14.2 ± 10.4 vs. 21.6 ± 17.4 %, p<0.00) but significantly lower monounsaturated and saturated fatty acids.

Finally, as the correlations with the nutrients and were examined we noticed that tHcy was positively correlated with intakes of protein (r = 0.267, p<0.00), saturated fatty acids (r = 0.334, p<0.00) and cholesterol (r = 0.265, p<0.05) as illustrated in table 4. Plasma homocysteine levels were also correlated with dietary sodium and zinc intakes. Thiolactonase activity was negatively associated with proteins (r = -0.345, p<0.05) and cholesterol intakes (r = -0.313, p<0.05). Ox LDL levels were positively correlated with lipid intakes in the diabetic patients (r = 0.324, p<0.05).

	Healthy subjects	Diabetics
Proteins (%)	12.4 ± 1.9	13.7 ± 3.8*
A/V	1.06 ± 0.27	1.1 ± 0.48
Carbohydrates (%)	56.8 ± 5.4	50.7 ± 7.7**
Fats (%)	30.8 ± 5.9	35.9 ± 7.5 **
SFA	23.2 ± 9.4	16.8 ± 8.1**
MUFA	46.9 ± 9.4	32.9 ± 14.8**
PUFA	14.2 ± 10.4	21.6 ± 17.4*
Cholesterol (mg)	188.2 ± 154	507.4 ± 206
Calcium(mg)	483.1 ± 154.3	507.4 ± 206
Vitamin B1 (mg)	0.49 ± 0.12	0.48 ± 0.16
Fiber (g)	16.3 ± 4.7	34.2 ± 15.5
Vitamin C (mg)	77.5± 30.4	82.7 ± 50.5
Vitamin E (mg)	7.1 ± 3.4	9.9 ± 10
Folates (µg)	134.4 ± 54.9	157.4 ± 71.2

A/V: percentage of Animal protein/ percentage of vegetal protein;
SFA: Saturated fatty acids,
MUFA: Monounsaturated fatty acids,
PUFA: Polyunsaturated fatty acids and.
*: p<0.05; **: p<0.001

Table 3. Daily nutrient intakes of the healthy and diabetic patients

	Proteins (%)	Fats (%)	SFA	Cholesterol	Sodium	Zinc
tHcy £	**.267****	-.138	**.334****	**.265***	**.324***	**.272***
HTase	**-.345***	.226	-.012	**-.313***	-.261	.211
ox-LDL	-.091	**.324***	-.028	-.038	-.234	-.260

*: p<0.05; **: p<0.001
£: tested with the Spearman's test of correlation

Table 4. Correlations between thiolactonase activity, plasma total homocysteine and oxidized LDL levels with selected nutrients in the diabetic patients

4. Discussion

Diabetic subjects constitute a patient population at high risk for cardiovascular disease, due to the influence of a clustering of risk factors. Plasma tHcy is considered as an emerging independent nontraditional risk factor for atherosclerotic vascular disease, which may enhance the effect of the traditional risk factors (Graham, 1997; Hackam & Anand, 2003). It is also a strong predictor of cardiovascular and all-cause mortality (Bostom et al., 1999). Therefore, it is important to know if dietary habits and lifestyle can affect plasma tHcy levels in this population, and eventually select the patients who would be at a higher risk for developing such complications. In the present study, tHcy levels were higher in the diabetic patient's group. Plasma tHcy levels have been studied extensively in diabetic, as well as in non-diabetic subjects. A number of studies did not find any differences in plasma tHcy values between diabetic and control subjects (Salarde et al., 2000; Lanfredini et al., 1998; Pavia et al. 2000, Diakoumopoulou et al., 2005). Some investigators demonstrated lower levels of tHcy in diabetics versus controls (Matteucci et al., 2002; Wollesen et al., 1999; Salardi et al., 2000). However, our findings are in accordance with other reports where tHcy were higher in the diabetic patients (Passaro et al., 2000; Yeromenko et al., 2000). Furthermore, homocysteine increases the production of ox-LDL and enhances their uptake by macrophages leading to the formation of foam cells that play a crucial role in atherosclerotic lesions (Tsai et al.,). Ox-LDL are considered as biochemical markers of coronary artery disease (Toshima et al., 2000 ; Holvoet et al, 2001). Accordingly, we found high levels of ox-LDL in diabetic patients exhibiting the highest levels of tHcy, which confirms the oxidative effect of homocysteine in the type 2 DM patients. Every 5 µM/L increase in the Hcy concentration increases the risk of CVD by 50%, and TC levels by 20 mg/dL. (Castro et al., 2006; Wald et al., 2002; Nygard et al., 1998; Genset et al., 1990). The mechanisms possibly responsible for causing endothelial dysfunction include changes in LDL, and Ox- LDL. The oxidation of LDL is increased by the combination of thiolactone and apo B's free lysyl epsilon amino residue (Rocchi et al., 2007; Mansoor et al., 1993, 2000). When LDL is reacted with Hcythiolactone in methionine, which is an explicit initiator of arteriosclerosis, LDL-binding thiol is increased by 250 nM per mg of LDL protein (Ferguson et al. 1999). The free amino- or thiol-adducted LDL causes aggregation, and increases LDL uptake in macrophages and atheroma production by lipids (Perna et al., 2003). Another mechanism by which Hcy may cause LDL oxidation is a possible deformation of LDL through Hcy autoxidation, which causes the oxidation of side chains of LDL such as fatty acids or apo B- 100 (Young & Woodside , 2000). Both Hcy and Ox-LDL could participate in thrombosis by increasing VCAM-1 and ICAM-1, caused by endothelial cell activation due to fibrinogen-platelet GPIIb-IIIa formation. Ox-LDL affects both initial and progressive stages of arteriosclerosis (Jakubowski, 2000; Dardik et al., 2000; Vadachkoria et al., 2004; Erl et al., 2000). On the other hand, circulating Hcy reduces NO-induced detoxification, vasodilation, and endothelial function (Rocchi et al., 2007). NO participates in a metabolic pathway (S-nitroso-HCY) that is able to protect against Hcy-induced endothelial oxidative damage. Paraoxonase plays also a key role in reducing Hcy endothelial damages. In our previous results, we found a decline in endogenous antioxidant defense system capability in type 2 DM patients indicating their high oxidative stress (Smaoui et al., 2006). Antioxidant status of enzymes in DM patients is controversial. Several authors have reported that lipid peroxides level increases in type 2 DM patients (Mooradian, 1991); on the other hand, other studies found no significant increase in these patients (Velazquez et al., 1991). Among the numerous antioxidant enzymes, we focused in the present study on the thiolactonase activities which were decreased in the diabetic patients. Most studies evaluated the paraoxonase activity in Type I and Type II diabetic patients and found a decreased activity in these patients (Boemi et al., 2001; Kordonouri et al., 2001; Letellier et al., 2002; Mackness B et al., 1998; 2002; Agachan et al., 2004). Paraoxonase is a multifunctional antioxidant enzyme that not only can detoxify paraoxon, destroy oxidized low-density lipoprotein (ox-LDL) but also can hydrolyze homocysteine thiolactone.

The mechanism by which PON1 is reduced in diabetes is poorly understood, but may be associated with an increase in blood glucose concentration. Glycation can both inactivate PON1 and increase lipid peroxidation in HDL (Hedrick et al., 2000). Glycated HDL also has a reduced ability to protect against oxidation (Ferretti et al., 2001). PON1 activity and concentration were decreased also in studies of healthy subjects with elevated fasting glucose levels (Leviev et al., 2001; Kordonouri et al., 2001). Our finding showed a negative association between HTase activities, tHcy levels and oxidized LDL levels. These levels were associated with higher triglycerides, total cholesterol and also higher Apo B levels. Apo B is superior to cholesterol and triglycerides as a coronary syndrome risk factor due to the heterogeneity of lipoprotein particle composition. In fact, plasma Apo B concentrations reflect the number of atherogenic lipoprotein particles including LDL, and chylomicron remnants which contain variable amounts of triglycerides and cholesterol, but each of these particles contain 1 molecule of Apo B as structural protein. Then, higher levels of Apo B found in the diabetic patients reflects their higher risk for developing cardiovascular diseases (Sniderman et al., 1997).

The SBP and DBP were also increased in the diabetic patients. The association between homocysteine and chronic complications of diabetes mellitus could be explained by different mechanisms; direct toxic effect on vascular endothelial and indirect effect on the normal methylation in endothelial cells (Weir & Molloy, 2000). Direct toxic effect of homocysteine could be mediated by damage to vascular endothelial cells, resulting in vascular events, such as microvascular disease. In the study of Fiorina et al. (Fiorina et al., 1998), Caucasian patients with elevated tHcy levels had significantly higher diastolic pressure and mean arterial pressure. These results are similar to our data. Other populations (Indians) have shown correlation between homocysteine concentrations and body weight (Das et al., 1999). Our results did not show correlations among tHcy and different anthropometric parameters (body mass index, waist to hip ratio). Nevertheless, a positive correlation between ox-LDL levels and BMI was established in the diabetic patients. There was also a positive association between ox-LDL levels and creatinine levels in the diabetic patients. No correlation was found between creatinine and tHcy levels. Most studies have been able to show a positive correlation between plasma Hcy and plasma creatinine levels, suggesting the importance of the kidney in the regulation of plasma Hcy. Renal function in Type 2 diabetes appears to change with the progress of the disease: hyperfiltration in the early stages and progressive deterioration with the progression of diabetes. Diabetes therefore provides an interesting situation with changes in kidney functions being superimposed on the already existing changes in the metabolic milieu. Moreover, we found a negative association between HTase activities tHcy levels and the levels of total cholesterol and ox-LDL. In fact, in certain diseases e.g. diabetes where HDL size is reduced, secretion of PON1 is affected due to the fact that PON1 tends to bind to larger sized species of HDL both *in vivo* (Blatter et al.,1993) and *in vitro* (Deakin et al., 2002). In addition, *in vitro* studies demonstrated that PON1 was inactivated by oxidized lipids and oxidized LDL (Aviram et al., 1999). PON1 is highly susceptible to inactivation by oxidation. In vitro, PON1 activity is protected by the antioxidant polyphenols quercetin and glabridin (Aviram et al., 1999), suggesting that dietary antioxidants may play a similar role in vivo. Studies have shown that consumption of pomegranate juice, rich in polyphenols and other antioxidants, can raise PON1 activity up to 20% in both humans and apoE knockout mice (Kaplan et al., 2001). Polyphenols extracted from red wine also increase PON1 activity in mice (Hayek et al.,

1997). Recent work from Gou´edard et al. (Gou´edard et al., 2004) provides evidence that dietary polyphenols can influence PON1 gene expression. Clinical trials of the antioxidant vitamins C and E have, to date, been unsuccessful in showing a link between vitamin intake and CHD risk. Likewise, their effect, if any, on PON1 activity is not clear. Jarvik et al. (Jarvik et al., 2002) found that PON1 activity correlated positively with the quantity of vitamins C and E in the diet; however, another study in which vitamin E was given to volunteers showed no change in PON1 activity (Arrol et al., 2000). In contrast, oleic acid from olive oil is associated with increased activity (Tomas et al., 2001; Wallace et al., 2001). Meals rich in used cooking fat, which contains a high content of oxidized lipids, were followed by a significant fall in PON1 activity when fed to healthy men (Sutherland et al., 1999). These correlations were not confirmed by our results. The thiolactonase activities were correlated negatively with protein and cholesterol intakes. Plasma homocysteine levels were in opposite positively correlated to protein intakes, the relative percentage of fats and saturated fatty acids in diet and sodium intakes. Accordingly, in the Hordaland study that included 5917 subjects, a higher intake of saturated fatty acids was positively associated with higher concentrations of plasma Hcy. Concentrations of Hcy were higher (by 8.8%) in the group with the highest intakes of saturated fatty acids compared to that with the lowest intake (Berstad et al., 2007). Food-based feeding trials have shown a reduction in blood Hcy in subjects who consume fortified cereals or whole grains in combination with fruits, vegetables and low fat dairy products (Lutsey et al., 2006; Appel et al., 2000). Several carefully studied populations in Mediterranean countries and in some areas in Asia, where traditional diets consist largely of foods of plant origin, exhibit low rates of many chronic diseases and long life expectancies. Many case-control and prospective studies have provided further evidence that high consumption of plant foods confers numerous health benefits. Although the mechanisms are not fully understood, carotenoids, folic acid, and fiber, all of which are abundant in the Mediterranean diet, appear to play important roles in the prevention of coronary artery disease (Kushi et al., 1995).

5. Conclusion

In conclusion, Hcy and thiolactonase activities and oxidized levels are interrelated in type 2 diabetic patients and are responsible, at least partly, of the vascular complications. Strong evidence suggested that excess of plasma homocysteine disturb lipid metabolism via the oxidation of LDL particle and its aggregation, and enhancing atherosclerosis progression. Another line of evidence suggested that thiolactonase activity is affect in diabetics partly by a glycation process that accentuates the endothelial damages of homocysteine. A very interesting aspect to be tested in future studies is the beneficial effect of certain nutriments on lipid parameters and plasma homocysteine levels. Future long-term studies on larger populations are needed for determining the exact role of homocysteine in the development of diabetes vascular complications and the metabolic ways of prevention.

6. Acknowledgment

This work was supported by a grant from the "Ministère de l'Enseignement Supérieur, de la Recherche Scientifique et de la Technologie" UR "Nutrition Humaine et Désordres Métaboliques" UR03ES08 and USCR-Spectrométrie de masse. We would like to thank

Alfresa Pharma Corporation, Japan for their assistance. We are also thankful to all the clinicians for their assistance with patients and controls recruitment.

7. References

Agachan, B., Yilmaz, H., Karaali, Z. and Isbir, T. (2004). Paraoxonase 55 and 192 polymorphism and its relationship to serum paraoxonase activity and serum lipids in Turkish patients with non-insulin dependent diabetes mellitus. *Cell. Biochem. Funct.* Vol.22, pp.163–168.

Appel, L., Moore, T., Obarzanek, E., Vollmer, W., Svetkey, L., Sacks, F., Bray, G.A., Vogt, T.M., Cutler, J.A., Windhauser, M,M., Lin, P.H., Karanja, N.A. (1997). Clinical trial of the effects of dietary patterns on blood pressure. *N Engl J Med.* Vol.336, pp.1117-24.

Appel, L.J., Miller, E.R., Jee, S.H., Stolzenberg-Solomon, R., Lin, P.H., Erlinger, T. (2000). Effect of dietary patterns on serum homocysteine: results of a randomized, controlled feeding study. *Circulation*. Vol.102, pp. 852-7.

Arnesen, E., Refsum, H., Bonaa, K.H., Ueland, P.M., Forde, O.H., Nordrehaug, J.E. (1995). Serum total homocysteine and coronary heart disease. *Int. J. Epidemiol*, vol.24, pp.704–709.

Arrol, S., Mackness, M. I. and Durrington, P. N. (2000). Vitamin E supplementaion increases the resistance of both LDL and HDL to oxidation and increases cholesteryl ester transfer activity. *Atherosclerosis*. Vol.150, pp.129–134.

Ascherio, A., Rimm, E.B., Giovannucci, E.L. (1992). A prospective study of nutritional factors and hypertension among US men. *Circulation*, vol.86, pp. 475-84.

Aviram, M., Rosenblat, M., Billecke, S. (1999). Human serum paraoxonase (PON1) is inactivated by oxidised low density lipoprotein and preserved by antioxidants. *Free Radicals Biol. Med.* Vol.26, pp.892–904.

Baynes JW, Thorpe SR. (1999). Role of oxidative stress in diabetic complications: a new perspective on an old paradigm. *Diabetes*, vol.48, pp.1-9.

Berstad, P., Konstantinova, S.V., Refsum, H., Nurk, E., Vollset, S.E, Tell, G.S., Ueland, P.M, Drevon, C.A, Ursin, G. (2007).Dietary fat andplasma total homocysteine concentrations in 2 adult age groups: the hordaland Homocysteine Study. *Am. J. Clin. Nutr.* Vol.85, pp.1598–1605.

Blatter, M.C., James, R. W., Messmer, S., Barja, F. and Pometta, D. (1993). Identification of a distinct human high-density lipoprotein subspecies defined by a lipoprotein-associated protein, K-45. Identity of K-45 with paraoxonase. *Eur. J. Biochem.* Vol. 211, pp. 871–879

Boemi, M., Leviev, I., Sirolla, C., Pieri, C., Marra, M. and James, R. W. (2001). Serum paraoxonase is reduced in type 1 diabetic patients compared to non-diabetic, first degree relatives; influence on the ability of HDL to protect LDL from oxidation. *Atherosclerosis*. Vol.155, pp.229–35.

Bostom, A.G., Silberhatz, H., Rosenberg, I.H., Selhub, J., D'Agostino, R.B., Wolf, P.A. (1999). Non-fasting plasma total homocysteine levels and all-cause and cardiovascular disease mortality in elderly Framingham men and women. *Arch Intern Med.* Vol.159, pp.1077-80.

Boushey, C.J., Beresford, S.A., Omenn, G.S. and Motulsky, A.G. (1995). A quantitative assessment of plasma homocysteine as a risk factor for vascular disease. Probable benefits of increasing folic acid intakes. *J. Am. Med. Assoc.* vol.274, pp. 1049–1057.

Castro, R., Rivera I, Blom, H.J., Jakobs, C., Tavares de Almeida, I. (2006). Homocysteine metabolism, hyperhomocystenemia and vascular disease: an overview. *J Inherit Metab Dis*, vol.29, pp.3-20.

Castro, R., Rivera, I., Blom, H.J., Jakobs, C., Tavares de Almeida, I. (2006). Homocysteine metabolism, hyperhomocystenemia and vascular disease: an overview. *J Inherit Metab Dis*. Vol.29, pp.3-20.

Dardik, R., Varon, D., Tamarin, I., Zivelin, A., Salomon, O., Shenkman, B. (2000). Homocysteine and oxidized low density lipoprotein enhanced platelet adhesion to endothelial cells under flow conditions: distinct mechanisms of thrombogenic modulation. *Thromb Haemost*. Vol.83, pp.338-44.

Deakin, S., Leviev, I., Gomaraschi, M., Calabresi, L., Franceschini, G. and James, R. W. (2002). Enzymatically active paraoxonase-1 is located at the external membrane of producing cells and released by a high affinity, saturable, desorption mechanism. *J. Biol. Chem*. Vol.277, pp.4301–4308.

Diakoumopoulou, E., Tentolouris, N., Kirlaki, E., Perrea, D., Kitsou, E., Psallas, M., Doulgerakis, D., Katsilambros N. (2005). Plasma homocysteine levels in patients with type 2 diabetes in a Mediterranean population: relation with nutritional and other factors. *Nutr Metab Cardiovasc Dis.* Vol.15, n.(2), pp.109-17

Erl, W., Weber, P.C., Weber, C. (1998). Monocytic cell adhesion to endothelial cells stimulated by oxidized low density lipoprotein is mediated by distinct endothelial ligands. *Atherosclerosis*. Vol.136, pp.297-303.

Ferguson, E., Hogg, N., Antholine, W.E., Joseph, J., Singh, R.J., Parthasarathy, S. (1999). Characterization of the adduct formed from the reaction between homocysteine thiolactone and low-density lipoprotein: antioxidant implications. *Free Radic Biol Med*. Vol.26, pp. 968-77.

Ferretti, G., Bacchetti, T., Marchionni, C., Caldarelli, L. and Curatola, G. (2001). Effect of glycation of high density lipoproteins on their physiochemical properties and on paraoxonase activity. *Acta Diabetol*. Vol.38, pp.163–169.

Frosst, P., Blom, H.J., Milos, R., Goyette, P., Sheppard, C.A., Metthews, R.G. (1995). A candidate genetic risk factor for vascular disease: a common mutation in methylenetetrahydrofolate reductase. *Nat Genet*. Vol.10, pp.111–3.

Fryer, R.H., Wilson, B.D., Gubler, D.B., Fitzgerald, L.A., Rodgers, G.M. (1993). Homocysteine, a risk factor for premature vascular disease and thrombosis, induces tissue factor activity in endothelial cells *Arterioscler. Thromb*. Vol.13, pp.1327–1333.

Furlong, C.E., Richter, R.J., Seidel, S.L., Motulsky, A.G. (1988). Role of genetic polymorphism of human plasma paraoxonase/arylesterase in hydrolysis of the insecticide metabolites chlorpyrifos oxon and paraoxon. *Am J Hum Genet*. Vol.43, pp.230–8.

Genest, J.J. Jr, McNamara ,J.R., Salem, D.N., Wilson, P.W., Schaefer, E.J., Malinow, M.R. (1990).Plasma homocyst(e)ine levels in men with premature coronary artery disease. *J Am Coll Cardiol*. Vol.16, pp.1114-9.

Gouedard, C., Barouki, R. and Morel, Y. (2004). Dietary polyphenols increase paraoxonase 1 gene expression by an aryl hydrocarbon receptor-dependant mechanism. *Mol. Cell. Biol.* Vol.24, pp.5209–5222.

Graham, I.M., Daly, L.E., Refsum, H.M., Robinson, K., Brattstrom, L.E., Ueland, P.M. (1997). Plasma homocysteine as a risk factor for vascular disease. The European Concerted Action Project. *J Am Med Assoc.* vol.277, n.(22), pp. 1775-81.

Hackam, D.G., Anand, S.S. (2003). Emerging risk factors for atherosclerotic vascular disease. *J Am Med Assoc.* vol.290, pp.932-40.

Harker, L.A., Harlan, J.M., Ross, R. (1983). Effect of sulfinpyrazone on homocysteine-induced endothelial injury and arteriosclerosis in baboons. *Circ. Res.* Vol.53, pp.731–739.

Hayek, T., Fuhrman, B., Vaya, J. et al. (1997). Reduced progression of atherosclerosis in the apolipoprotein E deficient mice following consumption of red wine, or its polyphenols quercetin, or catechin, is associated with reduced susceptibility of LDL to oxidation and to aggregation. *Arterioscler., Thromb., Vasc. Biol.* Vol.17, pp.2744–2752.

Hedrick, C. C., Thorpe, S. R., Fu, M. X. et al. (2000). Glycation impairs high-density lipoprotein function. *Diabetologia. Vol.*43, pp.312–320.

Holvoe,t P., Mertens, A., Verhamme, P. (2001). Circulating oxidized LDL is a useful marker for identifying patients with coronary artery disease. *Arterioscler Thromb Vasc Biol.* Vol.21, pp.844–8.

Jacobsen, D.W. (2001) in Homocysteine in Health and Disease (Carmel, R. and Jacobsen, D.W., eds), pp. 425–440, Cambridge University Press, Cambridge

Jakubowski, H. (1997). Metabolism of homocysteine thiolactone in human cell cultures. *J Biol Chem.* vol. 272, pp.1935-42.

Jakubowski, H. (2000). Homocysteine thiolactone: metabolic origin and protein homocysteinylation in humans. *J Nutr.* Vol.130, pp.377-81.

Jakubowski, H. (2004). Biochemical basis of homocysteine toxicity in humans. *Mol Cell Life Sci.* vol.61, pp.470–87. Jakubowski, H. (1999).Protein homocysteinylation: possible mechanism underlying pathological consequences of elevated homocysteine levels. *FASEB J.* vol.13, pp.2277–83.

Jakubowski, H. (2006). Pathophysiological consequences of homocysteine excess. *J Nutr.* Vol.136, pp.1741-9.

Jarvik, G. P., Tsai, N. T., McKinstry, L. A. (2002). Vitamin C and E intake is associated with increased paraoxonase activity. *Arterioscler., Thromb., Vasc. Biol.* Vol.22, pp.1329–1333

Kang, S.S., Wong, P.W., Malinow, M.R. (1992). Hyperhomocyst(e)inemia as a risk factor for occlusive vascular disease. *Annu. Rev. Nutr.* vol.12, pp.279–298.

Kannel, WB., McGee, DL. (1979). Diabetes and cardiovascular disease. The Framingham study. *JAMA*, vol.241, pp.2035–2038.

Kaplan, M., Hayek, T., Raz, A. et al. (2001). Pomegranate juice supplementation to atherosclerotic mice reduces macrophage lipid peroxidation, cellular cholesterol accumulation and development of atherosclerosis.*J. Nutr.* Vol.131, pp.2082–2089.

Kloor, D., Osswald, H. (2004) S-Adenosylhomocysteine hydrolase as a target for intracellular adenosine action. Trends Pharmacol. Sci. vol.25, pp. 294–297.

Kordonouri, O., James, R. W., Bennetts, B. (2001). Modulation by blood glucose levels of activity and concentration of paraoxonase in young patients with type 1 diabetes mellitus. *Metab. Clin. Exp.* Vol.50, pp. 657–660.

Koubaa, N., Hammami, S., Nakbi, A., Ben Hamda, K., Mahjoub, S., Kosaka, T. Hammami, M. (2008). Relationship between thiolactonase activity and hyperhomocysteinemia according to MTHFR gene polymorphism in Tunisian Behcet's disease patients. *Clin Chem Lab Med.* Vol. 46, n.(2), pp.187–192.

Koubaa, N., Nakbi, A., Smaoui, M., Abid, N., Chaaba, R., Abid, M., Hammami, M. (2007). Hyperhomocysteinemia and elevated ox-LDL in Tunisian type 2 diabetic patients: Role of genetic and dietary factors. *Clin Biochem.* Vol.40, pp.1007–1014.

Kushi, L.H., Lenart, E.B., Willett, W.C. (1995). Health implications of Mediterranean diets in light of contemporary knowledge. 1. Plant foods and dairy products. *Am J Clin Nutr.* Vol.61(suppl), pp.1407–15.

Lanfredini, M., Fiorina, P., Peca, M.G., Veronelli, A., Mello, A., Astorri, E., Dall'Aglio, P., Craveri, A. (1998). Fasting and post-methionine load homocyst(e)ine values are correlated with microalbuminuria and could contribute to worsening vascular damage in non-insulin-dependent diabetes mellitus patients. *Metabolism.* Vol.47, pp.915-21.

Letellier, C., Durou, M. R., Jouanolle, A. M., Le Gall, J. Y., Poirier, J. Y. and Ruelland, A. (2002). Serum paraoxonase activity and paraoxonase gene polymorphism in type 2 diabetic patients with or without vascular complications. *Diabetes Metab.* Vol.28, pp. 297–304.

Leviev, I., Kalix, B., Brulhart Meynet, M.-C. and James, R. W. (2001). The paraoxonase PON1 promoter polymorphism C(−107)T is associated with increased serum glucose concentrations in non-diabetic patients. *Diabetologia.* Vol. 44, pp.1177–1183.

Lutsey, P.L., Steffen, L.M., Feldman, H.A., Hoelscher, D.H., Webber, L.S., Luepker, R.V. (2006). Serum homocysteine is related to food intake in adolescents: the Child and Adolescent Trial for Cardiovascular Health. *Am J Clin Nutr.* Vol.83, pp.1380-6.

Mackness, B., Durrington, P. N., Boulton, A. J., Hine, D. and Mackness, M. I. (2002). Serum paraoxonase activity in patients with type 1 diabetes compared to healthy controls. *Eur. J. Clin. Invest.* Vol.32, pp. 259–256.

Mackness, B., Mackness, M. I., Arrol, S. et al. (1998) Serum paraoxonase (PON1) 55 and 192 polymorphism and paraoxonase activity and concentration in non-insulin dependent diabetes mellitus. *Atherosclerosis.* Vol.139, pp. 341–349.

Majors, A., Ehrhart, L.A., Pezacka, E.H. (1997). Homocysteine as a risk factor for vascular disease, enhanced collagen production and accumulation by smooth muscle cells. *Arterioscler Thromb Vasc Biol.* Vol.17, pp.2074–81.

Mansoor, M.A., Bergmark, C., Haswell, S.J., Savage, I.F., Evans, P.H., Berge, R.K. (2000). Correlation between plasma total homocysteine and copper in patients with peripheral vascular disease. *Clin Chem.* Vol.46, pp.385-91.

Mansoor, M.A., Ueland, P.M., Aarsland, A., Svardal, A.M. (1993). Redox status and protein binding of plasma homocysteine and other aminothiols in patients with homocystinuria. *Metabolism.* Vol. 42, pp.1481-5.

Matteucci, E., Rossi, L., Mariani, S., Fagnani, F., Quilici, V., Cinapri, V. (2002). Blood levels of total homocysteine in patients with type 1 diabetes (with no complications, diabetic nephropathy and/or retinopathy) and in their non-diabetic relatives. *Nutr Metab Cardiovasc Dis*. Vol.12, pp. 184-9.

Mooradian, A.D. (1991). Increased serum conjugated dienes in elderly diabetic patients. *J Am Geriatr Soc*. Vol. 39, pp.571–5.

Naruszewicz, M., Mirkiewicz, E., Olszewski, A.J. and McCully, K.S. (1994). *Nutr. Metab. Cardiovasc. Dis*. Vol.4, pp.70–77.

Nishinaga, M., Ozawa, T. and Shimada, K. (1993). Homocysteine, a thrombogenic agent, suppresses anticoagulant heparan sulfate expression in cultured porcine aortic endothelial cells. *J. Clin. Invest*. vol.92, pp.1381–1386.

Nishio, E., Watanabe Y. Br. (1997). Oxidized LDL induces apoptosis in cultured smooth muscle cells: a possible role for 7-ketocholesterol. *J. Pharmacol*. Vol.122, pp.269–274.

Nygård, O., Refsum, H., Ueland, P.M., Vollset, S.E. (1998). Major lifestyle determinants of plasma total homocysteine distribution: the Hordaland Homocysteine Study. *Am J Clin Nutr*. Vol.67, pp.263-70.

Parthasarathy. S., Santanam, N., Auge, N. (1998). Oxidised low-density lipoprotein: a two-faced Janus in coronary artery disease? *Biochem pharmacol*. Vol.56, pp.279–284.

Passaro, A., D'Ellia, K., Pareschi, P.L., Calzoni, F., Carantoni, M., Fellin, R. (2000). Factors influencing plasma homocysteine levels in type 2 diabetes. *Diabetes Care*. Vol.23, pp.420-1.

Pavia ,C., Ferrer, I., Valls, C., Artuch, R., Colome, C., Vilaseca, M.A. (2000). Total homocysteine in patients with type 1 diabetes. *Diabetes Care*. Vol.23, pp.84-7.

Perna, A.F., Ingrosso, D., Lombardi, C., Acanfora, F., Satta, E., Cesare, C.M. (2003). Possible mechanisms of homocysteine toxicity. *Kidney Int Suppl*. Vol.84, pp.137-40.

Price, J.F., Fowkes, F.G.R. (1997). Antioxidant vitamins in the prevention of cardiovascular disease. *Eur Heart J*. vol.18, pp.719-27.

Ratnoff, O.D. (1968). Activation of Hageman factor by L-homocystine. *Science*. Vol.162, pp.1007–1009.

Refsum, H., Nurk, E., Smith, A.D., Ueland, P.M., Gjesdal, C,G., Bjelland, I., Tverdal, A., Tell, G.S., Nygard, O., Vollset, S.E. (2006).The Hordaland Homocysteine Study: a community-based study of homocysteine, its determinants, and associations with disease. *J Nutr*. Vol.136, pp. 1731–1740.

Rocchi, E., Bursi, F., Ventura, P., Ronzoni, A., Gozzi, C., Casalgrandi, G. (2007). Anti- and pro-oxidant factors and endothelial dysfunction in chronic cigarette smokers with coronary heart disease. *Eur J Intern Med*. Vol.18, pp.314-20.

Salardi, S., Cacciari, E., Sassi, S., Grossi, G., Mainetti, B., Dalla Casa, C. (2000). Homocysteinemia, serum folate and vitaminB12 in very young patients with diabetes mellitus type 1. *J Pediatr Endocrinol Metab*. Vol.13, pp.1621-7.

Shih, D.M., Gu, L., Xia, Y.R., Navab, M., Li, W.F., Hama, S. (1998). Mice lacking serum paraoxonase are susceptible to organophosphate toxicity and atherosclerosis. *Nature*. Vol.394, pp.284-7.

Smaoui, M., Koubaa, N., Hammami, S., Abid, N., Feki, M., Chaaba, R., Attia, N., Abid, M., Hammami, M. (2006). Association between dietary fat and antioxidant status of Tunisian type 2 diabetic patients. Prostaglandins,*Leukot Essent Fat Acids*. Vol.74, pp.323–9.

Sniderman, A.D., Pedersen, T., Kjekshus, J. (1997). Putting low-density lipoproteins at center stage in atherogenesis. *Am J Cardiol.* Vol.79, n.(1), pp.64-67.

Stampfer, M.J., Malinow, M.R., Willett, W.C., Newcomer, L.M., Upson, B., Ullmann, D., Tishler, P.V, Hennekens, C.H. (1992). A prospective study of plasma homocyst(e)ine and risk of myocardial infarction in US physicians. *J. Am.Med. Assoc.* vol. 268 pp. 877–881.

Steinberg, D., Witztum, J.L. (2002). Is the oxidative modifications hypothesis relevant to human atherosclerosis? Do the antioxidant trials conducted to date reflect the hypothesis?. *Circulation.* Vol.105, pp.2107–2111.

Sutherland, W. H., Walker, R. J., de Jong, S. A., van Rij, A. M., Phillips, V. and Walker, H. L. (1999). Reduced postprandial serum paraoxonase activity after a meal rich in used cooking fat. *Arterioscler., Thromb., Vasc. Biol.* Vol.19, pp.1340–1347.

Tomas, M., Senti, M., Eluosa, R. (2001). Interaction between the Gln-Arg 192 variants of the paraoxonase gene and oleic acid intake as a determinant of high density lipoprotein cholesterol and paraoxonase activity. *Eur. J. Pharmacol.* Vol.432, pp.121–128.

Toshima, S., Hasegawa, A., Kurabayashi, M. (2000). Circulating oxidized low density lipoprotein levels: a biochemical risk marker for coronary heart disease. *Arterioscler Thromb Vasc Biol.* Vol.20, pp.2243–7.

Tsai, J.C., Perrella, M.A., Yoshizumi, M., Hsieh, C.M., Haber, E., Schlegel, R., Lee, M.E. (1994). Promotion of vascular smooth muscle cell growth by homocysteine: a link to atherosclerosis. *Proc. Natl. Acad. Sci. U.S.A.* vol.91, pp.6369–6373.

Tsai, M., Garg, U., Key, N.S. (1996). Molecular and biochemical approaches in the identification of heterozygotes for homocystinuria. *Atherosclerosis.* Vol.172, pp.69–77.

Upchurch, Jr, G.R., Welch, G.N., Fabian, A.J., Freedman, J.E., Johnson, J.L., Keaney, Jr, J.F. and Loscalzo, J. (1997). Homocyst(e)ine decreases bioavailable nitric oxide by a mechanism involving glutathione peroxidase. *J. Biol. Chem.* Vol.272, pp.17012–17017.

Vadachkoria, S., Sanchez, S.E., Qiu, C., Muy-Rivera, M., Malinow, M.R., Williams, M.A. (2004). Hyperhomocyst(e)inemia and elevated soluble vascular cell adhesion molecule-1 concentrations are associated with an increased risk of preeclampsia. *Gynecol Obstet Invest.* Vol.58, pp.133-9.

Velazquez, E., Winocour, P.H., Kesteven, P., Alberti, K.G., Laker, M.F. (1991). Relation of lipid peroxides to macrovascular disease in type 2 diabetes. *Diabet Med.* Vol.88, pp.752–8.

Wald D.S., Law M, Morris JK. (2004). The dose-response relation between serum homocysteine and cardiovascular disease: implications for treatment and screening. *Eur J Cardiovasc Prev Rehabil.* Vol.11, pp.250-3.

Wald D.S., Law, M., Morris, J.K. (2002). Homocysteine and cardiovascular disease: evidence on causality from a meta-analysis. *BMJ.* Vol.325, pp.1202.

Wald, D.S., Law, M., Morris, J.K. (2002). Homocysteine and cardiovascular disease: evidence on causality from a meta-analysis. *BMJ.* Vol. 325, pp.1202.

Wallace, A. J., Sutherland, W. H., Mann, J. I. and Williams, S. M. (2001). The effect of meals rich in thermally stressed olive and safflower oils on postprandial serum paraoxonase activity in patients with diabetes.*Eur. J. Clin. Nutr.* Vol.55, pp.951–958.

Welch, G.N. Loscalzo, J. (1998). Homocysteine and atherothrombosis. *N. Engl. J. Med.* Vol.338, pp.1042–1050.

Wollesen, F., Brattsrom, L., Refsum, H., Ueland, P.M., Berglund, L., Berne, C. (1999). Plasma total homocysteine and cysteine in relation to glomerular filtration rate in diabetes mellitus. *Kidney Int.* vol.55, pp.1028-35.

Yeromenko, Y., Lavie, L., Levy, Y. (2000). Homocysteine and cardiovascular risk in patients with diabetes mellitus. *Nutr Metab Cardiovasc Dis.* Vol.11, pp.108-16.

Part 3

Consequences of Obesity

10

Obesity-Induced Adipose Tissue Inflammation and Insulin Resistance

Po-Shiuan Hsieh
National Defense Medical Center/ Graduate Institute of Physiology Taipei, Taiwan

1. Introduction

Obesity-induced chronic systemic inflammation has been considered as a major risk factor for the development of type 2 diabetes mellitus (T2DM). In addition, the development of inflammation in adipose tissue has been speculated to be the main resource to initialize systemic inflammation and insulin resistance in the state of obesity. However, the molecular mechanisms underlying the development of adipose tissue inflammation are not yet completely characterized, which will be of clinical importance to clarify the potential drug targets for the prevention and treatment of obesity-associated T2DM. Thereby, the aim of this chapter will focus on reviewing the recent progress and prospective related to the understanding of obesity-induced adipose tissue inflammation and insulin resistance. The content of this chapter will highlight the possible contributing factors and interplay during the different developmental stages of obesity and associated insulin resistance. Accordingly, the possible roles of adipocytes, T cells, macrophages and endothelial cells in the initiation, propagation and exacerbation of adipose tissue inflammation will be further discussed. The cross-talk between cell types in the pathogenesis of inflamed adipose tissue and adipokine overproduction will also be extensively debated. Moreover, the important molecular mediators and/or chemokine and cytokine receptors in the development of obesity-induced adipose tissue inflammation and associated insulin resistance would also be added in the text. Finally, based on the recent advances in the relevant research field, the therapeutic strategies in the treatment of obesity-associated insulin resistance and T2DM will be discussed in this chapter.

2. Obesity, adipose tissue inflammation and insulin resistance

Obesity has reached epidemic proportions in most of the industrialized countries, resulting in an increasing prevalence of the metabolic syndrome characterized by visceral obesity, dyslipidemia, and insulin resistance. Obese adipocytes characterize as the important source of inflammation mediators by producing a large number of inflammatory cytokines and chemokines, such as TNF-alpha, IL-6, monocyte chemoattractant protein-1 (MCP-1), and dysregulated production of anti-inflammatory adipokines (e.g. adiponectin). Indeed, obesity-induced adipose tissue inflammation is the key process underlying activation of proinflammatory pathways known to interfere insulin signalling and induce insulin resistance. On the other hand, activation of inflammatory pathways in adipocytes impairs triglyceride storage and increases release of free fatty acids (FFAs), an excess of which known to induce insulin resistance in muscle and liver (Guilherme & Virbasius, 2008). In addition, it has been demonstrated that increased expression of MCP-1 in adipose tissue associated with obesity plays an important role in the pathogenesis of adipose macrophage infiltration and insulin resistance (Kanda, 2006). The infiltrated macrophages secrete a variety of chemokines and other cytokines that further promote a local inflammatory response resulting in subsequent systemic insulin resistance.

3. Immune system and obesity-induced adipose tissue inflammation

3.1 Innate immune system and the development of inflammation in adipose tissue

Macrophages are the fundamental part of the immediate innate defense mechanisms, which can promote specific adaptive immunity by inducing T-cell recruitment and activation while the body is disturbed. Macrophages have attracted considerable recent attention in adipose tissue biology following the discovery that they infiltrate the tissue in obesity and appear to play a substantial role in the inflammatory process (Haiyan, 2003; Weisberg, 2003). The majority of macrophages in obese adipose tissue aggregate in "crown- like structure" completely surrounding dead (necrotic-like) adipocytes and scavenging adipocyte debris (Cinti et al. 2005). The number of macrophages positively correlates with body mass and adipocyte size in both subcutaneous and visceral fat depots, even though macrophage infiltration is more prominent in the latter. Accumulated macrophages are considered to be the critical link between obesity and adipose tissue inflammation since they are the major source of pro- inflammatory cytokine production, notably TNF-alpha and IL-6, in adipose tissue (Cancello, 2005; Haiyan, 2003). Interestingly, the process appears reversible since macrophage infiltration and pro-inflammatory marker expression in the adipose tissue of obese subjects can be significantly reduced after weight loss (Brun, 2006; Cancello, 2005). Similarly to any immune and inflammatory responses, macrophage infiltration in expanding adipose tissue results from blood monocytes influx, likely attracted by the chemokine MCP-1 (Kanda, 2006). Indeed, it has been reported that MCP-1 secretion is markedly enhanced locally and in plasma in obese rodents and human patients. Mice with targeted deletion in the genes for monocyte MCP-1 and its receptor CCR2 both could attenuate adipose tissue macrophages (ATMs) infiltration and decrease inflammation in fat. It would subsequently protect these mice from high fat diet-induced insulin resistance (Kanda, 2006; Weisberg, 2006). Conversely, MCP-1 overexpressed mice have increased numbers of ATMs along with insulin resistance (Kamei et al., 2006). Moreover, some mechanistic insights to explain how macrophages are associated with inflammation in obesity, have emerged from the characterization of ATM activation state. Macrophage population and function have been revealed to be highly heterogeneous and dependent on the surrounding environment, which has led to their characterization and classification following the well-known classification of T-cell activation state into Th1/Th2 sub-types (Gordon, 2007). Typically, macrophages can be distinguished between the M1 phenotype, identified as the pro- inflammatory or "classifically"- activated state, secreting various cytokines (e.g. TNF-alpha, IL-6), and the M2 phenotype referred as to the anti- inflammatory or "alternatively"- activated state, which produces IL-10. Following a pulse dye labelling of ATMs to discriminate newly infiltrated ATMs from the resident ATMs, it has been shown that recruited ATMs during a diet- induced obesity exhibit an inflammatory M1 profile compared to already settled ATMs (Lumeng et al., 2007). Moreover, the same research group has also demonstrated that ATMs from lean mice retain the typical gene expression pattern of the M2 activation state, while ATMs from obese mice are characterized by enhanced expression levels of TNF-alpha and NOS2, both markers of the M1 activated state. This study supports that diet-induced obesity either converts or promotes the replacement of initial M2- polarized ATMs by M1- polarized ATMs, thereby contributing to the development of insulin resistance (Lumeng, 2007). In conclusion, ATMs are the major source of pro- inflammatory mediators in obese adipose tissue and contribute both to the local and systemic metabolic alterations and the general inflammatory state. Their number and activation states are likely crucial in the onset of obesity-associated adipose tissue inflammation and in the development of insulin resistance.

3.2 Adaptive immune system and the development of inflammation in adipose tissue

Macrophages infiltrating into adipose tissue during obesity could be largely extended by providing convincing evidence for an early participation of various cells from the adaptive immune system in the development of obesity (Kintscher, 2008; Rocha, 2008; Wu, 2007). For instance, T cells are also actively regulated in adipose tissue and contribute to obesity-induced inflammation. Previous studies have shown that specific rearrangements in the T cell receptor (TCR) are selected in adipose tissue, suggesting that antigens in fat may communicate with adaptive immune system (Nishimura et al., 2009). Several studies have pointed out that dietary (Rocha, 2008; Wu, 2007) or genetic obesity (Rausch et al., 2007) is associated with T- cell infiltration including both CD4+ and CD8+ T cells. The assessment of immune cell composition at early stage of high fat diet-induced obesity suggests that T-cell entry in adipose tissue precedes monocyte attraction and, therefore, might represent one of the processes initiating adipose tissue inflammation (Kintscher et al., 2008). Indeed, both the secretion of the chemokine C-C motif chemokine ligand (CCL) 5/ Regulated on Activation, Normal T Cell Expressed and Secreted (RANTES) and the expression level of its receptor CCR5 are enhanced in adipose tissue of obese male mice (Wu et al., 2007). Moreover, RANTES neutralization reduces T- cell migration *in vitro*. RANTES expression is not only restricted to T- cells but is also detected in mature adipocytes, more prominently in presence of TNF- alpha (Wu et al., 2007). CD4+ T cells in adipose tissue can be classified into pro-inflammatory Th1 polarized T cells secreting IFN- gamma and anti- inflammatory Th2 polarized T cells secreting IL-4 and IL-13. In lean mice, Th1 and Th2 polarized T cells are higher in visceral than in subcutaneous adipose tissue with both T- cell type being present at approximately equal amounts (Winer et al., 2009). In addition, the role of the Th1- type cytokine IFN- gamma in adipose tissue inflammation has been explored (Rocha et al., 2008). IFN- gamma mRNA expression was up-regulated in mouse adipose tissue after high fat diet feeding. 3T3-L1 adipocytes incubated with IFN- gamma exhibited a marked enhancement of the expression levels of various cytokines and chemokines. Moreover, IFN- gamma deficiency partly prevented the diet-induced increases of both ATM number and pro-inflammatory marker expression (TNF- alpha and MCP-1) in adipose tissue. On the other hand, several studies have also observed an increase in adipose tissue CD8+ T cells in the course of obesity (Nishimura, 2009; Winer, 2009). The infiltration of CD8+ T cells precedes the recruitment of macrophages in the development of adipose tissue inflammation (Nishimura et al., 2009). Depletion of CD8+ T cells before inducing obesity in mice prevents M1 macrophage infiltration into adipose tissue without changing adiposity or the number of

M2 macrophages residing in fat. In obese mice with existing inflammation, an antibody-mediated reduction of CD8+ T cells improved glucose tolerance and insulin sensitivity along with adipose tissue inflammation, providing evidence for a role of these CD8+ T cells not only in the initiation but also preservation of inflammation in adipose tissue. Furthermore, adoptive transfer of CD8+ T cells to CD8- deficient mice lead to increase adipose tissue inflammation. In summary, adipose tissue expansion is associated with changes in the number and various phenotype of lymphocytes. A pathological role of Th1 polarized T cells and CD8+ T cells in adipose could be described in the state of obesity correlating with adipose tissue inflammation and subsequent insulin resistance.

4. Adipokine dysregulation in obesity and insulin resistance

4.1 Obesity-induced upregulation of potentially deleterious adipokines

4.1.1 Leptin

Leptin is almost exclusively expressed and produced by white adipose tissue. Plasma Leptin concentration and mRNA expression in adipose tissue are directly related to the severity of obesity. An increase of fat mass is associated with the elevation of leptin (Considine et al., 1996). In animal models, expression of leptin is increased in conditions that are associated with release of pro- inflammatory cytokines such as TNF- alpha and IL-6 in monocytes and macrophages. Vice versa, TNF- alpha and IL-6 are capable of stimulating adipocyte leptin production (Antuna-Puente et al., 2008). Leptin also has significant effect on adaptive immunity, such as inducing a switch toward Th1-cell immune responses by increasing IFN-gamma, TNF- alpha secretion, and the suppression of Th2- cell responses in adipose tissue (Matareseet al., 2002). On the other hand, leptin has also been reported to improve insulin sensitivity through activation of AMP-activated protein kinase (AMPK) (Minokoshi et al., 2002). However, in human obesity, the high circulating leptin levels is exhibited secondary to the development of leptin resistance. Leptin administration has little or no effect on insulin resistance. Moreover, the leptin-signaling pathway as shown to, activate suppressor of cytokine signaling (SOCS)-3, which might opposite effect to inhibit insulin signaling (Howard & Flier, 2006). Taken together, it is suggested that leptin has proinflammatory effects and is involved in the pathogenesis of insulin resistance. However, the underlying mechanism of leptin in the etiology of obesity- associated adipose tissue inflammation and insulin resistance needs to be further elucidated.

4.1.2 Resistin

Resistin received its name from the original observation that it induced insulin resistance in mice (Steppan et al., 2001). Resistin expression has demonstrated to be increased in obese animals and has been implicated in the pathogenesis of obesity- associated insulin resistance and type 2 diabetes mellitus in mouse model (Steppan et al., 2001). Accordingly, administration of recombinant resistin to normal animal produced insulin resistance, whereas neutralizing resistin with specific antibody improved insulin sensitivity in obese animals with insulin resistance. This work was the first to illustrate resistin as a link between obesity and insulin resistance (Kim et al., 2001). On the other hand, studies indicate that stimulation of macrophages *in vitro* with endotoxin or proinflammatory cytokines leads to a marked increase in resistin production. Furthermore, administration of endotoxin to human volunteers is associated with an dramatical increase in circulating resistin levels

(Lehrke et al., 2004). Previous report regarded to the effects of resistin in the modulation of inflammatory responses has shown that resistin could upregulate expression of MCP-1 as well as cell adhesion molecule ICAM-1 in endothelial cell (Kawanami et al., 2004). However, subsequent human studies failed to link resistin to insulin resistance. In addition, this protein is not produced by human adipocytes. Further investigation is needed to characterize the role of resistin in the pathogenic link between obesity-induced adipose tissue inflammation and insulin resistance in human.

4.1.3 Visfatin

Visfatin has recently been identified as an adipokine that is secreted by adipocytes in visceral fat, decreases insulin resistance (Fukuhara et al., 2005). In both genetic and nutritional obese animal models, visfatin expression is induced predominantly in visceral adipose tissue. Similarly to insulin, visfatin could enhance glucose uptake in myocytes and adipocytes, and also inhibit hepatocyte glucose production (Fukuhara et al., 2005). Its insulin- like effects are also reported that visfatin could induce tyrosine phosphorylation of insulin receptors insulin receptor substrate-1 and 2 (IRS-1, IRS-2), and activation of PI3K. The pro-inflammatory effect of visfatin has been demonstrated in unstable lesions in patients with coronary heart disease. It showed that visfain can increase matrix metalloproteinase-9 activity in monocytes, and TNF- alpha and IL 8 in peripheral blood mononuclear cells (Dahl et al., 2007). All these studies strongly suggest that visfatin could be primarily regarded as an inflammatory mediator involved in several obesity-related pathological processes. Nevertheless, the molecule of visfatin has turned out to be previously identified as a growth factor for early B-lymphocytes termed pre-B cell colony enhancing factor(PBEF) (Samal et al., 1994). The role of visfatin in human T2DM remains debated (Chen, 2006; Sandeep, 2007).

4.1.4 TNF-alpha

TNF-alpha is a proinflammatory cytokine produced by numerous cells, but mainly by macrophages, lymphocytes and monocytes. In addition, adipocytes also produce TNF-alpha in humans and rodents. TNF-alpha is the first inflammatory cytokine shown to be produced by adipocytes (Hotamisligil et al., 1993). TNF-alpha level is increased in adipose tissue and plasma of obese patients and has been related to obesity- associated complications (Kern et al., 2001). TNF-alpha has been considered to be crucially involved in the pathophysiology of insulin resistance (Hotamisligil et al., 1993). Disruption of IRS-1 phosphorylation by TNFα has been reported to one of the possible mechanisms to interfere insulin signaling. Moreover, TNF-alpha has been shown to inhibit the conversion of pre-adipocytes to mature adipocytes, allowing further recruitment of uncommitted cells and thus possible expansion of adipose tissue mass (Kras et al., 2000). Therefore TNF-alpha is considered a likely mediator of the insulin resistance and T2DM associated with high visceral adiposity.

4.1.5 IL-6

Like TNF-alpha, the levels of IL-6 positively correlates with body mass index, especially in the state of obesity (Kern et al., 2001). It has been estimated that white adipose tissue contributes about 30% of circulating IL-6. Visceral white adipose tissue (WAT) produces. Higher levels of IL-6 compared with those in subcutaneous WAT (Fain, 2004; Fried, 1998). Most of the IL-6 comes from the stromal vascular fraction of adipose tissue. There is a positive relationship between IL-6 levels in adipose tissue and circulating C-reactive protein levels (Maachi et al., 2004), which is an important cardiovascular risk factor. Moreover, IL-6 produced by intra-abdominal adipose tissue has been documented to directly link to visceral obesity- related hypertriglyceridaemia by stimulating hepatic secretion of triglycerides (Nonogaki et al., 1995).

4.2 Obesity-induced downregulation of potentially beneficial adipokines

4.2.1 Adiponectin

Adiponectin is a protein highly expressed in adipose tissue. In contrast to other adipokines, adiponectin is underexpressed in obese patients with insulin resistance or T2DM. Adiponectin could enhance insulin sensitivity through activation of AMPK (Yamauchi et al., 2002). In addition to its effects on insulin sensitivity, adiponectin has an anti-inflammatory effect through its anti- TNF-alpha action. For example, the in vitro study has demonstrated that macrophage activity and TNF-alpha production were significantly diminished in macrophages while cotreated with adiponectin (Ouchi et al., 2000). The anti-inflammatory activities of adiponectin extend to inhibition of IL-6 production accompanied by induction of the endogenous anti- inflammatory cytokines IL-10 and IL-1 receptor antagonist (Kumada et al., 2004). On the basis of all the above-mentioned studies, adiponectin appears to act as an anti- inflammatory molecule in adipose tissue.

5. Cellular cross- talk and molecular mediators in the development of adipose tissue inflammation

5.1 Adipocyte dysfunction and inflammation

In obesity, excessive adipose tissue growth is associated with hypertrophy and hyperplasia of adipocytes. Excess energy intake or decreased expenditure results in excess TG accumulation and adipocyte hypertrophy in adipose tissue. Adipocyte size is related to dysregulated adipokines expression and secretion in humans. The hypertrophic adipocytes change their immune balance towards the production of pro- inflammatory, atherogenic and diabetic adipokines. Reportedly, the enlarged adipocytes appear to initiate macrophages infiltration which occurs secondarily in obesity through their dysregulated adipokine production (Jiao et al., 2009). Moreover, Nishimura et al showed that CD8+ T cells accumulated in obese adipose tissue, but not presence of greater number of CD8+ T cells in the systemic circulation in the state of obesity. The findings suggested that CD8+ T cells are activated by local stimulation in the adipose tissue (Nishimura et al., 2009). It implicates that obese adipose tissue activates CD8+ T cells via dysregulated adipokine expression. Adipocyte hypertrophy is associated with altered intracellular signaling. An increase in constitutive NF-κB activity has been reported in 3T3-L1 cell line during adipocyte differentiation and hypertrophy, which may potentially lead to adipokine overproduction (Berg et al., 2004). 3T3-L1 adipocyte hypertrophy could be artificially induced by preloading with palmitate, which in turn enhance oxidative stress and increase MCP-1 production through JNK and NF-κB signaling (Takahashi et al., 2008). In brief, adipose tissue might be regarded as an important source of inflammatory products *in vivo* (e.g. TNF-alpha, IL-6, leptin and adiponectin), which are regulated by the interactions among infiltrated immune cells and residual cells, i.e. adipocytes, endothelial cells in adipose tissue. Therefore, it could actively participate to initiate and regulate immune responses in local adipose tissue and whole body.

5.2 Hypoxia

It has been speculated that the dysregulation of the production of inflammation-related adipokines in obesity, linked to the development of the metabolic syndrome and other obesity-associated disorders, is a specific response to relative hypoxia in clusters of adipocytes distant from the vasculature as adipose tissue mass expands. Hypoxia is exhibited in adipose tissue of obese individuals where oxygen partial pressure and blood flow are reduced. Moreover, the expression of hypoxia- inducible factor- 1 alpha (HIF-1 alpha)-the master regulator of oxygen homeostasis" is higher in subcutaneous adipose tissue of obese vs. lean subjects (Cancello et al., 2005). In mouse model, hypoxia indicated by elevated HIF-1 alpha protein levels in WAT has also been demonstrated in both *ob/ob* mice and in diet- induced obese mice (Rausch, 2007; Ye, 2007). The presence of immunoreactive HIF-1 alpha, its induction by hypoxia and hypoxia mimetics have been demonstrated in several cell-based studies employing either the 3T3-F422A or 3T3-L1 adipocyte clonal cell lines (Chen, 2006; Lolmedet, 2003). Recent report has first showed that the production of angiogenic factors such as VEGF, leptin and matrix metalloproteinases are increased in 3T3-F422A adipocytes in response to low O2 tension (5% O2) or chemical hypoxia. The downregulation of adiponectin gene expression by hypoxia in 3T3-L1 adipocytes has subsequently been confirmed (Hosogai et al., 2007), and occurs also in human adipocytes (Wang et al., 2007). The context of macrophage involved in adipose tissue function, with the induction of IL-6, MIF, TNF- alpha and VEGF gene expressions under hypoxia has been demonstrated in peritoneal macrophages (Ye et al., 2007). These observations suggest that there is a link between pockets of inflammation within WAT and the recruitment of macrophages into these same areas of the tissue through the hypoxia-mediated signaling and relevant adipokine production.

5.3 Inflammatory fatty acids

Obesity and insulin resistance are associated with high circulating concentrations of free fatty acids. A potential link between adipose tissue fatty acid composition and obesity has been high-lighted in several studies (Decsi, 1996; Williams, 2007). Arachidonate is the primary source of fatty acids that mediate inflammatory responses. In obese children from the Mediterranean region, arachidonate levels were increased in adipose tissue compared to those in lean children (Savvas et al., 2004). These findings link arachidonate levels in adipose tissue with obesity. Since arachidonate and fatty acid products in adipose tissue are important in regulating lipolysis, lipogenesis and adipogenesis, it is speculated that phospholipase A2 enzymes that release arachidonate from membrane phospholipids may be directly involved in these three processes. In fact, it has been demonstrated that knockout of the gene that encodes adipose-tissue specific phospholipase A2 enzyme (Group XVI phospholipase A2 or AdPLA) in mice increased the rate of lipolysis by markedly reducing prostaglandin E2 levels. These mice also showed reduced tissue mass, triglyceride levels, insulin resistance and increased fatty acid oxidation in obese adipocytes induced by either a high-fat feeding or leptin deficiency (Jaworski et al., 2009). Phospholipase A2 may also be important in releasing arachidonate from inflammatory cells to be later metabolized by other cells such as adipocytes. As a result, adipocytes may become chronically energy over-loaded, which may alter their secretory profiles. Secretory phospholipase such as secretory Phospholipase A2 from inflammatory cells could act to release arachidonate from neighboring cells including adipocytes. The cyclooxygenase 1 and cyclooxygenase 2 are essential steps in the synthesis of prostanoids from arachidonate. Several studies have suggested that prostanoids modulate adipocyte differentiation and maturation (Shillabeer et al., 1998). The elevation in both prostaglandin E2 and prostaglandin I2 levels have been shown to induce adipocyte dysfunction (Kim & Moustaid-Moussa, 2000). Prostaglandin E2 acts on EP3 receptors to decrease lipolysis by decreasing cAMP concentration and, thereby, contributes to the hypertrophic development of adipocyte (Jaworski et al., 2009). In addition, it has been demonstrated that cyclooxygenase (COX)-2 mediated inflammation in fat plays a pivotal role in the development of adipose tissue inflammation, insulin resistance and fatty liver in high fat- induced obese rats (Hsieh et al., 2009, 2010). The time- dependent increases in plasma insulin, glucose, leptin levels and homeostasis model assessment of insulin resistance (HOMA-IR) shown in high- fat induced obese rats were significantly reversed in those co-treated with a selective COX2 inhibitor (Celecoxib or Mesulid). COX2 inhibition also significantly reversed adipocyte hypertrophy, macrophage infiltration and decreased in markers of adipocyte differentiation shown in high fat diet- induced obese rats, especially in visceral fat rather than those in subcutaneous fat (Hsieh et al., 2009, 2010). In addition, in the COX2 deficient mouse model, PPAR-gamma (an adipocyte differentiation marker) mRNA expression in epididymal adipose tissue was reduced (Ghoshal et al., 2010). Recently, COX2 has been shown to contribute to the differentiation of brown adipocytes in mice, following cold or adrenergic stimulation (Madsen, 2010 ; Vegiopoulos, 2010). They demonstrated that activating the COX2- mediated pathway in adipose tissue could trigger formation of lipid-burning brown adipose tissue and induce weight loss to treat obesity. But, the coming challenge is how to boost the pathway in adipose tissue without increasing COX2- related fat inflammation.

6. Potential therapeutic drugs and immunotherapy in the treatment of obesity -induced adipose tissue inflammation and insulin resistance

Various pharmacological interventions affect obesity-associated cardiometabolic abnormalities. The effects of these interventions depend on weight loss, changes in fat distribution and/or direct effects on adipose tissue inflammation. Furthermore, several pharmacological agents commonly used in patients with vascular diseases or diabetes mellitus also affect adipose tissue function by diverse mechanisms. Although the effects of these drugs on adipose tissue function are unintended, improving adipose tissue function of these treatments may causally link with their improving effects on vascular disease and T2DM.

6.1 Salicylates and COX2 inhibitors

Salicylates are one of the most commonly used nonsteroidal anti- inflammation drugs and have their main actions through COX inhibition. Selective COX2 inhibitors may improve obesity-associated adipose tissue abnormalities (Hsieh et al., 2009, 2010). Besides COX inhibiton, salicylates also act through inhibition of the activity of inhibitor of nuclear factor kappa-B kinase subunit beta (IKK-β) leading to a reduction in translocation of NF-kB to the nucleus, which action is crucially involved in the anti-diabetic effect of aspirin (Yin et al., 1998; Yuan et al., 2001). Accordingly, salicylate in doses of 3 and 4.5 grams per day improved insulin resistance as measured by using a hyperinsulinemic euglycemic clamp. It also decreased free fatty acid and increased adiponectin levels by 35~45% in patients with type 2 diabetes (Goldfine et al., 2008).

6.2 Beta- blockers

Several recent investigations have focused on the effects of the beta-blockers on adipose tissue dysfunction (Gress et al., 2000; Pollare et al., 1989). However, it still remains debated. For instance, a combined β1 and β2- adrenoceptor agonist is capable of downregulating adiponectin and upregulating TNF-alpha mRNA in murine adipocytes (Sharma et al., 2001). Conversely, some of the recent developed β- blockers do have beneficial effects on insulin resistance and adipokines without changes in weight. Nebivolol (5 mg daily), which has β2 intrinsic sympaticomimetic action, increases plasma adiponectin levels in overweight patients with hypertension (Celik et al., 2006). Celipprolol (up to 400 mg daily), a combined β1 antagonist and β2 agonist reduces plasma leptin levels without a change in body weight in patients with dyslipidemia (Malminiemi, 2000).

6.3 Aldosterone antagonists

Adipose tissue is capable of producing an unidentified mineralcorticoid releasing factor that may stimulate aldosterone production (Lamounier-Zepter & Ehrhart-Bornstein, 2006). In obese diabetic mice, blocking the mineralcorticoid receptor reduced the expression of pro-inflammatory cytokines in adipose tissue while it lead to an increased expression of adiponectin in cardiac and adipose tissue (Guo et al., 2008). Additional evidence for an important role of the mineralcorticoid receptor in adipose tissue comes from a study in obese mice. It showed that blocking the mineralcorticoid receptor with eplerone ameliorated insulin resistance, decreased the number of hypertrophic adipocytes and infiltrating macrophages (Hirata et al., 2009).

6.4 Angiotensin converting enzyme inhibitors (ACEI)

Angiotensin converting enzyme inhibitors (ACEI) could affect insulin resistance by reducing plasma concentration of angiotensin Ⅱ, which increases serine phosphorylation of the insulin receptor, insulin receptor substrate 1 and phosphadidylinositol-3-kinase leading to a state of insulin resistance (Folli et al., 1997). Angiotensin Ⅱ might also influence insulin resistance via a direct pro- inflammatory effect on adipocyte and subsequently change in MCP-1, IL-6 and IL-8 production via the NF-kB pathway and increase production of leptin via an ERK1/2 dependent pathway in a murine model (Skurk et al., 2004; Tsuchiya et al., 2006).

6.5 Statins

Statins might alleviate adipose tissue inflammation by inhibiting Toll- like receptor-4 triggered IFN-γ expression in macrophages, which are abundant in adipose tissue and by increasing PPAR-γ expression (Abe et al., 2008; Desjardins et al., 2008). Murine 3T3-L1 adipocytes incubated with blood samples from patients treated with parvastatin have been demonstrated to induce adiponectin production (Takagi et al., 2008). Moreover, atorvastatin, which is more lipophylic than pravasatin increases adiponectin levels in patients with coronary artery disease (CAD) or at high risk for CAD while having no effect on adiponectin in patients with diabetes (Ichida et al., 2006). Simvastatin, the most lipophylic statin, decreases adiponectin (Devaraj et al., 2007). These observations suggest that hydrophilic statins have more beneficial effect than those of lipophylic statins on adipose tissue dysfunction.

6.6 Thiazolidinediones

Thiazolidinediones (TZDs) such as pioglitazone and rosiglitazone have been suggested to be the potential drugs in preventing T2DM. Treatment with rosiglitazone for 3 years have been reported to lower the incidence of T2DM (Gerstein et al. 2006). TZDs may directly increase insulin sensitivity in the liver and adipose tissue where it is of critical importance for adipocyte differentiation. PPAR-γ agonists are thought to promote the uptake and storage of free fatty acids in adipocytes and may therefore protect the liver and muscle from the attacks of excess free fatty acids and their toxic effects. Also, PPAR-γ agonists such as pioglitazone have been shown to increase high molecular weight adiponectin and decrease TNF-αand RBP-4 levels in patients with T2DM (Aso et al., 2007).

6.7 Metformin

Apart from affecting glucose uptake in the liver and peripheral tissues, metformin has anti-inflammatory properties by inhibiting NF-kB and blocking the PI3K- Akt pathway in human vascular cells (Isoda et al., 2006). Recent study suggests that the effect of metformin on AMP-activated protein kinase (AMPK) dependent lipolysis in adipocytes may lead to lower plasma levels of fatty acids and improve adipose tissue function (Bourron et al., 2010). Moreover, metformin has been reported to reduce subcutaneous adipose tissue, total body fat percentage, BMI and waist circumference but not affect the amount of visceral adipose tissue in obese children and adolescents (Srinivasan et al., 2006). However, in a study with lean and obese patients with and without diabetes, metformin did not result in a reduction of BMI, nor did it affect plasma adiponectin levels after 4 months of treatment (Phillips et al., 2003). Thererby, the clinical implication of metformin on treatment of obesity remains controversial.

6.8 Immunotherapy

Nishimura and colleagues have shown that $CD8^+$ T cells play the important role in macrophage recruitment and adipose tissue inflammation. They found that large numbers of $CD8^+$ T cells infiltrated into obese epididymal adipose tissue and preceded the accumulation of macrophages in fat tissue of high-fat induced obese mice. In addition, the immunological and genetic depletion of $CD8^+$ T cells have been reported to lower macrophage infiltration, adipose tissue inflammation and ameliorate systemic insulin resistance (Nishimura et al., 2009). Besides, Winer and colleagues demonstrated that immunotherapy with $CD4^+$ T cell transfer into lymphocyte-free obese mice reversed weight gain and insulin resistance. Short-term treatment with CD3-specific antibody markedly reversed insulin resistance for months, despite continuation of a high-fat diet (Winer et al., 2009). Taken together, these observations not only demonstrate the importance of immune response in the development of obesity, but also identify a number of novel targets and strategies that could be harnessed to treat obesity in manners similar to the treatment of other immunological abnormalities.

7. Conclusion

Obesity-induced inflammation in adipose tissue has been considered as one of the main contributors to the development of insulin resistance and subsequent T2DM in the state of obesity. Both of the innate and adaptive immune systems have been documented to be crucially involved in the initiation and regulation of adipose tissue inflammation. In the meantime, the adipokine dysregulation and hypoxia-mediated signaling during the development of adipocyte hypertrophy are also actively participate into the pathogenesis of adipose tissue inflammation. Recently, the role of inflammatory fatty acids such as arachidonate in the etiology of adipogenesis and lipogenesis has also been the subject of intensive investigation. Although the detail mechanisms remain incompletely understood, it could be a promising therapeutic target for prevention and treatment of obesity-induced insulin resistance and T2DM in the prospective future. Besides, several therapeutic drugs used in the patients with vescular diseases or diabetes and immunotherapy have also been shown to reduce the risk of developing insulin resistance and T2DM.

8. Acknowledgment

The author appreciates Ms. Yen-Ju Hsieh, Ph.D. and Ms. Pei-Chi Chan, M.S. for the assistance of manuscript preparation and book chapter formation.

9. References

Abe, M.; Matsuda, M.; Kobayashi, H.; Miyata, Y.; Nakayama, Y.; Komuro, R.; Fukuhara, A.; Shimomura, I. (2008). Effects of statins on adipose tissue inflammation: their inhibitory effect on MyD88-independent IRF3/IFN-beta pathway in macrophages. *Arteriosclerosis, Thrombosis, and Vascular Biology*, Vol.28, No.5, pp. 871-877, ISSN 1079-5642

Antuna-Puente, B.; Feve, B.; Fellahi, S.; Bastard, J.P. (2008). Adipokines: the missing link between insulin resistance and obesity. *Diabetes & Metabolism*, Vol.34, No.1, pp. 2-11, ISSN 1262-3636

Aso, Y.; Yamamoto, R.; Suetsugu, M.; Matsumoto, S.; Wakabayashi, S.; Matsutomo, R.; Takebayashi, K.; Inukai, T. (2007). Comparison of the effects of pioglitazone and voglibose on circulating total and high-molecular-weight adiponectin, and on two fibrinolysis inhibitors, in patients with Type 2 diabetes. *Diabetic Medicine*, Vol.24, No.9, pp. 962-968, ISSN 0742-3071

Berg, A.H.; Lin, Y.; Lisanti, M.P.; Scherer, P.E. (2004). Adipocyte differentiation induces dynamic changes in NF-kappaB expression and activity. *American Journal of Physiology - Endocrinology and Metabolism*, Vol.287, No.6, pp. E1178-1188, ISSN 0193-1849

Bourron, O.; Daval, M.; Hainault, I.; Hajduch, E.; Servant, J.M.; Gautier, J.F.; Ferré, P.; Foufelle, F. (2010). Biguanides and thiazolidinediones inhibit stimulated lipolysis in human adipocytes through activation of AMP-activated protein kinase. *Diabetologia*, Vol.53, No.4, pp. 768-778, ISSN 0012-186X

Bruun, J.M.; Helge, J.W.; Richelsen, B.; Stallknecht, B. (2006). Diet and exercise reduce low-grade inflammation and macrophage infiltration in adipose tissue but not in skeletal muscle in severely obese subjects. *American Journal of Physiology - Endocrinology and Metabolism*, Vol.290, No.5, pp. E961-967, ISSN 0193-1849

Cancello, R.; Henegar, C.; Viguerie, N.; Taleb, S.; Poitou, C.; Rouault, C.; Coupaye, M.; Pelloux, V.; Hugol, D.; Bouillot, J.L.; Bouloumié, A.; Barbatelli, G.; Cinti, S.; Svensson, P.A.; Barsh, G.S.; Zucker, J.D.; Basdevant, A.; Langin, D.; Clément, K. (2005). Reduction of macrophage infiltration and chemoattractant gene expression changes in white adipose tissue of morbidly obese subjects after surgery-induced weight loss. *Diabetes*, Vol.54, No.8, pp. 2277-86, ISSN 0012-1797

Celik, T.; Iyisoy, A.; Kursaklioglu, H.; Kardesoglu, E.; Kilic, S.; Turhan, H.; Yilmaz, M.I.; Ozcan, O.; Yaman, H.; Isik, E.; Fici, F. (2006). Comparative effects of nebivolol and metoprolol on oxidative stress, insulin resistance, plasma adiponectin and soluble P-selectin levels in hypertensive patients. *Journal of Hypertension*, Vol.24, No.3, pp. 591-596, ISSN 0263-6352

Chen, M.P.; Chung, F.M.; Chang, D.M.; Tsai, J.C.; Huang, H.F.; Shin, S.J.; Lee, Y.J. (2006). Elevated plasma level of visfatin/pre-B cell colony-enhancing factor in patients with type 2 diabetes mellitus. *The Journal of Clinical Endocrinology & Metabolism*, Vol.91, No.1, pp. 295-299, ISSN 0021-972X

Chen, B.; Lam, K.S.; Wang, Y.; Wu, D.; Lam, M.C.; Shen, J.; Wong, L.; Hoo, R.L.; Zhang, J.; Xu, A. (2006). Hypoxia dysregulates the production of adiponectin and plasminogen activator inhibitor-1 independent of reactive oxygen species in adipocytes. *Biochemical and Biophysical Research Communications*, Vol.341, No.2, pp. 549-556, ISSN 0006-291X

Cinti, S.; Mitchell, G.; Barbatelli, G.; Murano, I.; Ceresi, E.; Faloia, E.; Wang, S.; Fortier, M.; Greenberg, A.S.; Obin, M.S. (2005). Adipocyte death defines macrophage localization and function in adipose tissue of obese mice and humans. *The Journal of Lipid Research*, Vol.46, No.11, pp. 2347-2355, ISSN 0022-2275

Considine, R.V.; Sinha, M.K.; Heiman, M.L.; Kriauciunas, A.; Stephens, T.W.; Nyce, M.R.; Ohannesian, J.P.; Marco, C.C.; McKee, L.J.; Bauer, T.L. (1996). Serum immunoreactive-leptin concentrations in normal-weight and obese humans. *The New England Journal of Medicine*, Vol.334, No.5, pp. 292-295, ISSN 0028-4793

Dahl, T.B.; Yndestad, A.; Skjelland, M.; Øie, E.; Dahl, A.; Michelsen, A.; Damås, J.K.; Tunheim, S.H.; Ueland, T.; Smith, C.; Bendz, B.; Tonstad, S.; Gullestad, L.; Frøland, S.S.; Krohg-Sørensen, K.; Russell, D.; Aukrust, P.; Halvorsen, B. (2007). Increased expression of visfatin in macrophages of human unstable carotid and coronary atherosclerosis: possible role in inflammation and plaque destabilization. *Circulation*, Vol.115, No.8, pp. 972-980, ISSN 0009-7322

Decsi, T.; Molnár, D.; Koletzko, B. (1996). Long-chain polyunsaturated fatty acids in plasma lipids of obese children. *Lipids*, Vol.31, No.3, pp. 305-311, ISSN 0024-4201

Desjardins, F.; Sekkali, B.; Verreth, W.; Pelat, M.; De, K. D.; Mertens, A.; Smith, G.; Herregods, M.C.; Holvoet, P.; Balligand, J.L. (2008). Rosuvastatin increases vascular endothelial PPARgamma expression and corrects blood pressure variability in obese dyslipidaemic mice. *European Heart Journal*, Vol.29, No.1, pp. 128-137, ISSN 0195-668X

Devaraj, S.; Siegel, D.; Jialal, I. (2007). Simvastatin (40 mg/day), adiponectin levels, and insulin sensitivity in subjects with the metabolic syndrome. *The American journal of cardiology*, Vol.100, No.9, pp. 1397-1399, ISSN 0002-9149

Fain, J.N.; Madan, A.K.; Hiler, M.L.; Cheema, P.; Bahouth, S.W. (2004). Comparison of the release of adipokines by adipose tissue, adipose tissue matrix, and adipocytes from visceral and subcutaneous abdominal adipose tissues of obese humans. *Endocrinology*, Vol.145, No.5, pp. 2273-2282, ISSN 0013-7227

Folli,F.; Kahn, C.R.; Hansen, H.; Bouchie, J.L.; Feener, E.P. (1997). Angiotensin II inhibits insulin signaling in aortic smooth muscle cells at multiple levels. A potential role for serine phosphorylation in insulin/angiotensin II crosstalk. *The Journal of Clinical Investigation*, Vol.100, No.9, pp. 2158-2169, ISSN 0021-9738

Fried, S.K.; Bunkin, D.A.; Greenberg, A.S. (1998). Omental and subcutaneous adipose tissues of obese subjects release interleukin-6: depot difference and regulation by glucocorticoid. *The Journal of Clinical Endocrinology & Metabolism*, Vol.83, No.3, pp. 847-850, ISSN 0021-972X

Fukuhara, A.; Matsuda, M.; Nishizawa, M.; Segawa, K.; Tanaka, M.; Kishimoto, K.; Matsuki, Y.; Murakami, M.; Ichisaka, T.; Murakami, H.; Watanabe, E.; Takagi, T.; Akiyoshi, M.; Ohtsubo, T.; Kihara, S.; Yamashita, S.; Makishima, M.; Funahashi, T.; Yamanaka, S.; Hiramatsu, R.; Matsuzawa, Y.; Shimomura, I. (2005). Visfatin: a protein secreted by visceral fat that mimics the effects of insulin. *Science*, Vol.307, No.5708, pp. 426-430, ISSN 0036-8075

Gerstein, H.C.; Yusuf, S.; Bosch, J.; Pogue, J. (2006). Effect of resiglitazone on the frequency of diabetes in patients with impaired glucose tolerence or impaired fasting glucose: a randomised controlled trial. The Lancet, Vol.368, No9541, pp. 1096-1105, ISSN 0140-6736

Ghoshal, S.; Trivedi, D.B.; Graf, G.A.; Loftin, C.D. (2011). Cyclooxygenase-2 deficiency attenuates adipose tissue differentiation and inflammation in mice. *The Journal of Biological Chemistry*, Vol.286, No.1, pp. 889-898, ISSN 0021-9258

Goldfine, A.B.; Silver, R.; Aldhahi, W.; Cai, D.; Tatro, E.; Lee, J.; Shoelson, S.E. (2008). Use of salsalate to target inflammation in the treatment of insulin resistance and type 2 diabetes. *Clinical and Translational Scienc*, Vol.1, No.1, pp. 36-43, ISSN 1752-8054

Gordon, S. (2007). Macrophage heterogeneity and tissue lipids. *The Journal of Clinical Investigation*, Vol.117, No.1, pp. 89-93, ISSN 0021-9738

Gress, T.W.; Nieto, F.J.; Shahar, E.; Wofford, M.R.; Brancati, F.L. (2000). Hypertension and antihypertensive therapy as risk factors for type 2 diabetes mellitus. Atherosclerosis Risk in Communities Study. *New England Journal of Medicine*, Vol.342, No.13, pp. 905-912, ISSN 0028-4793

Guilherme, A.; Virbasius, J.V.; Puri, V.; Czech, M.P. (2008). Adipocyte dysfunctions linking obesity to insulin resistance and type 2 diabetes. *Nature Reviews Molecular Cell Biology*, Vol.9, No.5, pp. 367-377, ISSN 1471-0072

Guo, C.; Ricchiuti, V.; Lian, B.Q.; Yao, T.M.; Coutinho, P.; Romero, J.R.; Li, J.; Williams, G.H.; Adler, G.K. (2008). Mineralocorticoid receptor blockade reverses obesity-related changes in expression of adiponectin, peroxisome proliferator-activated receptor-gamma, and proinflammatory adipokines. *Circulation*, Vol.117, No.17, pp. 2253-2261, ISSN 0009-7322

Hirata, A.; Maeda, N.; Hiuge, A.; Hibuse, T.; Fujita, K.; Okada, T.; Kihara, S.; Funahashi, T.; Shimomura, I. (2009). Blockade of mineralocorticoid receptor reverses adipocyte dysfunction and insulin resistance in obese mice. *Cardiovascular Research*, Vol.84, No.1, pp. 164-172, ISSN 0008-6363

Hotamisligil, G.S.; Shargill, N.S.; Spiegelman, B.M. (1993). Adipose expression of tumor necrosis factor-alpha: direct role in obesity-linked insulin resistance. *Science*, Vol.259, No.5091, pp. 87-91, ISSN 0036-8075

Hosogai, N.; Fukuhara, A.; Oshima, K.; Miyata, Y.; Tanaka, S.; Segawa, K.; Furukawa, S.; Tochino, Y.; Komuro, R.; Matsuda, M.; Shimomura, I. (2007). Adipose tissue hypoxia in obesity and its impact on adipocytokine dysregulation. *Diabetes*, Vol.56, No.4, pp. 901-911, ISSN 0012-1797

Howard, J.K. & Flier, J.S. (2006). Attenuation of leptin and insulin signaling by SOCS proteins. *Trends in Endocrinology and Metabolism*, Vol.17, No.9, pp. 365-371, ISSN 1043-2760

Hsieh, P.S.; Jin, J.S.; Chiang, C.F.; Chan, P.C.; Chen, C.H.; Shih, K.C. (2009). COX-2-mediated inflammation in fat is crucial for obesity-linked insulin resistance and fatty liver. *Obesity*, Vol.17, No.6, pp. 1150-1157, ISSN 20900708

Hsieh, P.S.; Lu, K.C.; Chiang, C.F.; Chen, C.H. (2010). Suppressive effect of COX2 inhibitor on the progression of adipose inflammation in high-fat-induced obese rats. *European Journal of Clinical Investigation*, Vol.40, No.2, pp. 164-171, ISSN 0014-2972

Ichida, Y.; Hasegawa, G.; Fukui, M.; Obayashi, H.; Ohta, M.; Fujinami, A.; Ohta, K.; Nakano, K.; Yoshikawa, T.; Nakamura, N. (2006). Effect of atorvastatin on in vitro expression of resistin in adipocytes and monocytes/macrophages and effect of atorvastatin treatment on serum resistin levels in patients with type 2 diabetes. *Pharmacology*, Vol.76, No.1, pp. 34-39, ISSN 0031-7012

Isoda, K.; Young, J.L.; Zirlik, A.; MacFarlane, L.A.; Tsuboi, N.; Gerdes, N.; Schönbeck, U.; Libby, P. (2006). Metformin inhibits proinflammatory responses and nuclear factor-kappaB in human vascular wall cells. *Arteriosclerosis, Thrombosis, and Vascular Biology*, Vol.26, No.3, pp. 611-617, ISSN 1079-5642

Jaworski, K.; Ahmadian, M.; Duncan, R.E.; Sarkadi-Nagy, E.; Varady, K.A.; Hellerstein, M.K.; Lee, H.Y.; Samuel, V.T.; Shulman, G.I.; Kim, K.H.; de Val, S.; Kang, C.; Sul, H.S. (2009). AdPLA ablation increases lipolysis and prevents obesity induced by high-fat feeding or leptin deficiency. *Nature Medicine*, Vol.15, No.2, pp. 159-168, ISSN 1078-8956

Jiao, P.; Chen, Q.; Shah, S.; Du, J.; Tao, B.; Tzameli, I.; Yan, W.; Xu, H. (2009). Obesity-related upregulation of monocyte chemotactic factors in adipocytes: involvement of nuclear factor-kappaB and c-Jun NH2-terminal kinase pathways. *Diabetes*, Vol.58, No.1, pp. 104-115, ISSN 0012-1797

Kamei, N.; Tobe, K.; Suzuki, R.; Ohsugi, M.; Watanabe, T.; Kubota, N.; Ohtsuka-Kowatari, N.; Kumagai, K.; Sakamoto, K.; Kobayashi, M.; Yamauchi, T.; Ueki, K.; Oishi, Y.; Nishimura, S.; Manabe, I.; Hashimoto, H.; Ohnishi, Y.; Ogata, H.; Tokuyama, K.; Tsunoda, M.; Ide, T.; Murakami, K.; Nagai, R.; Kadowaki, T. (2006). Overexpression of monocyte chemoattractant protein-1 in adipose tissues causes macrophage recruitment and insulin resistance. *The Journal of Biological Chemistry*, Vol.281, No.36, pp. 26602-26614, ISSN 0021-9258

Kanda, H.; Tateya, S.; Tamori, Y.; Kotani, K.; Hiasa, K.; Kitazawa, R.; Kitazawa, S.; Miyachi, H.; Maeda, S.; Egashira, K.; Kasuga, M. (2006). MCP-1 contributes to macrophage infiltration into adipose tissue, insulin resistance, and hepatic steatosis in obesity. *The Journal of Clinical Investigation*, Vol.116, No.6, pp. 1494-505, ISSN 0021-9738

Kawanami, D.; Maemura, K.; Takeda, N.; Harada, T.; Nojiri, T.; Imai, Y.; Manabe, I.; Utsunomiya, K.; Nagai, R. (2004). Direct reciprocal effects of resistin and adiponectin on vascular endothelial cells: a new insight into adipocytokine-endothelial cell interactions. *Biochemical and Biophysical Research Communications*, Vol.314, No.2, pp. 415-419, ISSN 0006-291X

Kern, P.A.; Ranganathan, S.; Li, C.; Wood, L.; Ranganathan, G. (2001). Adipose tissue tumor necrosis factor and interleukin-6 expression in human obesity and insulin resistance. *American Journal of Physiology - Endocrinology and Metabolism*, Vol.280, No.5, pp. E745-51, ISSN 0193-1849

Kim, K.H.; Lee, K.; Moon, Y.S.; Sul, H.S. (2001). A cysteine-rich adipose tissue-specific secretory factor inhibits adipocyte differentiation. *The Journal of Biological Chemistry*, Vol.276, No.14, pp. 11252-11256, ISSN 0021-9258

Kim, S. & Moustaid-Moussa, N. (2000). Secretory, endocrine and autocrine/paracrine function of the adipocyte. *Journal of Nutrition*, Vol.130, No.12, pp. 3110S-3115S, ISSN 0022-3166

Kintscher, U.; Hartge, M.; Hess, K.; Foryst-Ludwig, A.; Clemenz, M.; Wabitsch, M.; Fischer-Posovszky, P.; Barth, T.F.; Dragun, D.; Skurk, T.; Hauner, H.; Blüher, M.; Unger, T.; Wolf, A.M.; Knippschild, U.; Hombach, V.; Marx, N. (2008). T-lymphocyte infiltration in visceral adipose tissue: a primary event in adipose tissue inflammation and the development of obesity-mediated insulin resistance. *Arteriosclerosis, Thrombosis, and Vascular Biology*, Vol.28, No.7, pp. 1304-1310, ISSN 1079-5642

Kras, K.M.; Hausman, D.B.; Martin, R.J. (2000). Tumor necrosis factor-alpha stimulates cell proliferation in adipose tissue-derived stromal-vascular cell culture: promotion of adipose tissue expansion by paracrine growth factors. *Obesity Research*, Vol.8, No.2, pp. 186-193, ISSN 1071-7323

Kumada, M.; Kihara, S.; Ouchi, N.; Kobayashi, H.; Okamoto, Y.; Ohashi, K.; Maeda, K.; Nagaretani, H.; Kishida, K.; Maeda, N.; Nagasawa, A.; Funahashi, T.; Matsuzawa, Y. (2004). Adiponectin specifically increased tissue inhibitor of metalloproteinase-1 through interleukin-10 expression in human macrophages. *Circulation*, Vol.109, No.17, pp. 2046-2049, ISSN 0009-7322

Lamounier-Zepter, V. & Ehrhart-Bornstein, M. (2006). Fat tissue metabolism and adrenal steroid secretion. *Current Hypertension Reports*, Vol.8, No.1, pp. 30-34, ISSN 1522-6417

Lehrke, M.; Reilly, M.P.; Millington, S.C.; Iqbal, N.; Rader, D.J; Lazar, M.A. (2004). An inflammatory cascade leading to hyperresistinemia in humans. *PLoS Medicine*, Vol.1, No.2, pp. e45, ISSN 1549-1277

Lolmède, K.; Durand, de S. F. V.; Galitzky, J.; Lafontan, M.; Bouloumié, A. (2003). Effects of hypoxia on the expression of proangiogenic factors in differentiated 3T3-F442A adipocytes. *International Journal of Obesity and Related Metabolic Disorders*, Vol.27, No.10, pp. 1187-1195, ISSN 0307-0565

Lumeng, C.N.; Bodzin, J.L.; Saltiel, A.R. (2007). Obesity induces a phenotypic switch in adipose tissue macrophage polarization. *The Journal of Clinical Investigation*, Vol.117, No.1, pp. 175-184, ISSN 0021-9738

Lumeng, C.N.; Deyoung, S.M.; Bodzin, J.L.; Saltiel, A.R. (2007). Increased inflammatory properties of adipose tissue macrophages recruited during diet-induced obesity. *Diabetes*, Vol.56, No.1, pp. 16-23, ISSN 0012-1797

Maachi, M.; Piéroni, L.; Bruckert, E.; Jardel, C.; Fellahi, S.; Hainque, B.; Capeau, J.; Bastard, J.P. (2004). Systemic low-grade inflammation is related to both circulating and adipose tissue TNFalpha, leptin and IL-6 levels in obese women. *International*

Journal of Obesity and Related Metabolic Disorders, Vol.28, No.8, pp. 993-997, ISSN 0307-0565

Madsen, L.; Pedersen, L.M.; Lillefosse, H.H.; Fjaere, E.; Bronstad, I.; Hao, Q.; Petersen, R.K.; Hallenborg, P.; Ma, T.; De, M. R.; Araujo, P.; Mercader, J.; Bonet, M.L.; Hansen, J.B.; Cannon, B.; Nedergaard, J.; Wang, J.; Cinti, S.; Voshol, P.; Døskeland, S.O.; Kristiansen, K. (2010). UCP1 induction during recruitment of brown adipocytes in white adipose tissue is dependent on cyclooxygenase activity. *PLoS One*, Vol.5, No.6, pp. e11391, ISSN 1932-6203

Malminiemi, K. (2000). Long-term celiprolol therapy lowers fasting plasma leptin levels. Celiprolol Multicenter Study Group. *Cardiovascular Drugs and Therapy*, Vol.14, No.1, pp. 67-75, ISSN 0920-320

Matarese, G.; La Cava. A; Sanna, V, Lord, G.M.; Lechler, R.I,; Fontana, S.; Zappacosta, S. (2002). Balancing susceptibility to infection and autoimmunity: a role for leptin? *Trends Immunology,*Vol.23, No.4, pp. 182-7, ISSN 1471-4906.

Minokoshi, Y.; Kim, Y.B.; Peroni, O.D.; Fryer, L.G.; Müller, C.; Carling, D.; Kahn, B.B. (2002). Leptin stimulates fatty-acid oxidation by activating AMP-activated protein kinase. *Nature*, Vol.415, No.6869, pp. 339-343, ISSN 0027-8424

Nishimura, S.; Manabe, I.; Nagasaki, M.; Eto, K.; Yamashita, H.; Ohsugi, M.; Otsu, M.; Hara, K.; Ueki, K.; Sugiura, S.; Yoshimura, K.; Kadowaki, T.; Nagai, R. (2009). $CD8^+$ effector T cells contribute to macrophage recruitment and adipose tissue inflammation in obesity. *Nature Medicine*, Vol. 15, No.8, pp. 914-920, ISSN 1078-8956

Nonogaki, K.; Fuller, G.M.; Fuentes, N.L.; Moser, A.H.; Staprans, I.; Grunfeld, C.; Feingold, K.R. (1995). Interleukin-6 stimulates hepatic triglyceride secretion in rats. *Endocrinology*, Vol.136, No.5, pp. 2143-2149, ISSN 0013-7227

Ouchi, N.; Kihara, S.; Arita, Y.; Okamoto, Y.; Maeda, K.; Kuriyama, H.; Hotta, K.; Nishida, M.; Takahashi, M.; Muraguchi, M.; Ohmoto, Y.; Nakamura, T.; Yamashita, S.; Funahashi, T.; Matsuzawa, Y. (2000). Adiponectin, an adipocyte-derived plasma protein, inhibits endothelial NF-kappaB signaling through a cAMP-dependent pathway. *Circulation*, Vol.102, No.11, pp. 1296-1301, ISSN 0009-7322

Phillips, S.A.; Ciaraldi, T.P.; Kong, A.P.; Bandukwala, R.; Aroda, V.; Carter, L.; Baxi, S.; Mudaliar, S.R.; Henry, R.R. (2003). Modulation of circulating and adipose tissue adiponectin levels by antidiabetic therapy. *Diabetes*, Vol.52, No.3, pp. 667-674, ISSN 0012-1797

Pollare, T.; Lithell, H.; Selinus, I.; Berne, C. (1989). Sensitivity to insulin during treatment with atenolol and metoprolol: a randomised, double blind study of effects on carbohydrate and lipoprotein metabolism in hypertensive patients. *British Medical Journal*, Vol.298, No.6681, pp. 1152-1157, ISSN 0959-8138

Rausch, M.E.; Weisberg, S.; Vardhana, P.; Tortoriello, D.V. (2008). Obesity in C57BL/6J mice is characterized by adipose tissue hypoxia and cytotoxic T-cell infiltration. *International Journal of Obesity*, Vol.32, No.3, pp. 451-463, ISSN 0307-0565

Rocha, V.Z.; Folco, E.J.; Sukhova, G.; Shimizu, K.; Gotsman, I.; Vernon, A.H.; Libby, P. (2008). Interferon-gamma, a Th1 cytokine, regulates fat inflammation: a role for adaptive immunity in obesity. *Circulation Research*, Vol.103, No.5, pp. 467-476, ISSN 0009-7300

Samal, B.; Sun, Y.; Stearns, G.; Xie, C.; Suggs, S.; McNiece, I. (1994). Cloning and characterization of the cDNA encoding a novel human pre-B-cell colony-enhancing factor. *Molecular and Cellular Biology*, Vol.14, No.2, pp. 1431-1437., ISSN 0270-7306

Sandeep, S.; Velmurugan, K.; Deepa, R.; Mohan, V. (2007). Serum visfatin in relation to visceral fat, obesity, and type 2 diabetes mellitus in Asian Indians. *Metabolism*, Vol.56, No.4, pp. 565-570

Sharma, A.M.; Pischon, T.; Hardt, S.; Kunz, I.; Luft, F.C. (2001). Hypothesis: Beta-adrenergic receptor blockers and weight gain: A systematic analysis. *Hypertension*, Vol.37, No.2, pp. 250-254, ISSN 0914-911X

Shillabeer, G.; Kumar, V.; Tibbo, E.; Lau, D.C. (1998). Arachidonic acid metabolites of the lipoxygenase as well as the cyclooxygenase pathway may be involved in regulating preadipocyte differentiation. *Metabolism*, Vol.47, No.4, pp. 461-466

Skurk, T.; van Harmelen, V.; Hauner, H. (2004). Angiotensin II stimulates the release of interleukin-6 and interleukin-8 from cultured human adipocytes by activation of NF-kappaB. *Arteriosclerosis, Thrombosis, and Vascular Biology*, Vol.24, No.7, pp. 1199-1203, ISSN 1079-5642

Srinivasan, S.; Ambler, G.R.; Baur, L.A.; Garnett, S.P.; Tepsa, M.; Yap, F.; Ward, G.M.; Cowell, C.T. (2006). Randomized, controlled trial of metformin for obesity and insulin resistance in children and adolescents: improvement in body composition and fasting insulin. *Journal of Clinical Endocrinology & Metabolism*, Vol.91, No.6, pp. 2074-2080, ISSN 0021-972X

Steppan, C.M.; Bailey, S.T.; Bhat, S.; Brown, E.J.; Banerjee, R.R.; Wright, C.M.; Patel, H.R.; Ahima, R.S.; Lazar, M.A. (2001). The hormone resistin links obesity to diabetes. *Nature*, Vol.409, No.6818, pp. 307-312, ISSN 0028-0836

Takagi, T.; Matsuda, M.; Abe, M.; Kobayashi, H.; Fukuhara, A.; Komuro, R.; Kihara, S.; Caslake, M.J.; McMahon, A.; Shepherd, J.; Funahashi, T.; Shimomura, I. (2008). Effect of pravastatin on the development of diabetes and adiponectin production. *Atherosclerosis*, Vol.196, No.1, pp. 114-121, ISSN 0021-9150

Takahashi, K.; Yamaguchi, S.; Shimoyama, T.; Seki, H.; Miyokawa, K.; Katsuta, H.; Tanaka, T.; Yoshimoto, K.; Ohno, H.; Nagamatsu, S.; Ishida, H. (2008). JNK- and IkappaB-dependent pathways regulate MCP-1 but not adiponectin release from artificially hypertrophied 3T3-L1 adipocytes preloaded with palmitate in vitro. *American Journal of Physiology - Endocrinology and Metabolism*, Vol.294, No.5, pp. E898-909, ISSN 0193-1849

Tsuchiya, K.; Yoshimoto, T.; Hirono, Y.; Tateno, T.; Sugiyama, T.; Hirata, Y. (2006). Angiotensin II induces monocyte chemoattractant protein-1 expression via a nuclear factor-kappaB-dependent pathway in rat preadipocytes. *American Journal of Physiology - Endocrinology And Metabolism*, Vol.291, No.4, pp. E771-778, ISSN 0193-1849

Vegiopoulos, A.; Müller-Decker, K.; Strzoda, D.; Schmitt, I.; Chichelnitskiy, E.; Ostertag, A.; Berriel, D.M.; Rozman, J.; Hrabe, de A. M.; Nüsing, R.M.; Meyer, C.W.; Wahli, W.; Klingenspor, M.; Herzig, S. (2010). Cyclooxygenase-2 controls energy homeostasis in mice by de novo recruitment of brown adipocytes. *Science*, Vol.328, No.5982, pp. 1158-1161, ISSN 0036-8075

Wang, B.; Wood, I.S.; Trayhurn, P. (2007). Dysregulation of the expression and secretion of inflammation-related adipokines by hypoxia in human adipocytes. *Pflügers Archiv European Journal of Physiology*, Vol.455, No.3, pp. 479-492, ISSN 0031-6768

Weisberg, S.P.; McCann, D.; Desai, M.; Rosenbaum, M.; Leibel, R.L.; Ferrante, A.W. Jr. (2003). Obesity is associated with macrophage accumulation in adipose tissue. *The Journal of Clinical Investigation*, Vol.112, No.12, pp. 1796-1808, ISSN 0021-9738

Weisberg, S.P.; Hunter, D.; Huber, R.; Lemieux, J.; Slaymaker, S.; Vaddi, K.; Charo, I.; Leibel, R.L.; Ferrante, A.W. Jr. (2006). CCR2 modulates inflammatory and metabolic effects of high-fat feeding. *The Journal of Clinical Investigation*, Vol. 116, No.1, pp.115-124, ISSN 0021-9738

Williams, E.S.; Baylin, A.; Campos, H. (2007). Adipose tissue arachidonic acid and the metabolic syndrome in Costa Rican adults. *Clinical Nutrition*, Vol.26, No.4, pp. 474-482, ISSN 1938-3207

Winer, S.; Chan, Y.; Paltser, G.; Truong, D.; Tsui, H.; Bahrami, J.; Dorfman, R.; Wang, Y.; Zielenski, J.; Mastronardi, F.; Maezawa, Y.; Drucker, D.J.; Engleman, E.; Winer, D.; Dosch, H.M. (2009). Normalization of obesity-associated insulin resistance through immunotherapy. *Nature Medicine*, Vol. 15, No.8, pp. 921-929, ISSN 1078-8956

Wu, H.; Ghosh, S.; Perrard, X.D.; Feng, L.; Garcia, G.E.; Perrard, J.L.; Sweeney, J.F.; Peterson, L.E.; Chan, L.; Smith, C.W.; Ballantyne, C.M. (2007). T-cell accumulation and regulated on activation, normal T cell expressed and secreted upregulation in adipose tissue in obesity. *Circulation*, Vol.115, No.8, pp. 1029-1038, ISSN 0009-7322

Xu, H.; Barnes, G.T.; Yang, Q.; Tan, G.; Yang, D.; Chou, C.J.; Sole, J.; Nichols, A.; Ross, J.S.; Tartaglia, L.A.; Chen, H. (2003). Chronic inflammation in fat plays a crucial role in the development of obesity-related insulin resistance. *The Journal of Clinical Investigation*, Vol.112, No.12, pp. 1821-1830, ISSN 0021-9738

Yamauchi ,T.; Kamon, J.; Minokoshi, Y.; Ito, Y.; Waki, H.; Uchida, S.; Yamashita, S.; Noda, M.; Kita, S.; Ueki, K.; Eto, K.; Akanuma, Y.; Froguel, P.; Foufelle, F.; Ferre, P.; Carling, D.; Kimura, S.; Nagai, R.; Kahn, B.B.; Kadowaki, T. (2002). Adiponectin stimulates glucose utilization and fatty-acid oxidation by activating AMP-activated protein kinase. *Nature Medicine*, Vol.8, No.11, pp. 1288-1295, ISSN 1078-8956

Ye, J.; Gao, Z.; Yin, J.; He, Q. (2007). Hypoxia is a potential risk factor for chronic inflammation and adiponectin reduction in adipose tissue of ob/ob and dietary obese mice. *American Journal of Physiology - Endocrinology and Metabolism*, Vol.293, No.4, pp. E1118-1128, ISSN 0193-1849

Yin, M.J.; Yamamoto, Y.; Gaynor, R.B. (1998). The anti-inflammatory agents aspirin and salicylate inhibit the activity of I(kappa)B kinase-beta. *Nature*, Vol.396, No.6706, pp. 77-80, ISSN 0028-0836

Yuan, M.; Konstantopoulos, N.; Lee, J.; Hansen, L.; Li, Z.W.; Karin, M.; Shoelson, S.E. (2001). Reversal of obesity- and diet-induced insulin resistance with salicylates or targeted disruption of Ikkbeta. *Science*, Vol.293, No.5535, pp. 1673-1677, ISSN 0036-8075

zis, C.; Kyriakakis, M.; Tsimbinos, G.; Tornaritis, M.; Kafatos, A. (2004). Association of adipose tissue arachidonic acid content with BMI and overweight status in children from Cyprus and Crete. *British Journal of Nutrition*, Vol.91, No.4, pp. 643-649, ISSN 0007-1145

11

Assessment of Abdominal Adiposity and Organ Fat with Magnetic Resonance Imaging

Houchun H. Hu[1], Michael I. Goran[2] and Krishna S. Nayak[1]
[1]Ming Hsieh Department of Electrical Engineering, Viterbi School of Engineering
[2]Childhood Obesity Research Center, Department of Preventive Medicine, Keck School of Medicine
University of Southern California, Los Angeles, California
United States of America

1. Introduction

As the prevalence of obesity and type II diabetes continues to rise, accurate tools for quantifying abdominal body and organ fat are critically needed to assist researchers investigating therapeutic and preventive measures against obesity and its comorbidities. Fat accumulation in the liver, pancreas, and skeletal muscles are indicators of diabetes, the metabolic syndrome, and obesity. In addition to organ fat, the distribution of abdominal subcutaneous and visceral adipose tissue play critical roles in determining one's metabolic profile and health risks. Rapid comprehensive human body fat quantification remains an unsolved problem and unmet need. Magnetic resonance imaging (MRI) is the most promising modality to address such challenge. MRI is non-invasive, utilizes no ionizing radiation, provides 3D visualization of the anatomy, has immense flexibility in tissue contrast mechanisms, is safely repeatable across longitudinal studies without restrictions, and is applicable to cohorts of all ages, particularly children and adolescents.

This chapter provides the reader with an overview of MRI techniques for measuring abdominal adiposity and organ fat. The described methods are useful in preventive medicine for early detection of health risks, in studies for identifying changes in subcutaneous and visceral adipose tissue volumes due to intervention, such as bariatric surgery and diet, and in comparing trends between gender and ethnicity groups. The chapter is divided into several sections. It begins with a description of MRI principles. This provides the reader with basic knowledge and familiarizes them with terminology. Next, emphasis is placed on specific MRI approaches such as T_1-weighted imaging and magnetic resonance spectroscopy (MRS) as well as state-of-the-art chemical shift imaging (CSI) techniques that are used to assess body and organ fat. Each technique is discussed in detail and compared to its counterparts. Following this description of imaging methodologies, post-processing and image analysis procedures for extracting adipose tissue depot volumes and percent organ fat content from abdominal MRI data using commercially available software are explained. The advantages and disadvantages of each MRI approach with respect to imaging parameters, spatial resolution, subject motion, scan time, and appropriate fat quantitative endpoints are emphasized. The benefits and challenges of contiguous 3D acquisitions over 2D multi-slice approaches are reviewed. Finally, practical considerations in implementing these methods in the clinical setting are offered, along with an outlook on future fat imaging research. Throughout the chapter, illustrative figures accompany each section to highlight the topics.

2. Basic principles of magnetic resonance imaging

Detailed MRI physics are available for the casual (Hashemi & Bradley, 1999) and technical readers (Bernstein et al., 2004; Haacke et al., 1999; Vlaardingerbroek & den Boer, 1999).

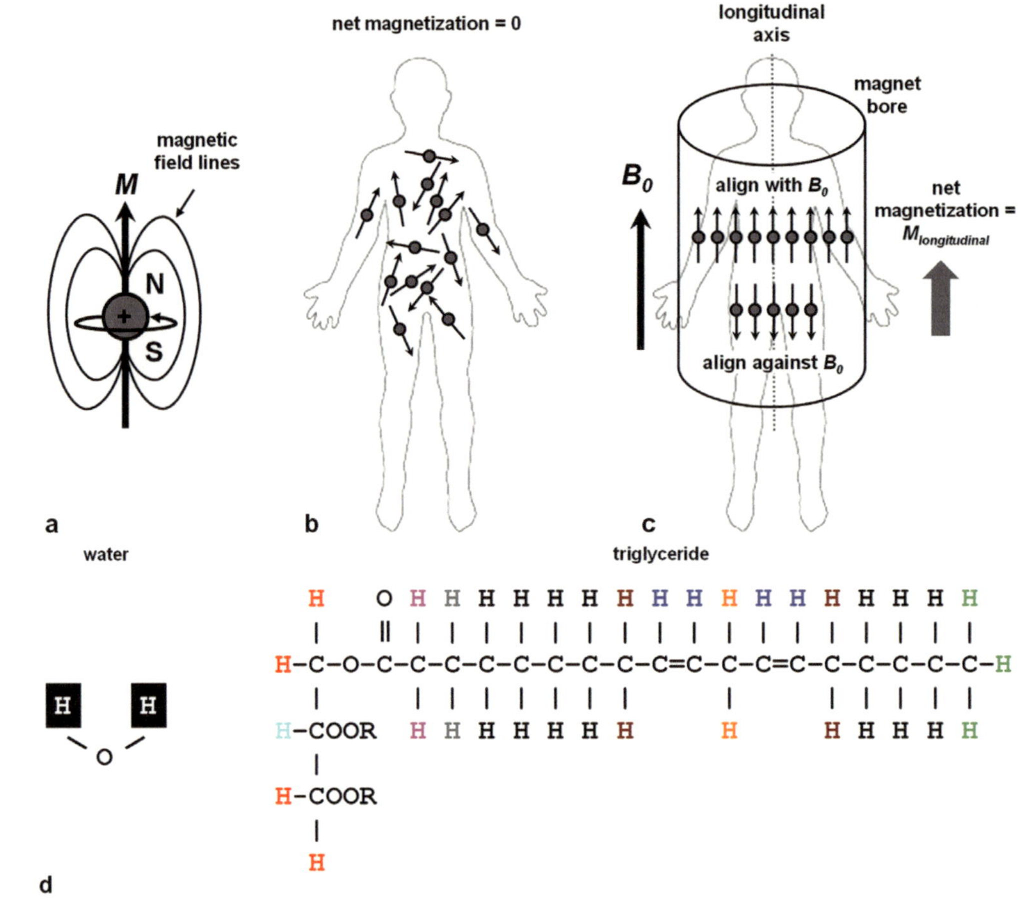

Fig. 1. Magnetization. (a) A hydrogen atom, or proton spin, exhibits a magnetic dipole *M*, due to the spinning motion of its positive nucleus. The dipole is similar to a bar magnet with "North (N)" and "South (S)" poles. (b) Spins are randomly oriented without the presence of a B_0 field and gives rise to no net magnetization. (c) Dipoles either align with or against the B_0 field in its presence, with a slight preference for the former. A measurable magnetization, $M_{longitudinal}$, is thus generated. (d) Water and fat (triglycerides) are the most common hydrogen-containing molecules. For fat, colors represent hydrogens with different local chemical environments. Figure (d) courtesy of G. Hamilton, Ph.D., University of California San Diego. Schematic presented for illustration only and is not drawn to scale.

2.1 Signal origin, magnetization, and precession: The "M"

The signal in MRI arises from the nucleus of an atom, which consists of one or more positively charged protons. Figure 1a illustrates a naturally spinning nucleus, which can be considered as a charged particle in motion (e.g. an electric current). The movement of this electric current, albeit an infinitesimally small one, produces a magnetic dipole M about the nucleus. While the inherent magnetic dipole of a single atom is small, a large population of atoms in an object or human body can be significant and detectable. The magnetization of hydrogen whose nucleus consists of a single proton (^1H) is frequently measured in MRI, due primarily to its high natural abundance in organic life forms. The two most common hydrogen-containing molecules are water and fat (e.g. triglycerides), as shown in Figure 1d. Their magnetization signals within an imaging object or patient are detected, excited, measured, and reconstructed into diagnostic images.

The superconducting MRI magnets used for human imaging generates a magnetic field (B_0) strength between 0.5 and 3.0 Tesla (T). Routine imaging is performed at 1.5T, and in more recent years at 3.0T. By comparison, these strengths are much greater than the natural North-South magnetic fields of Earth's poles, which varies between 0.3 and 0.6 Gauss (G), where 1T=10,000G. The B_0 field is oriented along the longitudinal axis of the magnet bore, as shown in Figure 1c. Prior to placing a subject within the magnet bore, each proton spin within a population has its magnetic dipole oriented in a random direction (Fig. 1b). The net magnetization of this population is zero and not detectable. Figure 1b illustrates spin behaviors after the subject enters the B_0 field. The magnetic field forces the individual dipoles to either align with or against B_0. Only a small fraction of spins preferentially align with B_0 than against it. Nevertheless, it is this slightly greater population of dipoles that align with B_0 and the abundance of hydrogen atoms *in vivo* that is responsible for producing a measurable net signal. Since this net magnetization is oriented along the longitudinal axis of the magnet bore, it is referred to as $M_{longitudinal}$. With higher B_0 fields, the proportion of aligned spins increases and gives rise to a larger $M_{longitudinal}$ and hence a stronger signal.

Interactions between the magnetization and the B_0 field causes precession. The Larmor frequency or rate of precession f_{Larmor} is determined by Equation 1, where $\gamma/(2\pi)$ is the gyromagnetic ratio of the nuclei of interest. For protons, it is 4,257 Hz/G.

$$f_{Larmor} = \gamma / (2\pi) \cdot B_0 \quad (1)$$

The Larmor frequency is nuclei specific and linearly proportional to B_0. At B_0 = 1.5T, proton f_{Larmor} is 63.86 MHz; at 3.0T, it doubles to 127.6 MHz (1MHz = 10^6 Hz, 1Hz=1 cycle/second). It is precession, the continuous motion of spin magnetization M at the Larmor frequency that induces signals needed for image generation. Thus, analogous to a radio transmitter and receiver, MRI signal detection is based on frequency, and as will be discussed later, it is precisely the Larmor frequency difference between hydrogens in water and fat that underpins several approaches to body and organ fat quantification.

2.2 Radiofrequency excitation and relaxation: the "R"

Once $M_{longitudinal}$ is generated, it must be tipped, or nutated, into the orthogonal transverse plane in order for signals from precessing spins to be detected by local receiver coil(s). This is shown in Figure 2. The nutation from $M_{longitudinal}$ to $M_{transverse}$ is accomplished through radiofrequency (RF) pulses that are applied on resonance at the Larmor frequency. In the figure, a 90° nutation or excitation is shown. However, an arbitrary value can be used. The angle of nutation is denoted by α and is referred to as the flip angle. Just as the RF excitation pulse is applied on resonance at the Larmor frequency to most efficiently nutate $M_{longitudinal}$, the receiver coil(s) are similar tuned to the Larmor frequency to detect $M_{transverse}$.

After $M_{transverse}$ is created and the RF pulse is turned off, the spins will gradually begin to "relax". Two simultaneous and independent relaxation processes occur. First, the signal will recover towards the longitudinal axis, progressively restoring the $M_{longitudinal}$ vector to its original state prior to RF excitation. The rate recovery is denoted by the T_1 spin-lattice term, an exponential constant. Second, spins in the transverse plane will gradually lose signal coherence. This causes a progressive reduction of $M_{transverse}$ at an exponential decay rate of T_2, also known as spin-spin relaxation. T_1 and T_2 values are material, tissue, and B_0 dependent (De Bazelaire et al., 2004; Stanisz et al., 2005).

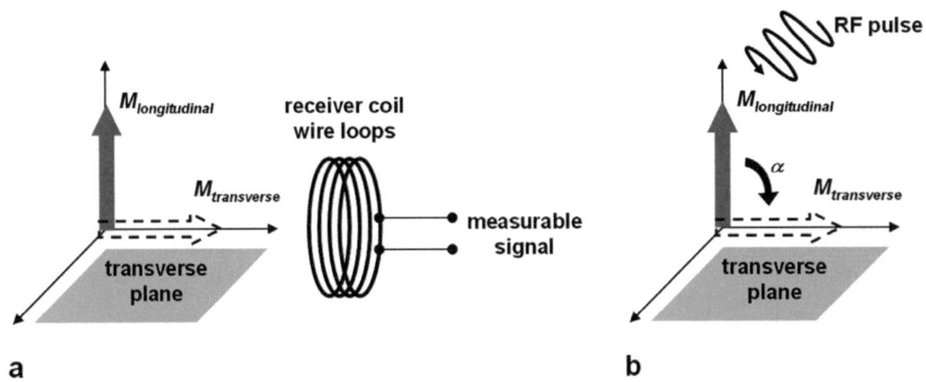

Fig. 2. RF excitation. (a) $M_{longitudinal}$ does not induce a signal in the receiver coil. In order for a measurable signal to be generated, $M_{longitudinal}$ must be nutated into the orthogonal plane (dashed arrow) to form $M_{transverse}$. (b) Nutation is accomplished via excitation by an RF pulse applied on resonance at the Larmor frequency. The duration and amplitude of the pulse determines the angle of nutation, or flip angle α. A 90° example is shown.

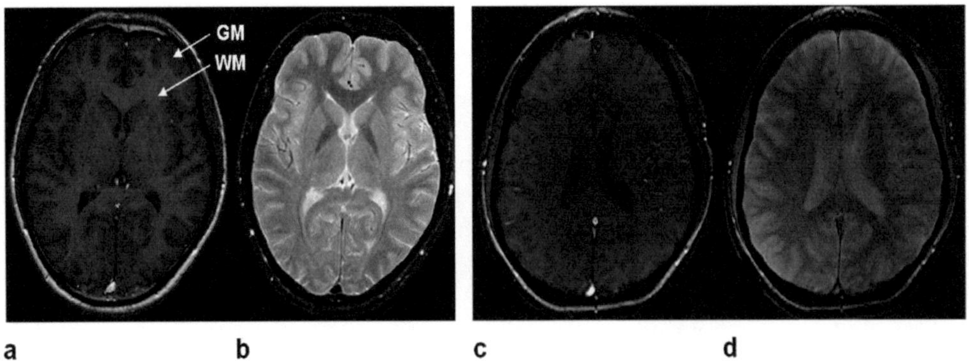

Fig. 3. Tissue contrast. Axial brain sections acquired with (a) TR=400 msec, TE=14 msec; (b) TR=2000 msec, TE=80 msec in one subject while keeping the flip angle constant. (a) A T_1-weighted image where gray matter (GM) is darker than white matter (WM). (b) A T_2-weighted image, where tissue contrast has been inverted and GM is brighter than WM. Axial brain sections acquired with (c) flip angle of 30 degrees and (d) 5 degrees in another subject, while keeping TR and TE constant. Note again differences in tissue contrast.

In an MRI experiment, RF pulses are repeated in the form of a pulse sequence to gather adequate data for each imaging slice of interest. After each RF excitation, a signal or echo is measured at a specified echo time (TE). The time between successive RF excitations is the repetition time (TR). By varying the flip angle, TR, and TE, an operator has immense flexibility over tissue signal contrast in the resultant image. Figure 3 illustrates two axial sections of a human brain, acquired with different pairs of TR and TE values. Note that the signal contrast between gray and white matter changes. TR and TE pairs that exploit the difference in T_1 values between tissues yield T_1-weighted images (Fig. 3a), where white matter (shorter T_1, faster recovery) is brighter than gray matter (longer T_1, slower recovery). On the contrary, TR/TE pairs that exploit differences in T_2 yield T_2-weighted images (Fig. 3b), where white matter (shorter T_2, faster decay) is darker than gray matter (longer T_2, slower decay). Similar tissue contrasts can be achieved by changing only the flip angle (Fig. 3c, d).

2.3 Magnetic gradients, k-space, and the Fourier transform: the "I"

In a pulse sequence, each echo gathers signal contrast and spatial information about the imaging object and its spin ensemble. A pulse sequence (Fig. 4) contains not only the RF component, but also three magnetic gradients, G_{slice}, G_{phase}, and G_{read}. These gradients perturb the B_0 field linearly as a function of distance. In synchrony with G_{slice}, a RF pulse can excite an isolated section of the imaging object (e.g. the head, abdomen, or knee). This is known as volume or slice-selection. G_{phase} and G_{read} then provide information on the spatial locations of spins from the excited section by establishing a one-to-one relationship between their locations and their unique precessing frequencies and phases (spatial-encoding). Aligning the three gradients in various combinations yields the desired image orientation.

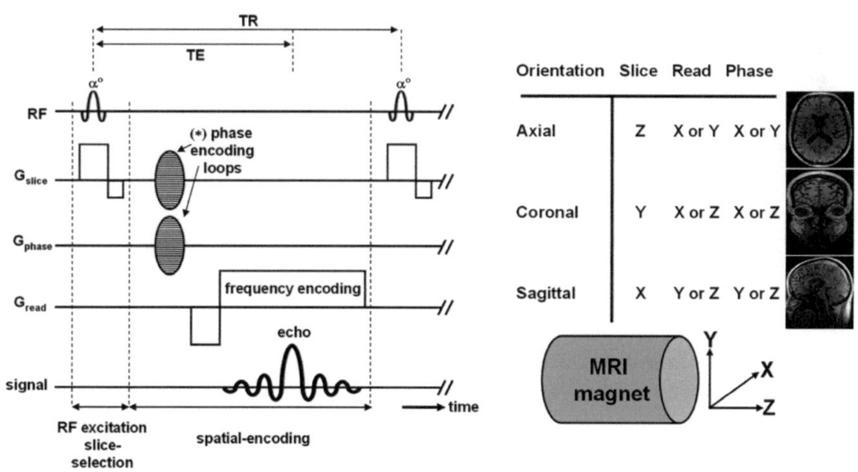

Fig. 4. A pulse sequence diagram. Gradient G_{slice} is applied in conjunction with the RF pulse to specifically excite a desired section of the imaging object at a given orientation. This is followed by 2D or 3D spatial-encoding (*), where locations of spins are determined based on their precessing frequency and their phase accrual in the presence of G_{read}, G_{phase}, and G_{slice}.

Each acquired echo provides a snapshot, or "view" of the underlying image. By iterating through multiple spatial (frequency and phase) encoding loops, differential "views" of the imaging object are obtained. Each echo is an oscillatory function that represents the sum of a spin ensemble observed from a particular "view", and each of the involved spins are precessing at a slightly different gradient-tuned frequency and phase. To separate the signal into its individual components, each echo is first stored as a line of data points in the spatial frequency domain, or *k*-space. Once all echoes are acquired, a Fourier Transform (FT) operation generates the image (Fig. 5).

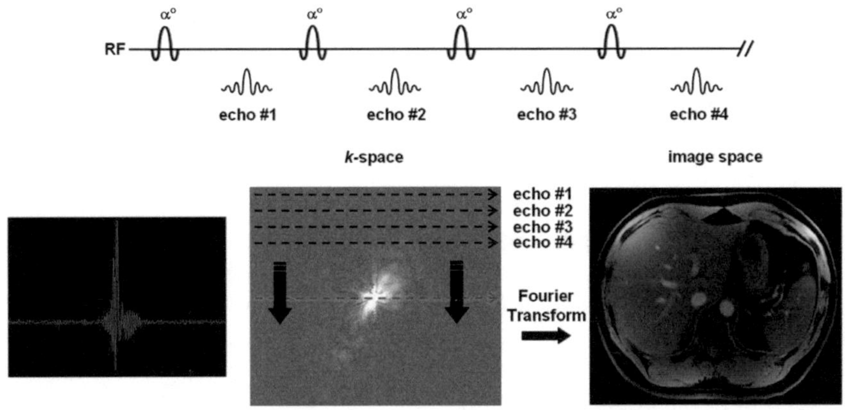

Fig. 5. Image formation. A pulse sequence collects echoes and fills the data in *k*-space after each RF pulse. A Fourier Transform yields the net image result after the pulse sequence iterates through multiple spatial-encoding "view" loops. An echo example is shown in red.

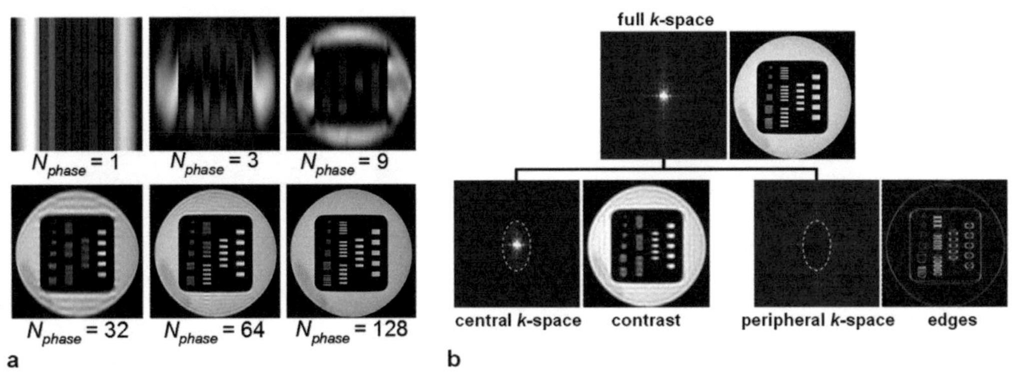

Fig. 6. *k*-space and resolution. (a) A set of images with varying numbers of "views". Resolution improves with more "views". (b) *k*-space can be considered in two parts, a central region containing low-spatial-frequency data inside the dashed ellipse, and a high-spatial-frequency region outside the ellipse. Images show that low-spatial-frequencies give rise to gross contrast, while high-spatial-frequencies contribute to edges and details. When an echo is acquired, it samples both central and peripheral *k*-space.

2.4 Field of view, spatial resolution, and acquisition time

Field of view (FOV) describes the size of the imaging volume and is set by the MRI operator. Spatial resolution refers to the physical dimensions of each 2D pixel or 3D voxel. Smaller dimensions provide greater spatial resolution and resolving power to delineate fine structures. Spatial resolution is determined by the number of acquired *k*-space data samples (*N*), and can be computed as the ratio of FOV and *N* along each axis. Higher resolution usually demands a greater number of samples, which consequently implies a longer acquisition time of the MRI experiment. This is because it typically takes one TR repetition to acquire each of the N_{phase} and N_{slice} phase-encoding "views". Figure 6a illustrates a series of images of a circular object. N_{read} was set constant (horizontal axis) while N_{phase} (vertical axis) was varied. With only one phase-encoding "view", vertical spatial resolution is non-existent. With nine "views", the circular outline and embedded parallel bars become visible. With 32, 64, and 128 "views", the detail of the bars are improved. Figure 6b illustrates a key property of *k*-space. A full *k*-space data set is shown along with its image. If only central *k*-space is reconstructed, the resultant image exhibits the overall shape and signal contrast of the object, but is blurry and lacks spatial detail. Conversely if only the peripheral data points are reconstructed, the resultant image is devoid of any signal contrast, but shows edge detail. Thus, both central and peripheral *k*-space are critical for high image quality.

3. Magnetic resonance imaging of fat

As the prevalence of obesity and type II diabetes continue to rise (Flegal et al., 2010), evidence has attributed obesity-related health risks to the accumulation of subcutaneous and visceral adipose tissue (SAT, VAT) and ectopic organ fat (Choudhary et al., 2007; Despres et al., 2008). Non-invasive assessment of body and organ fat has become an important component in obesity research and fat measures are useful as biomarkers to stratify risks and evaluate the efficacy of therapies.

Many methods have been historically available for body fat assessment (Ellis, 2000; Mattsson, 2006). Anthropometry, hydrodensitometry, air displacement plethysmography (ADP), bioelectric impedance (BIA), and dual energy X-ray absorptiometry (DEXA) have been widely used. The first four are indirect techniques because they measure body density or resistance, which are then converted into percent body fat using generalized equations (Jackson, 1982). Hydrodensitometry and ADP are limited to estimating total body fat, while BIA and DEXA are limited to total and regional body fat measures. Most importantly, these indirect methods are not able to differentiate between SAT and VAT or identify ectopic fat.

An increased utilization of computed tomography (CT) (Goodpaster et al., 2000, Kvist et al., 1988; Seidell et al., 1990), quantitative magnetic resonance (QMR) (Napolitano et al., 2008), and particularly MRI for body fat assessment (Abate et al., 1997; Berglund et al., 2010; Brix et al., 1993; Kullberg et al., 2009; Lancaster et al., 1991; Machann, et al., 2005; Ross et al., 2000; Schick et al., 2002; Siegel et al., 2007; Thomas et al., 2005;) has been reported in recent years. Along with DEXA, CT, QMR, and MRI are direct techniques because they identify fat based on the tissue's unique properties and signals in each modality. QMR does not yield images and is limited to measuring total body fat. In contrast, CT and MRI can differentiate SAT and VAT with multi-dimensional images. However, only MRI, with its sensitive contrast mechanisms for water and fat-based tissues, can accurately quantify ectopic fat. MRI is emerging as a comprehensive tool for fat quantification. The following sections describe fundamental MRI concepts that underpin T_1-weighted imaging, MR spectroscopy (MRS), and state-of-the-art chemical shift imaging (CSI).

3.1 T_1-Weighted MRI

As discussed in Section 2.2, MRI signal intensities are influenced by many factors including proton density, tissue-specific relaxation rates, the flip angle, and pulse sequence timings.

The T_1 of fat is one of the shortest amongst tissues *in vivo*. This indicates a very rapid recovery of its longitudinal magnetization between successive RF excitations. Therefore, by using a T_1-weighted sequence, strong tissue contrast can be achieved between short-T_1 fat tissues and muscles and organs with longer T_1 values (Fig. 7). Bright fat can thus be easily identified and delineated by simple signal intensity thresholding (e.g. cutoff) from darker structures. T_1-weighted sequences are very common in clinical MRI and are a part of nearly every protocol and anatomy. They have been used by several investigators as the standard workhorse tool for assessing SAT and VAT distributions (Machann et al., 2005; Ross et al. 2000; Siegel et al., 2007). T_1-weighted sequences are available as standard software on all commercial MRI scanners (GE, Philips, Siemens, Hitachi, and Toshiba) and can be easily implemented by the operator. Tissue T_1 values increase slightly with B_0 field, such that optimization in pulse sequence parameters are needed to maintain comparable tissue contrast between magnetic field strengths.

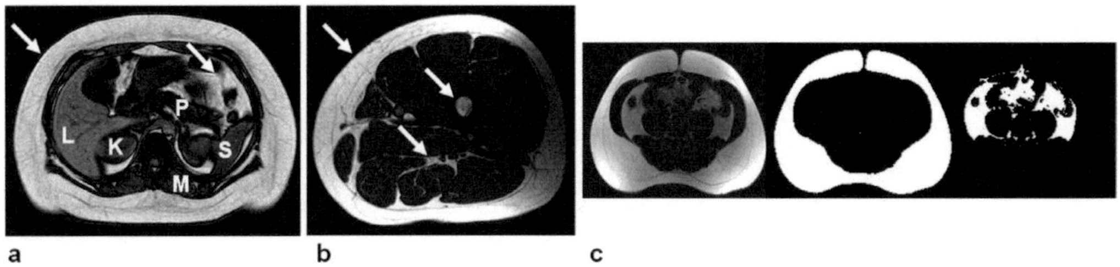

Fig. 7. T_1-weighted MRI. Examples in the (a) abdomen and (b) thigh, demonstrating the high signal intensities of fat *in vivo* (arrows: SAT, VAT, bone marrow, intermuscular fat) in contrast to darker muscles and organs (L: liver, P: pancreas, K: kidneys, M: muscle, S: spleen). (c) A high signal intensity threshold of an abdominal T_1-weighted image easily identifies fat pixels. Intensities with values below the set threshold are "discarded" and set to zero. For well-optimized T_1-weighted pulse sequences, this simple step can be quite robust in identifying abdominal SAT (middle) and VAT depots (right).

3.2 Single-voxel magnetic resonance spectroscopy

Single-voxel MRS has been the gold-standard for ectopic fat quantification (Hamilton et al., 2009; Kim et al., 2008; Lingvay et al., 2009; van Werven et al., 2009; Weis et al., 2008). Unlike MRI, MRS usually does not provide anatomical information in the form of an image. It instead yields a precise spectrum of chemical composition within one voxel. MRS relies on chemical shift, which refers to differences in the Larmor frequencies of water and fat protons (Fig. 8). Water protons from (-OH) hydroxyl groups are characterized by a spectral peak at 4.7 ppm (parts-per-million). In contrast, the predominant protons of triglycerides are from the $(-CH_2)_n$ methylene groups (black H in Fig. 1d). Due to different chemical environments surrounding the protons (oxygen in water versus carbon in triglycerides), methylene protons have a slightly lower resonant frequency. The frequency separation between water and the methylene fat peak is linearly proportional to B_0, such that larger chemical shift separations are achieved with increasing field strengths. At 1.5 and 3.0 Teslas and body temperature, the water-fat chemical shift is approximately 220 and 440 Hz, respectively (Brix et al., 1993; Cassidy et al., 2009; Ren et al., 2008). Note that this frequency difference is miniscule in comparison to the MHz Larmor values. Nevertheless, water-fat chemical shift is detectable via MRS and the resulting spectrum provides an intuitive visualization of the presence and relative quantity of chemical species. MRS packages are available on most commercial MRI scanners and typically require some operator expertise to implement.

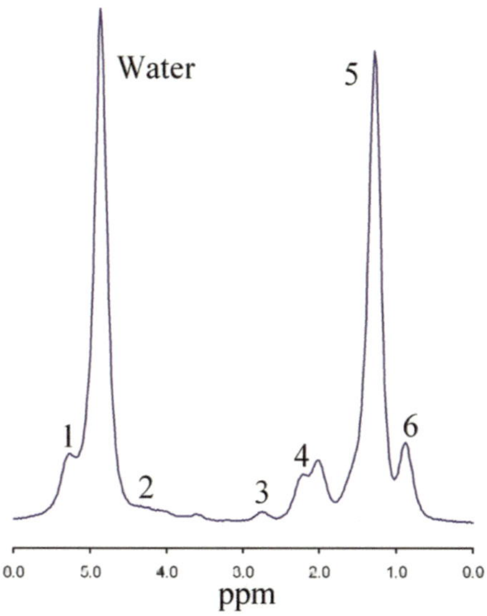

Peak	ppm	Assignment
1	5.3	-CH=CH- -CH-O-CO-
Water	4.7	H_2O
2	4.2	$-CH_2-O-CO-$
3	2.75	$-CH=CH-CH_2-CH=CH-$
4	2.1	$-CO-CH_2-CH_2-$ $-CH_2-CH=CH-CH_2-$
5	1.3	$-CO-CH_2-CH_2-$ $-(CH_2)_n-$
6	0.9	$-(CH_2)_n-CH_3$

Fig. 8. Example of a spectrum from ^{1}H MRS containing water and fat. The water peak is at 4.7 ppm. The fat methylene peak (#5) is shifted 3.4 ppm downfield, at 1.3 ppm. While water is a symmetrical molecule and has a true single peak, fat exhibits additional minor peaks from other moieties, some of which are in close proximity to the water peak. The area under each peak represents the amount of each species present, such that a fat:water ratio (e.g. a fat fraction) can be measured. The Larmor frequency separation between water and fat can be computed by multiplying the ppm difference by the right-side of Equation 1. Color notation corresponds to Figure 1. Figure courtesy of G. Hamilton, Ph.D., University of California San Diego.

3.3 Frequency-selective MRI

Since MRI involves RF pulses tuned to specific resonant frequencies, a novel technique that exploits the Larmor difference between water and fat to quantify SAT, VAT, and intermuscular fat has been developed (Kaldoudi et al., 1993; Machann J et al., 2003; Peng et al., 2007, Schick et al., 2002). One approach is to selectively excite fat spins by tuning a narrow bandwidth RF pulse specifically to fat's resonant frequency. As a result, only fat protons are nutated and detected by signal receivers while those of water remain in the longitudinal plane. The encoded data and image exhibit only signals from fat and the appearance resemble T_1-weighted contrast where fat appears recognizably bright (Fig. 9). The sharp contrast between water and fat-dominant tissues and organs readily facilitates thresholding and fat volume quantification. Selective-fat-excitation and water-suppression are terms used interchangeably to refer to this technique in literature.

A disadvantage of selective-fat-excitation is that the narrow bandwidth RF pulse can only account for the methylene fat peak and minor peaks that are in its close proximity. The fat peaks near water are neglected. This issue limits the applicability of frequency-selective MRI to SAT and VAT quantification only, and not ectopic fat content. Frequency-selective techniques can be implemented on all commercial scanners. The method works well at 1.5T, but can be unreliable at higher fields due to its sensitivity to B_0 inhomogeneities. B_0 inhomogeneity refers to unknown object-dependent and spatially-varying deviations of the magnetic field from its intended value, and can cause unintentional resonant frequency drifts on the order of 10^2 - 10^3 Hz. Inhomogeneities arise from manufacturing imperfections, perturbations by metals, and the mere placement of a human inside the magnet bore. They are quite significant around air-tissue-bowel interfaces. B_0 inhomogeneity, also known as off-resonance, globally shifts the ppm locations (and Larmor frequencies) of water and fat peaks such that they are no longer at 4.7 and 1.3 ppm, respectively. However, the difference between them remains unchanged at 3.4 ppm. In the presence of significant B_0 inhomogeneity, an RF pulse intended for fat's resonance can erroneously excite water's resonance. Although higher field strength leads to greater water-fat peak separation, the worsening B_0 inhomogeneity counteracts the benefit and degrades overall performance.

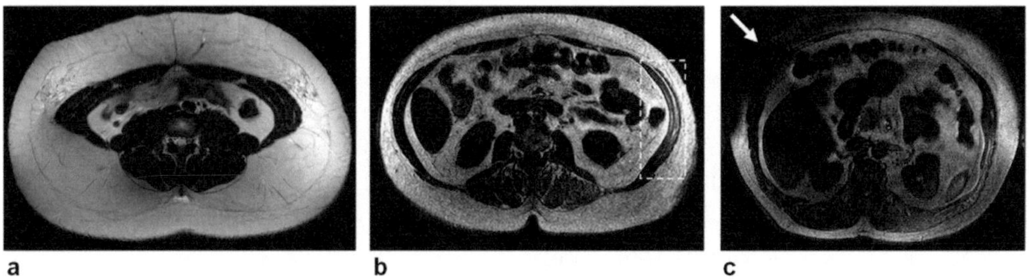

Fig. 9. Frequency-selective MRI. Three slices are shown acquired at (a) 1.5T, and (b, c) 3.0T. In (a), SAT and VAT exhibit high signal intensity, in contrast to water-dominant muscles and organs. In (b), the dashed box encloses the left oblique and transversus abdominis muscles. There is appreciable signal from the muscles, in comparison to the darker right side. Due to B_0 inhomogeneity, selective-fat-excitation was ineffective in this region. In (c), performance is severely hindered in the right anterior SAT region (arrow). Significant B_0 inhomogeneity has caused the selective-fat-excitation RF pulse to *suppress* fat signal.

3.4 Chemical shift MRI

Chemical shift imaging (CSI) integrates sensitive water-fat spectral detection from MRS with imaging (Bley et al., 2010; Hood & Ho, 1999; Ma, 2008). CSI consists of a family of approaches that have been developed over the past 25 years. Dixon was the first to demonstrate that by controlling the echo time when data was acquired after RF excitation, the net detected MRI signal can comprise either of water and fat in-phase (IP=W+F, aligned, phase=0 degrees) or out-of-phase (OP=W-F, anti-aligned, phase=180 degrees), as illustrated in Figure 10 (Dixon, 1984). Dixon recognized that by using this two-point (IP and OP) approach, separated water and fat images could be obtained by image algebra (Cassidy et al., 2009). By reconstructing separated water and fat images, a subsequent percent fat fraction map (fat:water ratio) can be computed, which would facilitate measurement of fat accumulation in organs on a voxel-by-voxel basis. Intuitively, one can realize that for a voxel containing only water or fat, its net signal will be the same on IP and OP acquisitions as one component's signal will be zero. In contrast, a voxel containing both water and fat will have different signals from the two acquisitions (Fig. 11). Recent developments in water-fat separation and image reconstruction algorithms have advanced the traditional two-point

Dixon method beyond IP/OP to arbitrary echo time choices (Berglund et al., 2011; Bydder et al., 2011; Eggers et al., 2011; Ma, 2008; Xiang, 2006).

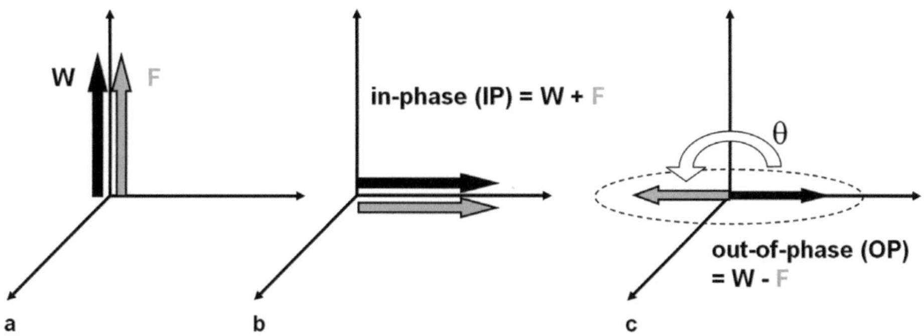

Fig. 10. Two-point Dixon MRI. (a) Before RF excitation, water (W) and fat (F) magnetizations are along the longitudinal axis. (b) Immediately after RF excitation, the transverse magnetizations are in-phase. An echo acquired at this point would reflect a net signal of W+F. (c) With the signal receivers tuned to the Larmor frequency of water, the slower precessing chemically-shifted fat signal will accrue a phase of 180 degrees, or OP, with respect to water after some time. An echo acquired at this point would reflect a net signal of W-F. As time proceeds, the signal will become IP and OP periodically. At 1.5T, the periodicity is 2.4 msec; at 3.0T, it is 1.2 msec. For this approach, only the methylene fat peak is considered. Note in (c) that both vectors are smaller in amplitude, due to T_2 relaxation.

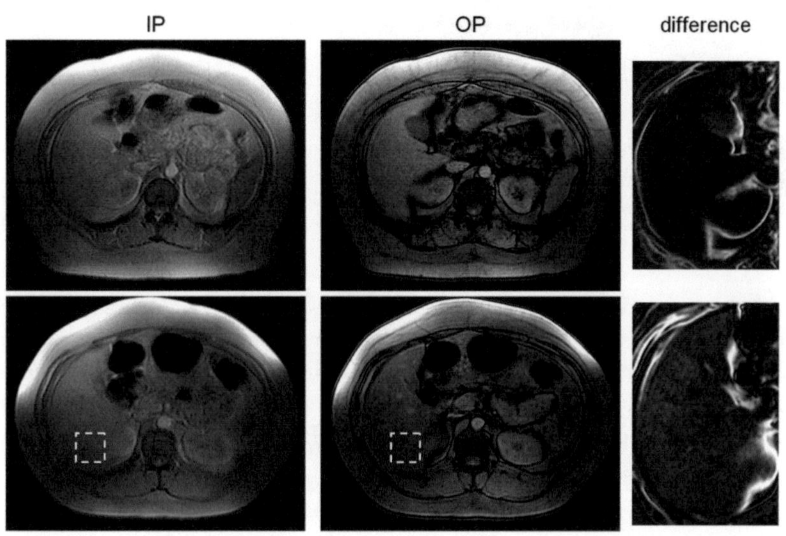

Fig. 11. Two-point Dixon MRI. In-phase (IP) and out-of-phase (OP) images from two subjects are shown. In the first subject (top row), the signal intensities within the liver between IP and OP images are similar. This signifies very little presence of hepatic fat. In the second subject (bottom row), the liver signal intensities is lower in the OP image (dashed regions). This indicates presence of hepatic fat. The difference image of the top subject is nearly zero in the liver, whereas the lower subject shows appreciable signal. As determined by MRS, the hepatic fat fractions of the subjects were 3.4% and 21.2%, respectively.

CSI has evolved significantly over the past decade due to strong motivation by clinical interest and research in obesity and its comorbidities, particularly fatty liver disease (Bley et al., 2010; Cassidy et al., 2009; Ma, 2008). More robust and improved techniques have been developed to incorporate B_0 inhomogeneity estimation into the water-fat separation algorithm. These variants typically require three or more TE measurements (e.g. three-point Dixon). Modern CSI approaches have also addressed the problem of water-fat signal ambiguity (Hussain et al., 2005), which refers to the inability of early two-point methods to determine whether fat or water is the predominant specie present in a voxel. In other words, a voxel contain x% fat and (100-x)% water can be indiscernible from a voxel containing x% water and (100- x)% fat (e.g. there is ambiguity about the 50% fat fraction apex). Many recent literature reports have validated CSI in measuring liver fat fraction (Kim et al., 2008; Guiu et al., 2009; Hussain et al, 2005; Hu et al., 2010; Meisamy et al., 2011; O'Regan et al., 2008; Yokoo et al., 2009). While CSI pulse sequences are not difficult to implement, they often require technician involvement and manufacturer support in establishing appropriate protocols. CSI software is available on new commercial MRI platforms as clinical or research-dedicated software.

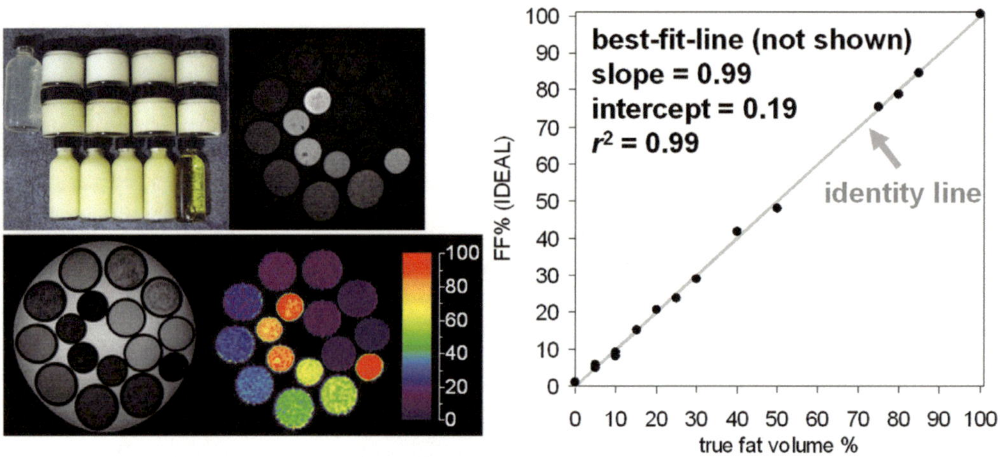

a b

Fig. 12. IDEAL fat fraction (FF) MRI. (a) Oil-water emulsions, ranging in percent volume oil from 0% (clear bottle) to 100% (transparent yellow bottle) are shown. IDEAL reconstructed fat-only and water-only images in the upper right and bottom left panels, respectively, along with the colorized FF map. The bottles are in a water-filled dish. (b) Correlation of true fat volume fraction against the mean FF from IDEAL. Excellent agreement is achieved.

Recent advances in CSI have led to the development of comprehensive methods such as IDEAL (Iterative Decomposition with Echo Asymmetry and Least squares) (Reeder et al., 2007). IDEAL is a generalization of the multi-echo Dixon model (a three to six-point Dixon approach) and has been successfully demonstrated at both 1.5 and 3.0 Tesla. At both field strengths, IDEAL is robust to B_0 inhomogeneity, addresses water-fat signal ambiguity such that percent fat fractions can be determined across the 0–100% range without ambiguity (Bernard et al., 2008; Hines et al., 2009), accounts for T_1 and T_2 relaxation of water and fat (Bydder et al., 2008; Chebrolu et al., 2010; Liu et al., 2007), and models the multiple peaks of fat with an accurate spectrum (Hernando et al., 2010; Yu et al., 2008). The latter is a critical methodological advancement in accurate ectopic fat quantification (percent organ fat fraction) as it accounts for nearly all of the minor fat spectral peaks in addition to the primary methylene peak. A single IDEAL acquisition yields not only reconstructed fat-only and water-only images and accurate fat fraction maps [*F*/(*F*+*W*)], but also IP and OP series that are useful for anatomical definition. IDEAL has been rigorously validated against MRS and other CSI methods in the liver (Hu et al., 2010; Reeder et al., 2009; Reeder & Sirlin, 2010; Meisamy et al. 2011). IDEAL and its variants have been used to study brown and white adipose tissues (Hu et al., 2010) and fat accumulation in the heart (Kellman et al., 2010). IDEAL is a patented and proprietary software that is commercially available from GE Healthcare. Figures 12-14 highlight the robustness and utility of IDEAL in visualizing and quantifying tissue fat fraction and organ fat content.

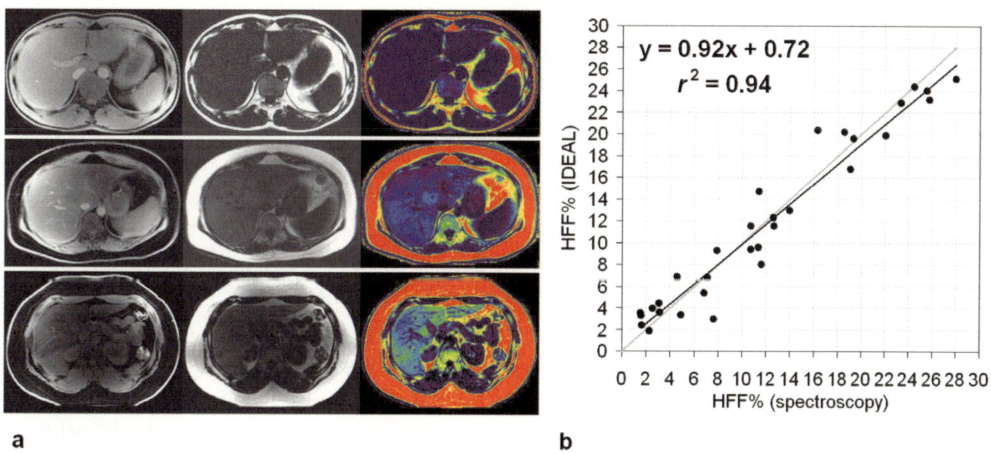

Fig. 13. IDEAL fat fraction (FF) MRI. (a) IDEAL-reconstructed water-only, fat-only, and colorized FF maps of the liver in three subjects are shown. Same color bar as Fig. 12. It is evident that the three subjects have varying degrees of fat accumulation in the liver, beginning with a low 3% in the top case (dark purple), to approximately 23% in the middle case (dark blue), to more than 40% (light blue, green) in the lower case. Note also greater SAT volumes in the middle and lower cases. (b) Excellent correlation in hepatic FF was achieved between IDEAL MRI and reference MRS (n=31). The identity line is in gray.

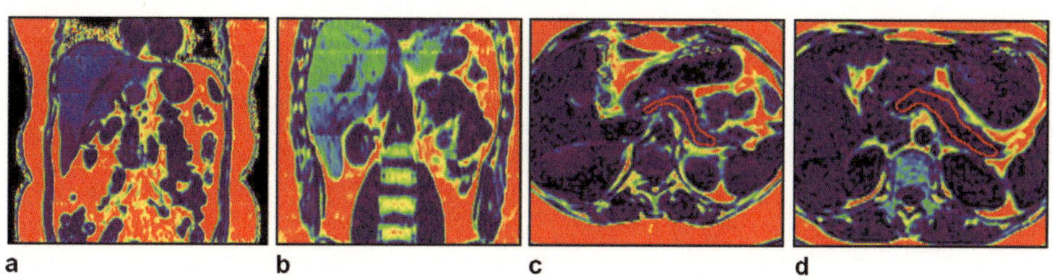

Fig. 14. IDEAL fat fraction (FF) MRI. (a, b) IDEAL-reconstructed FF maps of the liver in two subjects, shown in the coronal orientation. The 3D nature of IDEAL data facilitates visualization of the FF map from any perspective. Same color bar as Fig. 12. Note that SAT and VAT distributions can be clearly seen, along with varying degrees of fat accumulation in the liver. (c, d) Two examples of pancreas (red outline), with an average 11% and 5.1% percent FF within the traced regions, respectively.

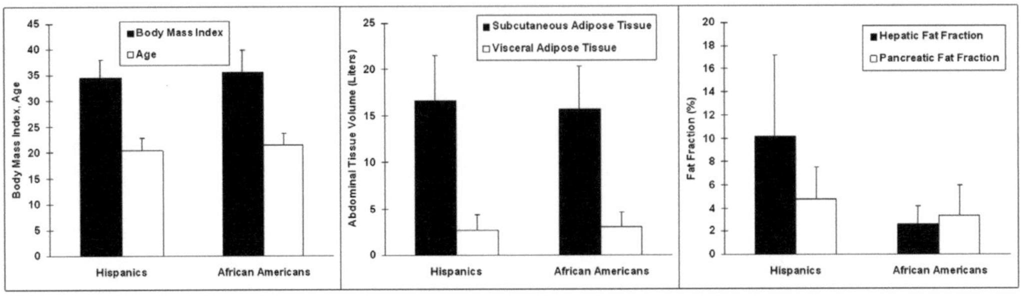

Fig. 15. Data from a cohort of age- and BMI-matched Hispanics and African Americans (n=13 in each group) using IDEAL MRI. Hispanics have significantly higher hepatic fat fractions (HFF) and slightly higher pancreatic fat fractions (not significant) than African Americans. However, the two groups have similar abdominal adipose tissue volumes. Due to their high HFFs, Hispanics are likely at a greater risk of obesity-related comorbidities.

At the University of Southern California, 3D IDEAL-MRI has been developed into a routine protocol and has been used by investigators to assess abdominal subcutaneous and visceral adipose tissue depot volumes and hepatic and pancreatic fat fraction in adolescents. The center has focused on comparing and contrasting these quantitative measures between genders and ethnicities. Figure 15 showcases results from a pilot study.

In summary, MR imaging and spectroscopy provide sensitive methods for detecting and quantifying adipose tissue volumes and ectopic fat fractions. Table 1 summarizes these methodologies and their principles. The quantitative fat endpoints achievable with each method are also listed. The reader is referred to three extensive review articles for additional details (Bley, 2010; Cassidy et al, 2009; Ma, 2008).

	Basis of Fat–Water Differentiation	Typical Dimensionality	Advantages	Disadvantages	Quantitative Endpoints
T_1-weighted MRI	T_1 relaxation	2D and 3D	strong fat-water tissue contrast, standard on all scanners, easy to implement, rapid scans	T_1 contrast varies with B_O field strength, requires protocol optimization	SAT and VAT volumes
Frequency-Selective MRI	chemical shift	2D and 3D	strong fat-water tissue contrast, option on most scanners, rapid scans	performance varies with B_O field strength and magnet inhomogeneity	SAT and VAT volumes
MR Spectroscopy (MRS)	chemical shift	single voxel	high spectral resolution of chemical profile, very accurate measure of fat to water fractions	limited coverage, requires expertise in protocol prescription, data collection and spectral analysis	ectopic fat fraction
Chemical Shift MRI	chemical shift	2D and 3D	complete fat-water tissue separation with accuracy comparable to MRS	not available on all scanners, requires special image reconstruction algorithms and protocol optimization for different B_O field strengths	SAT and VAT volumes, ectopic fat fraction

Table 1. Summary of MR imaging and spectroscopy methods for fat quantification.

4. Image analysis

In this section, procedures for extracting adipose tissue volumes and organ fat fractions from abdominal MRI data are discussed and illustrated using SliceOmatic software. The materials are presented in the context of abdominal imaging, but can be easily translated to other anatomies. The workflow for extracting fat measures from MRI data remains a daunting and costly task. It requires substantial data post-processing and analysis by an experienced operator. The steps involve the transfer of images to an offline workstation, followed by the use of dedicated software that typically require user involvement (Bonekamp et al., 2008). Free packages such as ImageJ, Osirix, and jMRUI (Naressi et al., 2001) and commercial programs such as SliceOmatic (Tomovision, Inc.), Analyze (AnalyzeDirect, Inc.) and Matlab (The Mathworks, Inc.) are commonly used for MRS analysis and image segmentation. Based on the author's experience, post-processing of a 3D abdominal MRI volume consisting of 60-80 slices can take approximately 45–60 minutes.

4.1 Subcutaneous and visceral adipose tissue

Since adipose tissue (SAT and VAT) is composed primarily of fat and its composition can be quite uniform, their identification and quantification in T_1-weighted, frequency-selective, and CSI data is straightforward. Single-voxel MRS can not be used since it does not provide anatomical data. For T_1 and frequency-selective approaches, a binary threshold is applied to the signal intensity of each voxel. Since fat is brighter, those voxels with intensities greater than the threshold are labeled as fat while those with lower intensities are excluded. Due to intensity variations that may arise across the image, the local threshold may need to be adjusted accordingly from region to region (Fig. 16). For CSI, the analysis can utilize the fat-only images and apply a similar threshold procedure. Alternatively, the analysis can exploit the fat fraction map where the signal intensity range is consistently fixed from 0–100%. Only voxels with fat fractions greater than a set value (e.g. 85%) are labeled as fat (Fig. 17).

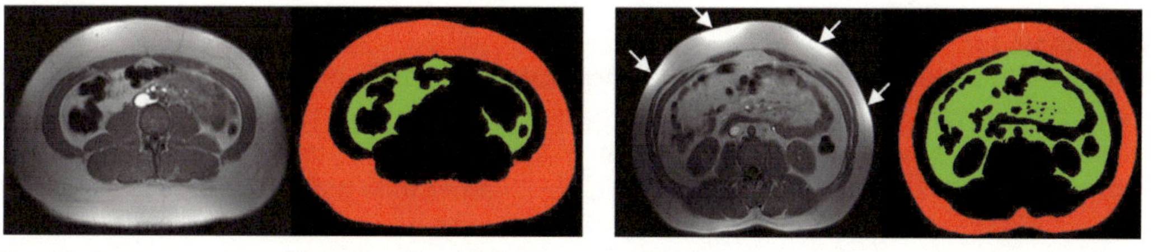

Fig. 16. Segmentation of SAT (red) and VAT (green) depots. Note the evident difference in VAT quantity between the two subjects. T_1-weighted images are shown. Arrows highlight artificial bright intensities caused by close proximity of the anatomy to receiver coils.

Regardless of the MRI technique, the operator usually needs to delineate the intra-abdominal boundary that separates SAT and VAT and the perimeter of the abdomen to exclude background air during segmentation. Additional exclusions of bowel contents, inter- and intra- muscular fat, spine and vertebrae, blood vessels, and other non-relevant structures are also required since some of these can have signal intensities that mimic fat. An area or volume measure is then computed for 2D multi-slice and contiguous 3D data based on the identified fat pixels/voxels, respectively. With the exception of CSI fat fraction data that is always normalized between 0% and 100%, the operator must determine suitable thresholds on a subject-to-subject basis. This is necessary since signal intensities vary across anatomy, subjects, examinations, and equipment and is usually not consistent. In SliceOmatic and Analyze, the operator has control over a sliding threshold and an interface that provides real time visual feedback on the performance of the chosen threshold.

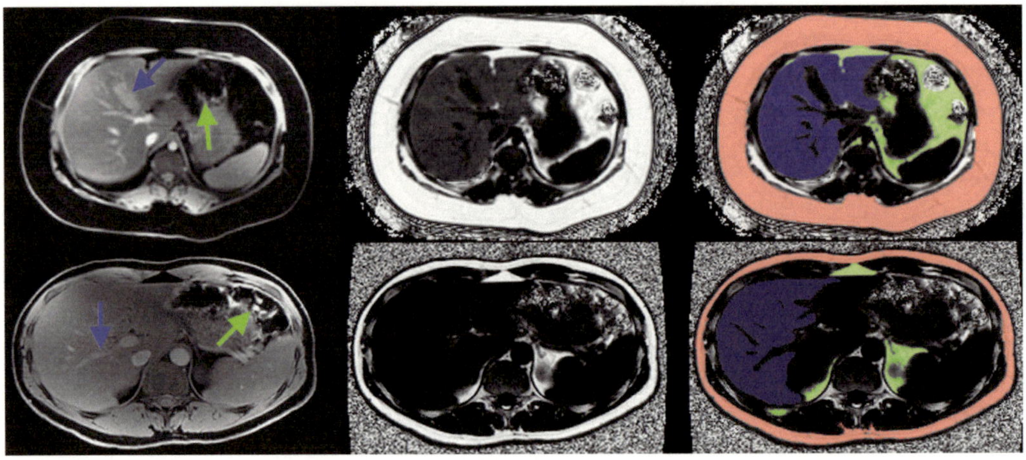

Fig. 17. IDEAL-based segmentation from two subjects, one with a fatty (top row) and one with a non-fatty (bottom row) liver. Water-only, fat fraction (0% black, 100% white) and overlay of segmentation (red: SAT, green: VAT, blue: liver) are shown in the left, middle, and right columns, respectively. The fuzzy noisy background in the fat fraction images has not been removed. In the fatty liver subject, note that hepatic vessels and the gall bladder (blue arrows) are well delineated in both water and fat fraction images, whereas in the non-fatty liver subject, such structures are only observable in the water image. Note that segmentation labels of the liver exclude these non-liver structures. VAT labels do not include erroneous signals from empty bowels (green arrows).

4.2 Ectopic fat

Ectopic fat quantification requires approaches that can separate water and fat signals within each voxel. Fat accumulation in organs and muscles can also be heterogenous. Therefore, the aforementioned binary threshold approach of "all fat" or "no fat" voxel classification is inadequate and only CSI methods are appropriate. Rather than measuring area or volume, a fraction of water and fat is computed. For MRS, the areas under the water and fat peaks can be calculated with software such as jMRUI. The MRS fat fraction is defined as the ratio of area under the fat peaks to the combined area of the water and fat peaks. CSI provides a fat fraction map across the imaging volume. The map is computed from the ratio of the reconstructed fat-only images to the sum of the water and fat images. To determine the fat fraction at a particular location, the operator simply draws a region-of-interest (ROI). The mean and standard deviation within the ROI is then computed. To quantify an organ, the operator must perform manual segmentation. Unlike single-voxel MRS, a volumetric fat fraction map affords immense flexibility. One can determine the average fat fraction across arbitrary ROI, including different lobes of the liver and the head and the tail of the pancreas. For accurate fat fractions, operator expertise is required for drawing ROIs and segmenting organs. In some cases, the fat fraction signal contrast surrounding abdominal organs may be poor, limiting an operator's ability to directly segment structures from the fat fraction maps and visualize organ-muscle boundaries. This is particularly true for liver, pancreas, and kidneys with low fat content that appear visually similar to surrounding muscles. In these instances, the water-only, fat-only, in-phase, and out-of-phase data are used to provide anatomical landmarks and guide the segmentation. The operator can first segment from these images and transfer the ROIs to the corresponding fat fraction data (Fig. 18). The analysis of organ fat can account for more than 70% of post-processing time. The pancreas and the kidneys are also in close proximity to fat-rich VAT depots. An inaccurately drawn ROI meant to enclose only the organs may contain erroneous VAT voxels. In such cases, the high VAT fat fractions will significantly impact the apparent measured organ fat fraction.

In summary, post-processing by a trained operator is needed for computing quantitative fat endpoints. For SAT and VAT volumes, strong tissue contrast can facilitate intensity-based thresholding. The measurement of ectopic fat requires MRS and CSI. Manual segmentation demands familiarity with software and anatomy, as well as significant operator input.

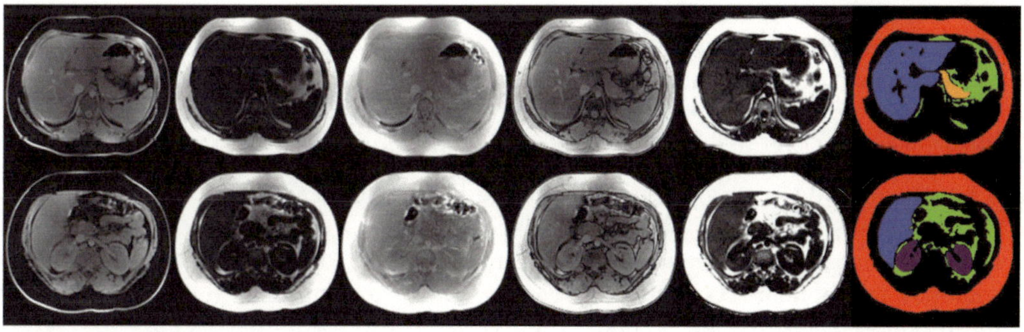

Fig. 18. Manual image segmentation from the full spectrum of IDEAL MRI data to delineate red: SAT, green: VAT, blue: liver, yellow: pancreas, purple: kidneys. Left to right: water-only, fat-only, in-phase, out-of-phase, fat fraction, and segmented labels from SliceOmatic.

5. Discussion

An investigator has several choices in MRI methods for body and organ fat assessment. In addition to selecting the appropriate technique, one must also consider tradeoffs between spatial resolution, scan time, and the need for breath-holds to minimize subject motion (Fig. 19). For MRS, 1–8 cm^3 voxels are commonly used. MRS requires a large voxel and several signal averages to yield a clean spectrum. Prescription of MRS voxels during an examination requires operator expertise such that placement of the voxel does not contain any undesired tissues. Motion from the subject or shifting of organs due to respiration or peristalsis after voxel placement can lead to spatial misalignments and unrealistic measurements (Hu et al., 2010). Respiration should be monitored with a bellows transducer for data synchronization. Alternatively, multiple and consistent breath-holds can be used with clear instructions given to the patient. In practice, these MRS approaches may not be possible in subjects with a large abdominal circumference or who have difficulties with breath-holds.

Resolutions for imaging approaches are on the order of millimeters. While small voxels are desirable for visualizing anatomical detail, it leads to increased scan times and lowers image signal-to-noise ratio. Long scan times also increase the risk of motion and blurring artifacts. In CSI, blurring artifacts from respiration can further cause unrealistic fat fraction distributions within organs and at organ-fat interfaces. High spatial resolution scans also necessitate breath-holding, which may not be well-tolerated by children, uncooperative or obese subjects. Spatial resolution is determined by the FOV and the acquisition matrix, the number of slices, the slice thickness, and the inter-slice gap, if any. These parameters are freely chosen by the operator, can impact scan time, and are dependent on body habitus.

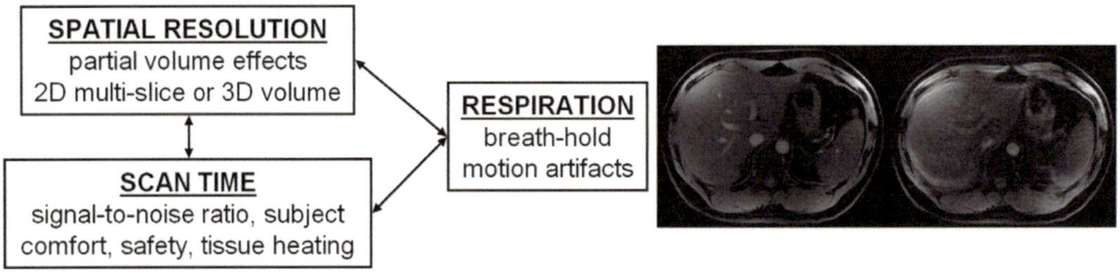

Fig. 19. Practical imaging parameters and considerations in MRI. In designing an appropriate protocol, one must consider the desired quantitative endpoints and leverage spatial resolution, scan time, patient safety, and the need for breath-holding. Image pair shows a slice of the liver in the same subject with (left) and without breath-holding (right).

The investigator and operator must also choose between 2D multi-slice or 3D volumetric pulse sequences. With 2D techniques, data are acquired on a slice-by-slice format such that data obtained for one slice is independent of any other slice. Subject motion and artifacts are generally not an issue in 2D methods. The time needed to acquire each slice is very short, requiring sub-seconds to a few seconds. The technique also allows the operator to specify a gap between non-contiguous adjacent slices. While this appears attractive in terms of scan efficiency, large inter-slice gaps and thick (~10 mm) slices can lead to partial volume errors and impact quantitative accuracy, especially in SAT and VAT depots. They are also difficult to generate subsequent 3D rendered visualizations (Fig. 20).

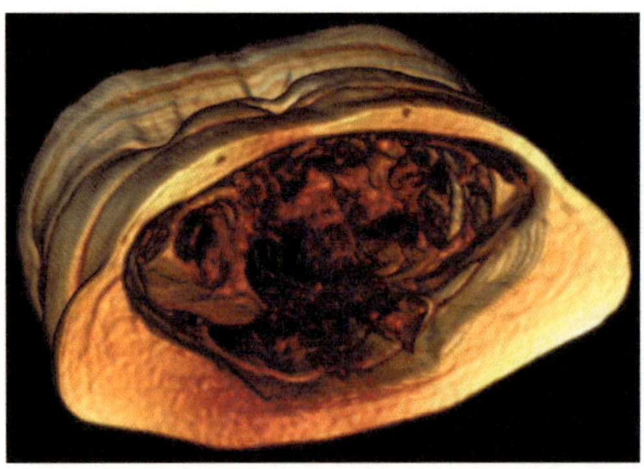

Fig. 20. Volume-rendered IDEAL MRI fat series, illustrating the contiguous 3D data set. The volume consists of 36 native 5-mm axial slices, obtained with three 15-sec breath-holds.

In contrast, 3D approaches acquire data that represent the entire volume. Volumetric imaging implies contiguous coverage and no inter-slice gaps. Given similar imaging parameters and coverage, 3D protocols often contain more slices, have longer scan times, and are more susceptible to motion than 2D approaches. However, since signals arise from a larger volume rather than a smaller slice, 3D methods exhibit greater signal-to-noise ratios. Breath-holding or respiratory gating is often required for abdominal 3D sequences. Three-dimensional approaches also offer intrinsic advantages over 2D methods, such as greater parallel imaging acceleration rates and more robust parallel imaging performance to reduce scan time. Parallel imaging is a topic beyond the scope of this chapter, and the reader is referred to the literature for details (Margolis et al., 2004). Other 3D benefits include thinner slices (sub-millimeter) and the ability to accommodating preparatory RF pulses that further enhance T_1 and fat to lean tissue contrast.

Lastly, for a given set of spatial resolutions and imaging parameters used in abdominal imaging, scan times in T_1-weighted, frequency-selective, MRS, and CSI approaches should be comparable between 1.5 and 3 Tesla protocols. In some instances, safety and RF tissue heating limits may lengthen 3 Tesla protocol durations over their 1.5 Tesla counterparts. At higher B_0 field strengths, greater chemical shift differences can also cause CSI sequences to increase in scan time due to shorter in-phase and out-of-phase echo periodicities.

In the literature, 2–4 mm in-plane resolution and a slice thickness between 5–10 mm have been reported for SAT and VAT quantification. For 2D multi-slice approaches inter-slice gaps as wide as 10 mm have been reported. Since the determination of volumes rely on thresholding and an "all fat" or "no fat" labeling each voxel, any incorrect labeling can lead to substantial quantification errors when using large voxels. Large voxels also generate partial volume effects where many can encompass both fat and lean tissues. These voxels exhibit ambiguous signal intensities that can cause threshold errors. Similarly, low spatial resolution and thick slices containing both organ and adjacent fat can exhibit unrealistic CSI fat fractions. There has been a transition in recent studies to adopt contiguous 2D multi-slice approaches with thin slices (Siegel et al., 2007) and 3D protocols (Berglund et al., 2010; Bornert et al., 2007; Kullberg et al., 2009).

For final consideration, modern MRI platforms are equipped with receiver arrays designed specifically for abdominal imaging. The array is strapped to the subject to provide high signal-to-noise ratios. However, they also create signal intensity variations across the imaging volume. If possible, these variations should be corrected with software from MRI vendors prior to image analysis. One attractive feature of CSI fat fraction maps is that they are generated as a ratio of water and fat images. While the individual source images may exhibit signal variations, their ratio removes the bias. The use of arrays may be limited in obese subjects as they are unable to fit within the magnet bore with the receivers strapped.

6. Future directions and conclusion

The design of appropriate MRI protocols for fat assessment requires considerations of the desired quantitative endpoints and tradeoffs in the imaging parameters. Other practical issues include body sizes of the cohort and the cost and throughput efficiency of the study. The usage cost associated with MRI can range from $300 to $600 per hour in a typical clinical radiology department. Regardless of the study, overhead time is always required for setup and for giving instructions to the subject. T_1-weighted and frequency-selective approaches are very fast and typically require only a few seconds per slice for data acquisition. Whole-abdomen coverage with these sequences takes only a few minutes of actual scan time and is generally considered as a first option for SAT and VAT quantification. In our experience, utilizing only these sequences, an exam can be comfortably completed in 10 minutes. If ectopic fat fractions are needed, either a MRS or CSI protocol is then added. The MRS sequence necessitates significant user interaction, preparation work, and operator time. In our experience, MRS per single voxel takes approximately 5 minutes. The further addition of a 3D whole-abdomen CSI protocol such as IDEAL will require 5–7 more breath-holds, bringing the total examination time from setup to patient removal to 30–45 minutes.

% difference in volume	SAT	VAT	Liver	Pancreas
Intra-Rater Comparison (11 subjects, 4 segmentations)				
Mean	-0.86	1.41	-0.13	-0.40
Range	-4.97 to 1.53	-8.34 to 4.47	-5.48 to 6.18	-6.66 to 5.00
Inter-Rater Comparison (7 subjects, 2 segmentations)				
Mean	1.32	1.20	-0.84	1.23
Range	-1.30 to 5.48	-6.05 to 5.64	-6.07 to 5.69	-5.21 to 9.95

Table 2. Percent difference in segmented volumes of fat depots and organs in two scenarios, as part of routine quality control performed at our institution. In the first, a single operator segmented 11 data sets, each 4 times, in random order. In the second, two independent operators, in a blinded format, segmented 7 data sets in random order. Note that the mean differences are all less than 2%, signifying excellent segmentation consistency.

Despite its rapid growth, MRI remains an untapped resource in obesity research and has not yet reached its full potential. Many opportunities remain for future investigation. Several groups have recognized the time-consuming and labor-intensive work involved with manual image segmentation. This can be daunting in longitudinal studies, as the process must be performed for every scan at multiple time points across the same subject. Efficient semi-automated and automated algorithms have been proposed, but are usually limited to in-house usage (Armao et al., 2006; Demerath et al., 2007; Kullberg et al., 2010; Peng et al., 2007; Positano et al., 2004; Wilhelm Poll et al., 2003). Techniques that can automatically segment adipose tissue and organs from a subject's MRI data at subsequent time points while utilizing *a priori* information from the same subject's baseline segmentations are being explored. The capability of achieving rapid intra-subject 3D registration, segmentation, and quantification will provide investigators with detailed person-specific information reflecting the temporal change in fat distribution and volumes in response to intervention. Such capability will also exploit the richness of 3D MRI that is unavailable in gapped 2D multi-slice data. Quality control will be essential in assuring consistency and accuracy. Fat measurements should be routinely validated against phantoms, between multiple blinded observers, and between manual and automated segmentations (Table 2). There are only a few literature reports describing the accuracy and repeatability of quantitative fat MRI.

In conclusion, MRI is the most powerful and comprehensive imaging tool for fat quantification. With CSI methods, recent studies are beginning to demonstrate their usefulness and investigators are exploring new fat biomarkers and associations in obesity with MRI that were previously untapped. This chapter has provided introductory materials for investigators to survey, understand, and integrate MRI into their studies.

7. Acknowledgment

The authors are grateful to the faculty and staff of the Childhood Obesity Research Center at the University of Southern California for research assistance, particularly Sherryl Esplana Rosa Rangel, Christina Ayala, and Kami McClure. The authors acknowledge Huanzhou Yu, Ph.D., Ann Shimakawa, M.S., and Jean Brittain, Ph.D., from GE Healthcare for technical and research support. The authors thank Gavin Hamilton, Ph.D., from the University of California San Diego for assistance with MRS, and Mark Punyanitya and Wei Shen, M.D., from Columbia University, for assistance with SliceOmatic. Finally, the authors acknowledge Daniel L. Smith, Jr., Ph.D, and Timothy R. Nagy, Ph.D., from the University of Alabama at Birmingham for recognizing the potential of IDEAL with brown adipose tissue.

8. References

Abate N, Garg A, Coleman R, Grundy SM, & Peshock RM. (1997). Prediction of total subcutaneous abdominal, intraperitoneal, and retroperitoneal adipose tissue masses in men by single axial magnetic resonance imaging slice. *American Journal of Clinical Nutrition*, Vol. 65, No. 2, February 1997, pp. 403-408.

Armao D, Guyon JP, Firat Z, Brown MA, & Semelka RC. (2006). Accurate quantification of visceral adipose tissue (VAT) using water-saturation MRI and computer segmentation: preliminary results. *Journal of Magnetic Resonance Imaging*, Vol. 23, No. 5, May 2006, pp. 736-741.

Berglund J, Johansson L, Ahlstrom H, & Kullberg J. (2010). Three-point Dixon method enables whole-body water and fat imaging of obese subjects. *Magnetic Resonance in Medicine*, Vol. 63, No. 6, June 2010, pp. 1659-1668.

Berglund J, Ahlstrom H, Johansson L, & Kullberg J. (2011). Two-point Dixon method with flexible echo times. *Magnetic Resonance in Medicine*, Vol. 65, No. 4, April 2011, pp. 994-1004.

Bernard CP, Liney GP, Manton DJ, Turnbull LW, & Langton, CM. (2008). Comparison of fat quantification methods: a phantom study at 3.0T. *Journal of Magnetic Resonance Imaging*, Vol. 27, No. 1, January, pp. 192-197.

Bernstein MA, King K, & Zhou X. (2004). *Handbook of MRI pulse sequences* (1st edition), Elsevier Academic Press, ISBN 0-12-092861-2, Amsterdam.

Bley TA, Wieben O, Francois CJ, Brittain JH, & Reeder SB. (2010). Fat and water magnetic resonance imaging. *Journal of Magnetic Resonance Imaging*, Vol. 31, No. 1, January 2010, pp. 4-18.

Bonekamp S, Ghosh P, Crawford S, Solga SF, Horska A, Brancati FL, Diehl AM, Smith S, & Clark JM. (2008). Quantitative comparison and evaluation of software packages for assessment of abdominal adipose tissue distribution by magnetic resonance imaging. *International Journal of Obesity*, Vol. 32, No. 1, January 2008, pp. 100-111.

Bornert P, Keupp J, Eggers H, & Aldefeld B. (2007). Whole-body 3D water/fat resolved continuously moving table imaging. *Journal of Magnetic Resonance Imaging*, Vol. 25, No. 3, March 2007, pp. 660-665.

Brix G, Heiland S, Bellemann ME, Koch T, & Lorenz WJ. (1993). MR imaging of fat-containing tissue : valuation of two quantitative imaging techniques in comparison to localized proton spectroscopy. *Magnetic Resonance Imaging*, Vol. 11, No. 7, pp. 977-991.

Bydder M, Yokoo T, Hamilton G, Middleton MS, Chavez AD, Schwimmer JB, Lavine JE, & Sirlin CB. (2008). Relaxation effects in the quantification of fat using gradient echo imaging. *Magnetic Resonance in Medicine*, Vol. 26, No. 3, January 2008, pp. 347-359.

Bydder M, Yokoo T, Yu H, Carl M, Reeder SB, & Sirlin CB. (2011). Constraining the initial phase in water-fat separation. *Magnetic Resonance Imaging*, Vol. 29, No. 2, February 2011, pp. 216-221.

Cassidy FH, Yokoo T, Aganovic L, Hanna RF, Bydder M, Middleton MS, Hamilton G, Chavez AD, Schwimmer JB, & Sirlin CB. (2009). Fatty liver disease: MR imaging techniques for the detection and quantification of liver steatosis. *Radiographics*, Vol. 29, No. 1, January-February 2009, pp. 231-260.

Chebrolu VV, Hines CDG, Yu H, Pineda AR, Shimakawa A, McKenzie CA, Samsonov A, Brittain JH, & Reeder SB. (2010). Independent estimation of T2* for water and fat for improved accuracy of fat quantification. Vol. 63, No. 4, April 2010, pp. 849-857.

Choudhary AK, Donnelly LF, Racadio JM, & Strife JL. (2007). Diseases associated with childhood obesity. *Americain Journal of Roentgenology*, Vol. 188, No. 4, April 2007, pp. 1118-1130.

De Bazelaire CM, Duhamel GD, Rofsky NM, & Alsop DC. (2004). MR imaging relaxation times of abdominal and pelvic tissues measured in vivo at 3.0T : preliminary results. *Radiology*, Vol. 230, No. 3, March 2004, pp. 652-659.

Demerath EW, Ritter KJ, Couch WA, Rogers NL, Moreno GM, Choh A, Lee M, Remsberg K, Czerwinski SA, Chumlea WC, Siervogel RM, & Towne B. (2007). Validity of a new automated software program for visceral adipose tissue estimation. *International Journal of Obesity*, Vol. 31, No. 2, February 2007, pp. 285-291.

Despres JP, Lemieux I, Bergeron J, Pibarot P, Mathieu P, Larose E, Rodes-Cabau J, Bertrand OF, & Poirier P. (2008). Abdominal obesity and the metabolic syndrome : contribution to global cardiometabolic risk. *Arteriosclerosis, Thrombosis, and Vascular Biology*, Vol. 28, No. 6, June 2008, pp. 1039-1049.

Eggers H, Brendel B, Duijndam A, & Herigault G. (2011). Dual-echo Dixon imaging with flexible choice of echo times. *Magnetic Resonance in Medicine*, Vol. 65, No. 1, January 2011, pp. 96-107.

Ellis KJ. Human body composition, in vivo methods. (2000). *Physiological Review*, Vol. 80, No. 2, April 2000, pp. 649-680.

Flegal KM, Caroll MD, Odgen CL, & Curtin LR. Prevalence and trends in obesity among US adults, 1999-2008. (2010). *Journal of the American Medical Association*, Vol. 303, No. 3, January 2010, pp. 235-241.

Goodpaster BH, Thaete FL, & Kelley DE. Composition of skeletal muscle evaluated with computed tomography. (2000). *Annals of New York Academy of Sciences*, Vol. 904, May 2000, pp. 18-24.

Guiu B, Petit JM, Loffroy R, Ben Salem D, Aho S, Masson D, Hillon P, Krause D, & Cercueil JP. (2009). Quantification of liver fat content: comparison of triple-echo chemical shift gradient-echo imaging and in vivo proton MR spectroscopy. *Radiology*, Vol. 250, No. 1, January 2009, pp. 95-102.

Haacke EM, Brown RW, Thompson MR, & Venkatesan R. (1999). *Magnetic resonance imaging, physical principles and sequence design* (1st edition), John Wiley and Sons, Inc., ISBN 0-471-35128-8, New York.

Hamilton G, Middleton MS, Bydder M, Yokoo T, Schwimmer JB, Kono Y, Patton HM, Lavine JE, & Sirlin CB. (2009). Effect of PRESS and STEAM sequences on magnetic resonance spectroscopic liver fat quantification. *Journal of Magnetic Resonance Imaging*, Vol. 30, No. 1, July 2009, pp. 145-152.

Hashemi RH, & Bradley, Jr. WG. (1997). *MRI the basics* (1st edition), Lippincott Williams and Wilkins, ISBN 0-683-18240-4, Philadelphia.

Hernando D, Liang ZP, Kellman P. (2010). Chemical shift-based water/fat separation : a comparison of signal models. *Magnetic Resonance in Medicine*, Vol. 64, No. 3, September 2010, pp. 811-822.

Hines CDG, Yu H, Shimakawa A, McKenzie CA, Brittain JH, & Reeder SB. (2009). T1 independent, T2* corrected MRI with accurate spectral modeling for quantification of fat: validation in a fat-water-SPIO phantom. *Journal of Magnetic Resonance Imaging*, Vol. 30, No. 5, November 2009, pp. 1215-1222.

Hood MN, & Ho VB. (1999). Chemical shift : the artifact and clinical tool revisited. *Radiographics*, Vol. 19, No. 2, March-April 1999, pp. 357-371.

Hu HH, Kim HW, Nayak KS, & Goran MI. (2010). Comparison of fat-water MRI and single-voxel MRS in the assessment of hepatic and pancreatic fat fractions in humans. *Obesity*, Vol. 18, No. 4, April 2010, pp. 841-847.

Hu HH, Smith DL, Jr., Nayak KS, Goran MI, & Nagy TR. (2010). Identification of brown adipose tissue in mice with fat-water IDEAL-MRI. *Journal of Magnetic Resonance Imaging*, Vol. 31, No. 5, May 2010, pp. 1195-1202.

Jackson AS, & Pollock ML. (1982). Steps toward the development of generalized equations for predicting body composition of adults. *Canadian Journal of Applied Sport Science*, Vol. 7, No. 3, September 1982, pp. 189-196.

Kaldoudi E, Williams SC, Barker GJ, & Tofts PS. (1993). A chemical shift selective inversion recovery sequence for fat-suppressed MRI: theory and experimental validation. *Magnetic Resonance Imaging*, Vol. 11, No. 3, March 1993, pp. 341-355.

Kellman P, Hernando D, & Arai AE. (2010). Myocardial fat imaging. *Current Cardiovascular Imaging Reports*, Vol. 3, No. 2, April 2010, pp. 83-91.

Kim H, Taksali SE, Dufour S, Befroy D, Goodman TR, Petersen KF, Shulman GI, Caprio S, & Constable RT. (2008). Comparative MR study of hepatic fat quantification using single-voxel proton spectroscopy, two-point Dixon and three-point IDEAL. *Magnetic Resonance in Medicine*, Vol. 59, No. 3, March 2008, pp. 521-527.

Kullberg J, Johansson L, Ahlstrom H, Courivaud F, Koken P, Eggers H, & Bornert P. (2009). Automated assessment of whole-body adipose tissue depots from continuously moving bed MRI: a feasibility study. *Journal of Magnetic Resonance Imaging*, Vol. 31, No. 1, July 2009, pp. 185-193.

Kullberg J, Brandberg J, Angelhed JE, Frimmel H, Bergelin E, Strid L, Ahlstrom H, Johansson L, & Lonn L. (2009). Whole-body adipose tissue analysis: comparison of MRI, CT and dual energy X-ray absorptiometry. *British Journal of Radiology*, Vol. 82, No. 974, February 2009, pp. 123-130.

Kullberg J, Karlsson AK, Stokland E, Svensson PA, & Dahlgren J. (2010). Adipose tissue distribution in children: automated quantification using water and fat MRI. *Journal of Magnetic Resonance Imaging,* Vol. 32, No. 1, July 2010, pp. 204-210.

Kvist H, Chowdhury B, Grangard U, Tylen U, & Sjostrom L. (1988). Total and visceral adipose-tissue volumes derived from measurements with computed tomography in adult men and women : predictive equations. *American Journal of Clinical Nutrition,* Vol. 48, No. 6, December 1988, pp. 1351-1361.

Lancaster JL, Ghiatas AA, Alyassin A, Kilcoyne RF, Bonora E, & DeForonzo RA. (1991). Measurement of abdominal fat with T_1-weighted MR images. *Journal of Magnetic Resonance Imaging,* Vol. 1, No. 3, May-June, pp. 363-369.

Lingvay I, Esser V, Legendre JL, Price AL, Wertz KM, Adams-Huet B, Zhang S, Unger RH, & Szczepaniak LS. (2009). Noninvasive quantification of pancreatic fat in humans. *Journal of Clinical Endocrinology and Metabolism,* Vol. 94, No. 10, October 2009, pp. 4070-4076.

Liu CY, McKenzie CA, Yu H, Brittain JH, & Reeder SB. (2007). Fat quantification with IDEAL gradient echo imaging: correction of bias from T1 and noise. *Magnetic Resonance in Medicine,* Vol. 58, No. 2, August, pp. 354-364.

Ma J, Slavens Z, Sun W, Bayram E, Estowski L, Hwang KP, Akao J, & Vu AT. (2008). Linear phase-error correction for improved water and fat separation in dual-echo Dixon techniques. *Magnetic Resonance in Medicine,* Vol. 60, No. 5, November 2008, pp. 1250-1255.

Ma J. (2008). Dixon techniques for water and fat imaging. *Journal of Magnetic Resonance Imaging,* Vol. 28, No. 3, September 2008, pp. 543-558.

Machann J, Bachmann OP, Brechtel K, Dahl DB, Wietek B, Klumpp B, Haring HU, Claussen CD, Jacob S, & Schick F. (2003). Lipid content in the musculature of the lower leg assessed by fat selective MRI: intra- and interindividual differences and correlation with anthropometric and metabolic data. *Journal of Magnetic Resonance Imaging,* Vol. 17, No. 3, March 2003, pp. 350-357.

Machann J, Thamer C, Schnoedt B, Haap M, Haring HU, Claussen CD, Stumvoll M, Fritsche A, & Schick F. (2005). Standardized assessment of whole body adipose tissue topography by MRI. *Journal of Magnetic Resonance Imaging,* Vol. 21, No. 4, April 2005, pp. 455-462.

Margolis DJ, Bammer R, & Chow LC. (2004). Parallel imaging of the abdomen. *Topics in Magnetic Resonance Imaging,* June 2004, Vol. 15, No. 3, pp. 197-206.

Mattsson S, & Thomas BJ. Development of methods for body composition studies. (2006). *Physics in Medicine and Biology,* Vol. 51, No. 13, July 2006, pp. R203-R228.

Meisamy S, Hines CD, Hamilton G, Sirlin CB, McKenzie CA, Yu H, Brittain JH, & Reeder SB. (2011). Quantification of hepatic steatosis with T1-independent, T2* corrected MR imaging with spectral modeling of fat : blinded comparison with MR spectroscopy. *Radiology,* Vol. 258, No. 3, March 2011, pp. 767-775.

Napolitano A, Miller SR, Murgatroyd PR, Coward WA, Wright A, Finer N, De Bruin TW, Bullmore ET, & Nunez DJ. Validation of a quantitative magnetic resonance method. (2008). *Obesity,* Vol. 16, No. 1, January 2008, pp. 191-198.

Naressi A, Couturier C, Castang I, de Beer R, & Graveron-Demilly D. (2001). Java-based graphical user interface for MRUI, a software package for quantitation of in vivo/medical magnetic resonance spectroscopy signals. *Computers in Biology and Medcine*, Vol. 31, No. 4, July 2001, pp. 269-286.

O'Regan DP, Callaghan MF, Wylezinska-Arridge M, Fitzpatrick J, Naoumova RP, Hajnal JV, & Schmitz SA. (2008). Liver fat content and T2*: simultaneous measurement by using breath-hold multiecho MR imaging at 3.0 T--feasibility. *Radiology*, Vol. 247, No. 2, May 2008, pp. 550-557.

Peng Q, McColl RW, Ding Y, Wang J, Chia JM, & Weatherall PT (2007). Automated method for accurate abdominal fat quantification on water-saturated magnetic resonance images. *Journal of Magnetic Resonance Imaging*, Vol. 26, No. 3, September 2007, pp. 738-746.

Positano V, Gastaldelli A, Sironi AM, Santarelli MF, Lombardi M, & Landini L. (2004). An accurate and robust method for unsupervised assessment of abdominal fat by MRI. *Journal of Magnetic Resonance Imaging*, Vol. 20, No. 4, October 2004, pp. 684-689.

Ren J, Dimitrov I, Sherry AD, & Malloy CR. (2008). Composition of adipose tissue and marrow fat in humans by 1H NMR at 7 Tesla. *Journal of Lipid Research*, Vol. 49, No. 9, September 2008, pp. 2055-2062.

Reeder SB, McKenzie CA, Pineda AR, Yu H, Shimakawa A, Brau AC, Hargreaves BA, Gold GE, & Brittain JH. (2007). Water-fat separation with IDEAL gradient-echo imaging. *Journal of Magnetic Resonance Imaging*, Vol. 25, No. 3, March 2007, pp. 644-652.

Reeder SB, Robson PM, Yu H, Shimakawa A, Hines CD, McKenzie CA, & Brittain JH. (2009). Quantification of hepatic steatosis with MRI: the effects of accurate fat spectral modeling. *Journal of Magnetic Resonance Imaging*, Vol. 29, No. 6, May 2009, pp. 1332-1339.

Reeder SB, & Sirlin CB. (2010). Quantification of liver fat with magnetic resonance imaging. *Magnetic Resonance Imaging Clinics of North America*, Vol. 18, No. 3, August 2010, pp. 337-357.

Ross R, Goodpaster B, Kelley D, & Boada F. (2000). Magnetic resonance imaging in human body composition research: from quantitative to qualitative tissue measurement. *Annals of New York Academy of Sciences*, Vol. 904, May 2000, pp. 12-17.

Seidell JC, Bakker CJ, & van der Kooy K. Imaging techniques for measuring adipose-tissue distribution—a comparison between computed tomography and 1.5T magnetic resonance. (1990). *American Journal of Clinical Nutrition*, Vol. 51, No. 6, June 1990, pp. 953-957.

Schick F, Machann J, Brechtel K, Strempfer A, Klumpp B, Stein DT, & Jacob S. (2002). MRI of muscular fat. *Magnetic Resonance in Medicine*, Vol. 47, No. 4, April 2002, pp. 720-727.

Siegel MJ, Hildebolt CF, Bae KT, Hong C, & White NH. (2007). Total and intraabdominal fat distribution in preadolescents and adolescents: measurement with MR imaging. *Radiology*, Vol. 242, No. 3, March 2007, pp. 846-856.

Stanisz GJ, Odrobina EE, Pun J, Escaravage M, Graham SJ, Bronskill MJ, & Henkelman RM. (2005). T1, T2 relaxation and magnetization transfer in tissue at 3T. *Magnetic Resonance in Medicine*, Vol. 54, No. 3, September 2005, pp. 507-512.

Thomas EL, Hamilton G, Patel N, O'Dwyer R, Dore CJ, Goldin RD, Bell JD, & Taylor-Robinson, SD. (2005). Hepatic triglyceride content and its relation to body adiposity: a magnetic resonance imaging and proton magnetic resonance spectroscopy study. *Gut*, Vol.54, No. 1, January 2005, pp. 122-127.

van Werven JR, Hoogduin JM, Nederveen AJ, van Vliet AA, Wajs E, Vandenberk P, Stroes ES, & Stoker J. (2009). Reproducibility of 3.0 Tesla magnetic resonance spectroscopy for measuring hepatic fat content. *Journal of Magnetic Resonance Imaging*, Vol. 30, No. 2, August 2009, pp. 444-448.

Vlaardingerbroek MT, & den Boer JA. (1999). *Magnetic resonance imaging* (2nd edition), Springer, ISBN 3-540-64877-1, Berlin.

Weis J, Johansson L, Ortiz-Nieto F, & Ahlstrom H. (2008). Assessment of lipids in skeletal muscle by high-resolution spectroscopic imaging using fat as the internal standard: Comparison with water referenced spectroscopy. *Magnetic Resonance in Medicine*, Vol. 59, No. 6, June 2008, pp. 1259-1265.

Wilhelm Poll L, Wittsack HJ, Koch JA, Willers R, Cohnen M, Kapitza C, Heinemann L, & Modder U. (2003). A rapid and reliable semi automated method for measurement of total abdominal fat volumes using magnetic resonance imaging. *Magnetic Resonance Imaging*, Vol. 21, No. 6, July 2003, pp. 631-636.

Xiang, QS. (2006). Two-point water-fat imaging with partially-opposed-phase (POP) acquisition: an asymmetric Dixon method. *Magnetic Resonance in Medicine*, Vol. 56, No. 3, September 2006, pp. 572-584.

Yokoo T, Bydder M, Hamilton G, Middleton MS, Gamst AC, Wolfson T, Hassanein T, Patton HM, Lavine JE, Schwimmer JB, & Sirlin CB. (2009). Nonalcoholic fatty liver disease: diagnostic and fat-grading accuracy of low-flip-angle multiecho gradient-recalled-echo MR imaging at 1.5 T. *Radiology*, Vol. 251, No. 1, April 2009, pp. 67-76.

Yu H, Shimakawa A, McKenzie CA, Brodsky E, Brittain JH, & Reeder SB. (2008). Multiecho water-fat separation and simultaneous R2* estimation with multifrequency fat spectrum modeling. *Magnetic Resonance in Medicine*, Vol. 60, No. 5, November 2008, pp. 1122-1134.

12

Non-Alcoholic Fatty Liver Disease (NAFLD), Adipocytokines and Diabetes Mellitus

Dhastagir Sultan Sheriff
Shri Sathya Sai Medical College and Research Institute, Tamilnadu
India

1. Introduction

Nonalcoholic fatty liver disease (NAFLD), which includes nonalcoholic steatosis and nonalcoholic steato- hepatitis (NASH), describes the clinicopathologic spectrum of alcohol-like liver disease in the nonalcoholic [Ludwig et al 1980].

Although it may be observed as an iatrogenic complication (due to drugs or anti-obesity surgery) or secondary to various other conditions (toxins, lipodystrophic syndromes, hypobetalipoproteinemia), NAFLD most commonly occurs as a primary (idiopathic) disease.

The clinical importance of primary NAFLD appears to rest on three main observations:

- It commonly occurs in the general population worldwide and among patients presenting with unexplained mild to moderate raised aminotransferase levels .
- It is not a sign or symptom of disease but it is a pathological condition that has the potential to progress to advanced hepatic and extrahepatic disease ,and to interact with other etiologies of liver disease .
- It may recur following orthotopic liver transplantation and poses a heavy burden of complications in the setting of major extrahepatic and liver-related surgery .

2. Reported risk factors

The conventional risk factors for the development of primary NAFLD include type II diabetes, insulin resistance, hyperlipidemia and obesity (Mezey,1998). NAFLD typically affects 50% of diabetics and 76% of obese patients (Bellantini et al 2000;Gupte et al.2004), and is the most common of all liver diseases. However, the prevalence of NASH is substantially less, affecting 18.5% of obese patients.

Other traditional risk factors include hyperuricemia, central obesity defined as waist circumference greater than 100 cm in males and greater than 88 cm in females, and hypertension.

Secondary causes of NAFLD include nutrition-related complications, such as total parenteral nutrition, rapid weight loss, and intestinal jejunoileal bypass surgery. Common causes of Steatosis is mention in Table.1.

Nonalcoholic fatty liver disease
Alcohol
Drugs—estrogens, coumadin, tamoxifen, valproic acid, methotrexate, isoniazid, corticosteroids, vitamin A, troglitazone, l-asparaginase, amiodarone, perhexiline, calcium channel blockers, nucleoside analogues
Hepatitis C (genotype 3)
Nutritional factors—rapid weight loss, total parenteral nutrition
Surgical considerations—gastrointestinal surgery for obesity, extensive small-bowel resection
Metabolic disorders—cystic fibrosis, abetalipoproteinemia, others
Syndromes associated with obesity, insulin resistance—lipodystrophies, hypopituitarism, Prader-Willi syndrome

Table 1. Conditions Associated With Macrovesicular Steatosis

Certain drugs are associated with NAFLD. Metabolic syndromes and pregnancy-related fatty liver diseases are also some of the secondary causes of NAFLD. Patients with normal body mass index (BMI) may develop NAFLD even in the absence of traditional risk factors. It is thought that the primary abnormality may be occult insulin resistance or central adiposity (Lee et al.1998).

The natural history of NAFLD still remains poorly defined. Mortality among NAFLD patients approaches 13%, which is greater than age- and sex-matched controls (6). Because these patients often have features of the metabolic syndrome, they are at high risk for cardiac-related death. Hence, both ischemic heart disease and malignancy are the leading causes of death in patients with NAFLD. However, liver disease is the third most common cause of mortality in this population, accounting for 13% of all deaths. This is significantly different than patients without NAFLD, in whom liver-related causes of mortality account for less than 1% of all deaths (Adams et al 2005). Clinical predictors of more advanced disease include people with diabetes, hypertriglyceridemia (Caldwell et al.1999) and those older than 40 years of age. Table.2. outlines the diagnostic criteria for NAFLD.

Parameter	Value
Impaired glucose tolerance	Fasting blood glucose l vel ≥110 mg/dL(5.6mmol/L)
High blood pressure	≥130/85 mm Hg
Elevated triglyceride levels	>250 mg/dL(1.7mmol/L)
Low high-density lipoprotein level	<40 mg/dL (1.00mmol/L)for men; <50 mg/dL(1.3mmol/L) for women
Abdominal obe ity	Waist: >102 cm (40 inches for men; >88 cm (35 inches) for women

Table 2. Diagnostic Criteria for the Metabolic Syndrome: Presence of Two or More of the Following Parameters

3. Diagnosis

Most patients with NAFLD are asymptomatic or suffer from nonspecific symptoms and signs such as fatigue, malaise or right upper quadrant pain. In most cases, the diagnosis is suspected in the context of the appropriate risk factor profile and incidental elevation of transaminases. Levels of aspartate aminotransferase and alanine aminotransferase are modestly elevated, although the ratio of aspartate aminotransferase to alanine aminotransferase is less than one, distinguishing NAFLD patients from those with alcohol-induced liver disease (Bacon et al.1994).

The International Federation of Clinical Chemistry and Laboratory Medicine established in 2002 a reference system for the measurement of enzyme activity of clinically important enzymes, including ALT, to be measured at 37 °C 23. Levels of 10-45 U/l are considered as normal, although reference values may still vary among laboratories.

The degree of elevation of transaminases does not reflect the underlying severity of the disease. The diagnosis of NAFLD can be suspected on the basis of radiological imaging such as ultrasound or magnetic resonance imaging.

However, the sensitivity of these modalities is low and often there is a significant degree of interobserver variability. A minimum of 30% of hepatocytes needs to be infiltrated by steatosis for the imaging techniques to detect fatty liver (Saadeh et al.2002).

Currently, the only method of distinguishing simple steatosis from NASH is the liver biopsy. Brunt et al (1999) proposed a grading and staging system for NASH. Grade 1 reveals mild steatosis, predominantly macrovesicular with minimal ballooning of hepatocytes and minimal inflammation. Grade 2 shows moderate steatosis, usually mixed macrovesicular and microvesicular with ballooning present in zone 3 hepatocytes, and some lobular inflammation. Grade 3 shows all the features of grade 2 plus the additional requirement of portalinflammation. Staging requires the presence of Masson trichrome stain. Stage 1 reveals zone 3 perivenular, perisinusoidal fibrosis, either focal or extensive. Stage 2 requires the features of stage 1, plus focal or extensive portal fibrosis. Stage 3, shows bridging fibrosis and stage 4 reveals cirrhosis with or without perisinusoidal fibrosis.

4. Pathogenesis

The progression from simple steatosis to steatohepatitis, fibrosis and cirrhosis is thought to be a two-hit hypothesis.

4.1 First hit

The first hit results in fat accumulation within the liver parenchyma. This occurs in abnormalities during uptake, synthesis and secretion of lipids resulting primarily from insulin resistance, which is quite common in patients with NAFLD (Marchesni et al.2001). Insulin resistance is often a primary abnormality in patients with NAFLD. There is often a genetic predisposition to insulin resistance, even in the absence of frank diabetes. Twenty per cent of the nondiabetic population may exhibit insulin resistance. Patients that exhibit more pronounced levels of insulin resistance exhibit a greater degree of steatosis (Angelico et al.2005). Central adiposity may contribute to the flow of excess free fatty acids (FFAs) to the liver by providing a direct route through the portal vein (Scheen and Luyckx. 2002). Patients with NAFLD often have risk factors such as type II diabetes, hyperlipidemia, hypertension and obesity, which are part of the insulin resistance syndrome.

Hyperinsulinemia promotes lipolysis in the adipocyte, resulting in increased FFAs delivered to the liver. In the hepatocyte, FFAs stimulate synthesis of more FFAs and inhibit oxidation of FFAs (Harrison et al.2002). The following figure 1. explains how expanded visceral mass leads to increased release of free fatty acids(FFA) from adipose tissue due to insulin resistance (IR)..

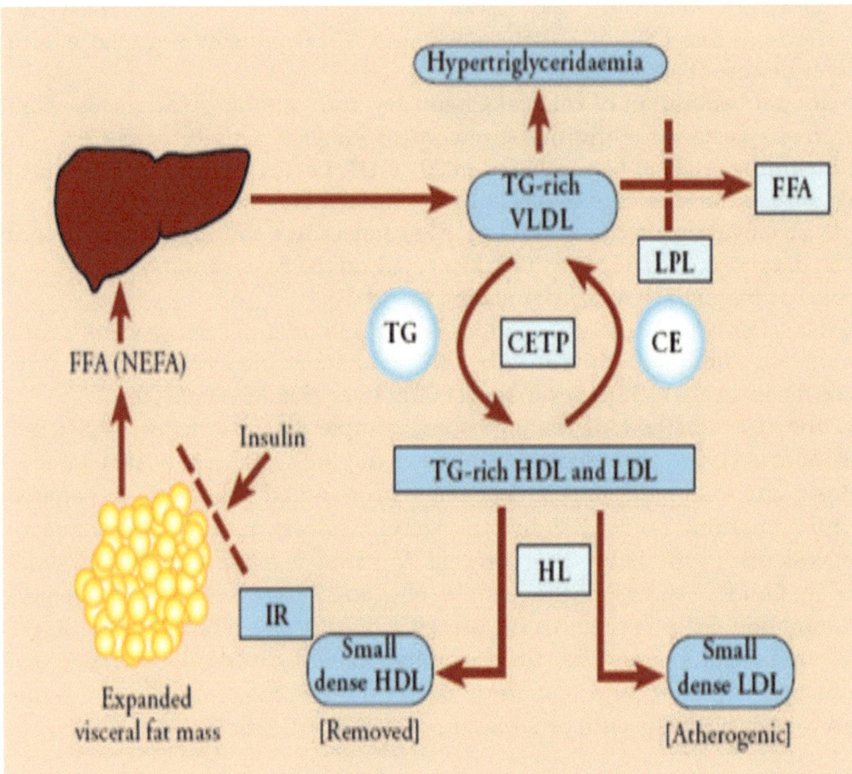

Fig. 1. Expansion of Visceral Fat Mass May Lead to Dyslipidemia and Insulin Resistance

The increased flux of free fatty acids into the liver results in the formation and secretion of very low density lipoprotein (VLDL)rich in Triglycerides. Inhibition or reduced activity of Lipoprotein lipase LPL) results in the distribution and formation of TG rich High density lipoprotein and Low density lipoprotein (LDL). Hepatic lipase acts on them to form small dense HDL and LDL (Dyslipidemia).

Insulin sensitivity is also influenced by peptide mediators, otherwise known as adipocytokines, such as tumour necrosis factoralpha (TNF-α), leptin and adiponectin and although the mechanisms by which this occurs remain largely unknown, theories are suggested. TNF-α influences steatosis by stimulating the release of FFAs from adipocytes into the liver.(Fig.2.)

TNF-α may directly induce apoptosis of hepatocytes promoting activation of hepatic stellate cells, stimulating fibrosis (Festi et al.2004). Leptin(Leptin resistance which is considered to be one of the possible third hit hypothesis) potentially may stimulate platelet-derived growth factor, ultimately leading to hepatic stellate cell proliferation resulting in fibrosis (Kejima et al.2005). Adiponectin may have a protective role against fatty liver. Recently it was shown that adiponectin levels were significantly reduced in patients with NAFLD compared with controls resulting in an inverse relationship between insulin resistance and adiponectin levels (Saargin et al.2005). This observation may result in a future therapeutic role in the pharmacological management of NAFLD.

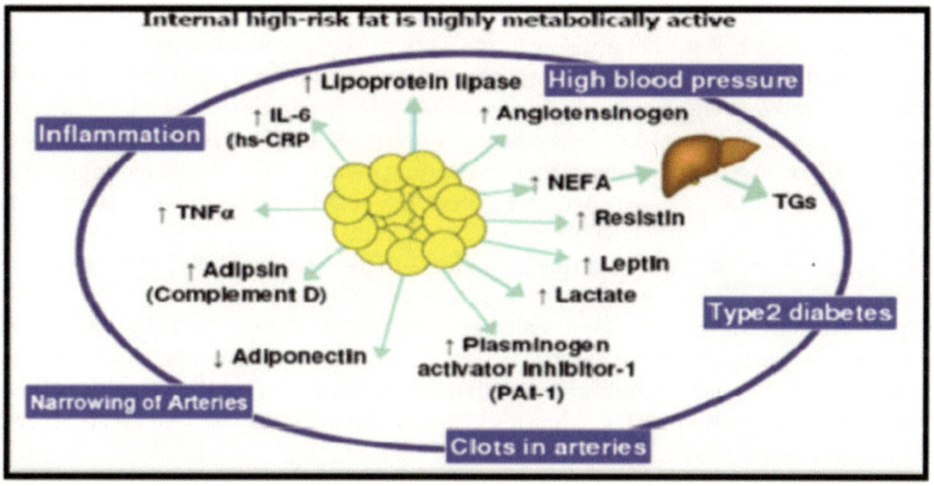

Fig. 2. Visceral Fat As a Major Site of Hormone Production, Inflammatory Markers and Its Possible Relationship including Type 2 Diabetes

4.2 Second hit

The second hit is hepatocellular injury that results from oxidative stress, lipid peroxidation and direct cellular toxicity from FFAs (hitture and Farrell 2001). Multiple mechanisms regarding hepatocyte injury have been proposed:

1. Increased expression of cytochrome P450 isoform CYP2E1 has been shown to occur in patients with NASH. CYP2E1 is a pro-oxidant, resulting in increased production of reactive oxygen species, capable of peroxidizing cell membranes.
2. Increased insulin leads to peripheral lipolysis resulting in excess fatty acids which catalyzes lipid peroxisomes. Peroxisomes are involved in the oxidation process of fatty acids. Oxidation, along with binding and export of fatty acids, is the primary method of protecting the liver from subsequent damage.
3. The peroxisome proliferators activated receptor-alpha (PPAR-α) is responsible for regulating the esterification and export of fatty acids in very low density lipoprotein, in the binding of fatty acids and in mitochondrial and peroxisomal oxidation. Reduced expression of PPAR-α may have an important role in the pathogenesis of NASH (Yeon et al.2004).
4. Mitochondrial abnormalities have been described in patients with NASH, but not in those with simple steatosis. These mitochondrial abnormalities lead to increased mitochondrial fatty acids beta-oxidation, eventually resulting in free radical formation hepatocyte injury and steatohepatitis. Patients who are insulin resistant but do not have mitochondrial abnormalities may develop fatty liver; however, generally they do not progress to steatohepatitis (Sanyal et al.2001).

5. Methods of managing the disease

Currently, management is aimed at lifestyle modification, primarily targeting weight loss achieved through dietary modification and exercise. Additionally, treatment of all other aspects of the metabolic syndrome must be instituted. Weight loss and exercise both improve insulin resistance (Cox et al.2004), which theoretically should improve steatosis. No randomized controlled study has been run to evaluate whether histological regression occurs in patients with steatohepatitis or fibrosis after weight loss, although case reports and open-label studies suggest improvement. Weight loss should not exceed more than 1 kg per week, because rapid weight loss can exacerbate steatosis. Similarly very low calorie diets that give less than 500 kcal/day and jejunoileal bypass surgery should be avoided as a method of weight loss, due to the risk of worsening fibrosis. The recommended target for weight loss is 10% of a person's body weight over a six-month period (Angulo,2002).Multiple popular diets exist as methods of weight loss). Some diets are founded on years of medical experience, while others have deviated substantially from mainstream medical advice The Weight Watchers program is one of the traditional models, restricting portion sizes and total calories consumed. Other popular diets include carbohydrate restriction without fat restriction (Atkins diet), macronutrient and glycemic load modification (Zone diet) and fat restriction (Ornish diet). The following figure gives an idea about the distribution of fat in various compartments and the markers that indicate these compartments respectively

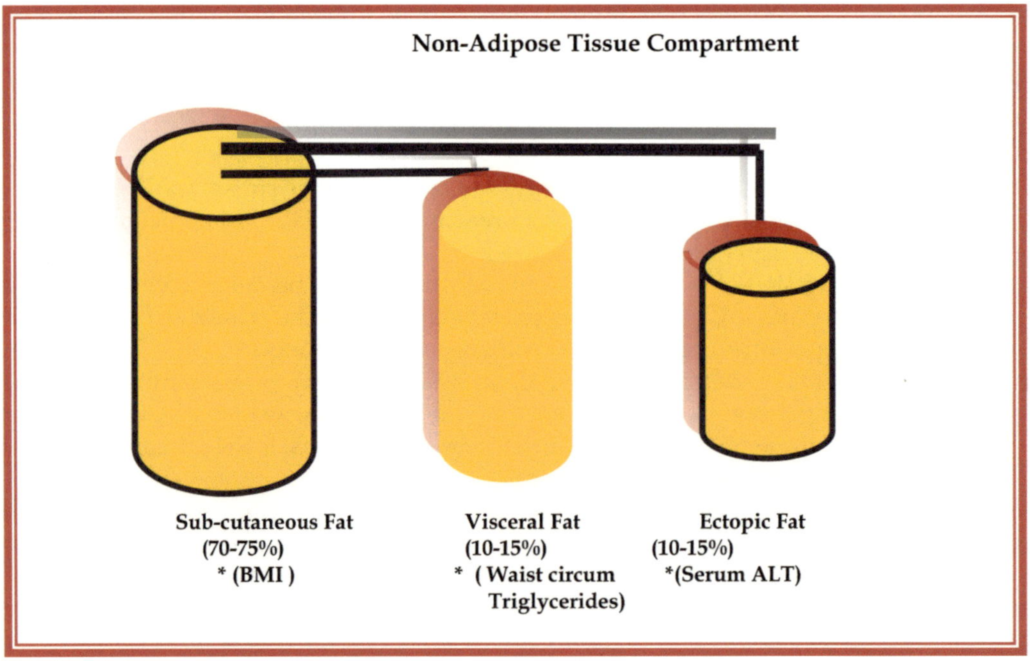

*As a Marker of Fat Measurement in various compartments BMI-Body Mass Index, Waist Circumference, Serum Alanine Aminotransferase (ALT)

Fig. 3. Distribution of Fat

In obese patients with BMI greater than 35 kg/m2, no significant differences were found regarding amount of weight lost at the end of one year (Dansinger et al.2005). Reduction of cardiovascular risk factors correlated with amount of weight loss. Weight loss of 3 kg to 6 kg over one year was achieved regardless of type of diet followed. Currently, no data exist regarding various types of diets in patients with NASH.

6. Medications that could induce weight loss

Medications to reduce weight are not routinely used in the treatment of NAFLD, and have not been studied in randomized clinical trials. One case series suggested that orlistat in patients with NASH was safe, and showed significant histological improvement in both degree of steatohepatitis and fibrosis after six to 12 months of therapy (Harrison et al.2003). Orlistat is a reversible inhibitor of gastric and pancreatic lipase, and is one of two agents that have been approved for the management of obesity. This medication forms a covalent bond with the active serine residue of gastric and pancreatic lipase in the stomach and small bowel, blocking the digestion and absorption of dietary triglycerides. Orlistat in combination with a controlled energy diet, rather than diet alone, significantly increased weight loss in obese adults after one year of therapy (Davidson et al.1999).
The second approved drug in the management of obesity is sibutramine. Sibutramine was evaluated in one nonrandomized study in patients with NASH (Sabuncu et al.2003). Sibutramine in combination with a low calorie diet-induced weight loss improved insulin resistance and transaminases, as shown by ultrasonographic regression in fatty liver, compared with diet alone. It is a noradrenaline-serotonin reuptake inhibitor and produces weight loss by a dual mechanism: reduction of food intake and increase in energy expenditure. Average weight loss is in the range of 5% to 8% from baseline. Recently, rimonabant, a selective cannabinoid-1 receptor blocker, has been shown to improve cardiovascular risk factor profile and reduce body weight(Despres et al.2005). Over 1000 overweight patients with BMIs between 27 kg/m2 and 40 kg/m2 participated in this study examining the effects of rimonabant and metabolic risk factors. Mean weight loss was 6.6 kg over 12 months at a dose of 20 mg.

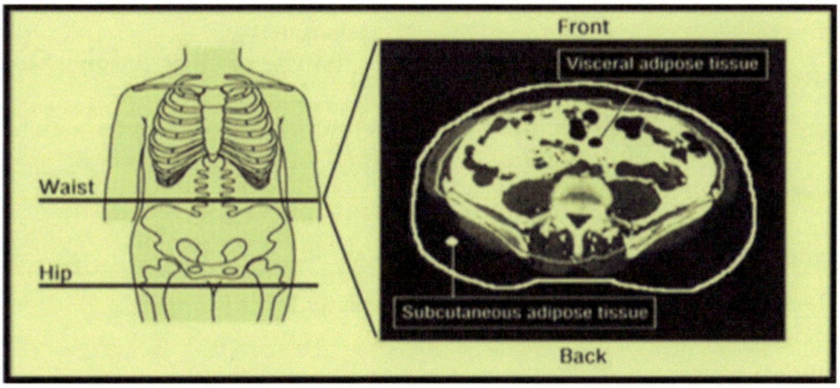

Fig. 4. WAIST HIP RATIO (WHR) AS A MEASURE OF Visceral Adiposity

Additionally, waist circumference was reduced, plasma high density lipoprotein levels increased, and plasma adiponectin levels were significantly higher in patients receiving rimonabant compared with placebo. This medication, and other weight reducing agents, may represent future therapeutic options for the pharmacological treatment of obese patients with NASH.

Certainly, diet should be combined with exercise to initiate and maintain weight loss. Exercise will enhance calorie deficit necessary for weight loss. A minimum of 30 min of moderate sustained activity five days per week is necessary to gain health benefits from exercise (28). Any fitness regimen should include a balance of aerobic exercise, strength and flexibility training

7. Pharmacotherapy for NAFLD

Currently, there are no approved pharmacological options for the treatment of NAFLD. Only three randomized controlled trials have been conducted to evaluate the efficacy of medical treatment in NAFLD (Table 3). The agents studied include antioxidants with vitamins E and C in combination, ursodeoxycholic acid and metformin. Although there was improvement in liver enzymes and steatosis in the trial evaluating metformin, there was no improvement in steatohepatitis or fibrosis at follow-up. The other two trials did not suggest any improvement in liver enzymes, steatosis, steatohepatitis or fibrosis. The remaining trials performed to date have been observational in design, had small sample size, and have had a short follow-up period. The thiazolidinediones are a class of insulin-sensitizing agents used to treat type II diabetes. Troglitazone was evaluated in an open-label trial involving 10 patients for duration of four to six months (Caldwell et al.2001). These patients had improvement in transaminases and liver histology. However, this medication was subsequently withdrawn from the market due to serious hepatic toxicity. Both rosiglitazone (Neuschwander-Tetri et al.2003) and pioglitazone (Promrat et al.2003) have been studied in open-label design, and have shown improvement in transaminases, steatosis and fibrosis. Recently VSL#3 was shown to lower markers of lipid peroxidation in patients with NASH (Loguercico et al.2005). However, larger randomized studies are needed before routine recommendation of these agents in the treatment of NASH.

Strategy	Treatment
Weight loss	Caloric restriction, exercise; sibutramine, orlistat; weight reduction surgery
Insulin-sensitizing agents	Metformin; peroxisome proliferator-activated receptor-gamma agonists (thiazolidinedione, rosiglitazone, pioglitazone)
Lipid-lowering drugs	Fibrates (gemfibrozil), fish oil
Antioxidants	*N*-acetylcysteine, vitamin E, betaine

Table. 3. Therapeutic Approaches for Nonalcoholic Fatty Liver Disease

8. Bariatric surgery

In the early age of bariatric surgery, jejunoileal bypass was the procedure most commonly performed.
A substantial proportion of patients developed advanced liver disease, presumably from bacterial overgrowth and endotoxemia in the bypassed intestine, resulting in bacterial translocation and liver disease. However, the jejunoileal bypass surgery has seldom been performed in recent years due to the multiple complications arising from this procedure. A

recent meta-analysis suggested that surgical therapy for weight loss was superior to other methods of weight loss in patients with BMI greater than 40 kg/m2 (Maggard et al.2005). This weight loss was sustained for a 10-year follow-up. Although there was a trend toward improved weight loss in patients with BMI between 35 kg/m2 and 39 kg/m2 in the surgically treated group, the data cannot be considered conclusive. Recently, one study evaluated laparascopic surgical weight loss via one of three techniques: roux-en-Y gastric bypass laparascopic adjustable gastric band and sleeve gastrectomy in patients with established NAFLD and metabolic syndrome.
Mean BMI was 56 kg/m2 (Mattar et al.2005). Patients had liver biopsies at the time of the bariatric surgery followed by a repeat biopsy after 15 months. Mean excess weight loss at the time of the second biopsy was 59%. There was a marked improvement in live steatosis, steatohepatitis and fibrosis. In fact, in some patients, inflammation and fibrosis completely resolved. Additionally, there was improvement in the metabolic risk factor profile.
Hence, as newer methods of bariatric surgery become more popular, there may be a future role for this type of surgery in morbidly obese patients with NASH.

9. Whether liver biopsy is mandatory?

Often, NAFLD is a diagnosis of exclusion. Patients are given advice regarding lifestyle modifications and re-evaluated clinically and biochemically several months later in routine follow-up. This may be a reasonable approach for the time being because there are no effective medications in the treatment of NAFLD. However, as pharmacotherapy becomes an option in the future, this line of thought may need to be revised. The distinction between pure fatty change and steatohepatitis can only be made histologically. This distinction is important because NAFLD has a benign prognosis, whereas NASH progresses toward cirrhosis. Because of the risk of NASH in patients suspected to have fatty liver, it could be argued that all patients should be offered a liver biopsy to stage the disease. However, in terms of logistics, cost and side effects, this may not be possible. Hence, it is reasonable to biopsy patients with risk factors for more advanced disease such as advancing age, obesity, hypertension and diabetes mellitus. Additionally, the liver biopsy may occasionally reveal unsuspected abnormalities indicating an alternate or additional diagnosis to fatty liver(Younossi, 2008).

10. Conclusions

Obesity epidemic is a global phenomena carrying with the risk of precipitating insulin resistant states including NAFLD which is shown to be on the rise. The primary abnormality for NAFLD reported is that of intrinsic insulin resistance. Therefore NAFLD could be one of the risk factors for the development of Type II Diabetes (Guido et al.2011). There seems to be no approved pharmacological therapies for the treatment of NASH. The major suggested treatment continues to be weight loss therapy through diet and exercise, and aggressive risk factor control.

11. References

[1] Ludwig J, Viggiano TR, McGill DB, Ott BJ. (1998)Nonalcoholic steatohepatitis. Mayo Clin Proc 1980;55:434-8.

[2] Mezey E] Dietary fat and alcoholic liver disease] Hepatology 28:901-5.

[3] Bellantani S, Saccoccio G, Masutti F, et al(2000) Prevalence of and risk factors for hepatic steatosis in northern Italy] Ann Intern Med 132:112-7.

[4] Gupte P, Amarapurkar D, Agal S, et al.(2004) Nonalcoholic steatohepatitis in type 2 diabetes mellitus] J Gastroenterol Hepatol 19:854-8.

[5] Lee JH, Rhee PL, Lee JK, et al.(1998) Role of hyperinsulinemia and glucose intolerance in the pathogenesis of nonalcoholic fatty liver in patients with normal body weight] Korean J Intern Med 13:12-4.

[6] Adams L, Lymp J, Sauver J, et al] (2005)The natural history of nonalcoholic fatty liver disease: A population-based cohort study] Gastroenterology 129:113-21.

[7] Caldwell SH, Oelsner DH, Iezzoni JC, Hespenheide EE, Battle EH, Driscoll CJ] (1999)Cryptogenic cirrhosis: Clinical characterization and risk factors for underlying disease] Hepatology 29:664-9.

[8] Bacon BR, Farahvash MJ, Janney CG, Neuschwander-Tetri BA.(1994) Nonalcoholic steatohepatitis: An expanded clinical entity] Gastroenterology 107:1103-9.

[9] Saadeh S, Younossi ZM, Remer EM, et al] (2002)The utility of radiological imaging in nonalcoholic fatty liver disease] Gastroenterology 123:745-50.

]10] Brunt EM, Janney CJ, Di Bisceglie AM, Neuschwander-Tetri BA, Bacon BR.(1999) Nonalcoholic steatohepatitis : A proposal for grading and staging the histology lesions] Am J Gastroenterol 94:2467-74.

[11] Marchesni G, Brizi M, Bianchi G, et al] (2001) Nonalcoholic fatty liver disease: A feature of the metabolic syndrome] Diabetes 50:1844-50.

]12] Angelico F, Del Ben M, Conti R, et al] Insulin resistance, the metabolic syndrome and nonalcoholic fatty liver disease] J Clin Endocrinol Metab 2005;90:1578-82.

[13] Scheen AJ, Luyckx FH.(2002) Obesity and liver disease] Best Pract Res Clin Endocrinol Metab 16:703-6.

[14] Harrison SA, Kadakia S, Lang KA, Schenker S.(2002) Nonalcoholic steatohepatitis: What we know in the new millennium] Am J Gastroenterol 97:2714-24.

[15] Festi D, Colecchia A, Sacco T, Bondi M, Roda E, Marchesini G.(2004) Hepatic steatosis in obese patients: Clinical aspects and prognostic significance] Obes Rev 5:27-42.

[16] Kejima K, Okumura K, Lang T, et al] (2005)The role of leptin in progression of nonalcoholic fatty liver disease] Hepatol Res 33:151-154.

[17] Sargin H, Sargin M, Gozu H, et al.(2005) Is adiponectin level a predictor of nonalcoholic fatty liver disease in nondiabetic male patients? World J Gastroenterol.11:5874-7.

[18] Chitturi S, Farrell GC] (2001)Etiopathogenesis of nonalcoholic steatohepatitis] Semin Liver Dis 21:27-41.

[19] Yeon J, Choi K, Baik S, et al.(2004) Reduced expression of peroxisome proliferators-activated receptor alpha may have an important role in the development of nonalcoholic fatty liver disease] J Gastr Hep 19:799-804.

]20] Sanyal AJ, Campbell-Sargent C, Mirshahi F, et al] (2001)Nonalcoholic steatohepatitis: Association of insulin resistance and mitochondrial abnormalities] Gastroenterology 120:1281-5.

[21] Cox KL, Burke V, Morton AR, Beilin LJ, Puddey IB.(2004) Independent and additive effects of energy restriction and exercise on glucose and insulin concentrations in sedentary overweight men] Am J Clin Nutr 80:308-16.

[22] Angulo P.(2003) Current best treatment for nonalcoholic fatty liver disease] Expert opin Pharmacother 4:611-23.

[23] Dansinger M, Gleason J, Griggith J, Selker H, Schaefer E.(2005) Comparison of the Atkins, Ornish, Weight Watchers, and Zone diets for weight loss and heart disease risk reduction] JAMA 93:43-53.

[24] Harrison S, Ramrakhiani S, Brunt E, Anbari M, Cortese C, Bacon B] (2003)Orlistat in the treatment of NASH: A case series] Am J Gastroenterol 98:926-30.

[25] Davidson MH, Hauptman J, DiGirolamo M, et al.(1999)Weight control and risk factor reduction in obese subjects treated for 2 years with orlistat: A randomized controlled trial] JAMA 281:235-42.

[26] Sabuncu T, Nazligul Y, Karaoglanoglu M, et al.(2003) The effects of sibutramine and orlistat on the ultrasonographic findings, insulin resistance and liver enzyme levels in obese patients with nonalcoholic steatohepatitis] Rom J Gastroenterol 12:189-92.

[27] Despres JP, Golay A, Sjostrom L et al.(2005) Effects of rimonabant on metabolic risk factors in overweight patients with dyslipidemia] N Engl J Med 353:2121-34.

[28] Centers for Disease Control and Prevention] Physical activity for everyone: Recommendations: How active do adults need to be to gain some benefit (2008) Physical Activity Guidelines for Americans] U.S] Department of Health and Human Services] 2010

[29] Caldwell SH, Hespenheide EE, Reddick JA, Iezzoni JC, Battle EH, Sheppard BL] (2001)A pilot study of a thiazolidinedione, troglitazone, in nonalcoholic steatohepatitis] Am J Gastroenterol 96:519-25.

[30] Neuschwander-Tetri BA, Brunt EM, Wehmeier KR, Oliver D, Bacon BR.(2003) Improved nonalcoholic steatohepatitis after 48 weeks of treatment with the PPAR-gamma ligand rosiglitazone] Hepatology 38:1008-17.

[31] Promrat K, Lutchman G, Uwaifo GI, et al.(2004) A pilot study of pioglitazone treatment for nonalcoholic steatohepatitis] Hepatology 39:188-96.

[32] Loguercico C, Federico A, Tuccillo, C, et al] (2005)Benefical effects of a probiotic VSL#3 on parameters of liver dysfunction in chronic liver diseases] J Clin Gastroenterol 39:540-3.

[33] Maggard MA, Shugarman LR, Suttorp M et al.(2005) Meta-analysis: Surgical treatment of obesity] Ann Intern Med 142:547-59.

[34] Mattar S, Velcu L, Rabinovitz M] Et al.(2005) Surgically-induced weight loss significantly improves nonalcoholic fatty liver disease and the metabolic syndrome] Ann Surg 242:610-7.

[35] Younossi Z.M.(2008) Current Management of Non-Alcoholic Fatty Liver Disease and Non-Alcoholic Steatohepatitis Alimentary Pharmacology & Therapeutics] 28(1):2-12]

[36] Guido L, Francesca R and Gianluca P(2008)Why Does NAFLD Predict Type 2 Diabetes? Current Diabetes Reports March 23m2011.DOI: 10.1007/s11892-011-0190-2

13

Disturbed Chylomicron Metabolism in Type 2 Diabetes - A Preventable Cause of Atherosclerosis?

Gerald H. Tomkin and Daphne Owens
Diabetes Institute of Ireland, Beacon, and Trinity College Dublin Ireland

1. Introduction

Diabetes remains a fascinating condition to observe and treat, at least for the authors. The rewards of observing patients who remain free of complications many, many years after diagnosis is however negated by seeing the terrible consequences of diabetic complications which occur, not only in patients who have had the disease for many years but also in those who are found to have the disease when they first present with complications. The evolution of diabetes care has been fueled by new pharmaceutical agents and the large trials that have followed demonstrating benefit. There have of course been occasional trials that have upset patients, diabetologists and people looking after diabetes as well as the pharmaceutical industry. An example early in my career as a diabetologist was the University Group diabetes program (UGDP) [1] which suggested harm rather than benefit from the sulphonylurea Tolbutamide and the biguanide Phenformin. The controversy which this trial caused was truly amazing involving the Supreme Court in the United States. Not many trials have been scrutinized by a national supreme court. A more recent example is the ACCORD study [2] which set out to examine the benefit of reducing blood sugar to below 6mmol/l. This study was stopped early because, although there was a reduction in myocardial infarction there was an increase in mortality. These trials have resulted in a magnificent increase in speculative literature and new consensus statements from lots of different bodies enthusiastic about giving advice through guidelines. The Annals of Internal Medicine is to be congratulated on publishing a paper written by Davidof "Music lessons; what Musicians can teach Doctors"[3]. The care of diabetes is certainly both an art and a science in 2011 and this article should re-enforce the diabetologist to be secure in practicing art as well as science in the management of diabetes.

Cardiovascular disease is unfortunately the major cause of death in patients with diabetes. For example in the San Antonia Heart Study Halfner et al [4] demonstrated the increased risk of cardiovascular mortality in patients with diabetes but without a previous MI was the same as that of non diabetic patients who already have had MI although another study disputed this [5]. A third prospective study in Finland demonstrated similar results to the San Antonia Study [6] and a metanalysis in 2009 confirmed this relationship [7]. Looking at the situation in a different way it has been shown that diabetic patients have a life expectancy 8-15 years less than non-diabetic people. Recently a prospective study of men aged 60 – 69 years followed up for 9 years was reported [8]. The authors found that only

men with early onset diabetes and a duration of 16.7 years showed cardiovascular risk similar to those with MI and no diabetes. Late onset diabetes was also associated with increase in coronary artery events and all cause mortality compared to non diabetic men who had no coronary heart disease (CHD), but the risk was less. Even more worryingly is the evidence that as blood sugar rises but is still within the pre-diabetes range the risk of cardiovascular disease increases [9-11]. Indeed the risk increase in percentage terms is greater in this group of patients than in those with diabetes.
Insulin resistance is a very early finding in the progression to diabetes and it has been suggested that abnormalities in fatty acid oxidation can be seen in close relatives of diabetic patients at an early age in adulthood [12,13] . A recent report from the Framingham Heart study has examined the effect of insulin resistance in subjects without diabetes. During a follow-up mean of 14 years the incidence of CHD was significantly greater in those with insulin resistance confirming previous studies that demonstrated that high insulin levels without hyperglycaemia was an important risk factor[14]. Hba1c has been shown to predict cardiovascular events and cardiovascular mortality independently of known cardiovascular disease [15-16]. These studies show a consistent and continuous relationship between glycaemia and cardiovascular risk even below diagnostic levels for diabetes. Chanman et al [17] have recently looked at non diabetic hyperglycaemia and cardiovascular risk and have demonstrated that in people with non-diabetic hyperglycaemia cardiovascular risk is highly dependent on the presence of other cardiovascular risk factors such as dyslipidaemia. These results are in keeping with the difficulty in demonstrating that lowering blood sugar improves cardiovascular outcome. There are of course some studies that show this ie Diabetes Control and complications/ Epidemiology of Diabetes Interventions and Complications (DCCT/EDIC) and UK Prospective Diabetes Study (UKPDS) follow-up [18.19]. However the original UKPDS did not show a significant effect on cardiovascular mortality [20]. A recent report from the FRENA registry [21] has shown in secondary prevention that patients with diabetes and HbA1c < 7% had a lower incidence of subsequent ischaemia and a lower mortality than those with HbA1c > 7%. These differences appeared only in patients with coronary artery disease (CAD). In this study more than 900 patients with type 2 diabetes were followed up over a mean period of 14 months [2, 21]. In the intensive care unit setting there was great excitement when studies showed that there was benefit from meticulous control of blood sugar but many studies since then have not confirmed these findings with regards to cardiovascular mortality [22,23].

2. Atherosclerosis in diabetes

Diabetes has been defined as an absolute or relative lack of insulin and it is therefore reasonable to consider the action of insulin and to recognize that deficiency in insulin does not lead only to hyperglycaemia but also to disturbance in fat and protein metabolism. Atherosclerosis is a condition of cholesterol and fat deposition in a vulnerable endothelium surface of an artery. It is not surprising therefore that attention has shifted, admittedly very slowly from the concept of dysglycaemia to dyslipidaemia for the cause of atherosclerosis in diabetes. Inspiration has come from the work of Shafrir and Guttman [24] who in 1965 demonstrated the relationship between free fatty acids and blood sugar. They divided into quartiles, people ranging from normal blood sugar to impaired glucose tolerance. They demonstrated that non-suppression of free fatty acids occurred as the blood sugars rose even in the normoglycaemic range. In a thought provoking review many years later Shafrir and Raz [25] made the suggestion and gave strong evidence to support the suggestion that Diabetes Mellitus should be renamed "Diabetes Lipidus".

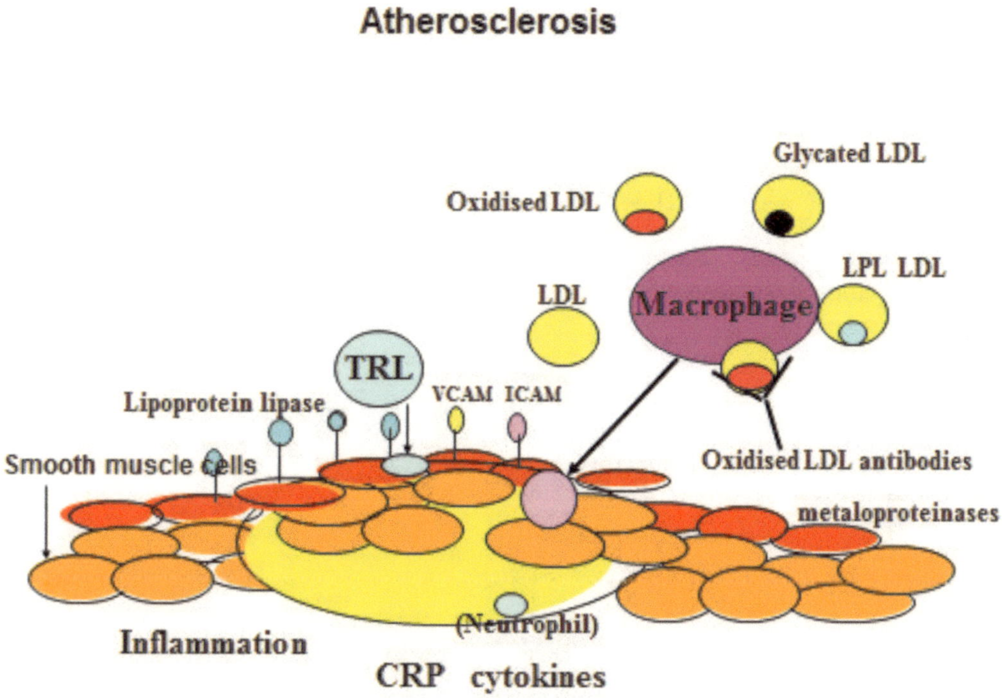

Fig. 1. LDL may become modified by oxidation, and glycation. The macrophage takes up modified LDL and enters the subendothelial space where it becomes a cholesterol laden foam cell. Macrophage uptake is facilitated by cytokines and chemotactic factors such as VCAM and ICAM. Uptake of cholesterol from triglyceride-rich lipoproteins is facilitated by lipoprotein lipase on the endothelial cell surface. Smooth muscle cells protect the plaque from rupture through metalloprotinases and thrombus formation.

Poorly controlled diabetes is usually associated with hypertriglyceridaemia which very often responds to hypoglycaemic therapy and normalization of blood sugars. The non-suppression of free fatty acids (FFA) results in excess free fatty acids reaching the liver from adipose tissue which in turn leads to an increase in very low density lipoprotein (VLDL) secretion in the postprandial phase. The cellular concentration of non esterified fatty acids (NEFA) is tightly controlled by the balance between triglyceride hydrolysis and NEFA esterification [26-28]. The hydrolysis of the primary and secondary ester bonds between long chain fatty acids and the glycerol backbone in triglyceride is called lypolysis and depends on specific hydrolases commonly designated lipases. Adipose triglyceride lipase (ATGL) selectively performs the first and rate limiting triacylglyceride hydrolysis to form diacylglycerol and NEFA [29, 30]. Hormone sensitive lipase hydrolyses tri-, di- and monoacylglycerol [31]. Monoglyceride lipase efficiently cleaves monoglycerols into glycerol and NEFAs. Thus lipoprotein lipase, together with adipose triglyceride lipase, hormone sensitive lipase and hepatic lipase are all involved in the storage and release of FFA and are all involved in the metabolism of the triglyceride-rich lipoproteins and the suppression of fatty acids within the adipocyte. Insulin has a direct effect in inhibition of hormone sensitive lipase and ATGL which releases fatty acids from the adipocyte and stimulates lipoprotein lipase which is involved in the delipidation of the triglyceride-rich lipoproteins necessary for lipoprotein clearance and FFA storage in the adipocyte. For review see Lass et al 2011 [32]. NEFA metabolism strongly effects glucose utilization and insulin resistance. ATGL affects glucose metabolism by different mechanisms and in a tissue specific manor ie measures of insulin signaling are increased in skeletal muscle and white adipose tissue but decreased in brown adipose tissue [33]. In pancreatic islets ATGL deficiency causes triglyceride accumulation and impairs fuel and non fuel stimulated insulin secretion suggesting that ATGL is required for the provision of NEFAs as energy source in the process of insulin secretion.

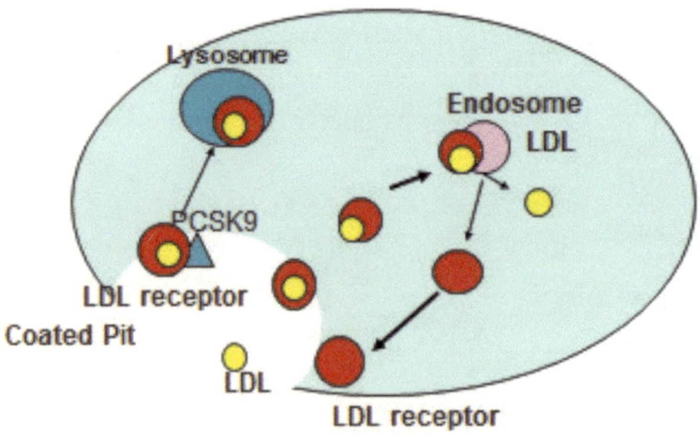

Fig. 2. LDL is cleared from the plasma by uptake by the apo B/E receptor in coated pits on the cell surface. The receptor is internalised and transported to the endosome where LDL is degraded and the cholesterol released. The receptor is normally recycled to the cell surface. PCSK9 is secreted into the pasma and binds to the LDL receptor inhibiting recycling of the receptor. Statins work by upregulating the LDL receptor and facilitating LDL clearance but they also upregulate PCSK9.

Cholesterol as a risk factor for atherosclerosis is so well documented that further confirmation seems unnecessary. The safety and efficacy of lowering cholesterol is also well established [34]. Long term prospective studies such as Framingham laid the foundations but examination of monogenetic hypercholesterolaemia, whether it be from apo B polymorphisms, the low density lipoprotein (LDL) receptor or the recent pro-protein convertase subtilism-like/kexin type 9 (PCSK 9) already had made the association between hypercholesterolaemia and atherosclerosis. PCSK9 is of particular interest since there are both loss of function and gain of function gene polymorphisms. In 2003 Abifidel et al [35] reported 23 families with autosomal dominant hypercholesterolaemia and premature CHD caused by missense mutations of PCSK9. Haughton et al in 2007 [36] demonstrated that over expression of PCSK9 in livers of mice reduced hepatic LDL receptor protein causing hyperchlesterolaemia suggesting that the mis sense mutations caused a gain of function to the mutant protein. They also showed that inactivation of PCSK9 resulted in hypocholesterolaemia. Loss of function mutations have also been identified in patients with hypocholesterolaemia. What is particularly interesting is that the reduction in cholesterol with these loss of function mutations is associated with much less coronary artery disease than would be expected with a similar reduction in cholesterol using statins. An explanation has been that the miss-sense mutation has been there since birth whereas statins are only used in middle age [37]. Statin therapy in heterozygous patients with this polymorphism has a much greater effect than would be associated with statins alone and these findings have been used to promote the idea that early statin use would increase benefit [37]. Statins upregulate sterol regulatory element binding protein (SREBP) which upregulates the LDL receptor but also causes a 45% increase in PCSK9 and a 70% increase when ezetimibe is added to the statin [38]. This is probably through regulation by SREBP thus development of cholesterol lowering drugs which do not increase PCSK9 would be very advantageous [39]. PCSK9 promotes LDL uptake by the LDL receptor but reduces the number of LDL receptors. Exciting animal studies suggest that inhibitors of PCSK9 may prove to be a powerful tool in cholesterol lowering particularly in conjunction with statins [40]. The Sammomys obesus (sand rat) has been very successfully used as a nutritionally-induced type 2 diabetes model [41]. Levy et al [42] investigated intestinal PCSK9 protein in this model and found that the protein was diminished and LDL receptor was raised in the diabetic compared to non-diabetic Sammomys. To investigate whether PCSK9 expression in diabetic patients played a part in diabetic dyslipidaemia, Brouwers et al [43] in the CODAM study measured PCSK9 in subjects with normal glucose metabolism with impaired glucose metabolism and type 2 diabetes. They found no difference in plasma PCSK9 between the 3 groups. Their study did suggest that the presence of type 2 diabetes may modify the relationship between plasma PCSK9 non-HDL cholesterol and apo B.

Early studies with statins such as the 4S study, demonstrated that diabetic patients responded better if anything than non-diabetic patients to statin therapy [44]. Other studies such as the Heart Protection Study [45.46] suggested that the response was similar in diabetic and non-diabetic patients. The role of hypertriglyceridaemia as a risk factor is less secure, perhaps because of the very strong inverse relationship between HDL cholesterol and the strong evidence that HDL protects against MI through various pathway [47]. Four years ago 2 important large studies demonstrated convincing evidence of the association between hypertriglyceridaemia and cardiovascular disease [48, 49]. Both these studies suggested that postprandial triglycerides are effective in predicting cardiovascular risk which fits in well with the concept of the atherogenicity of postprandial lipoproteins as will be discussed later. A recent examination of the diabetic patients in the Dutch and Potsdam contributions to the European Investigation into Cancer and Nutrition[50,51] was reported. The aims of the study were to examine the effects of postprandial time on the association and predictive value of non-fasting lipid levels and cardiovascular disease risk in participants with cardiovascular disease and diabetes. More than 1300 participants with diabetes at baseline were analysed. A cut off time between the groups of 3 hours was used in the assessment of cardiovascular risk prediction. The authors concluded that postprandial time did not influence the association of lipid concentrations with CVD in patients with diabetes nor did it effect a prediction of CVD risk [52]. The dramatic effects of cholesterol reduction with statins in reducing cardiovascular events has not been replicated using drugs such as fibrates which lower triglycerides although studies such as the DIAS study [53] did show significant lack of progression of coronary artery atherosclerosis using fenofibrate and the FIELD study [54] did show a significant reduction in the composit of CVD death, MI, stroke and coronary or carotid revascularization, even though many patients in that study had statins added to the treatment during that study and only 21% of patients enrolled had mixed dyslipidaemia, thus limiting its power. Also the Field Study [54] chose patients who did not have very elevated triglyceride levels which was anther problem with the study. A recent metanalysis systematically searched trials published between 1950 and 2010 and found that fibrates produced a 10% relative risk reduction for major cardiovascular events and a 13% relative risk reduction for coronary events ($p<0.001$) but had no effect on all risk or cardiovascular mortality[55]. Supporting the concept that fibrates may show more benefit in patients with hypertriglyceridaemia, Scott et al [56] on behalf of the Field Study Investigators explored whether the effect of fenofibrate on cardiovascular risk differed in subjects with and without metabolic syndrome. There were more than 9000 individuals with diabetes and components of the metabolic syndrome. They observed that the largest effect of fenofibrate on CVD risk was in patients with marked hypertriglyceridaemia (triglyceride >2.3) in whom a 27% risk reduction was observed with or without a low HDL cholesterol. From the above it becomes clear that diabetes is associated with an increased risk of atherosclerosis which can in part be reduced by either lowering LDL cholesterol or triglycerides.

3. The chylomicron in diabetes

The food we eat (quantity and quality) is responsible for the variation in an individuals lipoprotein profile accepting that the variation may be modified by exercise. This regulation is considerably disturbed in diabetes. It is important to recognize the role of the triglyceride-rich lipoproteins and in particular the chylomicron in modulating both VLDL and LDL quantity and composition [57]. High density lipoprotein (HDL) is also intimately linked to the triglyceride rich lipoproteins with a strong inverse correlation. Thus the chylomicron assumes dominance over all other lipoproteins particularly in diabetes and makes the study of chylomicron metabolism exciting and of major importance in the pathophysiology of diabetes, dyslipidaemia and atherosclerosis.

The chylomicron is defined by apolipoprotein (apo) B48 its solubilising protein. Many studies have shown an increase in the apo B48-containing lipoproteins both in the postprandial and fasting state in diabetes [58]. Originally it was thought that the problem was in clearance of the particles due to a relative lack of insulin which led to a reduction in lipoprotein lipase activity, slowing of lipolysis of the particle and delayed clearance by the liver. We demonstrated in an animal model of diabetes that chylomicron synthesis was also abnormal and confirmed that because of altered composition of the particle clearance was delayed perhaps due to insufficient apo E on the particle [59]. The regulation of chylomicron synthesis in the intestine is dependent on the amount of cholesterol that is available in the diet but chylomicron cholesterol also comes from the enterohepatic secretion of bile and the cholesterol that is excreted from the liver via this route as well as de novo cholesterol synthesis. The intestine is responsible for up to 25% of the cholesterol synthesized in the body. As an interesting aside at this stage it is useful to consider that people have been categorised into high and low absorbers of cholesterol and that cholesterol absorption is inversely related to cholesterol synthesis. As expected the high absorbers do less well on statin therapy but better on inhibition of cholesterol absorption by Ezetimibe, a drug that inhibits cholesterol absorption, compared to the people who are low absorbers of cholesterol. In the Framingham offspring study those patients with lower synthesis and higher absorption markers were more likely to develop cardiovascular disease [60,61]. These studies were confirmed by Silbernagel et al [62]. In 2440 participants of the LURIC study they found a modest association of high cholesterol absorption and low cholesterol synthesis with an increased severity of CAD. However Lakoskiet al [63] tested the hypothesis that individuals with high fractional absorption of cholesterol respond better to the cholesterol absorption inhibitor Ezetimibe than to simvastatin and visa versa. They did not find that baseline cholesterol absorption and synthesis predicted responsiveness to the above drugs rather they found that responsiveness to the two drugs was highly correlated. They suggest that factors downstream of the primary sites of action of these drugs are a major determinant of the response. In a subgroup analysis of the Scandinavian Simvastatin Survival Study (4S), Miettinen et al [64] showed that the baseline blood glucose level is related positively to cholesterol synthesis and negatively to that of absorption. Despite a marked glucose-related decrease in cholesterol synthesis with simvastatin, serum cholesterol reduction was not dependent on the baseline glucose level.

The discovery of Niemann Pick C1-like1(NPC1-L1) is an interesting story. The search for an explanation as to how cholesterol in the body is so finely regulated has been intensive. The finely tuned regulation of cholesterol was perhaps best illustrated by the report of the elderly gentleman who ate 25 eggs a day for many years but his cholesterol remained at just above 6mmol/l [65]. Altman and Davis in their search for molecules that might inhibit cholesterol absorption discovered by chance a compound which is now known as ezetimibe [66]. They discovered a putative gene, the NPC1L1. Elegant studies in mice demonstrated that knocking out this gene reduced cholesterol absorption by the same amount as happened when the wild mice were fed with ezetimibe. They showed that there was no further reduction in cholesterol absorption in the knockout mice when fed ezetimibe. The group went on to show that lack of Npc1L1 in apoE-/- mice results in a significant reduction in cholesterol absorption and plasma cholesterol levels, and causes nearly complete protection from the development of atherosclerosis, under both cholesterol-fed and non-cholesterol-fed conditions [67, 68]. Statins, which inhibit 3 Hydroxy 3 methylglutaryl co enzyme A (HMGCoA) reductase and cholesterol synthesis, have been shown to increase cholesterol absorption. It has also been shown that low absorbers of cholesterol respond better to statins than high absorbers. Ezetimibe potentiates the effect of statins, increasing their effectiveness by another 15 - 20% in relation to cholesterol lowering. Trembly et al [69] this year reported an increase in NPC1L1 by 19% in the small intestine in subjects on atorvastatin thus describing a mechanism whereby cholesterol absorption is increased in patients on statins. In animal studies we have demonstrated an increase in cholesterol absorption in diabetes [70] We asked the question as to whether diabetes might be associated with an increase in cholesterol absorption through stimulation of NPC1-L1. We demonstrated in animal models of diabetes that NPC1L1 was up-regulated [71] and in diabetic patients and we demonstrated an increase in mRNA [72] suggesting a mechanism for an increase in cholesterol absorption. In the Sammomas Obesus model of type 2 diabetes, the animals exhibiting weight gain, hyperinsulinaemia and hypercholesterolaemia, NPC1-L1 protein and gene expression were both significantly reduced in the intestine and the authors found a lower capacity to absorb cholesterol compared to controls [73,]. This may suggest interspecies variation but it is a surprising finding considering that this animal model of diabetes has been shown to have increased production of intestinal lipoprotein-containing apo B48 [74].

The mechanism whereby the body is almost completely unable to absorb plant sterols was a mystery until recently. Study of the familial condition, sitosterolaemia, unlocked the mystery [75]. Sitosterolaemia is a rare condition associated with early and severe atherosclerosis. The condition is associated with normal or slightly elevated cholesterol whereas total sterols are markedly increased. Search for polymorphisms in putative genes controlling plant sterol absorption or perhaps one should say blocking plant sterol absorption, identified ATP binding cassette proteins (ABC)G5 and G8 in the intestine [76]. Further work demonstrated that these two gene products work in tandem to re-excrete both plant sterols virtually completely and cholesterol to a lesser extent in a regulated way [77]. The genes were also found to be expressed in the liver where they are responsible for controlling cholesterol re-excretion into the bile [75-77]. It appears that these two genes are very important regulators of cholesterol and together with NPC1-L1 protein are responsible for cholesterol homeostasasis in the body. Polymorphisms of the ABCG5/G8 have not only been associated with increased serum sitosterol but also with increase in cholesterol. It has also been shown that polymorphisms in the ABCG5/G8 may influence cholesterol in weight reduction programs (the Q604E SNP in ABCG5 and the C54Y in ABC8) [78,79]. Gylling et al [80] examined polymorphisms in the ABCG5 and G8 genes and found that low serum cholesterol and cholesterol absorption were linked to a polymorphism (D19H) of the ABCG8 gene and characteristics of the insulin resistance syndrome in men was linked to Q604E polymorphism in the ABCG5 gene. The authors studied 263 mildly hypercholesterolaemic non-coronary subjects using colestanol to cholesterol ratio as a surrogate marker of cholesterol absorption efficiency. Since diabetes is so frequently associated with dyslipidaemia the ABCs became a target for research. Blocks et al [81] examined mRNA and protein expression of ABCG5 and G8 in the intestine of streptozotosin rats and found significant reduction in expression of both ABCG5 and G8. They found that levels were partially normalised on insulin supplementation. We have shown that ABCG5 and G8 were reduced by more than 50% in the intestine of zucker diabetic fa/fa rats compared with lean rats although this did not reach statistical significance [82]. Insulin treatment caused a non-significant increase in ABCG5 and G8 mRNA. In streptozotosin diabetic rats ABCG5 and G8 were both very significantly reduced in the intestine [83]. There was a negative correlation between both ABCG5 and G8 and chylomicron cholesterol [83]. In the Psamonas Obesus Levy et al [73,74] showed a reduction in ABC G5/G8 in the intestine. In the intestine of human subjects with type 2 diabetes, ABCG5 and G8 mRNA were both significantly lower compared to controls [71]. There was a negative correlation between ABCG5 and G8 and NCP1-L1 in the combined diabetic and control subjects [71]. There was a significant negative correlation between chylomicron cholesterol and both ABCG5 and G8 [71]. These two genes appear to play an important role in the dysregulation of cholesterol metabolism in diabetes

4. Microsomal triglyceride transfer protein

Intestinal microsomal triglyceride transfer protein (MTP) plays a major role in the assembly of the chylomicron particle and therefore of cholesterol and triglyceride metabolism. Intestinal MTP has become a hot topic since new inhibitors of intestinal MTP have been shown to lower triglyceride without causing hepatic steatosis at least in animal studies [84,85]. Although many polymorphisms of MTP have been described, some of which have considerable impact on LDL cholesterol in both non-diabetic and diabetic subjects [86,87], it is difficult to know whether the results mainly stemmed from the effect in the liver rather than the intestine. The intestinal inhibitors of MTP which have no effect on the liver, should answer this question in the future. In animal studies diabetes is associated with an increase in MTP mRNA with close correlation between MTP mRNA and chylomicron cholesterol[81,88-90]. In the rabbit increased MTP mRNA is associated with increase in chylomicron particle numbers [88] but in the rat it is associated with larger particles [89]. The fructose-fed insulin resistant hamster model, has an increase in MTP protein mass and this was associated with an increase in the triglyceride-rich intestinally derived lipoproteins [91]. Zolotowska et al [92] in 2003 examined the B48 containing lipoprotein assembly in the small intestine of *psamnonys obesus*, a model of nutritionally-induced diabetes and insulin resistance. De novo triglyceride synthesis, apo B48 biogenesis and triglyceride-rich lipoprotein assembly were all increased. MTP activity and protein expression however, were not altered. In the enterocyte of fructose fed golden hamster MTP mRNA and protein mass were increased by tumour necrosis factor(TNF)α but apo B levels in the enterocyte were not effected suggesting that there is considerable inter species variation [91]. In human studies in type 2 diabetes we demonstrated an increase in MTP mRNA in intestinal biopsies [71,90]. Diabetic patients who were on statin therapy had lower MTP mRNA compared to those not on statins [86,]. We found positive correlations between MTP mRNA and chylomicron fraction cholesterol and apo B48 [86]

5. Chylomicron and atherosclerosis

The circulating chylomicron has been the poor relation of the lipoproteins, at least until recently. There are many reasons for this ie post postprandial lipoprotein measurement is difficult to standardise. The amount of cholesterol that the chylomicron contains is very much less than that of the LDL particle and the statins have demonstrated such resounding success in reducing cholesterol and lowering cardiovascular risk. Those of us who champion the chylomicron as the most important lipoprotein do so in part because the number of chylomicrons, far exceeds that of LDL particles. Chylomicrons in fact carry as much cholesterol as LDL particularly in high cholesterol absorbers. They have a turnover in minutes whereas LDL has a half life of about 4 days. The lipoproteins are a transport mechanism for cholesterol and fat thus the shorter the half life the more the carrying power. The atherogenicity of the chylomicron particle depends on its ability to deliver cholesterol to the atherosclerotic plaque and studies both in animals and humans have demonstrated that indeed apo B48 is found in plaque demonstrating that the chylomicron can enter the endothelial space. The macrophage has a specific apo E receptor which enhances the uptake of the chylomicron particle. The composition of the chylomicron particle in diabetes has been difficult to define because separation of apo B48 particles from apo B100 particles is cumbersome. Using a monoclonal antibody against apo B48, Yoshimura et al [92] examined type 2 diabetic patients and non-diabetic patients. Although the separation of apo B48 from B100 was not complete the apo B48 containing chylomicrons had a higher content of triglyceride but there was no difference between those with diabetes and those without diabetes. They further confirmed a B48 receptor in TPH-1 cells (a human acute monocytic leukaemia cell line) and also in Hep G2 cells. The inflammatory process is at the centre of the atherosclerotic lesion. Chylomicron remnants induce macrophage foam cell formation [93,94]. The fatty acid composition of chylomicron remnants markedly influences the formation of macrophage foam cells. The group from the Royal Veterinary College in London has shown that enrichment with saturated fatty acids causes the remnants to be

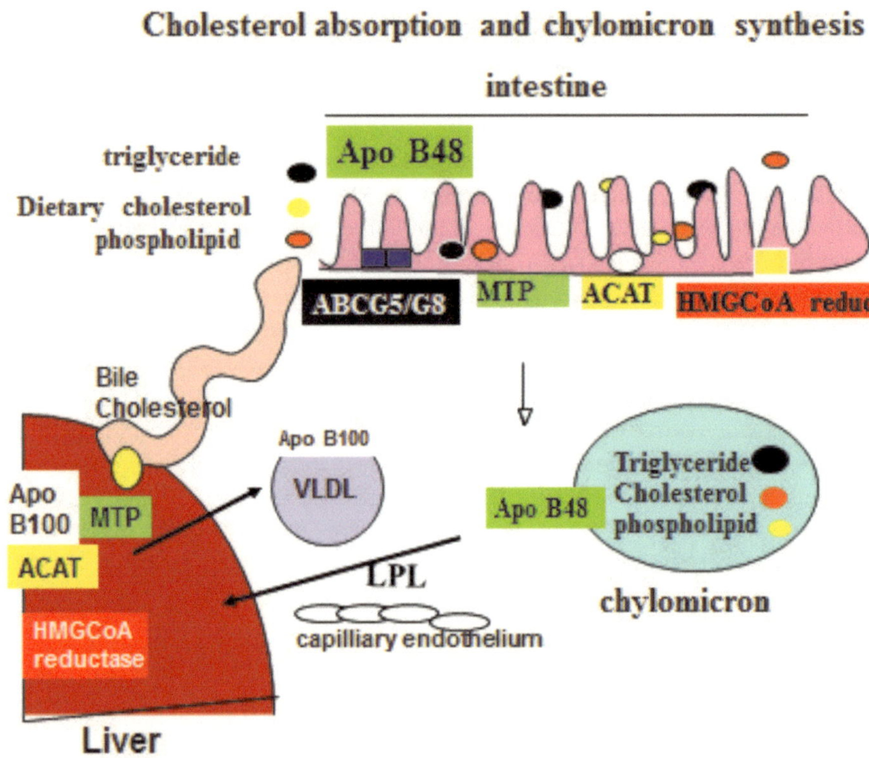

Fig. 3. The chylomicron is formed from dietary cholesterol, triglyceride, and phospholipid together with endogenously synthesised cholesterol for which HMGCoA reductase is the rate-limiting enzyme, and Some of the cholesterol is esterified by the enzyme ACAT. Intestinal cholesterol absorption is facilitated by NPC1L1 and opposed by ABCG5/G8. Intestinally produced apo B48 is the structural protein for the chylomicron and the particle is assembled under the influence of MTP. Most of the chylomicron triglyceride is hydrolised by lipoprotein lipase in the capiliaries prior to uptake of the particle by the liver where it is broken down and reassembled together with apo B100, again under the influence of MTP, and released as VLDL into the circulation.

taken up more quickly and cause greater cholesterol accumulation than those enriched with polyunsaturated fatty acids or monounsaturated fatty acids [95]. They further showed that the inflammatory process and the activity of nuclear factor-kB (NF-kB can be diminished if the Chylomicron remnants are enriched with polyunsaturated fatty acids [96]. This group had previously shown that oxidation of chylomicron remnants delayed uptake by the macrophage CD36 receptor in contrast to LDL where oxidation increases uptake in macrophages. The authors however do make the point that the CD36 receptor and phagocytosis play only a minor role in foam cell formation. The main uptake and internalisation being through the LDL receptor related protein (LRP) and the LDL receptor [97]. GLP-1-like agonists are now being widely used in the treatment of diabetes and have a beneficial effect on glycaemia and also lipidaemia [98]. Xiao et al 2011 [99] have recently shown in healthy men that glucagon acutely regulates hepatic but not intestinal lipoprotein metabolism both by decreasing lipoprotein particle production and inhibiting particle clearance. The classic diabetes fasting lipid indices of elevated LDL cholesterol, high triglyceride and low HDL in those with type 1 diabetes is often missing even if they have atherosclerosis[100]. However when adolescents with diabetes are compared to their non-diabetic siblings they have been shown to have higher triglycerides. LDL and lower HDL [101]. The SEARCH for diabetes in youth study (SEARCH) showed similar findings [102]. Guy [103] in a cross sectional study of 512 youths with type 1 diabetes mean duration 4.2 years and 188 healthy control subjects they found that those with HbA1c in the optimal range (<7.5%) were similar to controls whereas the poorly controlled subjects had raised total cholesterol, LDL cholesterol and non-HDL cholesterol together with significantly elevated apo B and more small dense LDL particles. The authors conclude that poor glycaemic control is an important mediator of abnormal lipoproteins. Very recently Mangat et al [104] examined the chylomicron in subjects with type 1 diabetes thus extending our knowledge of postprandial lipoprotein metabolism in diabetes. Just like in type 2 diabetes [105-107], Mangat et al show significantly higher concentrations both of fasting apo B48 and a total plasma apo B48 following a sequential meal challenge, than control subjects demonstrating impaired metabolism of chylomicron remnants. Interestingly they also demonstrated arterial retention of remnants ex vivo in type 1 diabetic rats and showed that remnants bound with significant affinity to human biglycan in vivo. They also showed a further 2.3 fold increased binding capacity when they used glycated biglycan.

6. Chylomicron turnover in diabetes

The chylomicron is mostly cleared by the liver through the B/E and LDL related protein (LRP) receptors. There is prolonged clearance in diabetes as shown by the length of time apo B48 remains in the circulation following a meal [105-107]. This is related both to compositional abnormalities in the chylomicron and to delay in lipolysis. As stated earlier apo E appears to be deficient on the particle [59]. Perhaps more importantly delipidation of the particle is abnormal. Lipoprotein lipase is an insulin dependent enzyme and in clinical practice treatment that normalises blood sugar is always associated with a reduction in triglyceride. The importance of the postprandial period in triglyceride metabolism and particularly in chylomicron metabolism is often overlooked with reliance on fasting blood sugar as being an indication of good diabetic control. The evidence that the postprandial blood sugar is a better indicator of cardiovascular risk than fasting blood sugar and the close relationship between hyperglycaemia and hypertriglyceridaemia suggests that normalisation of both blood sugar and triglycerides would reduce the atherosclerotic burden Cereillo [108]. Interest is growing in measurement and treatment of the postprandial phase but it is very demanding on both patient and physician. The increase in chylomicronaemia postprandially has a major impact on VLDL composition since the large triglyceride-rich lipoproteins generate small dense LDL [109 110]. Small dense LDL has been shown to be more easily oxidised and therefore has a greater capacity to be taken up by the macrophage. Small dense LDL is more common in diabetes. Many years ago the Scottish group were unable to show much in the way of a relationship between small dense LDL and atherosclerosis in diabetes [111] but more recently in a small study it has been reported LDL size was the stongest marker for clinically apparent as well as non apparent atherosclerosis In Type 2 diabetes [112]. Inhibition of cholesterol absorption with Ezetimibe improves the quality of VLDL, IDL and LDL by significantly reducing the triglyceride/cholesterol ratio in these lipoproteins [113] demonstrating the relationship between the chylomicron and the other apo B containing lipoproteins.

7. High density lipoprotein

The intimate inverse relationship between triglyceride-rich lipoproteins and HDL is well known and is particularly common in diabetes. The reason why this inverse correlation is so strong is due to the importance of apo A1 and apo E in the formation of HDL. Catabolism of the triglyceride-rich lipoproteins is necessary for the release of apo A1 and apo E, both intestinally and hepatically derived. The delayed catabolism of the triglyceride-rich lipoproteins in diabetes leads to a deficiency of apo A1 and apo E necessary for the formation of the nacent HDL particle with its specific detergent-like properties that can solublise vesicular phospholipid to create discoidal HDL particles [114]. Lipoprotein metabolism starting with the large chylomicron and ending with the small HDL particles is a closely interwoven dynamic milieu designed in times when food was in short supply. It is not surprising that disturbance of this intricate pathway occurs with over feeding or in diabetes when a lack of insulin relative or absolute disturbs energy metabolism.

8. Conclusion

The chylomicron is a major cholesterol carrying particle due to the large amount of chylomicrons produced postprandially. Chylomicron cholesterol is delivered to the atherosclerotic plaque and induces foam cell formation. Chylomicron clearance is delayed in diabetes but synthesis is also increased in diabetes. The other important cause of atherosclerosis in diabetes relates to the lipoprotein cascade, increased chylomicron production and decreased clearance leads to an atherogenic LDL (both small dense LDL and an LDL with an increase in esterified cholesterol) leading to increased oxidisability of the particle. Finally the increase in triglyceride-rich lipoproteins results in low HDL, an important atherosclerosis risk factor. Normalisation of the dyslipidaemia of diabetes and in particular chylomicronaemia should be a major goal in the prevention of the increased atherosclerosis found in diabetes

9. References

[1] Prout TE University Group Diabetes Program.. A progress report on the Int J Clin Pharmacol Biopharm. 1975;12:244-51.

[2] Action to Control Cardiovascular Risk in Diabetes Study Group, Gerstein HC, Miller ME, Byington RP, Goff DC Jr, Bigger JT, Buse JB, Cushman WC, Genuth S, Ismail-Beigi F, Grimm RH Jr, Probstfield JL, Simons-Morton DG, Friedewald WT. Effects of intensive glucose lowering in type 2 diabetes. N Engl J Med. 2008;12;358:2545-59.

[3] Davidoff F.Music Lessons: What Musicians Can Teach Doctors (and Other Health Professionals). Ann Intern Med. 2011;154:426-9.

[4] Haffner SM, Lehto S, Rönnemaa T, Pyörälä K, Laakso M. Mortality from coronary heart disease in subjects with type 2 diabetes and in nondiabetic subjects with and without prior myocardial infarction. N Engl J Med. 1998;339:229-34

[5] Evans JM, Wang J, Morris AD: Comparison of cardiovascular risk between patients with type 2 diabetes and those who had had a myocardial infarction: cross sectional and cohort studies. BMJ 324 : 939 –942,2002

[6] Juutilainen A, Lehto S, Rönnemaa T, Pyörälä K, Laakso M. Type 2 diabetes as a "coronary heart disease equivalent": an 18-year prospective population-based study in Finnish subjects. Diabetes Care. 2005;28:2901-7

[7] Bulugahapitiya U, Siyambalapitiya S, Sithole J, Idris I. Is diabetes a coronary risk equivalent? Systematic review and meta-analysis. Diabet Med. 2009;26:142-8.

[8] Wannamethee SG, Shaper AG, Whincup PH, Lennon L, Sattar N Impact of diabetes on cardiovascular disease risk and all-cause mortality in older men: influence of age at onset, diabetes duration, and established and novel risk factors. Arch Intern Med. 2011 14;171:404-10.

[9] Tominaga M, Equchi H, Manaka H, Igarashi K, Kato T, Sekikawa A: Impaired glucose tolerance is a risk factor for cardiovascular disease, but not impaired fasting glucose: the Funagata Diabetes Study. Diabetes Care 22:920–924,

[10] Meigs JB, Nathan DM, Wilson PW, Cupples LA, Singer DE: Metabolic risk factors worsen continuously across the spectrum of nondiabetic glucose tolerance: the Framingham Offspring Study. Ann Intern Med 1998;128: 524– 533

[11] The DECODE study group. European Diabetes Epidemiology Group. Diabetes Epidemiology: Collaborative analysis of Diagnostic criteria in Europe Glucose tolerance and mortality: comparison of WHO and American Diabetes Association diagnostic criteria.. Lancet 1999;354:617–621

[12] Lowell BB. Shulman GL Mitocondrial dysfunction in type 2 diabetes Science 2005; 307;384-387

[13] Weiss R, Dufour S, Taksali SE, Tamborlane WV, Petersen KF, Bonadonna RC, Boselli L, Barbetta G, Allen K, Rife F, Savoye M, Dziura J, Sherwin R, Shulman GI, Caprio S. Prediabetes in obese youth: a syndrome of impaired glucose tolerance, severe insulin resistance, and altered myocellular and abdominal fat partitioning. Lancet.2003;362;951-7

[14] Robins SJ, Lyass A, Zachariah JP, Massaro JM, Vasan RS. Insulin Resistance and the Relationship of a Dyslipidemia to Coronary Heart Disease: The Framingham Heart Study. Arterioscler Thromb Vasc Biol. 2011 Feb 10. [Epub ahead of print]PMID: 21311041

[15] Khaw KT, Wareham N, Bingham S, Luben R, Welch A, Day N. Association of hemoglobin A1c with cardiovascular disease and mortality in adults: the European Prospective Investigation into Cancer in Norfolk. Ann Intern Med. 2004;141:413-20

[16] Selvin E, Marinopoulos S, Berkenblit G, Rami T, Brancati FL, Powe NR, Golden SH. Meta-analysis: glycosylated hemoglobin and cardiovascular disease in diabetes mellitus. Ann Intern Med. 2004 ;141:421-31

[17] Chamnan P, Simmons RK, Jackson R, Khaw KT, Wareham NJ, Griffin SJ Non-diabetic hyperglycaemia and cardiovascular risk: moving beyond categorisation to individual interpretation of absolute risk. Diabetologia. 2011 ;54:291-9.

[18] Polak JF, Backlund JY, Cleary PA, Harrington AP, O'Leary DH, Lachin JM, Nathan DM; DCCT/EDIC Research Group.Progression of carotid artery intima-media thickness during 12 years in the Diabetes Control and Complications Trial/Epidemiology of Diabetes Interventions and Complications (DCCT/EDIC) study.Diabetes. 2011;60:607-13

[19] Rury R. Holman RR, Sanjoy KP,. Bethel AB, Matthews DR, Neil HAW, 10-Year Follow-up of Intensive Glucose Control in Type 2 Diabetes N Engl J Med 2008; 359:1577-1589

[20] UK Prospective Diabetes Study (UKPDS) Group Intensive blood-glucose control with sulphonylureas or insulin compared with conventional treatment and risk of complications in patients with type 2 diabetes (UKPDS 33). *Lancet.* 1998;352;837–853.

[21] Camafort M, Alvarez-Rodríguez LR, Muñoz-Torrero JF, Sahuquillo JC, López-Jiménez L, Coll R, Monreal M; FRENA Investigators Glucose control and outcome in patients with stable diabetes and previous coronary, cerebrovascular or peripheral artery disease. Findings from the FRENA Registry.Diabet Med. 2011;28:73-80..

[22] van den Berghe G, Wouters P, Weekers F, Verwaest C, Bruyninckx F, Schetz M, Vlasselaers D, Ferdinande P, Lauwers P, Bouillon R. Intensive insulin therapy in the critically ill patients. N Engl J Med. 2001;345:1359-67.

[23] Kavanagh BP, McCowen KC Glycemic control in the ICU. N Engl J Med. 2010 ;363:2540-6. Review.

[24] Shafrir E, Gutman A. Patterns of decrease of free fatty acids during glucoose tolerence tests Diabetes.1965;14:77-83.

[25] Shafrir E, Raz I. Diabetes: mellitus or lipidus? Diabetologia. 2003;46:433-40.

[26] Haemmerle G, Lass A, Zimmermann R, Gorkiewicz G, Meyer C, Rozman J, Heldmaier G, Maier R, Theussl C, Eder S, Kratky D, Wagner EF, Klingenspor M, Hoefler G, Zechner R. Defective lipolysis and altered energy metabolism in mice lacking adipose triglyceride lipase. Science. 2006;312;734-7

[27] Osuga J, Ishibashi S, Oka T, Yagyu H, Tozawa R, Fujimoto A, Shionoiri F, Yahagi N, Kraemer FB, Tsutsumi O, Yamada N Targeted disruption of hormone-sensitive lipase results in male sterility and adipocyte hypertrophy, but not in obesity. Proc Natl Acad Sci USA. 2000;97:787-92

[28] Karlsson M, Contreras JA, Hellman U, Tornqvist H, Holm C. cDNA cloning, tissue distribution, and identification of the catalytic triad of monoglyceride lipase. Evolutionary relationship to esterases, lysophospholipases, and haloperoxidases. J Biol Chem. 1997 ;272: 27218-23

[29] Zimmermann R, Strauss JG, Haemmerle G, Schoiswohl G, Birner-Gruenberger R, Riederer M, Lass A, Neuberger G, Eisenhaber F, Hermetter A, Zechner R. Fat mobilization in adipose tissue is promoted by adipose triglyceride lipase. Science. 2004;306;1383-6.

[30] Schoiswohl G, Schweiger M, Schreiber R, Gorkiewicz G, Preiss-Landl K, Taschler U, Zierler KA, Radner FP, Eichmann TO, Kienesberger PC, Eder S, Lass A, Haemmerle G, Alsted TJ, Kiens B, Hoefler G, Zechner R, Zimmermann R. Adipose triglyceride lipase plays a key role in the supply of the working muscle with fatty acids. J Lipid Res. 2010;51:490-9.

[31. Haemmerle G, Zimmermann R, Hayn M, Theussl C, Waeg G, Wagner E, Sattler W, Magin TM, Wagner EF, Zechner R.Hormone-sensitive lipase deficiency in mice causes diglyceride accumulation in adipose tissue, muscle, and testis. J Biol Chem. 2002;277: 4806-15.

[32] Lass A, Zimmermann R, Oberer M, Zechner R. Lipolysis - a highly regulated multi-enzyme complex mediates the catabolism of cellular fat stores. Prog Lipid Res. 2011 50:14-27. Review

[33] Yang Q, Graham TE, Mody N, Preitner F, Peroni OD, Zabolotny JM, Kotani K, Quadro L, Kahn BB. Serum retinol binding protein 4 contributes to insulin resistance in obesity and type 2 diabetes. Nature. 2005;436:356-62

[34] Cholesterol Treatment Trialists' (CTT) Collaboration, Baigent C, Blackwell L, Emberson J, Holland LE, Reith C, Bhala N, Peto R, Barnes EH, Keech A, Simes J, Collins R. Efficacy and safety of more intensive lowering of LDL cholesterol: a meta-analysis of data from 170,000 participants in 26 randomised trials. Lancet 2010 376;1670-81

[35] Abifadel M, Varret M, Rabès JP, Allard D, Ouguerram K, Devillers M, Cruaud C, Benjannet S, Wickham L, Erlich D, Derré A, Villéger L, Farnier M, Beucler I, Bruckert E, Chambaz J, Chanu B, Lecerf JM, Luc G, Moulin P, Weissenbach J, Prat A, Krempf M, Junien C, Seidah NG, Boileau C.Mutations in PCSK9 cause autosomal dominant hypercholesterolemia. Nat Genet. 2003;34:154-6

[36] Horton JD, Cohen JC, Hobbs HH. PCSK9: a convertase that coordinates LDL catabolism. J Lipid Res. 2009;50 Suppl:S172-7..

[37] Steinberg and Witztum Inhibition of PCSK9. A powerful weapon for achieving ideal cholesterol levels. PNAS 2009 106; 9546-9547

[38] Davignon J, Dubuc G. Statins and ezetimibe modulate plasma proprotein convertase subtilisin kexin-9 (PCSK9) levels. *Trans Am Clin Climatol Assoc.* 2009;120:163–73.

[39] Konrad RJ, Troutt JS, Cao G. Effects of currently prescribed LDL-C-lowering drugs on PCSK9 and implications for the next generation of LDL-C-lowering agents. Lipids Health Dis. 2011;10:38

[40] Chan JC, Piper DE, Cao Q, Liu D, King C, Wang W, Tang J, Liu Q, Higbee J, Xia Z, Di Y, Shetterly S, Arimura Z, Salomonis H, Romanow WG, Thibault ST, Zhang R, Cao P, Yang XP, Yu T, Lu M, Retter MW, Kwon G, Henne K, Pan O, Tsai MM, Fuchslocher B, Yang E, Zhou L, Lee KJ, Daris M, Sheng J, Wang Y, Shen WD, Yeh WC, Emery M, Walker NP, Shan B, Schwarz M, Jackson SM. A proprotein convertase subtilisin/kexin type 9neutralizing antibody reduces serum cholesterol in mice and nonhuman primates. Proc Natl Acad Sci U S A. 2009;106:9820-5.

[41] Shafrir E. Animal models of non-insulin-dependent diabetes. Diabetes Metab Rev. 1992;8:179-208. Review.

[42] Levy E, Lalonde G, Delvin E, Elchebly M, Précourt LP, Seidah NG, Spahis S, Rabasa-Lhoret R, Ziv E.Intestinal and hepatic cholesterol carriers in diabetic Psammomys obesus.Endocrinology. 2010;151:958-70.

[43] Brouwers MC, Troutt JS, van Greevenbroek MM, Ferreira I, Feskens EJ, van der Kallen CJ, Schaper NC, Schalkwijk CG, Konrad RJ, Stehouwer CD. Plasma proprotein convertase subtilisin kexin type 9 is not altered in subjects with impaired glucose metabolism and type 2 diabetes mellitus, but its relationship with non-HDL cholesterol and apolipoprotein B may be modified by type 2 diabetes mellitus: The CODAM study. Atherosclerosis. 2011 Mar 25. [Epub ahead of print]

[44] Pyörälä K, Ballantyne CM, Gumbiner B, Lee MW, Shah A, Davies MJ, Mitchel YB, Pedersen TR, Kjekshus J; Scandinavian Simvastatin Survival Study (4S). Reduction of cardiovascular events by simvastatin in nondiabetic coronary heart disease patients with and without the metabolic syndrome: subgroup analyses of the Scandinavian Simvastatin Survival Study (4S). Diabetes Care. 2004;27:1735-40.

[45] Heart Protection Study Collaborative Group. MRC/BHF Heart Protection Study of cholesterol lowering with simvastatin in 20536 high-risk individuals: a randomised placebo-controlled trial. Lancet 2002;360:7-22.

[46] Heart Protection Study Collaborative Group. Randomized trial of the effects of cholesterol-lowering with simvastatin on peripheral vascular and other major vascular outcomes in 20,536 people with peripheral arterial disease and other high-risk conditions. J Vasc Surg. 2007;45:645-654;

[47] Kontush A, Chapman MJ. Antiatherogenic function of HDL particle subpopulations: focus on antioxidative activities. Curr Opin Lipidol. 2010;21:312-8. Review

[48] Nordestgaard BG, Benn M, Schnohr P, Tybjaerg-Hansen A Nonfasting triglycerides and risk of myocardial infarction, ischemic heart disease, and death in men and women. JAMA. 2007;298:299-308

[49] Bansal S, Buring JE, Rifai N, Mora S, Sacks FM, Ridker PM Fasting compared with non-fasting triglycerides and risk of cardiovascular events in women. JAMA.2007;298:309-16.

[50] Sluijs I, van der Schouw YT, van der A DL, Spijkerman AM, Hu FB, Grobbee DE, Beulens JW. Carbohydrate quantity and quality and risk of type 2 diabetes in the European Prospective Investigation into Cancer and Nutrition-Netherlands (EPIC-NL) Study. Am J Clin Nutr. 2010;92:905-11.

[51] Haubrock J, Nöthlings U, Volatier JL, Dekkers A, Ocké M, Harttig U, Illner AK, Knüppel S, Andersen LF, Boeing H; on behalf of the European Food Consumption Validation Consortium. Estimating Usual Food Intake Distributions by Using the Multiple Source Method in the EPIC-Potsdam Calibration Study. J Nutr. 2011 Mar 23.

[52] van Dieren S, Peelen LM, Nöthlings U, van der Schouw YT, Rutten GE, Spijkerman AM, van der A DL, Sluik D, Boeing H, Moons KG, Beulens JW. External validation of the UK Prospective Diabetes Study (UKPDS) risk engine in patients with type 2 diabetes. Diabetologia. 2011;54:264-70.

[53] No authors listed]Effect of fenofibrate on progression of coronary-artery disease in type 2 diabetes: the Diabetes Atherosclerosis Intervention Study, a randomised study. Lancet. 2001;357;905-10.

[54] Keech A, Simes RJ, Barter P, Best J, Scott R, Taskinen MR, Forder P, Pillai A, Davis T, Glasziou P, Drury P, Kesäniemi YA, Sullivan D, Hunt D, Colman P, d'Emden M, Whiting M, Ehnholm C, Laakso M; FIELD study investigatorsEffects of long-term fenofibrate therapy on cardiovascular events in 9795 people with type 2 diabetes mellitus (the FIELD study): randomised controlled trial. Lancet. 2005;366;1849-61.

[55] Jun M, Foote C, Lv J, Neal B, Patel A, Nicholls SJ, Grobbee DE, Cass A, Chalmers J, Perkovic V. Effects of fibrates on cardiovascular outcomes: a systematic review and meta- analysis. Lancet. 2010;375;1875-84

[56] Scott R, O'Brien R, Fulcher G, Pardy C, D'Emden M, Tse D, Taskinen MR, Ehnholm C, Keech A; Fenofibrate Intervention and Event Lowering in Diabetes (FIELD) Study Investigators. Effects of fenofibrate treatment on cardiovascular disease risk in 9,795 individuals with type 2 diabetes and various components of the metabolic syndrome: the Fenofibrate Intervention and Event Lowering in Diabetes (FIELD) study. Diabetes Care. 2009;32:493-8.

[57] Rizzo M, Rini GB, Berneis K The clinical relevance of LDL size and subclasses modulation in patients with type-2 diabetes. Exp Clin Endocrinol Diabetes. 2007 115:477-82. Review.

[58] Adiels M, Olofsson SO, Taskinen MR, Borén J. Diabetic dyslipidaemia. Curr Opin Lipidol. 2006;17:238-46. Review.

[59] Phillips C, Madigan C, Owens D, Collins P, Tomkin GH. Defective chylomicron synthesis as a cause of delayed particle clearance in diabetes? Int J Exp Diabetes Res. 2002;3:171-8

[60] Matthan NR, Pencina M, LaRocque JM, Jacques PF, D'Agostino RB, Schaefer EJ, Lichtenstein AH. Alterations in cholesterol absorption/synthesis markers characterize Framingham offspring study participants with CHD. J Lipid Res. 2009 Sep;50(9):1927-35. Epub 2009 May 12.PMID: 19436064 [PubMed - in process]

[61] Matthan NR, Resteghini N, Robertson M, Ford I, Shepherd J, Packard C, Buckley BM, Jukema JW, Lichtenstein AH, Schaefer EJ; PROSPER Group. Cholesterol absorption and synthesis markers in individuals with and without a CHD event during pravastatin therapy: insights from the PROSPER trial. J Lipid Res. 2010 ;51:202-9.

[62] Silbernagel G, Fauler G, Renner W, Landl EM, Hoffmann MM, Winkelmann BR, Boehm BO, März W. The relationships of cholesterol metabolism and plasma plant sterols with the severity of coronary artery disease. J Lipid Res. 2009;50:334-41.

[63] Lakoski SG, Xu F, Vega GL, Grundy SM, Chandalia M, Lam C, Lowe RS, Stepanavage ME, Musliner TA, Cohen JC, Hobbs HH. Indices of cholesterol metabolism and relative responsiveness to ezetimibe and simvastatin. J Clin Endocrinol Metab. 2010;95:800-9.

[64] Miettinen TA, Gylling H Blood glucose and the metabolism of cholesterol in coronary patients with and without simvastatin treatment. Subgroup analysis of Scandinavian Simvastatin Survival Study (4S).Clin Chim Acta. 2007 Apr;379(1-2):53-8.

[65] Kern F Jr. Normal plasma cholesterol in an 88-year-old man who eats 25 eggs a day. Mechanisms of adaptation. N Engl J Med. 1991;324:896-9.

[66] Altmann SW, Davis HR Jr, Zhu IJ, Yao X, Hoos LM, Tetzloff F, Iyer Sp, Maguire M, Golovko A, Zeng M, Wang L, Murgolo N, Graziano MP: Niemann-Pick C1 Like 1 protein is critical for intestinal cholesterol absorption. Science 2004;303:1201-4,

[67] Deficiency of Niemann-Pick C1 Like 1 prevents atherosclerosis in ApoE-/- mice. Davis HR Jr, Hoos LM, Tetzloff G, Maguire M, Zhu LJ, Graziano MP, Altmann SW. Arterioscler Thromb Vasc Biol. 2007;27:841-9.

[68] Davis HR Jr, Lowe RS, Neff DR. Effects of ezetimibe on atherosclerosis in preclinical models. Atherosclerosis. 2011;215:266-78.

[69] Tremblay AJ, Lamarche B, Lemelin V, Hoos L, Benjannet S, Seidah NG, Davis HR Jr, Couture P. Atorvastatin increases intestinal expression of NPC1L1 in hyperlipidemic men. J Lipid Res. 2011;52:558-65.

[70] Gleeson A, Owens D, Collins P, Johnson , Tomkin GH. The relationship between cholesterol absorption and intestinal cholesterol synthesis in the diabetic rat model. Internat J Exp Diab Res 2000;1;203-210

[71] Lally S, Tan CY, Owens D, Tomkin GH. Messenger RNA levels of genes involved in dysregulation of postprandial lipoproteins in type 2 diabetes: the role of Niemann-Pick C1-like 1, ATP-binding cassette, transporters G5 and G8, and of microsomal triglyceride transfer protein. Diabetologia. 2006;49:1008-16.

[72] Lally S, Owens D, Tomkin GH. Genes that affect cholesterol synthesis, cholesterol absorption and chylomicron assembly. The relationship between the liver and intestine in control and streptozotosin diabetic rats Metabolism 2007:56:430-438

[73] Intestinal and hepatic cholesterol carriers in diabetic Psammomys obesus. Levy E, Lalonde G, Delvin E, Elchebly M, Précourt LP, Seidah NG, Spahis S, Rabasa-Lhoret R, Ziv E. Endocrinology. 2010;151:958-70.

[74] Levy E, Spahis S, Ziv E, Marette A, Elchebly M, Lambert M, Delvin E. Overproduction of intestinal lipoprotein containing apolipoprotein B-48 in Psammomys obesus: impact of dietary n-3 fatty acids. Diabetologia. 2006;49:1937-45.

[75] Berge KE, Tian H, Graf GA et al. Accumulation of dietary cholesterol in sitosterolemia caused by mutations in adjacent ABC transporters. Science 2000;290:1771-5,

[76] Graf GA, Yu L, Li WP, Gerard R, Tuma PL, Cohen JC, Hobbs HH. ABCG5 and ABCG8 are obligate heterodimers for protein trafficking and biliary excretion. J Biol Chem 2003;278;48275-48282

[77] Kosters A, Kunne C, Looije N, Patel SB, Oude Elferink RP, Groen AK. The mechanism of ABCG5/ABCG8 in biliary cholesterol secretion in mice. J Lipid Res. 2006 47:1959-66.

[78] Wang HH, Patel SB, Carey MC, Wang DQ. Quantifying anomalous intestinal sterol uptake, lymphatic transport, and biliary secretion in Abcg8(-/-) mice. Hepatology. 2007;45:998-1006

[79] Santosa S, Demonty I, Lichtenstein AH, Ordovas JM, Jones PJ. Single nucleotide polymorphisms in ABCG5 and ABCG8 are associated with changes in cholesterol metabolism during weight loss. J Lipid Res. 2007;48:2607-13.

[80] Gylling H, Hallikainen M, Pihlajamäki J, Agren J, Laakso M, Rajaratnam RA, Rauramaa R, Miettinen TA. Polymorphisms in the ABCG5 and ABCG8 genes associate with cholesterol absorption and insulin sensitivity. J Lipid Res. 2004;45:1660-5

[81] Blocks VW, Bakker-Van Waarde WM, Verkade HJ, Kema IP, Wolters H, Vink E, Groen AK, Kuipers F. Down-regulation of hepatic and intestinal Abcg5 and Abcg8 expression associated with altered sterol fluxes in rats with streptozotocin-induced diabetes. Diabetologia. 2004;47:104-12.

[82] Lally S, Owens D, Tomkin GH The different effect of pioglitazone as compared to insulin on expression of hepatic and intestinal genes regulating post-prandial lipoproteins in diabetes Atherosclerosis. 2007;193:343-51.

[83] Lally S, Owens D, Tomkin GH. Genes that affect cholesterol synthesis, cholesterol absorption and chylomicron assembly. The relationship between the liver and intestine in control and streptozotosin diabetic rats Metabolism 2007:56:430-438

[84] Aggarwal D, West KL, Zern TL, Shrestha S, Vergara-Jimenez M, Fernandez ML. JTT-130, a microsomal triglyceride transfer protein (MTP) inhibitor lowers plasma triglycerides and LDL cholesterol concentrations without increasing hepatic triglycerides in guinea pigs. BMC Cardiovasc Disord. 2005 ;27;5:30.

[85] Kim E, Campbell S, Schueller O, Wong E, Cole B, Kuo J, Ferkany J, Ellis J, Sweetnam P. A Small Molecule Inhibitor of Enterocytic Microsomal Triglyceride Transfer Protein; SLx-4090, Biochemical, Pharmacodynamic, Pharmacokinetic and Safety Profile. J Pharmacol Exp Ther. 2011 Mar 15. [Epub ahead of print] PMID:2140654

[86] Phillips C, Mullan K, Owens D, Tomkin GH. A common microsomal triglyceride transfer protein polymorphism significantly reduces low density lipoprotein cholesterol in type 2 diabetic patients through its effect on the triglyceride-rich lipoproteins. QJM 2004;97;211-218

[87] Karpe F, Lundahl B, Ehrenborg E, Eriksson P, Hamsten A. A common functional polymorphism in the promoter region of the microsomal triglyceride transfer

protein gene influences plasma LDL levels. Atheroscler Thromb Vasc Biol 1998;18;756-761

[88] Phillips C, Anderton K, Bennett A et al. Intestinal rather than hepatic microsomal triglyceride transfer protein as a cause of postprandial dyslipidaemia in diabetes. Metabolism 2002;51:847–852.

[89] Gleeson A, Anderton K, Owens D, et al The role of microsomal triglyceride transfer protein and dietary cholesterol in chylomicron production in diabetes. Diabetologia 1999;42:944–949

[90] Lally S, Owens D, Tomkin GH. The different effect of pioglitazone as compared to insulin on expression of hepatic and intestinal genes regulating post-prandial lipoproteins in diabetes. Atherosclerosis 2007;193:343–51.

[91] Qin B, Qiu W, Avramoglu RK, Adeli K. Tumor necrosis factor-alpha induces intestinal insulin resistance and stimulates the overproduction of intestinal apolipoprotein B48-containing lipoproteins. Diabetes 2007;56:450–61.

[92] Zoltowska M, Ziv E, Delvin E, Sinnett D, Kalman R, Garofalo C, Seidman E, Levy E.Cellular aspects of intestinal lipoprotein assembly in Psammomys obesus: a model of insulin resistance and type 2 diabetes. Diabetes. 2003 Oct;52(10):2539-45.

[93] Yoshimura N, Kinoshita M, Teramoto T.Isolation and characterization of apolipoprotein B48-containing lipoproteins with a monoclonal antibody against apolipoprotein B48. J Atheroscler Thromb. 2009;16(6):740-7.

[94] Botham KM, Bravo E, Elliott J, Wheeler-Jones CP. Direct interaction of dietary lipids carried in chylomicron remnants with cells of the artery wall: implications for atherosclerosis development. *Curr Pharm Des.* 2005;11:3681–3695.

[95] Proctor SD, Vine DF, Mamo JC. Arterial retention of apolipoprotein B(48)- and B(100)-containing lipoproteins in atherogenesis. *Curr Opin Lipidol.* 2002;13:461–470.

[96] De Pascale C, Avella M, Perona JS, Ruiz-Gutierrez V, Wheeler-Jones CP, Botham KM. Fatty acid composition of chylomicron remnant-like particles influences their uptake and induction of lipid accumulation in macrophages. *FEBS J.* 2006;273:5632–5640.

[97] De Pascale C, Graham V, Fowkes RC, Wheeler-Jones CP, Botham KM.Suppression of nuclear factor-kappaB activity in macrophages by chylomicron remnants: modulation by the fatty acid composition of the particles.FEBS J. 2009 Oct;276(19):5689-702. Epub 2009 Sep 2

[98] Bejta F, Moore EH, Avella M, Gough PJ, Suckling KE, Botham KM Oxidation of chylomicron remnant-like particles inhibits their uptake by THP-1 macrophages by apolipoprotein E-dependent processes. Biochim Biophys Acta. 2007 Jul;1771(7):901-10.

[99] Bunck MC, Cornér A, Eliasson B, Heine RJ, Shaginian RM, Wu Y, Yan P, Smith U, Yki-Järvinen H, Diamant M, Taskinen MR. One-year treatment with exenatide vs. insulin glargine: effects on postprandial glycemia, lipid profiles, and oxidative stress. Atherosclerosis. 2010;212:223-9.

[100] Xiao C, Pavlic M, Szeto L, Patterson BW, Lewis GF. Effects of acute hyperglucagonemia on hepatic and intestinal lipoprotein production and clearance in healthy humans. Diabetes. 2011;60:383-90.

[101] Howard BV. Lipoprotein metabolism in diabetes mellitus. J Lipid Res.1987;28:613-28.

[102] Lopes-Virella MF, Wohltmann HJ, Loadholt CB, Buse MG. Plasma lipids and lipoproteins in young insulin-dependent diabetic patients: relationship with control. Diabetologia. 1981;21:216-23.

[103] James RW, Pometta D: Differences in lipoprotein subfraction composition and distribution between type I diabetic men and control subjects. Diabetes 39:1158–1164, 1990
[104] Guy J, Ogden L, Wadwa RP, Hamman RF, Mayer-Davis EJ, Liese AD, D'Agostino R Jr, Marcovina S, Dabelea D.Lipid and lipoprotein profiles in youth with and without type 1 diabetes: the SEARCH for Diabetes in Youth case-control study. Diabetes Care. 2009;32:416-20.
[105] Mangat R, Su JW, Lambert JE, Clandinin MT, Wang Y, Uwiera RR, Forbes JM, Vine DF, Cooper ME, Mamo JC, Proctor SDIncreased risk of cardiovascular disease in Type 1 diabetes: arterial exposure to remnant lipoproteins leads to enhanced deposition of cholesterol and binding to glycated extracellular matrix proteoglycans. Diabet Med. 2011;28:61-72.
[106] Curtin A, Deegan P, Owens D, Collins P, Johnson A, Tomkin GH. Elevated triglyceride- rich lipoproteins in diabetes. A study of apolipoprotein B-48. Acta Diabetol 1996;33:205- 10.
[107] Curtin A, Deegan P, Owens D, Collins P, Johnson A, Tomkin GH. Intestinally derived lipoprotein particles in non-insulin-dependent diabetic patients with and without hypertriglyceridaemia. Acta Diabetol. 1995;32:244-50.
[108] Curtin A, Deegan P, Owens D, Collins P, Johnson A, Tomkin GH. Alterations in apolipoprotein B-48 in the postprandial state in NIDDM. Diabetologia. 1994;37:1259-64.
[109] Ceriello A. Does postprandial blood glucose matter and why? Endocrinol Nutr. 2009;56 Suppl 4:8-11
[110] Watson TD, Caslake MJ, Freeman DJ, Griffin BA, Hinnie J, Packard CJ, Shepherd J: Determinants of LDL subfraction distribution and concentrations in young normo-lipidemic subjects. Arterioscler Thromb, 1994; 14: 902-910
[111] Gaw A, Packard CJ, Lindsay GM, Griffin BA, Caslake MJ, Lorimer AR, Shepherd J Overproduction of small very low density lipoproteins (Sf 20-60) in moderate hypercholesterolemia: relationships between apolipoprotein B kinetics and plasma lipoproteins. J Lipid Res. 1995;36:158-71.
[112] Colhoun HM, Otvos JD, Rubens MB, Taskinen MR, Underwood SR, Fuller JH.Lipoprotein subclasses and particle sizes and their relationship with coronary artery calcification in men and women with and without type 1 diabetes. Diabetes. 2002 ;51:1949-56
[113] Berneis K, Jeanneret C, Muser J, Felix B, Miserez AR. Low-density lipoprotein size and subclasses are markers of clinically apparent and non-apparent atherosclerosis in type 2 diabetes.Metabolism. 2005 ;54:227-34.
[114] Bozzetto L, Annuzzi G, Corte GD, Patti L, Cipriano P, Mangione A, Riccardi G, Rivellese AA. Ezetimibe beneficially influences fasting and postprandial triglyceride-rich lipoproteins in type 2 diabetes. Atherosclerosis. 2011 Mar 15. Epub ahead of print]
[115] Lund-Katz S, Phillips MC High density lipoprotein structure-function and role in reverse cholesterol transport. Subcell Biochem. 2010;51:183-227. Review.

14

The Role of Adipose Tissue in Diabetic Kidney Disease

Young Sun Kang, Jin Joo Cha, Young Youl Hyun,
Ji Eun Lee*, Hyun Wook Kim* and Dae Ryong Cha
Division of Nephrology, Department of Internal Medicine
Medical College of Korea University, Wonkwang University,*
Korea

1. Introduction

Chronic kidney disease has become an important global public health threat. There are currently approximately 387,000 patients with end-stage kidney disease in the United States and 1.8 million patients worldwide who require dialysis therapy or a transplant for survival (DuBose, 2007). Over 23 million children and adults have diabetes mellitus in the United States, representing nearly 8% of the population. Forty-three percent of end-stage kidney disease patients in the US have diabetes mellitus, and more than 90% of these diabetics have type 2 diabetes; these statistics are similar to the situation in Korea (ESRD Registry Committe, 2010). Type 2 diabetes mellitus, hypertension, obesity, and dyslipidemia are components of metabolic syndrome and are all major risk factors for cardiovascular disease. With the availability of excess food in many parts of the world, obesity is a growing problem that is increasing at an alarming rate in adults as well as in children. Obesity increases the risk for type 2 diabetes mellitus, cardiovascular disease, cancer, musculoskeletal disorders, and pulmonary disease (Kramer, 2006). Although obesity is an important risk factor for diabetes and hypertension, the two most common etiologies of chronic kidney disease, obesity itself may also potentiate kidney damage.

The important etiologic factor of metabolic syndrome is insulin resistance, which leads to hyperinsulinemia; activation of the renin-angiotensin-aldosterone system (RAAS); increased syntheses of transforming growth factor beta 1 (TGF-β1), insulin-like growth factor-1 (IGF-1) and connective tissue growth factor (CTGF); and collagen production in the kidney. These changes cause renal mesangial cell proliferation, extracellular matrix (ECM) expansion and renal fibrosis (Sarafidis & Ruilope, 2006). In addition to its proliferative actions in the kidney, insulin likely influences renal function at the tubular level because its sodium-retaining action results in hypertension. Insulin may also contribute to glomerulus injury by increasing the glomerular filtration rate (GFR), intraglomerular pressure and urinary albumin excretion. Moreover, insulin resistance and hyperinsulinemia are directly associated with low endothelial nitric oxide synthesis, altered endothelin-1 secretion and high oxidative stress production. Although the kidney is affected by hyperglycemia in patients with diabetes mellitus, the role of altered renal lipid metabolism has not yet been extensively studied in obesity-related kidney disease, including diabetic nephropathy. However, previous reports have revealed that abnormalities in lipid and glucose metabolism in the kidney are also important in the development of organ injury, as is adipose tissue (Drury et al., 1950; Rubenstein et al., 1975; Schoolwerth et al., 1988; Stumvoll et al., 1997).

Obesity is a risk factor for the development of hypertensive nephrosclerosis, and focal and segmental glomerular sclerosis is considered to be independent risk factors for the progression of renal disease. Recent experimental and human clinical trials suggest that obesity can influence renal injury through various mechanisms, including hemodynamic changes in the glomeruli, alteration of renal lipid metabolism, increased oxidative stress, and inflammation via alteration of adipocytokines induced by adipose tissue changes in obesity. Additionally, circulating adipocytokines can also positively or negatively influence systemic insulin resistance, leading to organ injury and endothelial dysfunction. Recent insights about adipose tissue biology suggest that adipose tissue is not an energy storage tissue but an active endocrine organ that interacts with major target organs of metabolic syndrome, such as the liver, muscles and kidneys. A better understanding of adipose tissue biology will help researchers develop new therapeutic strategies for managing metabolic syndrome as well as diabetic vascular complications.

2. Adipose tissue and kidney

2.1 Adipose tissue as an endocrine organ

During the development of obesity, multiple functional and structural changes occur in the adipose tissue (called "adiposopathy"), such as an increase in the number and size of adipocytes, an increase in the infiltration of mononuclear cells, rarefaction of blood vessels, and apoptosis (Wellen & Hotamisligil, 2003). Because leptin, the first identified adipocytokine, has a systemic effect in the body, adipose tissue is now considered to be an active endocrine organ (Zhang et al., 1994). While many adipocytokines have been proposed, few have been studied in detail, and even fewer have been investigated in the kidney. These adipocytokines include several active molecules released by adipocytes, such as leptin, resistin, adiponectin or visfatin, as well as cytokines released by inflammatory cells, such as tumor necrosis factor alpha (TNF-α), interleukine-6 (IL-6), monocyte chemoattractant protein-1 (MCP-1), and interleukine-1 (IL-1). Interestingly, the circulating levels of these adipocytokines have been found to be altered in experimental animals and patients with kidney disease, which is an independent risk factor for cardiovascular diseases. Moreover, the production, secretion and regulatory actions of these proteins are not limited only to adipose tissue but are also described in other organ tissues. It is now recognized that the kidney itself can alter the clearance of adipocytokines as well as produce them. Recent experimental and clinical evidence has demonstrated possible molecules that cross-talk between adipose tissue and the kidney in the pathogenesis of obesity-related renal disease.

2.2 Role of leptin in kidney disease

Leptin is a representative adipocytokine that is primarily produced in adipose tissue and that plays an important role in appetite control and regulation of energy expenditure. The plasma leptin concentration is positively increased according to the degree of adiposity (Friedman & Halaas, 1998), and hyperleptinemia has been reported to be an independent risk factor for cardiovascular disease (Ren, 2004; Soderberg et al., 1999). However, recent experimental data imply that leptin may directly influence renal function through the small isoform of the leptin receptor (Ob-Ra) in the kidney (Wolf & Ziyadeh, 2006). Infusion of leptin in normal rats induced glomerulosclerosis and proteinuria, and transgenic mice overexpressing leptin also showed increased renal expressions of fibronectin and type IV collagen (Wolf et al., 2002). Several *in vitro* experiments using glomerular endothelial and mesangial cells also demonstrated that leptin stimulates the proliferation of endothelial cells, increases glucose uptake into mesangial cells and finally increases the productions of TGF-β1 and collagen (Wolf et al., 1999). In addition, leptin plays an important role in the progression of atherosclerosis, such as platelet aggregation and thrombosis, production of inflammatory cytokines (including TNF-α and IL-6) and calcification of vascular smooth muscle cells (Konstantinides et al., 2001). Leptin is also associated with sympathetic activation and can lead to hypertension and renal injury (Henegar et al., 2001; Kambham et al., 2001). Collectively, these data suggest that leptin contributes to the development of renal injury through both direct and indirect effects.

2.3. Role of adiponectin in kidney disease

Adiponectin is an important anti-diabetic adipocytokine produced in adipose tissue (Scherer, 2006). A large body of evidence has shown that adiponectin improves insulin sensitivity and exerts an anti-inflammatory effect in vascular cells (Scherer, 2006; Axelsson, 2008; Goldstein & Scalia, 2004). Adiponectin-null mice show increased susceptibility to insulin resistance when fed a high-fat diet, and treatment with adiponectin improves insulin sensitivity (Maeda et al., 2002). Studies of the genetic modulation of adiponectin receptors also suggest that representative adiponectin receptors 1 and 2 are involved in insulin resistance through the activation of AMP-activated protein kinase (AMPK) and peroxisome proliferator-activated receptor (PPAR) (Kadowaki et al., 2008; Mao et al., 2006). Interestingly, serum levels of adiponectin are lower in obese patients compared with those in lean patients (Kanaya et al. 2006; Laughlin et al. 2007). Although the association between adiponectin level and renal disease is still controversial, recent clinical studies have reported that serum adiponectin and albuminuria levels were inversely correlated (Tsioufis et al., 2005; Sharma et al., 2008; Yano et al., 2007). Considering that adiponectin is produced in adipose tissue and shows an inverse relationship with the amount of adiposity, these findings support the possibility of adiponectin as a candidate molecule that connects obesity and kidney disease.

Sharma et al. first reported the link between adiponectin and albuminuria in an adiponectin-null mouse (Sharma et al., 2008). The C57BL/6 adiponectin-null mouse exhibits albuminuria and pathologic changes in foot process effacement of podocytes (Sharma et al., 2008). This study observed that podocytes express the adiponectin R1 receptor, and that treatment with adiponectin normalized the albuminuria and pathologic changes of the foot process through adiponectin stimulation of the AMPK pathway, a key regulator of intracellular energy status with potent anti-proliferative and anti-oxidative effects. In addition, renoprotective effects of adiponectin have also been reported in the subtotal renal ablation model of adiponectin-knockout mice (Ohashi et al., 2007). An increase in visceral fat increases the productions of proinflammatory adipocytokines, which leads to an increase in oxidative stress in various target organs. Furthermore, the increase in adipose tissue oxidative stress results in further aggravation of systemic oxidative stress and inflammation, which positively affect the development of insulin resistance. Taken together, these data suggest that adiponectin is a possible mechanistic link between adipose tissue and renal disease. However, it is not yet clear whether adiponectin receptor 2 has a role in obesity-related kidney disease.

2.4 Role of visfatin in kidney disease

Among the adipocytokines, visfatin is a ubiquitous intracellular enzyme; it is also known as nicotinamide phosphoribosyltransferase (NAMPT)/pre-B cell colony-enhancing factor (PBEF-1). Visfatin is a newly identified adipocytokine that is secreted by adipocytes and that mimics insulin in animals (Fukuhara et al., 2005); however, its role in kidney disease is not yet known. In humans, early data have suggested that visfatin concentrations are increased in patients with type 2 diabetes mellitus (Chen et al., 2006), but that it is not in itself a mediator of insulin resistance (Lopez-Bermejo et al., 2006). Plasma visfatin concentrations were recently found to increase in patients with diabetes mellitus compared with those in healthy control participants (Kang et al., 2010c). These data did not show any significant relationships between plasma visfatin concentration and metabolic parameters, including the homeostasis model assessment of insulin resistance (HOMA-IR), HbA1c, or body-mass index (BMI). However, plasma levels of visfatin were markedly increased in patients with diabetic nephropathy irrespective of the stage of nephropathy. Visfatin level was associated with systemic inflammatory markers (such as MCP-1), and its levels were positively associated with systolic blood pressure, fasting blood glucose and carotid intima-medial thickness (IMT). These findings suggest that the plasma concentration of visfatin is elevated when inflammatory conditions exist.

Another experiment reported that plasma concentration of visfatin was increased in animals as well as humans during the early stages of diabetic nephropathy in type 2 diabetics (Kang et al., 2010d). The present study found that visfatin expression was markedly up-regulated in both the glomeruli and proximal tubules of the diabetic kidney. In another experiment, the synthesis and physiological action of visfatin in renal cells (such as mesangial cells) were studied to investigate the role of visfatin in diabetic nephropathy (Song et al., 2008). Visfatin was found to be synthesized in renal mesangial cells as well as adipocytes and stimulated glucose uptake in glomerular mesangial cells mediated by glucose transporter-1 (GLUT-1). In glomerular podocytes and tubular cells as well as mesangial cells, high glucose stimulation up-regulated marked visfatin synthesis but did not increase the response to angiotensin II stimulation (Kang et al., 2010d; Song et al., 2008). Exogenous visfatin administration induced synthesis of pro-fibrotic molecules, including TGF-β1, PAI-1 and type I collagen. Endogenous visfatin produced from renal cells, such as mesangial cells, podocytes and tubular cells, seems to stimulate glucose uptake and intracellular metabolic abnormalities.

Hyperglycemia in diabetes is associated with increased glucose uptake into cells and causes intracellular metabolic alterations, which are considered an important pathogenesis for diabetic microvascular complications. Consistently, previous studies have suggested that glucose uptake into mesangial cells promotes mesangial extracellular matrix protein accumulation, which is characteristic of diabetic nephropathy (Ayo et al., 1991; Haneda et al., 1991; Heilig et al., 1995).

However, in diabetic animals, exogenous visfatin administration interestingly improved diabetic nephropathy (Song et al., 2008). These results were in opposition to previously obtained observational data of humans and animals. First, visfatin treatment improved urinary albumin excretion in diabetic animals irrespective of plasma glucose concentration. Second, dramatic improvements in plasma lipid concentration and insulin resistance were observed. Third, visfatin regulated the balance of lipid metabolism in the diabetic kidney as well as in the liver and adipose tissue. Several possibilities may explain these paradoxical results. Visfatin may have a compensatory effect via both the autocrine and paracrine pathways, resulting in improved insulin resistance and lipid metabolism. Long-term visfatin infusion may restore the decreased availability of insulin receptors in the kidney. The next possibility is the benefit of a more physiologic route of intra-peritoneal visfatin injection compared to vascular infusion, which directly accumulates in the liver and visceral adipose tissue (the main organs regulating lipid and glucose metabolism) before achieving adequate concentration levels in the systemic circulations of the plasma, heart and kidney. Therefore, the secondary beneficial effects (improving insulin resistance and dyslipidemia) of visfatin on the kidney may be more effective than the direct renal effects. However, it is equally possible that a difference in the models of insulin resistance may have accounted for this apparent discrepancy. Despite the paradoxical effect of visfatin in this study, visfatin was shown to have beneficial effects on lipid metabolism and insulin resistance in diabetic animal experiments (Song et al., 2008). Long-term therapy with intraperitoneal visfatin injection eventually induced various organ-protective effects in type 2 diabetic nephropathy. Based on these results, visfatin might play some crucial role in the pathogenesis of insulin resistance and diabetic nephropathy.

2.5 Role of Renin-Angiotensin-Aldosterone System (RAAS)

Several clinical trials of hypertension have demonstrated a lower incidence of diabetes mellitus among patients treated with renin-angiotensin-aldosterone system (RAAS) inhibitor compared to that of those given other classes of anti-hypertensive drugs (Dahlof et al., 2002; Hansson et al., 1999; Yusuf et al., 2000). Although these studies were mostly performed among patients with hypertension or congestive heart failure, a relative risk for new-onset diabetes mellitus was reduced in patients using RAAS in a meta-analysis of randomized controlled trials. Furthermore, the activity of RAAS is also associated with metabolic syndrome (Engeli, 2006). These findings suggest that RAAS may have an important role in the development of diabetes mellitus. Interestingly, mature adipocytes express all components of RAAS, including angiotensinogen, angiotensin-converting enzyme and angiotensin type 1 (AT1) and angiotensin type 2 (AT2) receptors (Engeli et al., 2000). For these reasons, the anti-diabetic effect of RAAS inhibition was recently evaluated, and the effects of these drugs on adipocyte function were observed to occur via the modulation of adipocytokines (Kang et al., 2010a; Lee et al., 2008). Administration of an AT receptor antagonist (ARB) improved insulin resistance simultaneous to an improvement in diabetic nephropathy in an animal experiment. ARB augmented lipid accumulation, differentiation of adipocytes and improvement in adipocytokine synthesis in type 2 diabetic animals. In animals with diabetic nephropathy, ARB improved alterations in renal lipid metabolism and subsequently reduced renal cholesterol and triglyceride contents with decreased albuminuria. Importantly, in both adipocytes and renal cells, AT2 increased the synthesis of pro-inflammatory molecules in adipose tissue, such as plasminogen activator inhibitor-1 (PAI-1), MCP-1, and nuclear factor kappa B (NF-κB) activation, and then their synthesis was suppressed by ARB treatment.

The mechanisms linking obesity to hypertension are important for identifying specific treatments for these patients, and some evidence suggests that obesity is associated with increased aldosterone levels. Obesity induces activation of the RAS system in adipose tissue, and weight reduction often restores RAS activity to basal levels in lean healthy participants (Engeli et al., 2005). Proposed mechanisms for these interesting findings are the role of adipose-tissue-derived products called mineralocorticoid stimulating factor (MSF) and free fatty acids. An *in vitro* experiment showed the presence of MSF in conditioned media of adipocytes, which increased the production of aldosterone in cultured adrenal gland cells. Increased fatty acid production (especially non-esterified fatty acids) from adipose tissue in obese patients might stimulate aldosterone production in the adrenal gland. Metabolic syndrome and the cardiovascular and renal abnormalities associated with insulin resistance are mediated in part by aldosterone activity on the mineralocorticoid receptor (MR). In addition, recent research has shown that aldosterone promotes adipocyte differentiation *in vitro* through specific activation of the MR; a pro-inflammatory role for MR activation in adipose tissue has also been reported (Hirata et al., 2009). Patients with primary hyperaldosteronism (PA) showed differences in glucose metabolism compared with that of essential hypertensive patients; patients with PA have a lower beta-cell function that is influenced by aldosterone levels. This association was initially described in individuals with primary hyperaldosteronism and impaired glucose tolerance (Conn, 1965). Increased plasma aldosterone levels are associated with insulin resistance. It is also of interest that plasma aldosterone levels appeared to be positively correlated with plasma glucose levels in diabetic rat models of our previous study (Han et al., 2006). Aldosterone impairs lipid metabolism and insulin signaling in cardiovascular and renal tissue, as well as in fat, skeletal muscle and the liver (Sowers et al., 2009). Since aldosterone is also associated with glucose metabolism and dyslipidemia, selective aldosterone blockade may represent a particularly attractive therapeutic strategy in obese patients who have a cluster of cardiovascular risk factors.

Recently, a new RAAS inhibitor, direct renin inhibitor (DRI), has been used to manage hypertensive patients. While DRI has been primarily been studied in diabetic nephropathy, its effects have been extended into insulin resistance and metabolic syndrome in animal experiments (Kang et al., 2010a). DRI, which is independent of blood pressure lowering effects, showed a beneficial influence on the diabetic vascular complications of renal and cardiac injury. More importantly, its direct effect on pro-inflammatory molecules, such as MCP-1, TGF-β1, type Ⅳ collagen, PAI-1, and vascular endothelial growth factor (VEGF), may occur in the presence of target organ injury and not via RAAS activation. Additional findings have also revealed that DRI improved lipid parameters and insulin resistance with no effect on blood glucose level in the modulation of lipid metabolism in adipose, hepatic and renal tissues. Therefore, the RAAS inhibitor improved insulin resistance and lipid metabolism via anti-inflammatory actions on adipose tissue and also improved diabetic nephropathy.

2.6 Role of the MCP-1/CCR2 pathway

The kidney has been regarded as a target organ of critical complications in patients with metabolic syndrome, obesity, hypertension, dyslipidemia, and type 2 diabetes mellitus. While its important role in altering energy and glucose metabolism has been reported in patients with chronic kidney disease (Rubenstein et al., 1975), there is also considerable evidence of renal glucose production and utilization in animal models (Drury et al., 1950; Mather and Pollock, 2011; Schoolwerth et al., 1988; Stumvoll et al., 1997). The kidney contributes to glucose homeostasis through gluconeogenesis, glucose filtration, glucose reabsorption, and glucose consumption (Gerich, 2010). The human liver and kidneys release approximately equal amounts of glucose via gluconeogenesis in the post-absorptive state. Traditionally, pharmacotherapeutic interventions have been aimed at stimulating insulin secretion or addressing peripheral insulin resistance. A novel drug class currently being studied targets another pathophysiological process in the kidney of type 2 diabetes mellitus (Mather & Pollock, 2010; Neumiller et al., 2010). Therefore, the development of glucose-lowering drugs involving inhibition of renal glucose reabsorption, such as the sodium-glucose co-transporter 2 (SGLT2) inhibitor, has recently begun for use in type 2 diabetes mellitus.

The pathophysiology of diabetic nephropathy is multifactorial; it involves metabolic factors including hyperglycemia, genetic factors and hemodynamic factors such as hypertension and glomerular hyperfiltration (Han et al., 2006; Kang & Cha, 2009; Kang et al., 2009). Diabetic nephropathy was initially considered a non-inflammatory glomerular disease, and the inflammatory process has been largely ignored as a mechanism of diabetic nephropathy. However, recent animal and human clinical studies have provided evidence of the important role of inflammation in the development and progression of diabetic nephropathy (Han et al., 2010; Han et al., 2006; Ko et al., 2008). Hyperglycemia induces monocyte/macrophage infiltration in the kidney and contributes to the deposition of fibrotic molecules, which can lead to glomerulosclerosis. Moreover, there is abundant experimental evidence that inhibiting macrophage recruitment or macrophage activation can ameliorate renal inflammation and fibrosis. The MCP-1/C-C chemokine receptor 2 (CCR2) pathway has been reported to be an important mediator for inflammatory glomerular disease. The act of MCP-1 binding to the CCR2 receptor induces infiltration of inflammatory cells and proliferation of resident glomerular cells, such as epithelial and endothelial cells (Kato et al., 1999; Viedt et al., 2002). In addition, glomerular podocytes are the major glomerular cells that express MCP-1 in various proteinuric conditions, including diabetic and membranous nephropathies (Hartner et al., 2005; Prodjosudjadi et al., 1995). Blockade or loss of MCP-1 has been shown to provide renoprotective effects in experimental diabetic nephropathy (Chow et al., 2006; Kanamori et al., 2007), which suggests an influential role of the MCP-1/CCR2 pathway for the inflammatory process in diabetic injury. In addition, urinary MCP-1 excretion is increased in patients with early diabetic nephropathy, and acute-phase markers of inflammation are associated with the nephropathic state in type 2 diabetic patients (Dalla Vestra et al., 2005; Wada et al., 2000). However, CCR2, a seven-transmembrane protein-coupled receptor, is a receptor for MCP-1 and is expressed by monocytes. Local recruitment of monocytes is considered to be the predominant mechanism by which MCP-1 contributes to renal damage.

Many tissues, such as the pancreas, liver, skeletal muscle, heart, and vessels, are adversely affected by obesity (Matsuzawa, 2006). Although multiple molecular mechanisms contribute to the development of obesity-related complications, recent data (Ferrante, 2007) suggest that inflammation, especially that involving monocytes and macrophages, is a central axis in the pathophysiology of many obesity-related disorders. Obesity is accompanied by infiltration and activation of macrophages in adipose tissue, leading to the chronic inflammation of adipose tissue. Adipose tissue has been reported to be an important organ of obesity-induced inflammation as determined by measurement of its expressions of pro-inflammatory molecules (Hotamisligil et al., 1993). Obesity induces phenotypic changes in adipocytes, such as hypertrophy, and also induces an inflammatory response in adipocytes in an autocrine or paracrine fashion, resulting in impaired adipocyte function, including insulin signaling (Hotamisligil et al., 1996).

Several studies have reported that overexpression of MCP-1 causes macrophage recruitment in adipose tissue and insulin resistance (Kamei et al., 2006; Kanda et al., 2006). Adipocytes express CCR2, the primary receptor for MCP-1, which causes the expressions of inflammatory genes and impaired uptake of insulin-dependent glucose (Charo & Ransohoff, 2006). Obese mice with a CCR2 deficiency have shown improved insulin resistance, attenuated hepatic steatosis, increased adiponectin expression, and reduced macrophage content in adipose tissue when the mice were induced into obesity by a high-fat diet (Weisberg et al., 2006). Several CCR2 antagonists also resulted in decreased macrophage accumulation in adipose tissue with an accompanying improvement in insulin resistance (Kang et al., 2010b; Tamura et al., 2008). These results propose the possibility of an expanded role of the CCR2 genotype in adipose and hepatic tissues against insulin resistance in metabolic syndrome. Therefore, the MCP-1/CCR2 pathway might have an important role in insulin resistance with macrophage infiltration into adipose tissue, leading to systemic inflammatory and metabolic consequences.

Considering that inflammation in both adipose tissue and the kidney has an important role in insulin resistance and metabolic syndrome, common mechanisms between adipose tissue and the kidney should be identified. There may be cross-talk between adipose tissue and the kidney with obesity-induced inflammatory injury in metabolic syndrome, particularly in diabetic nephropathy. We performed mutual epididymal fat transplantation between diabetic and non-diabetic animals to support this hypothesis (Kim et al., 2010). We observed that diabetic db/db mice who received epididymal fat from normal db/m mice showed a significant decrease in urinary albumin excretion. In addition, there was significant improvement in renal pathologic changes, including decreases in TGF-β1, type IV collagen and PAI-1 protein expressions. The beneficial effect of non-diabetic epididymal fat transposition into diabetic animals supports the possibility of this same type of cross-talk in type 2 diabetic nephropathy. Functional and phenotypic changes in adipose tissue in obesity might have an impact on renal function through the various mechanisms of metabolic and hormonal effects, such as the MCP-1/CCR2 pathway and those of numerous adipocytokines.

2.7 Role of the Vitamin D Receptor (VDR)

Vitamin D deficiency is known to be related to cardiovascular disease and chronic kidney disease. Vitamin D improves albuminuria and the progression of renal injury independent of its classic actions (de Zeeuw et al., 2010; Deb et al., 2010; Kang et al., 2010). These animal studies provide rationale for treatment with the vitamin D receptor (VDR) agonist, paricalcitol, in the improvement of type 2 diabetic nephropathy and lipid metabolism. In the present study, there were no differences in the basal characteristics of body weight, fasting plasma glucose, HbA1c, glucose tolerance test, insulin tolerance test, serum creatinine level, or systolic and diastolic blood pressure. However, paricalcitol improved cardiac left ventricular mass index and urinary albumin excretion. Moreover, paricalcitol-treated diabetic mice showed improved plasma lipid profiles of total cholesterol, triglycerides and LDL cholesterol. Interestingly, cholesterol and triglyceride contents in kidney tissue were dramatically decreased by paricalcitol, and a similar result was observed in fat and liver tissues. In addition, plasma and urinary 8-isoprostane levels were markedly inhibited by paricalcitol treatment. Tissue lipid peroxidase (LPO) levels in kidney, fat and liver tissues were significantly improved. Paricalcitol suppressed the pro-inflammatory molecular synthesis and improved the morphological changes in renal glomerulosclerosis, hepatic steatosis and adipose phenotypic change of diabetic mice. The *in vitro* experiment with cultured VDR-siRNA mesangial cells revealed changes in gene expression and protein synthesis of the enzymes related to the lipid metabolism of fatty acid synthase (FAS), 3-hydroxy-3-methylglutaryl-coenzyme A reductase (HMG-Co AR; inducing cholesterol synthesis) and sterol-regulatory element-binding protein-1c (SREBP-1c; inducing cholesterol synthesis). Paricalcitol may have a protective effect on diabetic nephropathy through an improvement of systemic and tissue lipid metabolism and an anti-oxidative effect.

3. Conclusions

The role of the kidney is not only as a target organ during the development of obesity and metabolic syndrome, but also as a regulatory organ that cross-talks with adipose tissue. A large body of evidence has demonstrated that various adipocytokines, RAAS and VDR of the kidney and adipose tissue are associated with one another; alterations of these substances can lead to many complications of metabolic syndrome that develop from obesity-induced inflammation. Eventually, the improvement of insulin resistance through an anti-inflammatory effect on adipose tissue could result in the improvement of diabetic nephropathy, which decreases cardiovascular complications in metabolic syndrome. A better understanding of adipose tissue biology will help researchers develop a new therapeutic strategy to manage metabolic syndrome, including diabetic vascular complications. Future studies should focus on the aforementioned potential targets to improve insulin resistance as well as diabetic nephropathy.

4. Acknowledgment

This work was supported by a Korea University grant.

5. References

Axelsson, J. (2008). The emerging biology of adipose tissue in chronic kidney disease: from fat to facts. *Nephrol Dial Transplant*, Vol.23, No.10, pp.3041-3046, ISSN 0931-0509

Ayo, S.H., Radnik, R., Garoni, J.A., Troyer, D.A., & Kreisberg, J.I. (1991). High glucose increases diacylglycerol mass and activates protein kinase C in mesangial cell cultures. *Am J Physiol,* Vol.261, No.4, pp.F571-577, ISSN 0363-6127

Charo, I.F., & Ransohoff, R.M. (2006). The many roles of chemokines and chemokine receptors in inflammation. *N Engl J Med,* Vol.354, No.6, pp.610-621, ISSN 0028-4793

Chen, M.P., Chung, F.M., Chang, D.M., Tsai, J.C., Huang, H.F., Shin, S.J., & Lee, Y.J. (2006). Elevated plasma level of visfatin/pre-B cell colony-enhancing factor in patients with type 2 diabetes mellitus. *J Clin Endocrinol Metab,* Vol.91, No.1, pp.295-299, ISSN 0021-972X

Chow, F.Y., Nikolic-Paterson, D.J., Ozols, E., Atkins, R.C., Rollin, B.J., & Tesch, G.H. (2006). Monocyte chemoattractant protein-1 promotes the development of diabetic renal injury in streptozotocin-treated mice. *Kidney Int,* Vol.69, No.1, pp.73-80, ISSN 0085-2538

Conn, J.W. (1965). Hypertension, the potassium ion and impaired carbohydrate tolerance. *N Engl J Med,* Vol.273, No.21, pp.1135-1143, ISSN 0028-4793

Dahlof, B., Devereux, R.B., Kjeldsen, S.E., Julius, S., Beevers, G., de Faire, U., Fyhrquist, F., Ibsen, H., Kristiansson, K., Lederballe-Pedersen, O., *et al.* (2002). Cardiovascular morbidity and mortality in the Losartan Intervention For Endpoint reduction in hypertension study (LIFE): a randomised trial against atenolol. *Lancet,* Vol.359, No.9311, pp.995-1003, ISSN 0099-5355

Dalla Vestra, M., Mussap, M., Gallina, P., Bruseghin, M., Cernigoi, A.M., Saller, A., Plebani, M., & Fioretto, P. (2005). Acute-phase markers of inflammation and glomerular structure in patients with type 2 diabetes. *J Am Soc Nephrol,* Vol.16, No.3, Suppl 1, pp.S78-82, ISSN 1046-6673

de Zeeuw, D., Agarwal, R., Amdahl, M., Audhya, P., Coyne, D., Garimella, T., Parving, H.H., Pritchett, Y., Remuzzi, G., Ritz, E., *et al.* (2010). Selective vitamin D receptor activation with paricalcitol for reduction of albuminuria in patients with type 2 diabetes (VITAL study): a randomised controlled trial. *Lancet,* Vol.376, No.9752, pp.1543-1551, ISSN 0099-5355

Deb, D.K., Sun, T., Wong, K.E., Zhang, Z., Ning, G., Zhang, Y., Kong, J., Shi, H., Chang, A., & Li, Y.C. (2010). Combined vitamin D analog and AT1 receptor antagonist synergistically block the development of kidney disease in a model of type 2 diabetes. *Kidney Int,* Vol.77, No.11, pp.1000-1009, ISSN 0085-2538

Drury, D.R., Wick, A.N., Mac, K.E., Hillyard, N., Fitch, R., Blackwell, M.E., Bancroft, R.W., & Dorough, M.E. (1950). Formation of glucose by the kidney. *Am J Physiol* , Vol.163, No.3, pp.655-661, ISSN 0002-9513

DuBose, T.D., Jr. (2007). American Society of Nephrology Presidential Address 2006: chronic kidney disease as a public health threat--new strategy for a growing problem. *J Am Soc Nephrol,* Vol.18, No.4, pp.1038-1045, ISSN 1046-6673

Engeli, S. (2006). Role of the renin-angiotensin- aldosterone system in the metabolic syndrome. *Contrib Nephrol,* Vol.151, pp.122-134, ISSN 0302-5144

Engeli, S., Bohnke, J., Gorzelniak, K., Janke, J., Schling, P., Bader, M., Luft, F.C., & Sharma, A.M. *(2005).* Weight loss and the renin-angiotensin-aldosterone system. *Hypertension,* Vol.45, No.3, pp.356-362, ISSN 0194-911X

Engeli, S., Negrel, R., & Sharma, A.M. (2000). Physiology and pathophysiology of the adipose tissue renin-angiotensin system. *Hypertension,* Vol.35, No.6, pp.1270-1277, ISSN 0194-911X

ESRD Registry Committe, Korean Soc Nephrol (2010). Current Renal Replacement Therapy in Korea. *Korean J Nephrol,* Vol.29, No.2, pp.525-551, ISSN 1975-9460

Ferrante, A.W., Jr. (2007). Obesity-induced inflammation: a metabolic dialogue in the language of inflammation. *J Intern Med,* Vol.262, No.4, pp.408-414, ISSN 0954-6820

Friedman, J.M., & Halaas, J.I. (1998). Leptin and the regulation of body weight in mammals. *Nature,* Vol.395, No.6704, pp.763–770, ISSN 0028-0836

Fukuhara, A., Matsuda, M., Nishizawa, M., Segawa, K., Tanaka, M., Kishimoto, K., Matsuki, Y., Murakami, M., Ichisaka, T., Murakami, H., *et al.* (2005). Visfatin: a protein secreted by visceral fat that mimics the effects of insulin. *Science,* Vol.307, No.5708, pp.426-430, ISSN 0036-8075

Gerich, J.E. (2010). Role of the kidney in normal glucose homeostasis and in the hyperglycaemia of diabetes mellitus: therapeutic implications. *Diabet Med*, Vol.27, No.2, pp.136-142, ISSN 0742-3071

Goldstein, B., & Scalia, R. (2004). Adiponectin: A novel adipokine linking adipocytes and vascular function. *J Clin Endocrinol Metab*, Vol.89, No.6, pp.2563–2568, ISSN 0021-972X

Han, K.H., Han, S.Y., Kim, H.S., Kang, Y.S., & Cha, D.R. (2010). Prolonged administration enhances the renoprotective effect of pentoxifylline via anti-inflammatory activity in streptozotocin-induced diabetic nephropathy. *Inflammation*, Vol.33, No.3, pp.137-143, ISSN 0360-3997

Han, K.H., Kang, Y.S., Han, S.Y., Jee, Y.H., Lee, M.H., Han, J.Y., Kim, H.K., Kim, Y.S., & Cha, D.R. (2006). Spironolactone ameliorates renal injury and connective tissue growth factor expression in type II diabetic rats. *Kidney Int*, Vol.70, No.1, pp.111-120, ISSN 0085-2538

Haneda, M., Kikkawa, R., Horide, N., Togawa, M., Koya, D., Kajiwara, N., Ooshima, A., & Shigeta, Y. (1991). Glucose enhances type IV collagen production in cultured rat glomerular mesangial cells. *Diabetologia*, Vol.34, No.3, pp.198-200, ISSN 0012-186X

Hansson, L., Lindholm, L.H., Niskanen, L., Lanke, J., Hedner, T., Niklason, A., Luomanmaki, K., Dahlof, B., de Faire, U., Morlin, C., *et al.* (1999). Effect of angiotensin-converting-enzyme inhibition compared with conventional therapy on cardiovascular morbidity and mortality in hypertension: the Captopril Prevention Project (CAPPP) randomised trial. *Lancet*, Vol.353, No.9153, pp.611-616, ISSN 0099-5355

Hartner, A., Veelken, R., Wittmann, M., Cordasic, N., & Hilgers, K.F. (2005). Effects of diabetes and hypertension on macrophage infiltration and matrix expansion in the rat kidney. *BMC Nephrol*, Vol.6, No.1, pp.6, ISSN 1471-2369

Heilig, C.W., Concepcion, L.A., Riser, B.L., Freytag, S.O., Zhu, M., & Cortes, P. (1995). Overexpression of glucose transporters in rat mesangial cells cultured in a normal glucose milieu mimics the diabetic phenotype. *J Clin Invest*, Vol.96, No.4, pp.1802-1814, ISSN 0021-9738

Henegar, J.R., Bigler, S.A., Henegar, I.K., Tyagi, S.C., & Hall, J.E. (2001). Functional and structural changes in the kidney in the early stages of obesity. *J Am Soc Nephrol*, Vol.12, No.6, pp.1211–1217, ISSN 1046-6673

Hirata, A., Maeda, N., Hiuge, A., Hibuse, T., Fujita, K., Okada, T., Kihara, S., Funahashi, T., & Shimomura, I. (2009). Blockade of mineralocorticoid receptor reverses adipocyte dysfunction and insulin resistance in obese mice. *Cardiovasc Res*, Vol.84, No.1, pp.164-172, ISSN 0008-6363

Hotamisligil, G.S., Peraldi, P., Budavari, A., Ellis, R., White, M.F., & Spiegelman, B.M. (1996). IRS-1-mediated inhibition of insulin receptor tyrosine kinase activity in TNF-alpha- and obesity-induced insulin resistance. *Science*, Vol.271, No.5249, pp.665-668, ISSN 0036-8075

Hotamisligil, G.S., Shargill, N.S., & Spiegelman, B.M. (1993). Adipose expression of tumor necrosis factor-alpha: direct role in obesity-linked insulin resistance. *Science*, Vol.259, No.5091, pp.87-91, ISSN 0036-8075

Kadowaki, T., Yamauchi, T., & Kubota, N. (2008). The physiological and pathophysiological role of adiponectin and adiponectin receptors in the peripheral tissues and CNS. *FEBS Lett*, Vol.582, No.1, pp.74–80, ISSN 0014-5793

Kambham, N., Markowitz, G.S., Valeri, A.M., Lin, J., & D'Agati, V.D. (2001). Obesity-related glomerulopathy: an emerging epidemic. *Kidney Int*, Vol.59, No.4, pp.1498–1509, ISSN 0085-2538

Kamei, N., Tobe, K., Suzuki, R., Ohsugi, M., Watanabe, T., Kubota, N., Ohtsuka-Kowatari, N., Kumagai, K., Sakamoto, K., Kobayashi, M., *et al.* (2006). Overexpression of monocyte chemoattractant protein-1 in adipose tissues causes macrophage recruitment and insulin resistance. *J Biol Chem*, Vol.281, No.36, pp.26602-26614, ISSN 0021-9258

Kanamori, H., Matsubara, T., Mima, A., Sumi, E., Nagai, K., Takahashi, T., Abe, H., Iehara, N., Fukatsu, A., Okamoto, H., *et al.* (2007). Inhibition of MCP-1/CCR2 pathway ameliorates the development of diabetic nephropathy. *Biochem Biophys Res Commun*, Vol.360, No.4, pp.772-777, ISSN 0006-291X

Kanaya, A.M., Wassel, F.C., Vittinghoff, E., Havel, P.J., Cesari, M., Nicklas, B., Harris, T., Newman, A.B., Satterfield, S., & Cummings, S.R. (2006). Serum adiponectin and coronary heart disease risk in older Black and White Americans. *J Clin Endocrinol Metab*, Vol.91, No.12, pp. 5044–5050, ISSN 0021-972X

Kanda, H., Tateya, S., Tamori, Y., Kotani, K., Hiasa, K., Kitazawa, R., Kitazawa, S., Miyachi, H., Maeda, S., Egashira, K., *et al.* (2006). MCP-1 contributes to macrophage infiltration into adipose tissue, insulin resistance, and hepatic steatosis in obesity. *J Clin Invest*, Vol.116, No.6, pp. 1494-1505, ISSN 0021-9738

Kang, Y.S., Hyun, Y.Y., Cha, J.J., Lee, J.E., Kim, H.W., Han, K.H., Kim, H.K., Cha, D.R. (2010). Paricalcitol, Vitamin D analogue, ameliorated renal injury through an improvement of lipid metabolism and an anti-oxidative effect in diabetic nephropathy. *J Am Soc Nephrol*, Vol.21, pp.690A(abstract), ISSN 1046-6673

Kang, Y.S., & Cha, D.R. (2009). Aldosterone and diabetic kidney disease. *Curr Diab Rep*, Vol.9, No.6, pp.453-459, ISSN 1534-4827

Kang, Y.S., Ko, G.J., Lee, M.H., Song, H.K., Han, S.Y., Han, K.H., Kim, H.K., Han, J.Y., & Cha, D.R. (2009). Effect of eplerenone, enalapril and their combination treatment on diabetic nephropathy in type II diabetic rats. *Nephrol Dial Transplant*, Vol.24, No.1, pp.73-84, ISSN 0931-0509

Kang, Y.S., Lee, M.H., Song, H.K., Hyun, Y.Y., Cha, J.J., Ko, G.J., Kim, S.H., Lee, J.E., Han, J.Y., & Cha, D.R. (2011) Aliskiren improves insulin resistance and ameliorates diabetic vascular complications in db/db mice. *Nephrol Dial Transplant*, Vol.26,35 No.4, pp.1194-1204, ISSN 0931-0509 (2011a)

Kang, Y.S., Lee, M.H., Song, H.K., Ko, G.J., Kwon, O.S., Lim, T.K., Kim, S.H., Han, S.Y., Han, K.H., Lee, J.E., *et al.* (2010b). CCR2 antagonism improves insulin resistance, lipid metabolism, and diabetic nephropathy in type 2 diabetic mice. *Kidney Int*,Vol.78, No.9, pp.883-894, ISSN 0085-2538

Kang, Y.S., Song, H.K., Lee, M.H., Ko, G.J., & Cha, D.R. (2010c). Plasma concentration of visfatin is a new surrogate marker of systemic inflammation in type 2 diabetic patients. *Diabetes Res Clin Pract*, Vol.89, No.2, pp.141-149, ISSN 0168-8227

Kang, Y.S., Song, H.K., Lee, M.H., Ko, G.J., Han, J.Y., Han, S.Y., Han, K.H., Kim, H.K., & Cha, D.R. (2010d). Visfatin is upregulated in type-2 diabetic rats and targets renal cells. *Kidney Int*, Vol.78, No.2, pp.170-181, ISSN 0085-2538

Kato, S., Luyckx, V.A., Ots, M., Lee, K.W., Ziai, F., Troy, J.L., Brenner, B.M., & MacKenzie, H.S. (1999). Renin-angiotensin blockade lowers MCP-1 expression in diabetic rats. *Kidney Int*, Vol.56, No.3, pp.1037-1048, ISSN 0085-2538

Kim, H.Y., Hyun, Y.Y., Lee, J.E., Han, K.H., Kang, Y.S., Cha, D.R. (2010). Effect of mutual epididymal fat transplantation between db/db mice and db/m mice on urinary albumin excretion level. *J Am Soc Nephrol*, Vol.21, pp.695A(abstract), ISSN 1046-6673

Ko, G.J., Kang, Y.S., Han, S.Y., Lee, M.H., Song, H.K., Han, K.H., Kim, H.K., Han, J.Y., & Cha, D.R. (2008). Pioglitazone attenuates diabetic nephropathy through an anti-inflammatory mechanism in type 2 diabetic rats. *Nephrol Dial Transplant*, Vol.23, No.9, pp.2750-2760, ISSN 0931-0509

Kramer, H. (2006). Obesity and chronic kidney disease. *Contrib Nephrol*, Vol.151, pp.1-18, ISSN 0302-5144

Lee, M.H., Song, H.K., Ko, G.J., Kang, Y.S., Han, S.Y., Han, K.H., Kim, H.K., Han, J.Y., & Cha, D.R. (2008). Angiotensin receptor blockers improve insulin resistance in type 2 diabetic rats by modulating adipose tissue. *Kidney Int*, Vol.74, No.7, pp.890-900, ISSN 0085-2538

Konstantinides, G., Sch¨afer, K., Koschnick, S., & Loskutoff, D.J. (2001). Leptin-dependent platelet aggregation and arterial thrombosis suggests a mechanism for atherothrombotic disease in obesity. *J Clin Invest*, Vol.108, No.10., pp.1533-1540, ISSN 0021-9738

Laughlin, G.A., Barrett-Connor, E., May, S., & Lan-genberg, C. (2007). Association of adiponectin with coronary heart disease and mortality: The Rancho Bernardo study. *Am J Epidemiol*, Vol.165, No.2, pp.164–174, ISSN 0002-9262

Lopez-Bermejo, A., Chico-Julia, B., Fernandez-Balsells, M., Recasens, M., Esteve, E., Casamitjana, R., Ricart, W., & Fernandez-Real, J.M. (2006). Serum visfatin increases with progressive beta-cell deterioration. *Diabetes*, Vol.55, No.10, pp.2871-2875, ISSN 0012-1797

Maeda, N., Shimomura, I., Kishida, K., Nishizawa, H., Matsuda, M., Nagaretani, H., Furuyama, N., Kondo, H., Takahashi, M., Arita, Y., Komuro, R., Ouchi, N., Kihara, S., Tochino, Y., Okutomi, K., Horie, M., Takeda, S., Aoyama, T., Funahashi, T., & Matsuzawa, Y. (2002). Diet-induced insulin resistance in mice lacking adiponectin/ ACRP30. *Nat Med*, Vol.8, No.7, pp.731–737, ISSN 1078-8956

Mao, X., Kikani, C.K., Riojas, R.A., Langlais, P., Wang, I., Ramos, F.J., Fang, Q., Christ-Roberts, C.Y., Hong, J.Y., Kim, R.Y., Liu, F., & Dong, L.Q. (2006). APPL1 binds to adiponectin receptors and mediates adiponectin signaling and function. *Nat Cell Biol*, Vol.8, No.5, pp.516–523, ISSN 1465-7392

Mather, A., & Pollock, C. (2010). Renal glucose transporters: novel targets for hyperglycemia management. *Nat Rev Nephrol*, Vol.6, No.5, pp.307-311, ISSN 1795-5061

Mather, A., & Pollock, C. (2011). Glucose handling by the kidney. *Kidney Int*, Vol.79, Suppl 120, pp. S1-6, ISSN 0085-2538

Matsuzawa, Y. (2006). The metabolic syndrome and adipocytokines. *FEBS Lett*, Vol.580, No.12, pp.2917-2921, ISSN 0014-5793

Neumiller, J.J., White, J.R., Jr., & Campbell, R.K. (2010). Sodium-glucose co-transport inhibitors: progress and therapeutic potential in type 2 diabetes mellitus. *Drugs*, Vol.70, No.4, pp.377-385, ISSN 0012-6667

Ohashi, K., Iwatani, H., Kihara, S., Nakagawa, Y., Komura, N., Fujita, K., Maeda, N., Nishida, M., Katsube, F., Shimomura, I., Ito, T., & Funahashi, T. (2007). Exacerbation of albuminuria and renal fibrosis in subtotal renal ablation model of adiponectin-knockout mice. *Arterioscler Thromb Vasc Biol*, Vol.27, No.9, pp.1910–1917, ISSN 1049-8834

Prodjosudjadi, W., Gerritsma, J.S., van Es, L.A., Daha, M.R., & Bruijn, J.A. (1995). Monocyte chemoattractant protein-1 in normal and diseased human kidneys: an immunohistochemical analysis. *Clin Nephrol*, Vol.44, No.3, pp.148-155, ISSN 0301-0430

Ren, J. (2004). Leptin and hyperleptinemia—from friend to foe for cardiovascular function. *J Endocrinol*, Vol.181, No.1, pp.1–10, ISSN 0022-0795

Rubenstein, A.H., Mako, M.E., & Horwitz, D.L. (1975). Insulin and the kidney. *Nephron*, Vol.15, No.3-5, pp.306-326, ISSN 0028-2766

Sarafidis, P.A., & Ruilope, L.M. (2006). Insulin resistance, hyperinsulinemia, and renal injury: mechanisms and implications. *Am J Nephrol*, Vol.26, No.3, pp.232-244, ISSN 0250-8095

Scherer, P. (2006). Adipose tissue: From lipid storage compartment to endocrine organ. *Diabetes*, Vol.55, No.6, pp.1537–1545, ISSN 0012-1797

Schoolwerth, A.C., Smith, B.C., & Culpepper, R.M. (1988). Renal gluconeogenesis. *Miner Electrolyte Metab*, Vol.14, No.6, pp.347-361, ISSN 0378-0392

Sharma, K., Ramachandrarao, S., Qiu, G., Usui, H.K., Zhu, Y., Dunn, S.R., Ouedraogo, R., Hough, K., McCue, P., Chan, L., Falkner, B., & Goldstein, B.J. (2008). Adiponectin regulates albuminuria and podocyte function in mice. *J Clin Invest*, Vol.118, No.5, pp.1645–1656, ISSN 0021-9738

Sŏderberg, S., Ahr´en, B., Jansson, J.H., Johnson, O., Hallmans, G., Asplund, K., & Olsson, T. (1999). Leptin is associated with increased risk of myocardial infarction. *J Intern Med*, Vol.246, No.4, pp.409–418, ISSN 0954-6820

Song, H.K., Lee, M.H., Kang, Y.S., Ko, G.J., Kwon, O.S., Kim, S.H., Lee, J.E., Shin, J.H., Han, J.Y., Kim, H.K., Cha, D.R. (2008). Chronic administration of visfatin ameliorated diabetic nephropathy in db/db mice. *J Am Soc Nephrol*, Vol.19, pp.51A(abstract), ISSN 1046-6673

Song, H.K., Lee, M.H., Kim, B.K., Park, Y.G., Ko, G.J., Kang, Y.S., Han, J.Y., Han, S.Y., Han, K.H., Kim, H.K., *et al.* (2008). Visfatin: a new player in mesangial cell physiology and diabetic nephropathy. *Am J Physiol Renal Physiol*, Vol.295, No.5, pp.F1485-1494, ISSN 0363-6127

Sowers, J.R., Whaley-Connell, A., & Epstein, M. (2009). Narrative review: the emerging clinical implications of the role of aldosterone in the metabolic syndrome and resistant hypertension. *Ann Intern Med*, Vol.150, No.11, pp.776-783, ISSN 0003-4819

Stumvoll, M., Meyer, C., Mitrakou, A., Nadkarni, V., & Gerich, J.E. (1997). Renal glucose production and utilization: new aspects in humans. *Diabetologia*, Vol.40, No.7, pp.749-757, ISSN 0012-186X

Tamura, Y., Sugimoto, M., Murayama, T., Ueda, Y., Kanamori, H., Ono, K., Ariyasu, H., Akamizu, T., Kita, T., Yokode, M., *et al.* (2008). Inhibition of CCR2 ameliorates insulin resistance and hepatic steatosis in db/db mice. *Arterioscler Thromb Vasc Biol*, Vol.28, No.12, pp.2195-2201, ISSN 1049-8834

Tsioufis, C., Dimitriadis, K., Chatzis, D., Vasiliadou, C., Tousoulis, D., Papademetriou, V., Toutouzas, P., Stefanadis, C., & Kallikazaros, I. (2005). Relation of microalbuminuria to adiponectin and augmented C-reactive protein levels in men with essential hypertension. *Am J Cardiol*, Vol.96, No.7, pp.946-951, ISSN 0002-9149

Viedt, C., Vogel, J., Athanasiou, T., Shen, W., Orth, S.R., Kubler, W., & Kreuzer, J. (2002). Monocyte chemoattractant protein-1 induces proliferation and interleukin-6 production in human smooth muscle cells by differential activation of nuclear factor-kappaB and activator protein-1. *Arterioscler Thromb Vasc Biol*, Vol.22, No.6, pp.914-920, ISSN 1049-8834

Wada, T., Furuichi, K., Sakai, N., Iwata, Y., Yoshimoto, K., Shimizu, M., Takeda, S.I., Takasawa, K., Yoshimura, M., Kida, H., *et al.* (2000). Up-regulation of monocyte chemoattractant protein-1 in tubulointerstitial lesions of human diabetic nephropathy. *Kidney Int*, Vol.58, No.4, pp.1492-1499, ISSN 0085-2538

Weisberg, S.P., Hunter, D., Huber, R., Lemieux, J., Slaymaker, S., Vaddi, K., Charo, I., Leibel, R.L., & Ferrante, A.W., Jr. (2006). CCR2 modulates inflammatory and metabolic effects of high-fat feeding. *J Clin Invest*, Vol.116, No.1, pp.115-124, ISSN 0021-9738

Wellen, K.E., & Hotamisligil, G.S. (2003). Obesity-induced inflammatory changes in adipose tissue. *J Clin Invest*, Vol.112, No.12, pp.1785–1788, ISSN 0021-9738

Wolf, G., Chen, S., Han, D.C., & Ziyadeh, F.N. (2002). Leptin and renal disease. *Am J Kidney Dis*, Vol.39, No.1, pp.1-11, ISSN 0272-6386

Wolf, G., Hamann, A., Gan, D.C., Helmchen, U., Thaiss, F., Ziyadeh, F.N., & Stahl, A.K. (1999). Leptin stimulates proliferation and TGF-β expression in renal glomerular endothelial cells: potential role in glomerulosclerosis. *Kideny Int*, Vol.56, No.3, pp.860-872, ISSN 0085-2538

Wolf., G & Ziyadeh., F.N. (2006). Leptin and renal fibrosis. *Contrib Nephrol*, Vol.151, pp.175-183, ISSN 0302-5144

Yano, Y., Hoshide, S., Ishikawa, J., Hashimoto, T., Eguchi, K., Shimada, K., & Kario, K. (2007). Differential impacts of adiponectin on low-grade albuminuria between obese and nonobese persons without diabetes. *J Clin Hypertens (Greenwich)*,Vol.9, No.10, pp.775–782, ISSN 1524-6175

Yusuf, S., Sleight, P., Pogue, J., Bosch, J., Davies, R., & Dagenais, G. (2000). Effects of an angiotensin-converting-enzyme inhibitor, ramipril, on cardiovascular events in high-risk patients. The Heart Outcomes Prevention Evaluation Study Investigators. *N Engl J Med*, Vol.342, No.3, pp.145-153, ISSN 0028-4793

Zhang, Y., Proenca, R., Maffei, M., Barone, M., Leopold, L., & Friedman, J.M. (1994). Positional cloning of the mouse obese gene and its human homologue. *Nature*, Vol.372, No.6505, pp.425-432, ISSN 0028-0836

15

The Role of the Endocannabinoid System in the Pathogeny of Type 2 Diabetes

Robert Dinu[1], Simona Popa[2] and Maria Mota[3]
[1]*Resident Doctor, Department of Diabetes, Nutrition and Metabolic Diseases, Emergency Clinical County Hospital Craiova, PhD Student, University of Medicine and Pharmacy Craiova,*
[2]*University Assistant, MD, PhD, Department of Diabetes, Nutrition and Metabolic Diseases, University of Medicine and Pharmacy Craiova,*
[3]*Professor, MD, PhD, Department of Diabetes, Nutrition and Metabolic Diseases, University of Medicine and Pharmacy Craiova, Romania*

1. Introduction

Diabetes mellitus is characterized by chronic hyperglycemia with disturbances of carbohydrate, fat, and protein metabolism resulting from defects in insulin secretion, insulin action, or both (Bennett & Knowler, 2005). The pathophysiology of type 2 diabetes mellitus (T2DM) includes three mechanisms: insulin deficiency due to insufficient pancreatic insulin production, excessive hepatic glucose release and insulinresistance in peripheral tissues and liver (Gurber, 2010).

Usually, T2DM is associated with a cluster of cardiovascular and metabolic risks including obesity (especially abdominal obesity), decreased levels of high-density lipoprotein cholesterol (HDL), high levels of triglycerides, elevated blood pressure and silent inflammation and diabetes itself is considered to be a cardiovascular disease risk equivalent (Task Force on Diabetes and Cardiovascular Diseases of the European Society of Cardiology and the European Society for the Study of Diabetes, 2007). Taking into account the fact that T2DM is associated with obesity and excess fat accumulation may be the main cause of T2DM, one can evaluate the role of the endocannabinoid system (ECS) assessing (1) its role in the pathogeny of obesity and (2) the role of ECS on hyperglycemia; this last part can be split in (a) the implication of ECS on insulin resistance and (b) its effects on insulin release.

2. The endocannabinoid system

ECS is a very important physiological system involved in appetite stimulation, food intake and energy balance. Besides its metabolic functions, the ECS has also implications upon individual behavior, regarding preferences for sweets or fats, different substances abuses etc.

2.1 The endocannabinoid system – a historical perspective

The history of the discovery of the endocannabinoid system is connected to the history of the human use of the cannabis. A special note is to be mentioned: at first there were discovered the exogenous substances that activate this system and then the receptors and finally the endogenous ligands of this system were described. The first evidence about human use of the plant *Cannabis sativa* comes from fragments of pottery from China almost 10,000 years BC. These fragments appear to have some imprints of a plant that is considered to be hemp. Other proofs come from the cloths found in the Chinese burial chambers of the Chou dynasty (1122-265 BC). Therefore, the first use of cannabis appears to be for the manufacture of cloths, ropes and nets. The first description of the therapeutical effect of cannabis are from the Chinese pharmacopoeia Pen-ts'ao, ca. 1-2 century AD (Iversen, 2000). Nevertheless, it was only in 1964 when Gaoni and Mechoulam described the structure of delta-9-tetrahydrocannabinol (Δ^9-THC), the main psychoactive substance found in the cannabis plant (Howlett et al., 2004).

The next step was the identification of specific sites for the action of Δ^9-THC. In 1990, Matsuda et al. cloned the CB1 receptor, the main receptor for THC binding (Di Marzo, 2006). It was obvious that human body did not create cell receptors for exogenous substances only, therefore the endogenous ones had to be found. In 1992, Mechoulam and Pertwee discovered the first CB1 receptor agonist, anandamide, and they proved its THC-like functions. In 1993, Munro et al. cloned the CB2 receptor and two years later Mechoulam et al. and Waku et al. independently identified the second endogenous agonist of the cannabinoid receptors, 2-arachidonoyglycerol (2-AG). In the same year, Vicenzo di Marzo named these endogenous substances "endocannabinoids", after the name given to endorphins and the name given to the entire system derived from here (Di Marzo, 2006).

2.2 The structure of the endocannabinoid system

ECS is composed of cannabinoid receptors CB1 and CB2, their endogenous ligands and the enzymes which mediate endogenous ligands' biosynthesis and degradation (Lutz, 2002).

2.2.1 The cannabinoid receptors

There were identified two types of cannabinoid receptors until now. CNR1 represents the gene coding CB1 and it is localized at 6q14-q15 level. There is a significant similitude between the human CB1 and the one identified in rats or in mice and CB1 receptors were cloned in other species including fish and invertebrates. This receptor has 472 aminoacids and it is a G-protein coupled receptor with seven trans-membrane domains (Demuth & Molleman, 2006).

CB1 receptors are expressed mainly in the brain, but also in other organs involved in energetic homeostasis: adipose tissue, liver, gastrointestinal tract, pancreas and skeletal muscle. There are several endogenous agonists of the cannabinoid receptors, anandamide (N-arachidonylethanolamine) and 2-arachidonoylglycerol (2-AG) being the two main important molecules (Demuth & Molleman, 2006).

ECS is considered to link emotional response to stress with appetite and energy balance and it functions like an after stress recovery system which remains inactive in repose physiologic conditions. Activation of the central CB1 receptors is believed to modulate satiety and increase sensitivity to rewarding stimuli, including food (Eggan & Lewis, 2007). On the other hand, activation of CB1 receptors in the adipose tissue and in the liver can regulate metabolism and lipids storage (Jbilo et al., 2005).

The gene of the CB2 receptor is located on gene 1 at p36.11 level and it codes for a protein with 360 aminoacids. It is involved mainly in immunomodulation and its polymorphisms have been associated with autoimmune diseases (Sipe et al., 2005) but also with osteoporosis.

Beside the two cannabinoid receptors, there are other possible targets for the cannabinoids: vanilloid receptors (*transient receptor potential vanilloid type 1 – TRPV1*), subtypes of CB1 receptor, CB2-like receptors and possibly other non-CB1, non-CB2, non-TRPV1 receptors that can interact with the cannabinoids (Pertwee, 2005).

2.2.2 The endocannabinoids and the cannabinoid receptor agonists

After the discovery of the two types of cannabinoid receptors the subsequent research focused on the isolation of the main endogenous substances that interact with these substrates. In 1993, anandamide was discovered followed soon after by the isolation of the 2-arachidonoylglycerol (2-AG) the endogenous compound with the most important cannabinoid receptor agonist activity (Lutz, 2002). After their isolation, it was noticed that the two substances were synthesized from the cell membrane-derived phospholipids and due to their lipophilic structure (Fig. 1), they are not needed to be stored in vesicles like other mediators. Anandamide has many biological *in vivo* and *in vitro* functions such as the activation numerous kinases like p38 mitogen-activated protein kinaze (p38 MAPK), c-Jun N-terminal kinase (JNK), protein kinase B, the stimulation of arachidonic acid release, appetite stimulation, memory inhibition, pain modulation, vasodilatation, blood pressure decrease and neuroprotection (Onaivi et al., 2005).

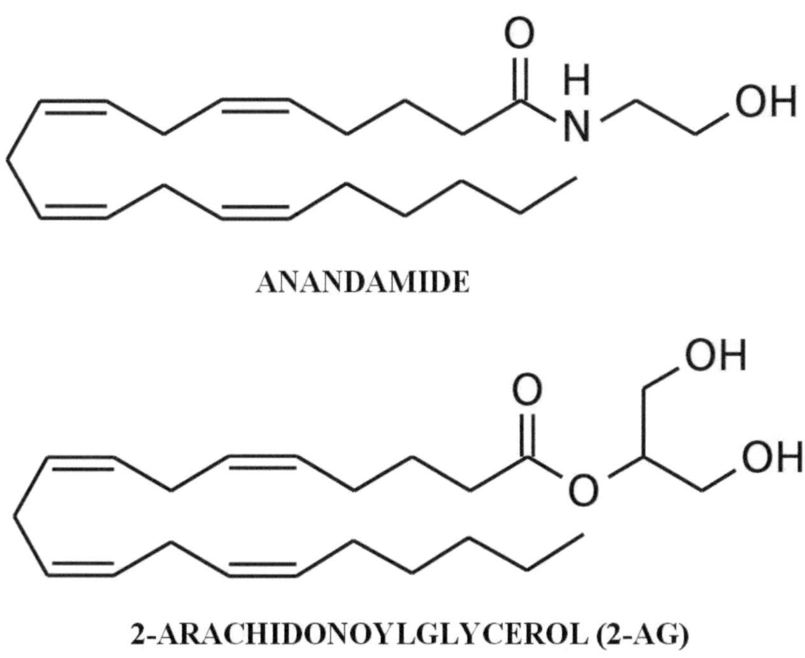

Fig. 1. The structure of anandamide and 2-AG (adapted from Doyle, 2011)

Like anandamide, 2-AG has been found in various concentrations in the brain depending on the studied area, age, physiological and pathological conditions. 2-AG has a reduced binding activity compared to anandamide but it acts on both cannabinoid receptors and only on them. This is why some consider it as the only endogenous agonist of the ECS.
Among the two substances, other products have been described as acting on the cannabinoid receptors. Oleamide, noladin ether (2-arachidonyl glyceryl ether), virodhamine and N-arachidonoyl-dopamine (NADA) can bind to one of the cannabinoid receptors. Their role in the physiology and physiopathology of the ECS has to be determined.

2.2.3 The metabolism of the endocannabinoids

The metabolic pathways of the two best described substances have many common features. Both compounds derive from the enzymatic hydrolysis of the products derived from the membrane phospholipids. Both substances are released and then taken back into the cell by diffusion and they are inactivated by intracellular hydrolysis. There are also some differences between the metabolic pathways of the two substances and this explains why the levels of these substances can vary depending on different physiological conditions (Pertwee, 2005).
The life cycle of the endogenous cannabinoids is different from the one of the other endogenous ligands. Neither anandamide, nor 2-AG is held in vesicles, but they are synthesized "on demand" following the Ca^{2+} influx that determines the activation of the Ca^{2+}-dependent biosynthetic enzymes (Di Marzo et al., 1998). It was shown that endocannabinoids are retrograde signaling molecules that suppress GABA release from presynaptic terminals following depolarization of a hippocampal CA1 pyramidal neuron. This process is known as depolarization-induced suppression of inhibition (DSI) (Wilson & Nicoll, 2001). The synthesis of endocannabinoids is not well understood. The enzymes that mediate this process are still being characterized and it is not possible to localize it to a particular subcellular compartment. Some studies indicate that the endocannabinoids are released from neuronal somata and dendrites (Egertova et al., 1998). Soon after their synthesis in the postsynaptic cell, the endogenous cannabinoids are secreted by simple diffusion or passive (energy-independent) carrier proteins may be required. Afterwards, they bind within the binding site crevice formed by the seven transmembrane helices of CB1 receptor of the presynaptic neuron (Fig. 2). The subsequent activation of CB1 by endocannabinoids results in the inhibition of Ca^{2+} channels in the presynaptic cell. Because the release of cationic neurotransmitters from vesicles (in the presynaptic cell) is Ca^{2+}-dependent, activation of CB1 results in the suppression of neurotransmitter release (Onaivi et al., 2005).
Little is known also about the subsequent events following receptor interaction. It has been proposed that endocannabinoids are released into the extracellular space and then transported by a specific transport protein on both neurons and glia that mediate endocannabinoid uptake (Piomelli et al., 1998). It has also been shown that an antagonist of this transporter, AM404, potentiates the effect of exogenous anadamide on cultured neurons. After being transported into the cell, anadamide is subsequently broken down into arachidonic acid and ethanolamine by a membrane-bound enzyme called fatty acid amide hydrolase (FAAH) (Di Marzo et al., 1998; Piomelli et al., 1998) that is localized to the endoplasmic reticulum (Fig. 3). An alternative mechanism proposed by Deutsch et al. is that anandamide uptake after receptor interaction is a process of simple diffusion (Glaser et al., 2003). The same authors indicated that transport inhibitors such as AM404 are actually inhibitors of FAAH *in vitro*. The mechanism of action for 2-AG appears to be similar.

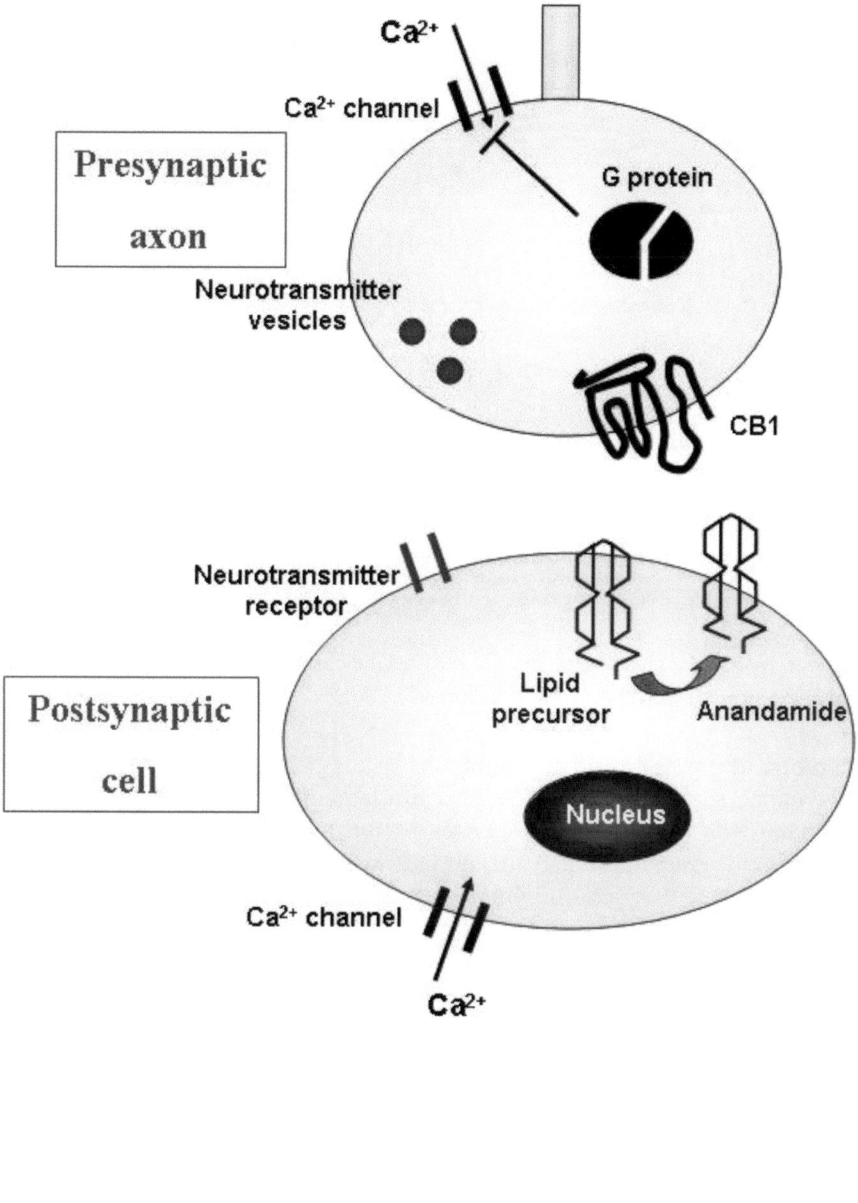

Fig. 2. The mechanism of action of anandamide

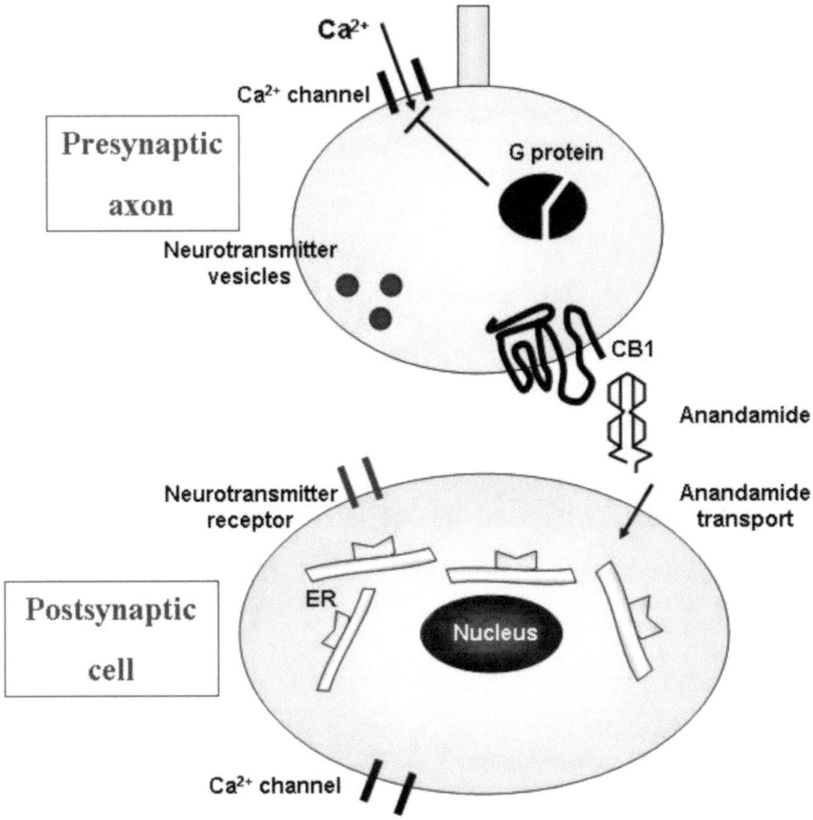

Fig. 3. The uptake and degradation of anandamide

2.2.4 The biology of cannabinoid signaling

Retrograde synaptic signaling is considered a fundamental feature of the nervous system and endocannabinoids are one of the classes of retrograde messengers involved in the regulation of synaptic transmission. Thus, endocannabinoids mediate the rapid retrograde suppression of both excitatory and inhibitory synapses. Functionally, endocannabinoids are released from depolarized postsynaptic neurons in a calcium-dependent manner and act retrogradely onto presynaptic CB receptors to suppress neurotransmitter release.

CB1 and CB2 receptors are coupled with G protein, negatively to adenylate cyclase and positively to mitogen-activated PK. CB1R couples to the G protein signal transduction pathways in presynaptic nerve terminals and transduces the cannabinoid stimulation of MAP kinase and the inhibition of adenylate cyclase, thereby attenuating the production of cyclic AMP. CB1Rs are also coupled to ion channels through G proteins, positively to A-type and inwardly rectifying potassium channels, and negatively to N-type and P/Q-type calcium channels and to D-type potassium channels (Howlett and Mukhopadhyay, 2000). The quantity of cAMP decreases and cAMP-dependent PK (PKA) is inhibited by CB1R activation. In the absence of cannabinoids, PKA phosphorylates the potassium channel protein and exerts decreased outward potassium current. In the presence of cannabinoids the phosphorylation of the channel by PKA is reduced, which increases the outward potassium current. Moreover, cannabinoids can close sodium channels, but whether or not this effect is receptor mediated has yet to be established. Other cellular responses triggered with CB1 receptor activation include other PK pathways such as the p38 MAKP, JUN N-terminal kinase, (JNK), focal adhesion kinase (FAK), and phosphoinositide-3 kinase (Akt) signaling, which might mediate effects on apoptosis (Molina-Holgado et al., 2002).

Acting on ion channels, the endocannabinoids mediate the rapid retrograde suppression of both excitatory and inhibitory synapses. Functionally, they are released from depolarized postsynaptic neurons in a calcium-dependent manner and act retrogradely onto presynaptic CBRs to suppress neurotransmitter release.

3. The role of ECS in obesity

The pathophysiological role of ECS has been documented on numerous studies involving animal models and also humans. Some of the animals used in the studies developed obesity as a result of leptin gene or leptin receptor gene mutations and others presented diet-induced obesity (DIO). These are the two main representative types of obesity: genetic or diet-induced.

It has been described that ECS plays an important role in the regulation o food intake by homeostatic and non-homeostatic (or hedonic) energy regulation pathways (Matias et al., 2008).

It was noticed that hypothalamic levels of endocannabinoids were increased in all models of leptin deficiency or defective leptin receptors signaling. This study proved the negative regulation of endocannabinoids by leptin. Moreover, leptin treatment for these mice leads to an important reduction of endocannabinoids levels (Engeli, 2008). It was also proved that hypothalamic endocannabinoid levels are decreased after systemic leptin administration in rats, and increased in rodent models of congenital hyperphagia and obesity, such as db / db mice and Zucker rats, where leptin signalling is defective, as well as in ob / ob mice, where leptin biosynthesis is defective and exogenous leptin can restore the normal (low) levels of endocannabinoids.

DIO also has an impact on ECS regulation. There were found increased levels of anandamide after feeding piglets a diet enriched in long-chain polyunsaturated fatty acids (LC-PUFA) like arachidonic acid and docosahexaenoic acid (DHA). These models also presented CB1 receptor downregulation in hypothalamus and the authors explained it as a result of increased levels of anandamide and 2-AG in extra-hypothalamic regions. Lower CB1 density was correlated with cumulative energy intake from the palatable, fat-enriched diet. In contrast, a fish-oil diet was associated with reduced 2-AG levels in the brain (Engeli, 2008).

After food deprivation, endocannabinoids act on CB1 receptors stimulating the central orexigenic system in the hypothalamus, therefore, controlling the homeostatic regulation of food imbalance (Di Marzo et al., 2001). Besides that, ECS may stimulate food intake by reinforcing the motivational processes involving the nucleus accumbens (Matias et al., 2008). Endocannabinoids, directly injected in the hypothalamus or the nucleus accumbens, can induce food-intake in satiated animals (Cota et al., 2006). Therefore, it appears that the ECS participates in the orexigenic hypothalamic network regulated by leptin. Moreover, CB1 receptors are distributed in the hypothalamus in a way suggesting that they regulate directly the expression of orexigenic signals such as agouti-related protein (AGRP), orexins and melanocyte-concentrating hormone (MCH) or anorexic signals such as those produced from pro-opiomelanocortin (POMC) and the cocaine-and amphetamine-regulated transcript (CART) (Cota et al., 2003).

The ECS is implicated in adipose tissue homeostasis also directly via CB1 receptors located in adipocytes. Cota et al. were the first that suggested the implication of ECS in energy balance regulation by acting directly on peripheral CB1 receptors (Cota et al., 2003). Many researchers started their work to discover the peripheral mode of action of the ECS as a system that reduces energy expenditure and directs energy balance towards energy storage into the adipose tissue. Other organs involved in the process of energy storage are the liver, the skeletal muscle and the pancreas. It is well known that dietary triglycerides are transported to the liver from the intestine via chylomicrons. In addition, hepatic triglyceride synthesis from fatty acids and glycerol takes place under the influence of insulin produced by the pancreas in the postprandial state. Triglycerides are then secreted into blood as very low density lipoproteins (VLDL) that go either to the adipose tissue to be store as re-esterified triglycerides, or are metabolized into fatty acids that will be used as energy source after mitochondrial β-oxidation. Another major energy source in the body is represented by the oxidisable glucose in the skeletal muscle. The muscle will contribute to energy balance also by regulating the circulating levels of nutrients, and in particular of glucose, which can also be transformed into fatty acid precursors in the adipose tissue and the liver.

Several studies demonstrated the presence of endocannabinoid receptors in both animal and human adipose tissue. CB1 receptors are present in white adipose tissue and coupled to stimulation of lipoprotein lipase. These findings suggested that the ECS tonically contributes to fat accumulation, independently from the amount of food ingested and by acting directly on the adipose tissue. Studies carried out in the mouse 3T3 adipocyte cell lines showed that the blockade of CB1 receptors arrests adipocyte proliferation (Gary-Bobo et al., 2006), suggesting that endocannabinoids might stimulate proliferation. Moreover the formation of endocannabinoids precedes pre-adipocyte differentiation into mature adipocytes and chronic stimulation of CB1 receptors during adipocyte differentiation accelerates the appearance of an early marker of differentiation, peroxisome proliferator- activated receptor-γ (PPAR-γ), while inducing accumulation of lipid droplets (Matias et al., 2006). Cota *et al.* showed that CB1 receptor null mice exhibited significantly lower amounts of fat mass and higher amount of lean mass than wild-type mice even when fed with the same amount of food (Matias et al., 2008). Also, CB1 receptor protein expression increased with increasing adipocyte size and adiposity while exercise training inhibited these receptors and the peroxisome proliferators-activated receptor-δ (PPARδ). PPARδ tonically inhibits the expression of CB1 in a mouse clonal adipocyte cell line (Yan et al., 2007). When speaking of human studies, one study showed increased levels of anandamide and 2-AG in the plasma of menopausal obese women when compared with lean women of the same age (Engeli, 2008). Anandamide and 2-AG were increased in plasma of obese subjects with diabetes too. In a study that compared lean and obese men and women with either subcutaneous or visceral adipose tissue accumulation, 2-AG plasma levels were clearly correlated with visceral adipose tissue mass and the group with subcutaneous adipose tissue did not differ from the lean control group with regard to 2-AG plasma concentration (Bluher et al., 2006). The same study indicated that women had higher anandamide plasma levels than men, but no relationship with obesity or body fat distribution was found. Another study to support these findings was performed in 62 men and the subjects in the highest tertile of 2-AG levels presented with markedly increased visceral adipose tissue mass despite having almost the same body mass index as those in the lower two tertiles of plasma 2-AG. On the other hand, anandamide was negatively correlated with visceral fat mass (Cote et al., 2007). Both studies showed that increased plasma 2-AG correlates with markers of metabolic syndrome (such as free fatty acids, triglycerides, HDL cholesterol, adiponectin), and is associated with decreased insulin sensitivity and enhanced glucose and insulin responses during an oral glucose load.

While the role of the brown adipose tissue in humans is less clear, it is known that it importantly contributes to thermogenesis and energy expenditure in small mammals. CB1 receptors are also present in mouse brown adipocytes (Perwitz et al., 2006) and the endocannabinoids might, therefore, regulate thermogenesis in this tissue. It has been demonstrated that CB1 inhibits the uncoupling protein-1 (UCP-1), a thermogenic, mitochondrial, proton translocating membrane protein (Perwitz et al., 2006).

Another mechanism may involve adiponectin, which is a cytokine that reduces the circulating levels of free fatty acids by inhibiting lipid storage stimulating fatty acid oxidation. It was proved that stimulation of CB1 receptors inhibits adiponectin expression in mature adipocyte while their blockade was associated with increased adiponectin expression (Matias et al., 2008). It is possible for CB1 receptors to induce lipogenesis by inhibition of cAMP formation. Matias et al. (Matias et al. 2006) found that, in mature adipocytes, a CB1 receptor agonist inhibited cAMP formation in a way that was significantly attenuated by CB1 receptor antagonists but not by a CB2 receptor antagonist. Inhibition of cAMP and, subsequently, protein kinase A (PKA) might stimulate lipogenesis by inhibiting the AMP-activated protein kinase (AMPK). This enzyme is stimulated by PKA-mediated phosphorylation and plays a key role in energy metabolism because it reduces fatty acid synthesis and stimulates fatty acid β-oxidation in several tissues. Interestingly, other studies demonstrated that Δ9- THC decreases AMPK phosphorylation both in subcutaneous and, particularly, visceral adipose tissue (Kola et al., 2005). Because adiponectin stimulates AMPK activity, the CB1-mediated inhibition of adiponectin expression in adipocytes might reinforce this effect (Matias et al. 2006).

Another way for ECS-enhanced lipogenesis in adipocytes might be through their ability to stimulate glucose uptake by these cells via the enhancement of both basal and insulin-induced translocation to the plasma membrane of the glucose transporter 4 (GLUT4) (Gasperi et al., 2007; Pagano et al., 2007). In mouse adipocytes this effect seems to be mediated by CB1-induced stimulation of nitric oxide synthesis (Gasperi et al., 2007), while in human adipocytes CB1 activates the phosphatidylinositol-3-kinase cascade (Pagano et al., 2007). Increased glucose uptake and, subsequently, glycolysis might be the way for *de novo* fatty acid biosynthesis, and this effect might underlie part of the pro-lipogenetic effect of CB1 receptor agonists in these cells (Matias et al., 2008).

A few studies tried to determine the effect of weight loss on ECS in obese subjects (Engeli et al., 2005, Engeli et al., 2008). Unfortunately, in all these studies, circulating anandamide and 2-AG, CB1 and FAAH gene expression in subcutaneous abdominal adipose tissue, were not influenced by weight loss, although metabolic parameters such as fasting insulin and blood pressure were significantly decreased as surrogates of successful therapy. The authors explained that weight loss might not have been large or fast enough and that, probably with a more rigid protocol, an influence on the ECS might have been seen. If weight loss does not influence the ECS in obese subjects, an alternative hypothesis is that genetic modifications could be the cause of dysregulation of the ECS in obesity.

There were several studies concerning the mutations of the CNR1 gene that encodes CB1 receptor. Russo et al. analyzed two variants of exon 4 of CNR1, scanning the gene for

polymorphisms rs12720071 (3813A/G) and rs806368 (4895A/G), in a study carried out on a group of European men. The results indicated that allele 3813G was associated with the growth of abdominal circumference (AC), subscapular cutaneous skinfold and body mass index (BMI). There have been observed no associations between rs806368 polymorphism and the determined variables. The haplotype's analysis consisted in the studying of 3 frequent haplotypes: A3813A4895 (AA), A3813G4895 (AG) and G3813G4895 (GG), haplotype GG being associated with the increase of the abdominal circumference and subscapular cutaneous skinfold (Russo et al., 2007).
The polymorphism rs1049353 (1422A/G) was associated in men with a significant increase of the abdominal circumference, waist to hip ratio and of adipose mass after the adjustment for age and BMI. Adipose mass percent was also associated with this polymorphism but the association disappeared after the adjustment for age and BMI (Peters et al., 2007). Another study carried out on Swedish and Danish subjects indicated that polymorphisms rs806381, rs2023239, rs6454674 and rs10485170 associated with an increased BMI (Benzinou et al., 2008).

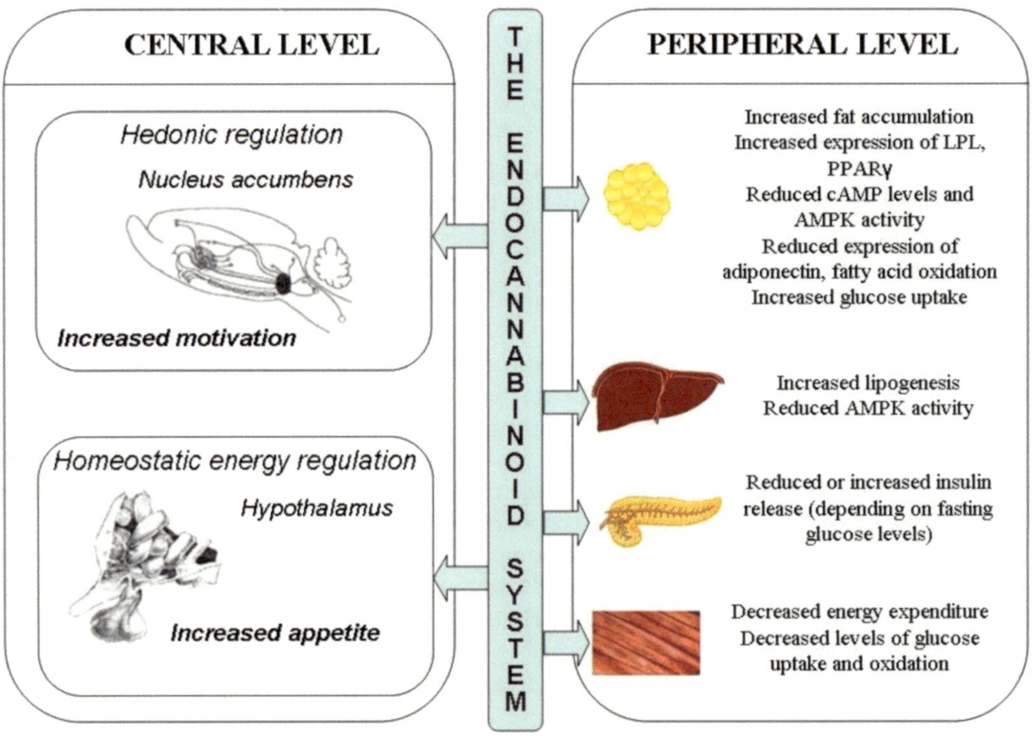

Fig. 4. The role of ECS in energy balance (adapted after Matias et al., 2008).

Muller et al. studied 8 polymorphisms in German children and adolescents: in region 5' (rs9353527, rs754387, rs6454676), in intron 2 (rs806379, rs1535255), exon 3 (rs2023239), intron 3 (rs806370) and in coding region (rs1049353), but they couldn't find any association with obesity (Muller et al., 2007).
Probably the most important proofs, that ECS is involved in obesity, come from the studies using selective CB1 receptors antagonists such as Rimonabant, where a significant reduction

of body fat was noticed. The Rimonabant in Obesity (RIO) study indicated that 1 year treatment with selective CB1 receptor antagonist, rimonabant 20mg, significantly reduced weight and abdominal circumference compared with diet and lifestyle therapy alone (Di Marzo et al., 2008). The figure 4 describes the ways by which ECS controls the energy balance.

4. The role of ECS in insulin sensitive organs

Adipose tissue. It is well known that adipose tissue is, beside the major energy depot, a very important source of adipokines that play a major role in insulin sensitivity and glucose homeostasis and the role of the ECS in modulating the adipose tissue was already discussed. Adiponectin is one of the adipokines involved in free fatty acid oxidation and hyperglycemia improvement (Kadowaki et al., 2006). It was already mentioned that overactivation of ECS is associated with low adiponectin levels and dysregulation of the adipose tissue.

Liver. Activation of CB1 receptors in mice leads to increased de novo fatty acid synthesis. One of the studies concerning the role of the ECS in the liver demonstrated, in rat hepatocytes, that anandamide inhibits acetyl-CoA-carboxylase activity leading to inhibition of de novo fatty acid synthesis. Furthermore, fatty acid oxidation was found to be increased since carnitine palmitoyltransferase-1 and the rate of ketogenesis from palmitate were stimulated by anandamde. Both effects on fatty acid synthesis and oxidation were prevented by an inhibitor of the anandamide enzymatic hydrolysis via FAAH (Guzman et al., 1995). This study, that presents the role of arachidonic acid originating from anandamide in stimulating the oxidation of fatty acids and inhibiting their synthesis, is of a great importance.

Activation of CB1 receptors in the liver also affects fatty acid homeostasis: CB1 receptors are expressed in hepatocytes, mainly around the centrilobular vein, and CB1-/- mice exhibit lower expression of the important transcription factor SREBP-1c that is implicated in the regulation of fatty acid synthesis (Osei-Hyiaman et al., 2005). Activation of CB1 receptors in the liver enhances the expression of SREBP-1c and of its targets. These effects may explain the stimulatory effect of a CB1 receptor agonist on fatty acid synthesis and lipogenesis in these cells. Measurement of the fatty acids production in the liver after pretreatment of mice with a cannabinoid receptor agonist indicated a twofold increase of fatty acid synthesis (Osei-Hyiaman et al., 2005). An increase of fatty acids synthesis was also noticed in hepatocytes isolated from mice and treated with tge same CB1 agonist. The increase in fatty acids synthesis was found neither in the liver nor in isolated hepatocytes from mice pretreated with rimonabant or CB1 receptor knockout (CB1-/-) mice. These mechanisms explain the lipogenetic action of CB1 receptors in these cells.

A great observation was that CB1-/- mice, unlike their wild-type littermates, do not develop hepatic steatosis after several weeks of a high-fat diet, a condition that leads to up-regulation of both hepatic anandamide and CB1 expression levels and down-regulation of FAAH.

In conclusion, the possible mechanism explaining the role of the ECS in the liver is the following: under normal energy homeostatic conditions, the low levels of CB1 receptors and high levels of FAAH increase the arachidonic-acid-mediated stimulation of fatty acid oxidation by anandamide. After several weeks of a high-fat diet the reduction of FAAH activity and the enhancement of CB1 receptors favour instead anandamide and CB1-

mediated hepatic lipogenesis (Matias et al., 2008). It is possible for the endocannabinoids to exert a function on glucose homeostasis in the liver also in healthy animals, because a CB1 receptor blocker was proven to stimulate glycogenolysis in liver in lean normoglycemic rats (Herling et al., 2007).

As it was mentioned, ECS might contribute o the development of diet induced obesity, which is found to be associated with an increase in the hepatic levels of the endocannabinoid anandamide and CB1-mediated fatty acid synthesis in mice (Nogueiras et al., 2008).

Muscle. One of the evidences of the involvement of the ECS in energy expenditure at the level of the skeletal muscle came from the observation that blood anandamide levels were significantly elevated in runners and cyclists but not in sedentary controls following 1h of moderate intensity exercise (Sparling et al., 2003). Other studies indicated that CB1 receptor knockout mice had higher energy expenditure, probably due to the energy combustion produced by fat or carbohydrate oxidation. Recent studies demonstrated that administration of a CB1 receptor antagonist increased energy expenditure in rats. A study about the chronic administration of rimonabant showed enhanced glucose uptake and oxidation by the isolated soleus muscle of genetically obese mice (Liu et al., 2005). Moreover, another study indicated that the very low density of CB1 receptors in the mouse soleus muscle increases when the animals are kept on a high-fat diet (Pagotto et al., 2006). Another study that dealed with the effect of a CB1 receptor antagonist AM251 in an in vitro model of skeletal muscle, indicated that this one increases the expression of AMPKα1 and decreases that of the pyruvate dehydrogenase kinase-(PDK)4 (Cavuoto et al., 2007). More importantly, anandamide blocked only the effect of AM251 on the expression of AMPKα1, and not that on PDK4, suggesting that only the former effect, and the subsequent likely activation of lipolysis and fatty acid oxidation, of the CB1 receptor antagonist is CB1 receptor-mediated.

PDK4 is known as an important inhibitor of the pyruvate dehydrogenase complex, which links glycolysis to ATP production and to the Krebs cycle and its inhibition by AM251 might stimulate glucose flux into the mitochondria and cause an increase of glucose oxidation in the muscle. The opposite is expected to occur with endocannabinoids (Cavuoto et al., 2007).

In leptin-deficient mice that exhibit hyperglycemia and insulinresistance, treatment with selective CB1 receptors antagonists increased basal oxygen consumption and glucose uptake in isolated soleus muscle preparations (Liu et al., 2005).

5. The ECS in the pancreas

Several findings suggest that ECS in involved not only in glucose uptake but also in the control of insulin levels. In pancreatic islets from mice, it was noticed that CB1 receptors are mainly expressed in non-β cells whereas CB2 are expressed in both β and non-β (Juan-Pico et al., 2006). There were seen differences between mice and rats, while in rats and humans both CB1 and CB2 receptors were noticed in both α- and β-cells (Matias et al., 2008; Di Marzo, 2008).

Juan-Pico et al. (Juan-Pico et al., 2006) observed co-localization of CB1 receptors with glucagons predominantly but some co-staining with insulin was also noticed particularly in human islets. Nakata and Yada (Nakata & Yada, 2008) observed co-localization of CB1 receptor with insulin in some but not all β-cells in mouse islets. Another study of Starowicz et al. indicated that CB1 receptors are highly co-expressed with glucagon in both mice and rats with a wider distribution of the CB2R throughout more of the islet cell types (Starowicz et al., 2008). On the other hand, Li et al. (Li et al., 2010a) showed co-expression of both CB1 and CB2 receptors with insulin but not with glucagons expressing cells in the mouse. A possible explanation for all these contrasting results came from a recent publication that proved that many commercial CB1 receptor antibodies exhibit nonspecific interactions (Grimsey et al., 2008).

There is evidence for the expression in the pancreatic islet of all the molecules requested for the synthesis and degradation of the endocannabinoids (Bermudez-Silva et al., 2008). In conditions of hyperglycemia, over-expression of biosynthetic endocannabinoid enzymes and low levels of degrading enzymes was noticed.

In insulinoma cell lines from rats and also humans islets there were noticed increased levels of the endocannabinoids in response to glucose stimulation (Bermudez-Silva et al., 2008). It is known that β-cells are depolarized and they release of calcium in response to glucose-stimulated insulin release. Therefore, the increased calcium levels stimulate their synthesis in the β-cells.

Two studies (Juan-Pico et al., 2006; Nakata & Yada, 2008) observed a decrease in the amplitude of glucose-induced calcium oscillations in mouse islets in response to treatment with 2-AG (10mmol/l) and anandamide (1mmol/l). A decrease in calcium oscillations would be expected to adversely affect insulin secretion. Juan-Pico et al. noticed a 30% reduction in static insulin secretion by the endocannabinoids and Nakata and Yada observed a concentration-dependent inhibition of insulin release by AEA (1–10mmol/l) in mouse islets. Moreover, Nakata and Yada also noticed a decrease in glucose-induced calcium oscillations and insulin secretion in response to a more specific CB1 receptor agonist. The same authors also showed that a general CB1/CB2 receptor agonist and a specific CB1 receptor agonist, arachidonyl-2-chloroethylamide (ACEA) (100 nmol/l) significantly decreased insulin secretion from mouse islets. All these initial in-vitro experiments in rodents indicate that endocannabinoids and CB1 receptor agonists have deleterious effects on insulin secretion.

Li et al. (Li et al., 2010a,b) showed that treatment with ACEA (10mmol/l) decreased cAMP production in a mouse clonal β-cell and mouse islets. However this same group showed a concurrent increase in calcium levels in, and insulin secretion from, mouse b-cells in response to these cannabinoid receptor agonists in the presence of glucose (Doyle, 2011).

The apparent contradiction to the previous published results and to the fact that cAMP and calcium oscillations following glucose-stimulated insulin secretion are highly interdependent and amplify each other (Ni et al., 2011) was explained by the same author by stating that the stimulatory effect of cannabinoid receptor agonism on intracellular calcium levels overrides the inhibitory effect on cAMP production (Doyle, 2011).

Because ECS appears to modulate glucose homeostasis in both glucose dependent insulin release and glucose uptake from tissues pathways, studies to evaluate the glucose homeostasis *in vivo* were performed. Systemic stimulation of CB1 receptors in lean normoglycemic rats determined slower blood glucose clearance while activation of CB2 receptors improved glucose clearance (Matias et al., 2008).

When anandamide or ACEA were administered acutely to Wistar rats prior to a glucose tolerance test, the rats developed severe glucose intolerance (Bermudez-Silva, 2006). The effect was reversed by the CB1 receptor antagonist AM251, suggesting direct effect on glucose tolerance through this receptor. In this study, the authors did not measure insulin secreted during the glucose tolerance test so it can not be estimated the direct effect on insulin secretion (Doyle, 2011). In another study, they examined glucose tolerance in response to specific CB1 and CB2 receptors agonists and antagonists and they confirmed the specific effect of the CB1 receptor on glucose intolerance with CB2 receptor imparting a degree of glucose tolerance (Bermudez-Silva et al., 2008).

Subchronic administration (18 days) of AM251 (6 mg/kg, interperitoneal) decreased circulating plasma glucose and increased glucose tolerance after a glucose load in ob/ob mice (Irwin et al., 2008).

Other studies observed that CB1 stimulation increased insulin secretion. Interestingly, CB1 agonists also enhanced glucagons release from human alpha cells and CB2 agonists reduce both insulin and glucagon release (Di Marzo, 2008). The possible explanation was that CB1 receptors inhibit glucose expenditure by inhibiting insulin utilization in skeletal muscle but enhancing it in the adipose tissue for energy storage into fats (Matias et al. 2008).

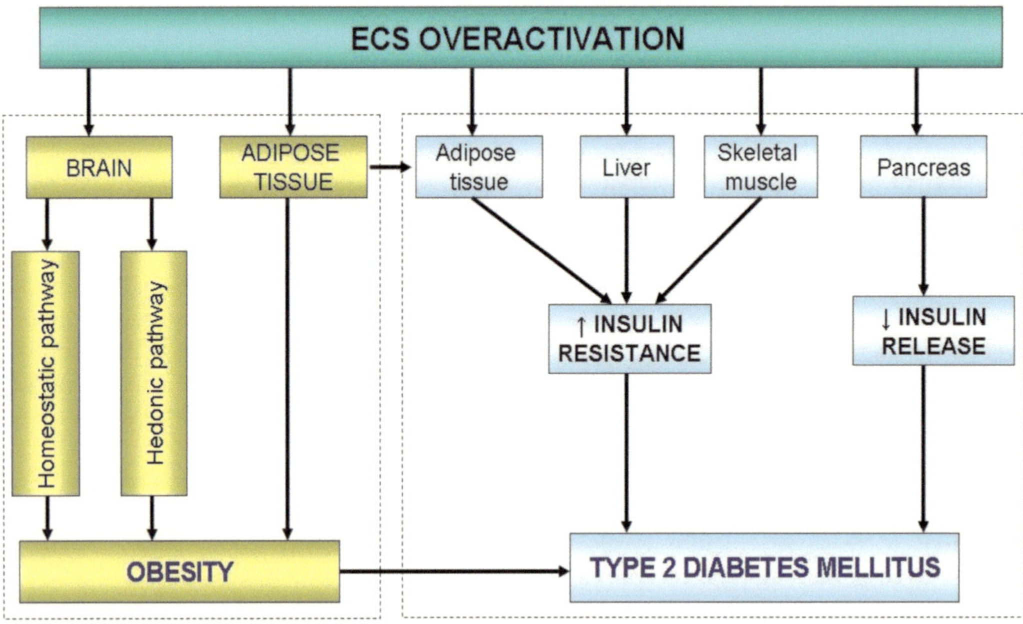

Fig. 5. The major mechanisms by which over-activation of ECS may lead to T2DM

The major evidence that dysregulated ECS is involved in glucose homeostasis comes from the clinical studies using CB1 receptor antagonists treatment. The Rimonabant in Obesity (RIO) study indicated that 1 year treatment with selective CB1 receptor antagonist, rimonabant 20mg, significantly reduced weight and abdominal circumference compared with diet and lifestyle therapy alone. The RIO-Lipids trial showed that subjects with dyslipidaemia and body mass index between 27 and 40kg/m^2 exhibited significant increase in HDL-cholesterol, reduction in plasma triacylglycerol and increase in plasma adiponectin levels. The RIO-Diabetes trial enrolled 1045 overweight/obese subjects with T2DM that received treatment with metformin or sulfonylurea treatment alone. The subjects receiving rimonabant showed significant body weight reduction improvement in glucose control. Approximately 50% of the improvements in HbA1c levels were independent of weight loss (Di Marzo, 2008). The results can be attributed in part to a reduction in insulin resistance in the liver, fat and skeletal muscle, and an increase in lipolysis and direct effects also on the pancreatic β-cell cannot be ruled out (Van Gaal et al., 2008). In October 2008, rimonabant was withdrawn from market in Europe and it was not approved for use in the USA due to the severe psychiatric side-effects including anxiety, depression, and suicidal ideation (Doyle, 2011).

The main mechanisms explaining the implication of the ECS in the pathogeny of T2DM are represented in Figure 5.

6. Future perspectives

Unfortunately, the withdrawal of rimonabant, due to the psychiatric side affects, diminished the interest for investigating the role of ECS in the pathogeny of T2DM.

But as previous studies and RIO trials indicated, the ECS has an important role in the pathogeny of T2DM and obesity proving the fact that it represents a physiological system implicated in energy storage, contributing together with other genes and systems at the "thrifty phenotype" that can lead to pathological conditions like T2DM and diabetes when over-activated.

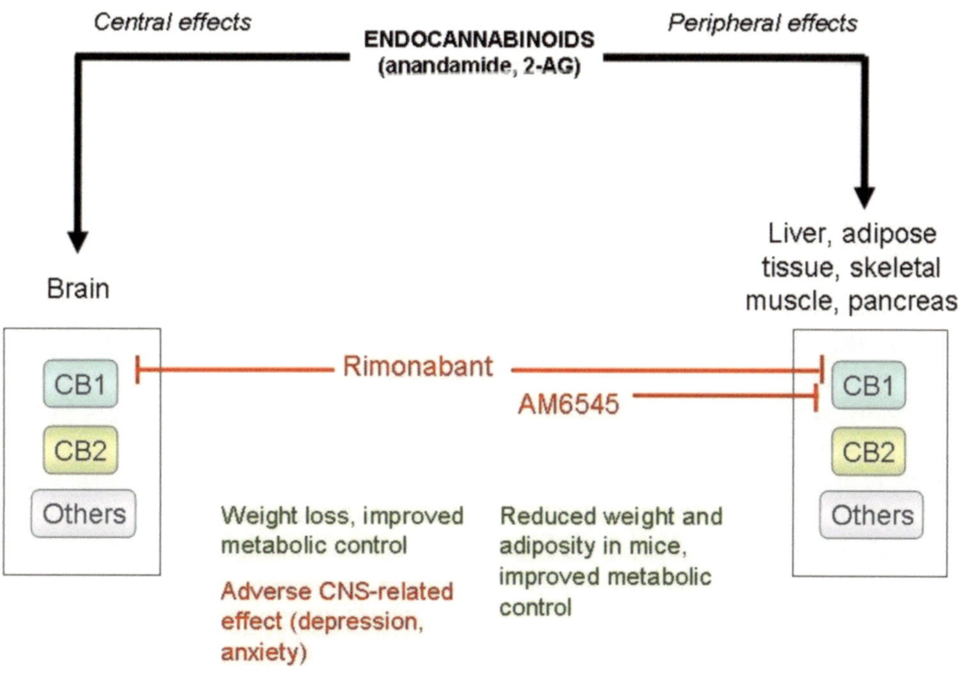

Fig. 6. The possible ways for targeting the ECS (adapted from Patti et al., 2010)

Nevertheless, emerging evidence supported the idea that interrupting endocannabinoid action selectively only in peripheral tissues may be an approach to treat the metabolic consequences of obesity and related diseases, including type 2 diabetes, without causing the undesirable CNS effects that occurred with rimonabant. The studies of Tam and colleagues brought back the attention to the ECS (Tam et al., 2010). Tam et al. first developed a CB1 antagonist (AM6545) that retained binding activity but could not penetrate the brain due to its reduced lipid solubility (Tam et al., 2010). Therefore, it could not block the CB1 receptors in the CNS. Remarkably, acting only on peripheral CB1 receptors AM6545 reduced body weight and adiposity in mice with diet-induced obesity and also improved systemic metabolism, as indicated by reduced fasting glucose, improved glucose tolerance, reduced insulin and leptin levels, increased adiponectin levels, and reduced hepatic triglyceride content in mice with diet-induced obesity (Patti et al., 2010) (Figure 6). The potency of AM6545 was a bit smaller probably due to additional centrally mediated effects of rimonabant on food intake or metabolism.

The discovery of the ECS represents a great step towards better understanding the pathogeny of obesity and T2DM. Due to its numerous interactions with other physiological systems, it remains an important target for the future treatments of T2DM and not only. In order to clearly elucidate the role of this system and for the development of peripheral selective, nonbrain penetrant, CB1 receptor antagonists, future studies are needed.

7. Acknowledgements

This study is part of research grant financed by the National University Research Council - MEDC - ANCS Grant, PN II - ID 711- No 234/01.10.2007. Project Director, Prof. Maria Mota.

8. References

Bennett, P.H. & Knowler W.C. (2005). Definition, Diagnosis, and Classification of Diabetes Mellitus and Glucose Homeostasis, In: *Joslin's Diabetes Mellitus*. Kahn, C.R., (Ed.), pp. 331-340, Lippincott Williams & Wilkins, ISBN 978-078-1727-96-9, Boston, MA, USA

Benzinou, M. et al. (2008). Endocannabinoid receptor 1 gene variations increase risk for obesity and modulate body mass index in European populations. *Hum Mol Genet*. Vol.17, No.13, pp. 1916-21

Bermudez-Silva, F.J. et al. (2006). Activation of cannabinoid CB1 receptors induces glucose intolerance in rats. *Eur J Pharmacol*. No.531, pp. 282–284

Bermudez-Silva, F.J. et al. (2008). Presence of functional cannabinoid receptors in human endocrine pancreas. *Diabetologia*. Vol.51, pp. 476–487

Bluher M, et al. (2006). Dysregulation of the peripheral and adipose tissue endocannabinoid system in human abdominal obesity. *Diabetes*. No.55, pp.3053–3060

Cavuoto, P,. et al. (2007). Effects of cannabinoid receptors on skeletal muscle oxidative pathways. *Mol Cell Endocrinol*. No.267, pp. 63–69

Cota, D. et al. (2003). The endogenous cannabinoid system affects energy balance via central orexigenic drive and peripheral lipogenesis. *J Clin Invest*. No.112, pp. 423–431

Cota, D. et al. (2006). Cannabinoids, opioids and eating behavior: the molecular face of hedonism? *Brain Res Rev*. No.51, pp. 85–107

Cote, M. et al. (2007). Circulating endocannabinoid levels, abdominal adiposity and related cardiometabolic risk factors in obese men. *Int J Obes* No.31, pp. 692–699

Demuth, D.G. & Molleman, A. (2006). Cannabinoid signaling. *Life Sci*, No.78, pp. 549-563

Di Marzo, V. et al. (1998) . Endocannabinoids: endogenous cannabinoid receptor ligands with neuromodulatory action. *Trends Neurosci*, No.21, pp. 521–528

Di Marzo, V. et al. (2001) Leptin-regulated endocannabinoids are involved in maintaining food intake. *Nature*. No.410, pp. 822–825

Di Marzo, V. (2006) A brief history of cannabinoid and endocannabinoid pharmacology as inspired by the work of British scientists. *Trends Pharmacol Sci*, Vol.27, No.3, pp. 134-40

Di Marzo, V. (2008). The endocannabinoid system in obesity and type 2 diabetes. *Diabetologia*. Vol.51, pp. 1356-1367

Doyle, M.E. (April 2011). The role of the endocannabinoid system in islet biology. *Curr Opin Endocrinol Diabetes Obes*. Vol.18, No.2, pp. 153-158

Egertova, M. et al. (1998). A new perspective on cannabinoid signalling: complementary localization of fatty acid amide hydrolase and the CB1 receptor in rat brain. *Proc R Soc Lond B Biol Sci*. No.265, pp. 2081–2085

Eggan, S.M. & Lewis, D.A. (2007). Immunocytochemical distribution of the cannabinoid CB1 receptor in the primate neocortex: a regional and laminar analysis. *Cereb. Cortex*, Vol.17, No.1, pp. 175–191

Engeli, S. et al. (2005). Activation of the peripheral endocannabinoid system in human obesity. *Diabetes*. No.54, pp. 2838–2843

Engeli, S (2008). Dysregulation of the endocannabinoid system in obesity. *J Neuroendocrinol*. No.20, pp. 110–115

Engeli, S. et al. (2008). Peripheral endocannabinoid system activity in patients treated with sibutramine. *Obesity*. Vol.16, No.5, pp. 1135-7

Garber, A.J. (2010). Incretin-based therapies in the management of type 2 diabetes: rationale and reality in a managed care setting. *Am J Manag Care*, Vol.16, No.7 Suppl, pp. S187-94.

Gary-Bobo, M. et al. (2006). The cannabinoid CB1 receptor antagonist rimonabant (SR141716) inhibits cell proliferation and increases markers of adipocyte aturation in cultured mouse 3T3 F442A preadipocytes. *Mol Pharmacol*. No.69, pp.471–478

Gasperi, V. et al. (2007). Endocannabinoids in adipocytes during differentiation and their role in glucose uptake. *Cell Mol Life Sci*. No.64, pp. 219–229

Glaser, S.T. et al. (2003) Evidence against the presence of an anandamide transporter. *Proc Natl Acad Sci USA* Vol.100, No.7, pp. 4269–74

Grimsey, N.L. et al. (2008). Specific detection of CB1 receptors; cannabinoid CB1 receptor antibodies are not all created equal! *J Neurosci Methods*. No.171, pp. 78–86

Guzman, M. et al. (1995). Effects of anandamide on hepatic fatty acid metabolism. *Biochem Pharmacol*. No.50, pp. 885–888

Herling, A.W. et al. (2007). CB1 receptor antagonist AVE1625 affects primarily metabolic parameters independently of reduced food intake in Wistar rats. *Am J Physiol Endocrinol Metab*. No.293, pp. E826–E832

Howlett, A.C. & Mukhopadhyay, S. (2000) Cellular signal transduction by anandamide and 2-arachidonoylglycerol. *Chem. Phys. Lipids*. No.108, pp. 53–70

Howlett, A.C. et al. (2004). Cannabinoid physiology and pharmacology: 30 years of progress. *Neuropharmacology*, No.47, pp. 345–358

Irwin, N. et al. (2008). Antidiabetic effects of sub-chronic administration of the cannabinoid receptor (CB1) antagonist, AM251, in obese diabetic (ob/ob) mice. *Eur J Pharmacol*. No.581, pp. 226–233

Iversen, L.L. (2000). *The science of Marijuana*. Oxford University Press, ISBN 0-19-513123-1, New York, USA

Jbilo, O. et al. (2005). The CB1 receptor antagonist rimonabant reverses the diet induced obesity phenotype through the regulation of lipolysis and energy balance. *FASEB J*, Vol.19, No.11, pp. 1567–1569

Juan-Pico, P. et al. (2006). Cannabinoid receptors regulate Ca($^{2+}$) signals and insulin secretion in pancreatic beta-cell. *Cell Calcium*. No.39, pp. 155–162

Kadowaki, T. et al. (2006). Adiponectin and adiponectin receptors in insulin resistance, diabetes, and the metabolic syndrome. *J Clin Invest*. No.116, pp. 1784–1792

Kola, B. et al. (2005). Cannabinoids and ghrelin have both central and peripheral metabolic and cardiac effects via AMP-activated protein kinase. *J Biol Chem*. No.280, pp. 25196–25201

Li, C. et al. (2010a). Expression and function of cannabinoid receptors in mouse islets. *Islets*. No.2, pp. 293–302

Li, C. et al (2010b). Cannabinoid receptors are coupled to stimulation of insulin secretion from mouse MIN6 beta-cells. *Cell Physiol Biochem*. No.26, pp.187–196

Liu, Y.L. et al. (2005). Effects of the cannabinoid CB1 receptor antagonist SR141716 on oxygen consumption and soleus muscle glucose uptake in Lep(ob)/Lep(ob) mice. *Int J Obes*. No.29, pp. 183–187

Lutz, B. (2002). Molecular biology of cannabinoid Receptors. *Prostaglandins. Leukotrienes and Essential Fatty Acids* Vol.66, No.2-3, pp. 123-142

Matias, I. et al. (2006). Regulation, function, and dysregulation of endocannabinoids in models of adipose and beta-pancreatic cells and in obesity and hyperglycemia. *J Clin Endocrinol Metab*. No.91, pp. 3171–3180

Matias, I. et al. (2008). Endocannabinoids: Some Like it Fat (and Sweet Too). *J Neuroendocrinol* No.20, pp. 100–109

Molina-Holgado, E. et al. (2002) Cannabinoids promote oligodendrocyte progenitor survival: Involvement of cannabinoid receptors and phosphatidylinositol-3 kinase/Akt signaling. *J. Neurosci*. No.22, pp. 9742–9753.

Müller, T.D. et al. (2007). No evidence for an involvement of variants in the cannabinoid receptor gene (CNR1) in obesity in German children and adolescents. *Mol Genet Metab*. Vol.90, No.4, pp. 429-3

Nakata, M. & Yadam T. (2008). Cannabinoids inhibit insulin secretion and cytosolic Ca($^{2+}$) oscillation in islet beta-cells via CB1 receptors. *Regul Pept*. No.145, pp. 49–53

Ni, Q. et al. (2011). Signaling diversity of PKA achieved via a Ca($^{2+}$)-cAMP-PKA oscillatory circuit. *Nat Chem Biol*. No.7, pp. 34–40

Nogueiras, R. et al. (2008). The endocannabinoid system and the control of glucose homeostasis. *J Neuroendocrinol*. Vol.20, Suppl 1, pp. 147-151

Onaivi, E.S. et al. (2006). Endocannabinoids: The Brain and Body's Marijuana and Beyond. CRC Press, 2005, ISBN: 978- 0-415-30008-7, Boca Raton, FL, USA

Osei-Hyiaman, D. et al. (2005). Endocannabinoid activation at hepatic CB1 receptors stimulates fatty acid synthesis and contributes to diet-induced obesity. *J Clin Invest*. No.115, pp. 1298–1305

Pagano, C. et al. (2007). The endogenous cannabinoid system stimulates glucose uptake in human fat cells via phosphatidylinositol 3-kinase and calcium-dependent mechanisms. *J Clin Endocrinol Metab.* No.92, pp. 4810–4819

Pagotto, U. et al. (2006). The emerging role of the endocannabinoid system in endocrine regulation and energy balance. *Endocr Rev.* No.27,pp. 73–100

Patti ME. (2010). Rehashing endocannabinoid antagonists: can we selectively target the periphery to safely treat obesity and type 2 diabetes? *J Clin Invest.* Vol.120, No.8, pp. 2646-2648

Peeters, A. et al. (2007). The G1422A variant of the cannabinoid receptor gene (CNR1) is associated with abdominal adiposity in obese men. *Endocrine.* Vol.31, No.2, pp. 138-41

Pertwee, R. (2005). *Cannabinoids.* Springer, ISBN 3-540-22565-X, Berlin Heidelberg New York

Perwitz, N. et al. (2006). Cannabinoid receptor signaling directly inhibits thermogenesis and alters expression of adiponectin and visfatin. *Horm Metab Res.* No.38, pp. 356–358

Piomelli, D. Et al. (1998) Endogenous cannabinoid signaling. *Neurobiol Dis* No.5, pp. 462–73

Russo, P. et al. (2007). Genetic variations at the endocannabinoid type 1 receptor gene (CNR1) are associated with obesity phenotypes in men. *J Clin Endocrinol Metab.* Vol.92, No.6, pp. 2382-6

Sipe, J.C. et al. (2005) Reduced endocannabinoid immune modulation by a common cannabinoid 2 (CB2) receptor gene polymorphism: possible risk for autoimmune disorders. *J Leukoc Biol.* No.78, pp. 231–8

Sparling, P.B. et al. (2003). Exercise activates the endocannabinoid system. *Neuroreport* No. 14, pp. 2209–2211

Starowicz, K.M. et al. (2008). Endocannabinoid dysregulation in the pancreas and adipose tissue of mice fed with a high-fat diet. *Obesity (Silver Spring).* No.16, pp. 553–565

Tam, J. et al. (2010). Peripheral CB1 cannabinoid receptor blockade improves cardiometabolic risk in mouse models of obesity. *J Clin Invest.* Vol.120, No.8, pp. 2953–2966

Task Force on Diabetes and Cardiovascular Diseases of the European Society of Cardiology (ESC) and the European Society for the Study of Diabetes (EASD), (2007). Guidelines on diabetes, prediabetes and cardiovascular diseases: executive summary. *European Heart Journal,* No.28, pp. 88-136

Van Gaal, L. et al. (2008). Efficacy and safety of rimonabant for improvement of multiple cardiometabolic risk factors in overweight/obese patients: pooled 1-year data from the Rimonabant in Obesity (RIO) program. *Diabetes Care.* Vol.31, Suppl 2, pp. S229-S240

Wilson, R.I. & Nicoll, R.A. (2001). Endogenous cannabinoids mediate retrograde signalling at hippocampal synapses. *Nature.* No.410, pp. 588–92

Yan, Z.C. et al. (2007). Exercise reduces adipose tissue via cannabinoid receptor type 1 which is regulated by peroxisome proliferatoractivated receptor-delta. *Biochem Biophys Res Commun*. No.354, pp. 427–433

Part 4

Treatments

16

Beyond Dietary Fatty Acids as Energy Source: A Point of View for the Prevention and Management of Type 2 Diabetes

Lourdes M. Varela, Almudena Ortega, Sergio Lopez, Beatriz Bermudez, Rocio Abia and Francisco J.G. Muriana
Laboratory of Cellular and Molecular Nutrition, Instituto de la Grasa, ***CSIC***
Spain

1. Introduction

Dietary fatty acids have been traditionally viewed as substrates for the generation of high-energy molecules and as precursors for the biosynthesis of macromolecules. However, accumulating data from multiple lines of evidence suggest that dietary fatty acids are linked to the pathogenesis of type 2 diabetes, which involves abnormalities in both insulin secretion and action (Lopez et al., 2010).

Dietary fatty acids are absorbed into epithelial cells of the small intestine, are assembled into nascent triglyceride-rich lipoproteins, enter the bloodstream, and are transported to peripheral tissues. Therefore, the main physiological — but sometimes pathological — contribution to plasma triglycerides and tissue fatty acids, in terms of both quantity and quality, occurs during the postprandial period (Miles & Nelson, 2007). Acute elevation in plasma triglycerides, which may produce local elevation of fatty acids in beta-cells, is related to the increase of glucose-induced insulin secretion (Lopez et al., 2008; Lopez et al., 2010). Adipose tissue serves as a triglyceride storage site and, when necessary, stored triglycerides in adipocytes can be hydrolyzed by their adipose triglyceride and hormone-sensitive lipases to release fatty acids into the bloodstream. Excessive rates of lipid turnover have been shown to precede the development of type 2 diabetes in subjects with a family history of type 2 diabetes and nondiabetic obese individuals (Cusi, 2009). Decreased insulin sensitivity in adipose tissue is characterized by the increase of lipolysis and plasma fatty acid levels despite hyperinsulinemia, and impaired suppression of plasma fatty acid levels by insulin. This elevation in the plasma fatty acids, if chronic, induces a decrease in hepatic and skeletal muscle insulin sensitivity and detrimental effects on beta-cell function, which has been referred to as lipotoxicity (Giacca et al., 2011). Here, we review studies in insulin-secreting cell lines, islet cells, animal models, and human beings that have informed our current understanding of the mechanistic links among dietary fatty acids, beta-cell function, and insulin sensitivity.

2. Types of major dietary fatty acids

A fatty acid is a carboxylic acid that often has a long unbranched aliphatic chain. Fatty acids are divided into SFA and unsaturated fatty acids based on structural and chemical properties (Fig. 1). SFA do not contain any double bonds or other functional groups along the chain, which is fully saturated with hydrogen atoms. Palmitic acid (16:0) is composed of 16 carbon atoms and is the principal SFA in the diet. SFA is found chiefly in animal products, including meats and dairy foods, but is also found in some plant sources, including coconut, cottonseed, and palm kernel oils. MUFA are unsaturated fatty acids that contain one pair of carbon atoms linked by a cis double bond. The major dietary MUFA is oleic acid (18:1n-9), which has 18 carbon atoms with the double bond occurring 9 carbon atoms away from the methyl end of the fatty acid molecule. Oleic acid is the primary component of olive oil, but also can be found in hazelnut, canola, and peanut oils. A carbon chain that contains two or more cis double bonds with the first double bond located between the third and fourth or sixth and seventh carbon atom from the methyl end of the fatty acid molecule characterises the families of n-3 or n-6 PUFA. These families cannot be

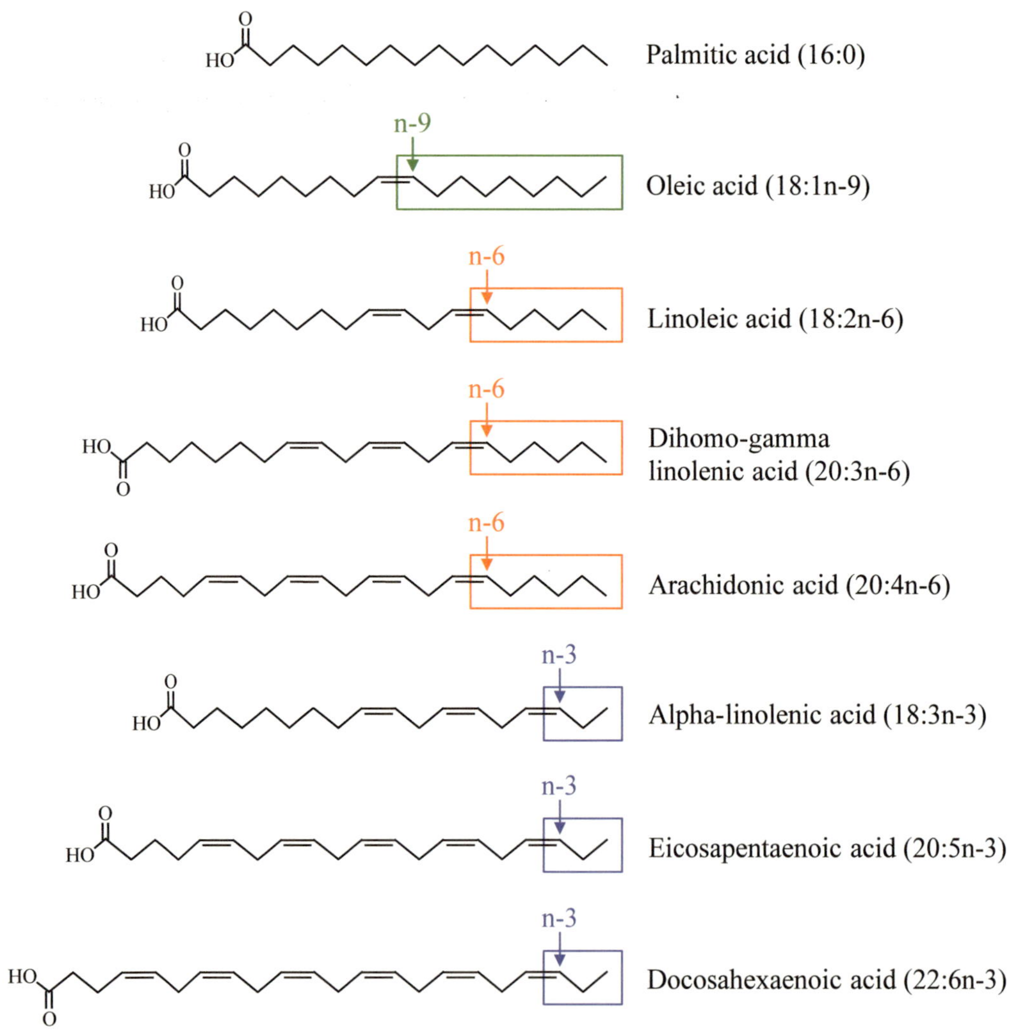

Fig. 1. The structure of the most significant dietary fatty acids.

synthesised by the human body (double bonds can be introduced into all positions of the fatty acid chain except for the n-3 and n-6 positions) and must be obtained from the diet either as alpha-linolenic acid (18:3n-3) and linoleic acid (18:2n-6), or their long-chain PUFA derivatives (Das, 2006). Of these fatty acids, eicosapentaenoic acid (20:5n-3), docosahexaenoic acid (22:6n-3), dihomo-gamma linolenic acid (20:3n-6), and arachidonic acid (20:4n-6) are the most metabolically significant. While conversion of linoleic acid to dihomo-gamma linolenic acid and arachidonic acid is typically very efficient, conversion of alpha-linolenic acid to eicosapentaenoic acid and docosahexaenoic acid is much less so (Brenna et al., 2009). This fact has particular importance in people with compromised alpha-linolenic acid availability or conversion enzyme activity. Therefore, not only alpha-linolenic acid and linoleic acid but also long-chain n-3 PUFA should be considered as essential fatty acids. Linoleic acid and alpha-linolenic acid can be found in vegetable oils, linoleic acid in safflower, sunflower, soybean, maize, and cottonseed oils, and alpha-linolenic acid in flaxseed, blackcurrant, walnut, rapeseed, and soybean oils. Eicosapentaenoic acid and docosahexaenoic acid are abundant in cold-water fatty fish, including herring, sardines, mackerel, salmon, tuna, and shellfish.

Requirements in MUFA, n-3 and n-6 PUFA are satisfied by the diet. MUFA can be synthesised from acetyl-CoA within mammalian tissues. However, it is unclear whether the entire MUFA requirement can be met by de novo metabolic machinery. MUFA, and specifically oleic acid, represent one of the core components of the Mediterranean diet (mainly due to the liberal use of virgin olive oil), which represents a prototypical dietary model associated with a long life expectancy and a low occurrence of chronic diseases, including type 2 diabetes (Lopez-Miranda et al., 2010).

3. Dietary fatty acids on insulin secretion

3.1 Acute and long-term in vitro or animal studies

Pancreatic beta-cells can respond to dietary fatty acids at the metabolic, signal transduction and transcriptional levels to promote or attenuate beta-cell function or survival (Torres et al., 2009). The ability of fatty acids to acutely induce insulin secretion spans a remarkably broad range, increasing and decreasing with chain length and degree of unsaturation, respectively. Oleic acid elicits half the insulinotropic potency of palmitic acid in perfused rat pancreas. Furthermore, acute exposure of rat insulinoma INS-1 cells to oleic acid enhances insulin production and even reverses the inhibitory effect of TNF-alpha (Vassiliou et al., 2009). This output of insulin from beta-cells can be mediated by different metabolic processes, which are activated once the fatty acids reach the cytoplasm and/or bind to cell surface platforms, including G protein-coupled receptor 40 (GPR40) (Morgan & Dhayal, 2009) and fatty acid translocase FAT/CD36 (Wallin et al., 2010). On the contrary, long-term (chronic) exposure of human islet cells to palmitic acid impairs glucose-stimulated insulin secretion, reduces insulin gene transcription and induces beta-cell apoptosis (lipotoxicity) (Giacca et al., 2011), whereas oleic acid is cytoprotective for beta-cells and even attenuates the proapoptotic effects of palmitic acid (Morgan, 2009). There are a growing number of proposed mechanisms regarding the toxicity of palmitic acid in beta-cells, ranging from physical and chemical rearrangement of lipid stores to transcriptional regulation of lipogenic genes (Poitout et al., 2009). Endoplasmic reticulum (ER) homeostasis is particularly affected by a sustained hypersecretory activity of beta-cells to fatty acids (Cnop et al., 2010). Other effects include direct ER Ca^{2+} depletion, an increase in phosphorylation of the ER Ca^{2+} sensor protein kinase R-like ER kinase (PERK), and an increase in the protein level of transcription factor C/EBP-homologous protein (CHOP) (Gwiazda et al., 2009). Palmitic acid-induced INS-1 beta-cell death involves the activation of the stress-related C-Jun N-terminal kinase (JNK) pathway through Toll-like receptor 4 (TLR4) (Lee et al., 2011). It is notable that the precise mechanisms by which oleic acid antagonizes the deleterious effects of palmitic acid in beta-cells remain unknown.

In a mouse model of haploinsufficiency of beta-specific glucokinase ($Gck^{+/-}$), where animals have a normal beta-cell mass but impair insulin secretion in response to glucose, dietary linoleic acid was recently found to exacerbate beta-cell ER stress and apoptosis (Shirakawa et al., 2011). An increase in CHOP-positive nuclei and terminal deoxynucleotidyltransferase-mediated dUTP-biotin nick-end labelling (TUNEL)-positive apoptotic nuclei were observed in pancreatic beta-cells of $Gck^{+/-}$ mice fed a diet rich in sucrose and linoleic acid, when compared with a diet rich in sucrose and oleic acid. These effects were not evident in euglycemic wild-type or insulin receptor substrate-1 deficient ($IRS\text{-}I^{-/-}$) mice, indicating that hyperglycemia amplifies fatty acid-induced beta-cell ER stress and lipotoxicity. Likewise, the expression levels of CHOP, activating transcription factor 4 (ATF-4), and cleaved caspase-3, and the Bax/Bcl-2 ratio significantly increase in pancreatic islets from wild-type mice or stably transformed insulinoma cell line MIN6 when exposed to linoleic acid or palmitic acid in comparison with oleic acid in the presence of high-glucose concentration.

3.2 Human postprandial studies: saturated fatty acids versus monounsaturated fatty acids

Exaggerated postprandial hypertriglyceridemia is an inherent feature of diabetic dyslipidemia and is frequently found even in diabetic patients with normal fasting triglycerides (Tentolouris et al., 2008). Such phenomena would be consistent with studies linking SFA-rich meals to dysfunctions in insulin secretion and the frequency of type 2 diabetes (Misra et al., 2010). It is probable that MUFA, PUFA, and SFA could compete at the level of the beta-cell (Fig. 2). The islet tissue, which expresses LPL, could access triglycerides from postprandial triglyceride-rich lipoproteins (TRL) as a source of free fatty acids, in which case, the type and concentration of the fatty acid in the immediate vicinity of the beta-cells is likely to be dependent on the nature of the dietary fatty acids (Lopez et al., 2010). As indicated above, the input of fatty acids into the beta-cell can be mediated by cell surface platforms (GPR40 and FAT/CD36), but apoE-dependent and independent recognition sites could also cooperate with LPL to selectively remove postprandial TRL and to immediately generate intracellular fatty acids via catabolic pathways (Lass et al., 2011; von Eckardstein & Sibler, 2011).

When compared to SFA (i.e., palmitic acid)-rich meals, MUFA (i.e., oleic acid)-rich meals induce a lower early postprandial insulin response in healthy subjects (Lopez et al., 2008). These findings are consistent with the notion that in comparison with palmitic acid, oleic acid might moderate the compensatory hyperactivity of beta-cells in the postprandial state, although whether this maintenance of glucose tolerance during feeding periods could prevent or delay the development of overt type 2 diabetes remains to be elucidated.

Fasting hypertriglyceridemia results from either overproduction of triglycerides by the liver, impaired lipolysis, or a combination of both. In hypertriglyceridemic patients, the overproduction of triglycerides is disproportionately greater than the increase in apoB100 production, resulting in the formation of large triglyceride-rich VLDL particles (Caslake &

Packard, 2004). Obesity and insulin resistance result in increased hepatic supply of fatty acids and overproduction of triglycerides. Insulin inhibits VLDL production in an effort to reduce the postprandial triglyceride response to a high-fat meal. A recent randomised and within-subject crossover study in volunteers who were newly diagnosed with type IIb or IV hyperlipoproteinemia revealed that postprandial beta-cell function is buffered with MUFA when compared to SFA (Lopez et al., 2011), therefore extending the relationship between MUFA-rich meals and the benefits on postprandial glucose homeostasis observed in subjects with normal fasting triglyceride levels (Lopez et al., 2008) to a population of subjects with high fasting triglyceride levels.

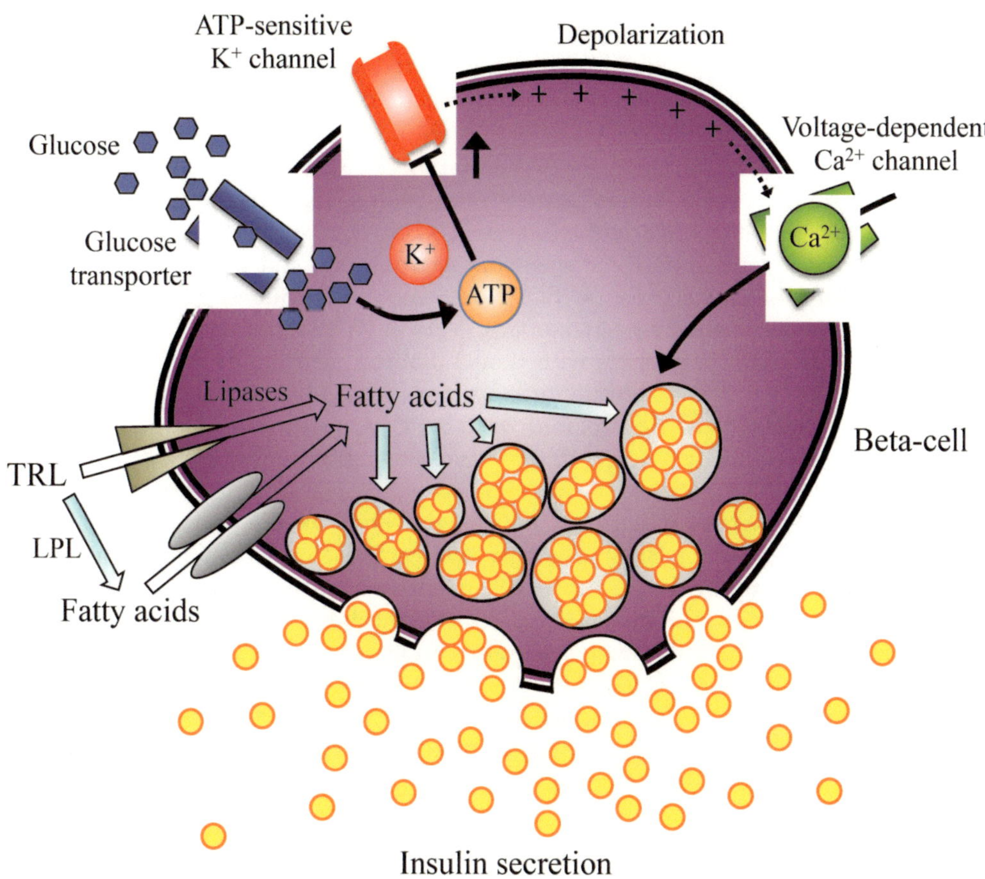

Fig. 2. The potential impact of dietary fatty acids on beta-cell function in the postprandial state.

4. Dietary fatty acids on insulin sensitivity

4.1 Long and short-term human controlled studies

Long-term habitual dietary fatty acids also relates to insulin sensitivity. However, food-frequency questionnaires do not provide reliable estimates of absolute amounts of dietary fatty acids, which may in part explain the inconsistency of long-term studies linking dietary fatty acids with beneficial or detrimental effects on glucose metabolism. There is only consensus that a fatty acid pattern associated with decreased insulin sensitivity is characterized by high consumption of palmitic acid. The diversity of dietary fatty acids is reflected in plasma lipids and tissues. For example, the fatty acid composition in adipose tissue partially reflects the consumption of dietary fatty acids over a considerable time, but also reflects the activities of enzymes responsible for fatty acid synthesis, desaturation, and elongation. In a recent observational study, palmitic acid in adipose tissue was negatively linked to insulin sensitivity in a large community-based cohort of elderly men (Iggman et al., 2010). It was also found a positive association between oleic acid, linoleic acid, and alpha-linolenic acid in adipose tissue and insulin sensitivity. Furthermore, decreased insulin sensitivity and type 2 diabetes are related to increased pancreatic cancer risk. A positive association of palmitic acid intake, mainly from red meat and dairy products, with pancreatic cancer has been recently described in men and women after a mean of 6.3 years of follow up (Thiebaut et al., 2009).

Despite the reasonable replacement for SFA in terms of risk factor for chronic diseases in general and type 2 diabetes in particular are MUFA, because the consumption of n-3 and n-6 PUFA is limited to less than 10% of the total daily calories, most studies have involved n-3 and n-6 PUFA for investigating the association between long and short-term dietary fatty acid consumption and insulin sensitivity. There is no clear evidence to suggest that n-3 PUFA improve insulin sensitivity in humans. Very high doses of n-3 PUFA may even impair insulin sensitivity in subjects with type 2 diabetes (Mostad et al., 2006). However, after only 5 weeks, the insulin sensitivity is improved in volunteers (healthy, obese, and type 2 diabetics) when SFA are replaced by n-6 PUFA (Summers et al., 2002). Similar findings are observed in overweight individuals after substitution of SFA with MUFA (Lovejoy et al., 2002).

The mechanisms by which dietary fatty acids influence insulin sensitivity have been previously reviewed (Riserus, 2008). The fatty acid composition of cell membrane may be affected by dietary fatty acids, and then cell membrane functions, e.g., translocation of glucose transporters, membrane fluidity, ion permeability, and/or insulin receptor binding/affinity. Dietary fatty acids can also improve hepatic insulin sensitivity by suppressing lipogenic gene expression and hepatic lipogenesis, and stimulating hepatic fatty acid oxidation. SFA, palmitic acid in particular, have a contrary effect. Different observational studies suggest that the level of palmitic acid intake may even independently predict type 2 diabetes (Hodge et al., 2007).

4.2 Human postprandial studies: saturated fatty acids versus monounsaturated fatty acids

Dietary fatty acid quality, rather than quantity, has been suggested to acutely influence insulin sensitivity in humans (Lopez et al., 2010). Compensatory hyperinsulinemia due to enhanced beta-cell function is considered to be an obligate accompanying feature in insulin resistance syndromes (Reaven, 2005). Euglycemic clamps or frequently sampled intravenous glucose tolerance tests are the reference methods to determine beta-cell sensitivity to glucose and the sensitivity of body tissues to insulin (Cobelli et al., 2007). However, these tests are far from physiological because insulin secretion or activity is only measured in the steady-state. Empirical and model-based indices based on the oral glucose tolerance test (OGTT) provide a reasonable approximation of postprandial beta-cell function and whole-body insulin sensitivity (Bartoli et al., 2011). An important caveat of the OGTT is that the events associated with the ingestion of a pure glucose solution are not wholly equivalent to the numerous metabolic events associated with eating a mixed high-fat meal when both carbohydrates and fatty acids are ingested.

It has been hypothesised that insulin resistance syndromes might be a postprandial phenomenon linked to the acute metabolism of dietary fatty acids (Pedrini et al., 2006). When mixed high-fat meals with different proportions of dietary fatty acids are administered to healthy subjects, they become less insulin resistant postprandially as the proportion of MUFA to SFA, and oleic acid to palmitic acid, in dietary fatty acids increase (Lopez et al., 2008). In subjects who were newly diagnosed with type IIb or IV hyperlipoproteinemia, postprandial insulin sensitivity is also improved with MUFA when compared to SFA (Lopez et al., 2011). Furthermore, with regard to resistance to insulin-mediated glucose disposal, SFA (i.e., palmitic acid) was found to stimulate additional insulin secretion to maintain postprandial glucose homeostasis, suggesting a mechanism of lipid-induced deterioration of insulin sensitivity coupled with compensatory insulin secretion that is distinctively modulated by dietary fatty acids.

5. Conclusion

Dietary fatty acids are nutrient signals that play a relevant role in modulating insulin secretion and action. SFA, particularly palmitic acid, are associated with damage of glucose-stimulated insulin secretion and lipotoxicity in beta-cells and with decline of insulin sensitivity. MUFA, particularly oleic acid, are cytoprotective for beta-cells, even attenuate the cytotoxic effects of palmitic acid, and improve insulin sensitivity in comparison with SFA. PUFA, either of n-3 or n-6 family, do not confer additional benefit over MUFA. Therefore, efforts to promote the consumption of MUFA in place of SFA should be relevant as part of a dietary lifestyle strategy to prevent or manage type 2 diabetes.

6. Acknowledgment

The work was supported by MICINN grants AGL2004-04958, AGL2005-03722, and AGL2008-02811, CSIC grants to L.M.V. and B.B., MICINN grants to A.O., and Marie Curie grant PERG07-GA-2010-268413. L.M.V., A.O, S.L., and B.B. are considered equal first authors.

7. References

Bartoli, E.; Fra, G.P. & Carnevale Schianca, G.P. (2011). The Oral Glucose Tolerance Test (OGTT) Revisited. *European Journal of Internal Medicine*, Vol. 22, No. 1, pp. 8-12.

Brenna, J.T.; Salem, N.Jr.; Sinclair, A.J.; Cunnane, S.C. & International Society for the Study of Fatty Acids and Lipids, ISSFAL. Alpha-Linolenic Acid Supplementation And Conversion To N-3 Long-Chain Polyunsaturated Fatty Acids In Humans. *Prostaglandins, Leukotrienes, and Essential Fatty Acids*, Vol. 80, No. 2-3, pp. 85-91.

Caslake, M.J. & Packard, C.J. Phenotypes, Genotypes And Response To Statin Therapy. *Current Opinion in Lipidology*, Vol. 15, No. 4, pp. 387-392.

Cnop, M.; Ladriere, L.; Igoillo-Esteve, M.; Moura, R.F. & Cunha, D.A. (2010). Causes And Cures For Endoplasmic Reticulum Stress In Lipotoxic B-Cell Dysfunction. *Diabetes, Obesity & Metabolism*, Vol. 12, No. 2, pp. 76-82.

Cobelli, C.; Toffolo, G.M.; Dalla Man, C.; Campioni, M.; Denti, P.; Caumo, A.; Butler, P. & Rizza, R. (2007). Assessment Of Beta-Cell Function In Humans, Simultaneously With Insulin Sensitivity And Hepatic Extraction, From Intravenous And Oral Glucose Tests. *American Journal of Physiology, Endocrinology and Metabolism*, Vol. 293, No. 1, pp. E1-E15.

Cusi, K. (2009). Lessons Learned From Studying Families Genetically Predisposed To Type 2 Diabetes Mellitus. *Current Diabetes Report*, Vol. 9, No. 3, pp. 200-207.

Das, U.N. (2006). Essential Fatty Acids - A Review. *Current Pharmaceutical Biotechnology*, Vol. 7, No. 6, pp. 467-482.

Giacca, A.; Xiao, C.; Oprescu, A.I.; Carpentier, A.C. & Lewis, G.F. (2011). Lipid-Induced Pancreatic B-Cell Dysfunction: Focus On In Vivo Studies. *American Journal of Physiology, Endocrinology and Metabolism*, Vol. 300, No. 2, pp. E255-E262.

Gwiazda, K.S.; Yang, T.L.; Lin, Y. & Johnson, J.D. (2009). Effects Of Palmitate On ER And Cytosolic Ca2+ Homeostasis In Beta-Cells. *American Journal of Physiology, Endocrinology and Metabolism*, Vol. 296, No. 4, pp. E690-E701.

Hodge, A.M.; English, D.R.; O'Dea, K.; Sinclair, A.J.; Makrides, M.; Gibson, R.A. & Giles, G.G. (2007). Plasma Phospholipid And Dietary Fatty Acids As Predictors Of Type 2 Diabetes: Interpreting The Role Of Linoleic Acid. *The American Journal of Clinical Nutrition*, Vol. 86, No. 1, pp. 189-197.

Iggman, D.; Arnlov, J.; Vessby, B.; Cederholm, T.; Sjogren, P. & Riserus, U. (2010). Adipose Tissue Fatty Acids And Insulin Sensitivity In Elderly Men. *Diabetologia*, Vol. 53, No. 5, pp. 850-857.

Lass, A.; Zimmermann, R.; Oberer, M. & Zechner, R. (2011). Lipolysis - A Highly Regulated Multi-Enzyme Complex Mediates The Catabolism Of Cellular Fat Stores. *Progress in Lipid Research*, Vol. 50, No. 1, pp. 14-27.

Lee, S.M.; Choi, S.E.; Lee, J.H.; Lee, J.J.; Jung, I.R.; Lee, S.J.; Lee, K.W. & Kang, Y. (2011). Involvement Of The TLR4 (Toll-Like Receptor4) Signaling Pathway In Palmitate-Induced INS-1 Beta Cell Death. *Molecular and Cellular Biochemistry*, Epub ahead of print.

Lopez, S.; Bermudez, B.; Abia, R. & Muriana, F.J.G. (2010). The Influence Of Major Dietary Fatty Acids On Insulin Secretion And Action. *Current Opinion in Lipidology*, Vol. 21, No. 1, pp. 15-20.

Lopez, S.; Bermudez, B.; Ortega, A.; Varela, L.M.; Pacheco, Y.M.; Villar, J.; Abia, R. & Muriana F.J.G. (2011). Effects Of Meals Rich In Either Monounsaturated Or Saturated Fat On Lipid Concentrations And On Insulin Secretion And Action In Subjects With High Fasting Triglyceride Concentrations. *The American Journal of Clinical Nutrition*, Vol. 93, No. 3, pp. 494-499.

Lopez, S.; Bermudez, B.; Pacheco, Y.M.; Villar, J.; Abia, R. & Muriana, F.J.G. (2008). Distinctive Postprandial Modulation Of Beta Cell Function And Insulin Sensitivity By Dietary Fats: Monounsaturated Compared With Saturated Fatty Acids. *The American Journal of Clinical Nutrition*, Vol. 88, No. 3, pp. 638-644.

Lopez-Miranda, J.; Perez-Jimenez, F.; Ros, E.; De Caterina, R.; Badimon, L.; Covas, M.I.; Escrich, E.; Ordovas, J.M.; Soriguer, F.; Abia, R.; de la Lastra, C.A.; Battino, M.;

Corella, D.; Chamorro-Quiros, J.; Delgado-Lista, J.; Giugliano, D.; Esposito, K.; Estruch, R.; Fernandez-Real, J.M.; Gaforio, J.J.; La Vecchia, C.; Lairon, D.; Lopez-Segura, F.; Mata, P.; Menendez, J.A.; Muriana, F.J.G.; Osada, J.; Panagiotakos, D.B.; Paniagua, J.A.; Perez-Martinez, P.; Perona, J.; Peinado, M.A.; Pineda-Priego, M.; Poulsen, H.E.; Quiles, J.L.; Ramirez-Tortosa, M.C.; Ruano, J.; Serra-Majem, L.; Sola, R.; Solanas, M.; Solfrizzi, V.; de la Torre-Fornell, R.; Trichopoulou, A.; Uceda, M.; Villalba-Montoro, J.M.; Villar-Ortiz, J.R.; Visioli, F. & Yiannakouris, N. (2010). Olive Oil And Health: Summary Of The II International Conference On Olive Oil And Health Consensus Report, Jaén And Córdoba (Spain) 2008. *Nutrition, Metabolism, and Cardiovascular Diseases*, Vol. 20, No. 4, pp. 284-294.

Lovejoy, J.C.; Smith, S.R.; Champagne, C.M.; Most, M.M.; Lefevre, M.; DeLany, J.P.; Denkins, Y.M.; Rood, J.C.; Veldhuis, J. & Bray, G.A. (2002). Effects Of Diets Enriched In Saturated (Palmitic), Monounsaturated (Oleic), Or Trans (Elaidic) Fatty Acids On Insulin Sensitivity And Substrate Oxidation In Healthy Adults. *Diabetes Care*, Vol. 25, No. 8, pp. 1283-1288.

Miles, J.M. & Nelson, R.H. (2007). Contribution Of Triglyceride-Rich Lipoproteins To Plasma Free Fatty Acids. *Hormone and Metabolic Research*, Vol. 39, No. 10, pp. 726-729.

Misra, A.; Singhal, N. & Khurana, L. (2010). Obesity, The Metabolic Syndrome, And Type 2 Diabetes In Developing Countries: Role Of Dietary Fats And Oils. *Journal of the American College of Nutrition*, Vol. 29, No. 3, pp. 289S-301S.

Morgan, N.G. (2009). Fatty Acids And Beta-Cell Toxicity. *Current Opinion in Clinical Nutrition and Metabolic Care*, Vol. 12, No. 2, pp. 117-122.

Morgan, N.G. & Dhayal, S. (2009). G-Protein Coupled Receptors Mediating Long Chain Fatty Acid Signalling In The Pancreatic Beta-Cell. *Biochemical Pharmacology*, Vol. 78, No. 12, pp. 1419-1427.

Mostad, I.L.; Bjerve, K.S.; Bjorgaas, M.R.; Lydersen, S. & Grill, V. (2006). Effects Of N-3 Fatty Acids In Subjects With Type 2 Diabetes: Reduction Of Insulin Sensitivity And Time-Dependent Alteration From Carbohydrate To Fat Oxidation. *The American Journal of Clinical Nutrition*, Vol. 84, No. 3, pp. 540-550.

Pedrini, M.T.; Niederwanger, A.; Kranebitter, M.; Tautermann, C.; Ciardi, C.; Tatarczyk, T. & Patsch, J.R. (2006). Postprandial Lipaemia Induces An Acute Decrease Of Insulin Sensitivity In Healthy Men Independently Of Plasma NEFA Levels. *Diabetologia*, Vol. 49, No. 7, pp. 1612-1618.

Poitout, V.; Amyot, J.; Semache, M.; Zarrouki, B.; Hagman, D. & Fontes, G. (2010). Glucolipotoxicity Of The Pancreatic Beta Cell. *Biochimica et Biophysica Acta*, Vol. 1801, No. 3, pp. 289-298.

Reaven, G.M. (2005). Insulin Resistance, The Insulin Resistance Syndrome, And Cardiovascular Disease. *Panminerva Medica*, Vol. 47, No. 4, pp. 201-210.

Riserus, U. (2008). Fatty Acids And Insulin Sensitivity. *Current Opinion in Clinical Nutrition and Metabolic Care*, Vol. 11, No. 2, pp. 100-105.

Shirakawa, J.; Amo, K.; Ohminami, H.; Orime, K.; Togashi, Y.; Ito, Y.; Tajima, K.; Koganei, M.; Sasaki, H.; Takeda, E. & Terauchi, Y. (2011). Protective Effects Of A Dipeptidyl Peptidase-4 (DPP-4) Inhibitor Against Increased {Beta} Cell Apoptosis Induced By Dietary Sucrose And Linoleic Acid In Mice With Diabetes. *The Journal of Biological Chemistry*, Epub ahead of print.

Summers, L.K.; Fielding, B.A.; Bradshaw, H.A.; Ilic, V.; Beysen, C.; Clark, M.L.; Moore, N.R. & Frayn, K.N. (2002). Substituting Dietary Saturated Fat With Polyunsaturated Fat Changes Abdominal Fat Distribution And Improves Insulin Sensitivity. *Diabetologia*, Vol. 45, No. 3, pp. 369-377.

Tentolouris, N.; Arapostathi, C.; Perrea, D.; Kyriaki, D.; Revenas, C. & Katsilambros, N. (2008). Differential Effects Of Two Isoenergetic Meals Rich In Saturated Or Monounsaturated Fat On Endothelial Function In Subjects With Type 2 Diabetes. *Diabetes Care*, Vol. 31, No. 12, pp. 2276-2278.

Thiebaut, A.C.; Jiao, L.; Silverman, D.T.; Cross, A.J.; Thompson, F.E.; Subar, A.F.; Hollenbeck, A.R.; Schatzkin, A. & Stolzenberg-Solomon, R.Z. (2009). Dietary Fatty Acids And Pancreatic Cancer In The NIH-AARP Diet And Health Study. *Journal of the National Cancer Institute*, Vol. 101, No. 14, pp. 1001-1011.

Torres, N.; Noriega, L. & Tovar, A.R. (2009). Nutrient Modulation Of Insulin Secretion. *Vitamins and Hormones*, Vol. 80, pp. 217-244.

Vassiliou, E.K.; Gonzalez, A.; Garcia, C.; Tadros, J.H.; Chakraborty, G. & Toney, J.H. Oleic Acid And Peanut Oil High In Oleic Acid Reverse The Inhibitory Effect Of Insulin Production Of The Inflammatory Cytokine TNF-Alpha Both In Vitro And In Vivo Systems. *Lipids in Health and Disease*, Vol. 8, No. 25, pp. 1-10.

von Eckardstein, A. & Sibler, R.A. (2011). Possible Contributions Of Lipoproteins And Cholesterol To The Pathogenesis Of Diabetes Mellitus Type 2. *Current Opinion in Lipidology*, Vol. 22, No. 1, pp. 26-32.

Wallin, T.; Ma, Z.; Ogata, H.; Jørgensen, I.H.; Iezzi, M.; Wang, H.; Wollheim, C.B. & Bjorklund, A. (2010). Facilitation Of Fatty Acid Uptake By CD36 In Insulin-Producing Cells Reduces Fatty-Acid-Induced Insulin Secretion And Glucose Regulation Of Fatty Acid Oxidation. *Biochimica et Biophysica Acta*, Vol. 1801, No. 2, pp. 191-197.

17

Minimizing Postprandial Oxidative Stress in Type 2 Diabetes: The Role of Exercise and Selected Nutrients

Richard J. Bloomer, Cameron G. McCarthy and Tyler M. Farney
Cardiorespiratory/Metabolic Laboratory, The University of Memphis, Memphis, United States of America

1. Introduction

Approximately 25.8 million Americans (8.3% of the population) are currently living with diagnosed (18.8 million) or undiagnosed (7.0 million) diabetes (World Health Organization, 2011), most of whom are type 2 in pathology. An additional 79 million Americans are estimated to have pre-diabetes (World Health Organization, 2011). Unfortunately, the overall prevalence of these conditions continues to rise, as indicated by the 1.9 million newly diagnosed cases of diabetes in 2010 within people aged 20 years and older (World Health Organization, 2011). A similar situation presents itself within other nations around the world, with an estimated 220 million individuals currently living with diabetes (World Health Organization, 2011).

The onset and progression of diabetic disorders, as well as the related complications, are linked to impairments in glucose and lipid metabolism (O'Keefe & Bell, 2007), both of which are strongly associated with increased production of reactive oxygen and nitrogen species (RONS) (Ceriello & Motz, 2004; Fisher-Wellman & Bloomer, 2009b). Increased RONS production coupled with impaired antioxidant defense (a common finding among patients with diabetes) promotes oxidation of specific biomolecules (e.g., lipids, proteins, DNA), which can lead to an exacerbation of diabetic complications (Giacco & Brownlee, 2010). While variables such as blood glucose and blood triglycerides have traditionally been measured in a fasted state, increasing evidence suggests that measurement of *postprandial* glycemia, lipemia, as well as oxidative stress biomarkers, may provide more important clinical information concerning an individual's susceptibility to both type 2 diabetes mellitus (T2DM) onset and disease progression—as well as related conditions (O'Keefe & Bell, 2007; Pastromas et al., 2008).

For example, increased postprandial oxidative stress has been implicated in the pathophysiology of diabetes (Wright et al., 2006) and cardiovascular disease (Ceriello, 2004), which may be linked to the strong association between the postprandial rise in blood glucose and triglycerides and the generation of RONS. Moreover, randomized controlled trials indicate that reducing postprandial triglycerides appears to slow atherosclerotic progression and may improve long-term cardiovascular prognosis (O'Keefe & Bell, 2007). Therefore, methods to reduce the postprandial rise in glycemia and lipemia may help to prevent oxidative stress related complications in T2DM patients.

Drugs to treat hyperglycemia (e.g., sulfonylureas) and hyperlipidemia (e.g., statins) have been reported in some studies to promote favorable outcomes related to minimizing the postprandial rise in blood glucose and triglycerides (Nakajima, 2010; O'Keefe et al., 2011). However, non-pharmacological approaches also exist and have been discussed previously (Davi et al., 2010; Tucker et al., 2008). In particular, both acute and chronic exercise, as well as specific nutrient *intake* (e.g., certain macronutrients, antioxidants, glucose regulatory and insulin mimetic agents, lipid lowering agents) or *proscription* (e.g., saturated fat and simple sugar) may be considered in an attempt to minimize postprandial oxidative stress.

Specific to the above, exercise and selective nutrient intake may aid in attenuating postprandial oxidative stress in three distinct ways. First, exercise stimulates an increase in endogenous antioxidant enzyme activity and other protective mechanisms (e.g., heat shock proteins (Geiger & Gupte, 2011)). Exogenous antioxidant intake in the form of whole foods and nutritional supplements may provide additional protection against RONS production following a meal (Neri et al., 2005; Neri et al., 2010). Second, exercise improves blood glucose clearance via enhanced glucose-4-transport protein (GLUT 4) translocation and protein content (McGee & Hargreaves, 2006; Rockl et al., 2008), as well as enhanced insulin-insulin receptor binding and post-receptor signaling (McGee & Hargreaves, 2006). Nutrients acting to minimize the rise in blood glucose (e.g., fiber (Sierra et al., 2002)) or to enhance glucose clearance (e.g., herbal extracts (Yin et al., 2008)) may also provide benefit. Third, exercise improves blood triglyceride clearance via enhanced lipoprotein lipase activity (Seip & Semenkovich, 1998) and a reduction in chylomicron-triglyceride half-life (J. C. Cohen et al., 1989). Nutrients acting to minimize the rise in blood triglycerides or to enhance triglyceride clearance may also prove beneficial (Cottin et al., 2011), as well as altering nutrient intake to favor lower intake of saturated fat and simple sugar and higher intake of "healthy" fats and dietary fiber (Bloomer, Kabir, Canale et al., 2010; Jenkins et al., 2007; Marin et al., 2011).

In this chapter we provide an overview of the role of RONS in diabetic complications and provide a rationale for the inclusion of both exercise and selected nutrients to combat postprandial oxidative stress in those with T2DM. It is likely that these non-pharmacological approaches may not only improve glycemic control in a rested and fasted state, but also in response to feeding. If so, these methods should be strongly considered and implemented into the clinical treatment plan of type 2 diabetics in an effort to not only considerably improve the long-term prognosis of such individuals, but also to significantly reduce the financial burden associated with the chronic treatment of this disease.

2. Diabetes overview

Diabetes is present in multiple forms, but most commonly diagnosed as type 2 in pathology (World Health Organization, 2011). Diabetes is associated with multiple medical complications ranging from increased risk of cardiovascular disease to amputations and blindness. As the incident rate continues to rise, the economic burden associated with this disease also continues to grow. For example, the combined direct and indirect cost associated with diabetes has been estimated at $174 billion in 2007 within the United States alone (World Health Organization, 2011), with estimated and projected future costs being considerably higher. Related to the direct costs of $116 billion, after adjusting for population age and sex differences, the average medical expenditures among individuals with diagnosed diabetes were 2.3 times higher than what expenditures would have been in the absence of diabetes. Indeed, diabetes is not only associated with significant impairments in both the quality and quantity of life in most patients, but poses a major burden to the healthcare economy.

3. Oxidative stress description

Oxidative stress is a term used to describe a condition of imbalance that exists between prooxidants and antioxidants, in such a way that prooxidant production overwhelms antioxidant defenses (Bloomer, 2008). This may lead to the oxidation of lipids, proteins, DNA, glutathione, and other molecules in ways that impair cellular function (Bloomer, 2008). Although excessive production of prooxidants (also referred to as reactive oxygen and nitrogen species [RONS]) may be problematic, RONS generation occurs in part as a consequence of normal cellular metabolism (Halliwell & Cross, 1994) and serves several vital functions *in vivo*. For example, RONS play an important role in cell signaling (Haddad, 2002), cellular immunity (Fialkow et al., 2007), apoptosis (Lee & Wei, 2007), and redox regulation of gene transcription (H. Liu et al., 2005). Hence, RONS are essential for normal physiological function. It is important to note that under normal physiologic conditions, the endogenous antioxidant defense system, in conjunction with exogenous antioxidants consumed through whole food and nutritional supplements, serve to protect small and large molecules from oxidative modification via RONS.

3.1 Association with disease

Increased biomarkers of oxidative stress have been noted in those living with disease (Dalle-Donne et al., 2006), as well as in various tissues extracted upon autopsy. It is possible that during repeated exposure to stressful conditions in which RONS production is increased, and during which time adequate protection is not available, the antioxidant defense system may be overwhelmed. The resultant oxidative stress may lead to progressive oxidation of cellular constituents, eventually leading to functional decline of vital components (e.g., vascular endothelium) and disease (Dalle-Donne et al., 2006). However, while associations between various oxidative stress biomarkers, impairments in cellular function, and frank disease have been noted in many studies, direct *cause and effect* data are scarce (Maiese et al., 2007). For example, in many cases the evidence consists only of observations of increased levels of oxidative stress biomarkers (e.g., lipid, protein, and DNA oxidation) in persons with a particular disease such as diabetes (Baynes & Thorpe, 1999) or cardiovascular disease (Tsimikas, 2006). In other cases, subjects with certain diseases such as T2DM have demonstrated improved markers of health following antioxidant therapy (Wu et al., 2007), suggesting that RONS may have been a possible cause of disease or disease progression. However, when considering the multi-factorial pathology of most disease states, it is likely that systems aside from those associated with RONS are also involved. Additional study is needed before conclusions can be made pertaining to the specific role of RONS in human disease—and whether RONS are a major cause of disease or merely a consequence of the disease process.

3.2 Formation of Reactive Oxygen and Nitrogen Species (RONS)

As discussed earlier, a state of "oxidative stress" is created when RONS production exceeds antioxidant defense. Both non-radical and radical species are considered to be RONS, the latter which are often referred to as "free radicals", defined as any species capable of independent existence containing one or more unpaired electrons (Halliwell, 1991). The majority of biological molecules are non-radicals and contain only paired electrons. However, if a single electron is unpaired within an orbital, it is said to be "free". Free radicals are typically regarded as highly reactive (hence the term "reactive" oxygen and nitrogen species), because they seek to accept electrons from other molecules. The donation of electrons can then produce additional free radicals, leading to a chain reaction of radical generation, which may continue until a chain terminating reaction occurs.

Although RONS are generated as a component of normal cellular metabolism, they can also be produced through exposure to a wide variety of stimuli. These include, but are not limited to exposure to environmental toxins (Matsuoka et al., 2010), cigarette smoke (Edirisinghe & Rahman, 2010), ozone (Bocci et al., 2009; Yang & Omaye, 2009), intense physical exercise (Bloomer, 2008; Fisher-Wellman & Bloomer, 2009a), and ingestion of certain nutrients (Sies, Stahl, & Sevanian, 2005). Specifically, a state of oxidative stress may be mediated through a disruption of the electron transport system leading to increased formation of superoxide radicals, an increase in the activity of RONS generating enzymes (e.g., xanthine oxidase), activation of cyclooxygenases, lipoxygenases, phagocytes, and phospholipases, as well as through an acute or chronic decrease in antioxidant protection (Jackson et al., 2007).

3.2.1 Exercise conditions

More than 300 original investigations have been performed in relation to exercise-induced oxidative stress (Fisher-Wellman & Bloomer, 2009a). The results of this work are mixed, with many studies documenting an acute oxidative stress, while others fail to demonstrate such findings. The opposing results are likely due to discrepancies in the exercise protocols, the training status and age of subjects, the biomarkers measured, and the timing of blood collection relative to the exercise bout (Fisher-Wellman & Bloomer, 2009a). Regardless, there are multiple potential sites for RONS formation in relation to an acute bout of exercise. These include primary sources in which RONS are generated in direct response to a given condition (e.g., formation of superoxide within the respiratory chain, prostanoid metabolism, catecholamine autoxidation, heightened xanthine oxidase activity), as well as secondary sources in which RONS production might occur in response to muscle damage (e.g., neutrophil respiratory burst activity, disruption of iron containing proteins) (Bloomer, 2008). It is important to note that despite the potential for oxidative stress arising from acute exercise, such a condition is generally short lived. That is, any post-exercise elevation in oxidative stress biomarkers typically returns to baseline within minutes to hours following the cessation of exercise. Moreover, this acute increase in RONS is necessary to allow for the up-regulation in antioxidant defense—in accordance with the principle of hormesis (Radak et al., 2008). For these reasons, concern over an acute increase in RONS as a consequence of strenuous exercise should be minimal.

3.2.2 Feeding conditions

The generation of RONS and the ensuing oxidative stress following a meal is referred to as *postprandial* oxidative stress. This appears directly linked with the rise in blood glucose (Monnier et al., 2006) and triglycerides (Bae et al., 2001) following feeding. Individuals with diabetes and pre-diabetes appear more susceptible to postprandial oxidative stress due to the fact that they experience prolonged periods of hyperglycemia (Ceriello et al., 2002; Y. Miyazaki et al., 2007; Schindhelm et al., 2007) and hypertriglyceridemia (Ceriello et al., 2002;

Nappo et al., 2002) following meals, as compared to those with normal blood glucose control. Elevations in both glucose and triglycerides are directly linked to superoxide production (Bae et al., 2001; Nishikawa et al., 2000), a potent RONS which is known to react with other molecules causing additional RONS generation (Brownlee, 2005). It is likely that superoxide is generated within the mitochondria during the process of substrate oxidation following the ingestion of energy dense meals—in particular those high in saturated fat (Fisher-Wellman & Bloomer, 2009b). Therefore, methods of attenuating postprandial glycemia and lipemia (e.g., ingestion of lower calorie meals, decreased intake of saturated fat and simple sugar) may be associated with a decrease in RONS generation. Moreover, because the blood glucose (Monnier et al., 2006) and triglyceride response (Bloomer, Ferebee et al., 2009) to feeding is at least partly mediated by the fasting levels of these variables, a decrease in fasting blood glucose or triglycerides should result in lower postprandial oxidative stress. A lifestyle approach of modifying dietary intake might be considered a "first line" defense to decrease both fasting and postprandial oxidative stress. It should be noted that unlike exercise, for which the oxidative stress response is typically short lived, the oxidative stress response following a high calorie, high fat meal may persist for several hours (e.g., 4-6) following feeding (Bloomer, Cole et al., 2009; Bloomer, Fisher-Wellman et al., 2009; Melton et al., 2009; Saxena et al., 2005), and the response is exacerbated in those who are obese (Bloomer & Fisher-Wellman, 2009).

3.2.2.1 Meal composition and size

It is evident that the dietary practices of many individuals are not ideal, with consumption of dietary fat and simple sugars meals being prevalent (Drewnowski, 2007; Livesey et al., 2008). The sheer size of individual meals is often larger than what is needed based on energy demands, which may exacerbate and prolong postprandial glycemia and lipemia (Zilversmit, 1979)—allowing for greater RONS production. The severity of the oxidative load imposed appears dependent on the magnitude and rate of glycemia and lipemia experienced post-feeding (O'Keefe & Bell, 2007). Indeed, moderate to strong correlations exist for both glucose (Monnier et al., 2006) and triglycerides (Bae et al., 2001; Bloomer, Ferebee et al., 2009; Bloomer & Fisher-Wellman, 2010; Fisher-Wellman & Bloomer, 2010; Saxena et al., 2005) and oxidative stress biomarkers post-feeding.

Studies have included a variety of meals to induce an oxidative stress, ranging from isolated protein, carbohydrate, and fat, to mixed meals involving some combination of macronutrients. However, in most postprandial oxidative stress studies, the meal of choice is predominantly lipids. Such a meal reliably induces a state of oxidative stress, with a corresponding increase in blood triglycerides. We have recently compared the oxidative response to four different isocaloric meals (protein, carbohydrate, lipid, and mixed) and found that the lipid meal resulted in the greatest increase in postprandial oxidative stress (Fisher-Wellman & Bloomer, 2010). We have replicated these findings with regards to the lipid meal compared to a carbohydrate meal (Bloomer, Kabir, Marshall et al., 2010), noting that the oxidative stress response is dependent on meal size (i.e., increased calories = greater oxidative stress). Taken together, these data indicate that both meal composition and size impact postprandial oxidative stress.

3.3 Cellular dysfunction

The rise in circulating glucose and triglycerides, and the ensuing postprandial oxidative stress, triggers a harmful biochemical cascade throughout the circulation, including inflammation, endothelial dysfunction, hypercoaguability, and sympathetic hyperactivity, all of which may promote further RONS generation and oxidative damage (Fisher-Wellman & Bloomer, 2009b). The specific mechanisms of RONS generation in the postprandial state have yet to be elucidated due to the complexity of the cellular signaling cascade that exits *in vivo*. However, it appears that RONS initiate pathways of gene transcription, inflammation, and cellular adhesion, which induce further RONS generation and cellular damage (Fisher-Wellman & Bloomer, 2009b). When an excess of substrate enters the mitochondria, an accumulation of superoxide is generated from the electron transport chain (E. J. Anderson et al., 2009; Brownlee, 2005; Koves et al., 2008).

Within the peripheral tissue, this oxidative disruption can activate several pro-inflammatory transcription factors (nuclear factor κB [NF- κB] and tumor necrosis factor α [TNF-α]), which may induce further RONS production and insulin resistance (Aljada et al., 2006; Sinha et al., 2004). It is proposed that this form of RONS mediated insulin resistance is a means for peripheral tissue to reduce the amount substrate after excessive nutrient intake (Ceriello & Motz, 2004). In turn, substrate may accumulate within the circulation leading to hyperglycemia and hyperlipidemia (Fisher-Wellman & Bloomer, 2009b).

Within the vasculature, the endothelium may produce RONS by similar mechanics as peripheral tissue under conditions of hyperglycemia and hyperlipidemia (Ceriello & Motz, 2004). The increased RONS generation leads to the migration of phagocytic cells (leukocytes and neutrophils) to the endothelium, which produce additional RONS via NADPH oxidase (Mohanty et al., 2000; Mohanty et al., 2002; Van Oostrom et al., 2003). Moreover, this can lead to the release of inflammatory cytokines (Aljada et al., 2006) and cellular adhesion molecules (Ceriello et al., 2004; Rubin et al., 2008), which may be contributing factors to atherosclerosis, myocardial infarction, and stroke (Aljada et al., 2006).

3.3.1 Methods of assessing RONS formation

Since radicals are highly reactive and short lived (e.g., 10^{-5} seconds for superoxide), they are difficult to measure in biological systems. However, direct measurement techniques do exist; the most common being electron spin resonance (ESR) spectroscopy involving spin traps (Knight, 1999). Unfortunately, the equipment needed for such measurements is sophisticated and costly and the procedures are labor intensive, making the analysis of large numbers of samples difficult. More common is the use of indirect methods to measure oxidized biomolecules such as lipids, proteins, and DNA—resulting from exposure to RONS. By measuring these oxidative stress biomarkers, the degree of RONS generation and antioxidant capacity can be inferred, although specific information related to the type and extent of RONS remains unknown.

Due to the vast growth in this area of study, a variety of analysis procedures have been used to measure oxidative stress biomarkers (Rimbach et al., 1999), ranging from spectrophotometric assays to procedures using gas chromatography-mass spectroscopy (GC-MS) and high performance liquid chromatography (HPLC) coupled with electrochemical or chemiluminescence detection. Several commercially available assay kits are now available, while some companies offer oxidative stress related reagents and assay kits exclusively—while also providing analytical services for these procedures. Analyses can be performed using several body fluids (e.g., blood, urine, saliva), as well as muscle and organ tissue.

3.3.2 Common biomarkers of oxidative stress

Numerous biomarkers have been used in oxidative stress related research. Although a complete discussion of these markers is beyond the scope of this chapter, the biomarkers indicated below appear most commonly used. It should be understood that due to the growing interest in this line of work, new biomarkers and assay procedures emerge each year.

With regards to lipids, the following assays are commonly used: isoprostanes, lipid hyroperoxides, malondialdehyde (MDA), thiobarbituric acid reactive substances (TBARS), oxidized low density lipoproteins (ox-LDL-C), conjugated dienes, and hexanoyl lysine. With regards to proteins, the following assays are commonly used: protein carbonyls, nitrotyrosine, individual oxidized amino acids, and advanced oxidation protein products. With regards to DNA, the following assays are commonly used: 8-hydroxy-2'-deoxyguanosine (8-OHdG) and individual oxidized DNA strand breaks (comet assay).

In addition to the above, numerous individual antioxidants (e.g., ascorbate, tocopherols), antioxidant enzymes (e.g., superoxide dismutase), and antioxidant capacity markers can be measured. In relation to the latter, the following four assays are common: Trolox equivalent antioxidant capacity (TEAC), Oxygen Radical Absorbance Capacity (ORAC), Ferric Reducing Ability of Plasma (FRAP), and Total Radical-Trapping Antioxidant Parameter (TRAP).

Enzymes such as xanthine oxidase and peroxides such as hydrogen peroxide can also be measured. Other biomarkers thought to be associated with oxidative stress (e.g., inflammatory markers, obesity markers) are often included in postprandial studies. Finally, markers of endothelial function such as nitrate and nitrite (surrogate markers of nitric oxide) and flow mediated dilation are often included in studies of postprandial oxidative stress—due to the association between increased RONS production, decreased nitric oxide bioavailability, and endothelial dysfunction.

4. Minimizing and protecting against postprandial RONS

In an attempt to decrease the potential harm of RONS following acute feedings, it appears most prudent to attempt to simply avoid any significant elevation in RONS to begin with. This may be best accomplished by decreasing the overall calorie load within any given meal (Bloomer, Kabir, Marshall et al., 2010), while reducing the amount of saturated fat and simple sugar and replacing such calories with "healthy" fat and dietary fiber (Jenkins et al., 2007). In addition, the use of selected micronutrients may prove helpful. Finally, the performance of regular exercise may act to minimize postprandial oxidative stress. Beyond this prophylactic approach involving alterations in both nutrient intake and physical activity, the plan becomes one of treatment (i.e., handling the increased production of RONS due to the spike in blood glucose and blood triglycerides).

The remainder of this chapter focuses on the role of exercise and selected nutrient intake in an attempt to attenuate postprandial oxidative stress. While some studies have focused exclusively on diabetic patients, many others have not. However, because the potential mechanisms of actions in relation to glucose and triglyceride uptake, as well as the up-regulation in antioxidant defense may be similar for diabetic and non-diabetic individuals, we have included studies specific to both populations. Where possible, distinctions are made between studies.

5. Exercise and postprandial oxidative stress

Aerobic exercise has been shown to ameliorate postprandial oxidative stress and hyperlipidemia, with consumption of a high fat meal (Clegg et al., 2007; McClean et al.,

2007); however few studies have been conducted to address this issue. This effect may be due to an acute improvement in both triglyceride and glucose clearance, as well as an increase in antioxidant enzyme activity resulting from the exercise bout (McClean et al., 2011). The following text outlines findings specific to these areas of investigation.

5.1 Acute exercise

5.1.1 Triglyceride metabolism

It is well documented that exercise improves multiple aspects of human health and reduces both morbidity and mortality. Over the past few decades, a great amount of attention has been given to exercise as a therapeutic tool to reduce circulating triglyceride levels, both at rest and following meal consumption. Although, the exact mechanisms involved in attenuation of postprandial lipemia with exercise are not fully understood (Katsanos, 2006), exercise has been shown to decrease circulating triglyceride levels (Pronk, 1993), as well as help to reduce the amount of triglyceride secretion by the liver (Borsheim et al., 1999; Gill et al., 2001).

As highlighted earlier, reducing postprandial triglyceride levels is of particular importance, as this rise in circulating lipids post-feeding may be associated to increased risk for cardiovascular disease, possibly linked to the formation of RONS (Bae et al., 2001). It is well documented that a positive correlation exists between postprandial triglyceride levels and oxidative stress biomarkers (Bae et al., 2001; Bloomer, Ferebee et al., 2009; Bloomer & Fisher-Wellman, 2010; Fisher-Wellman & Bloomer, 2010; Saxena et al., 2005). Therefore, if exercise is successful at reducing postprandial triglycerides, it may also be associated with a decrease in oxidative stress.

Exercise has been reported to increase the activity of lipoprotein lipase (LPL) (Seip & Semenkovich, 1998), and thus improve triglyceride clearance. Lipoprotein lipase is expressed on adipocytes and skeletal muscle cells, with a main function of removing triglyceride from circulating lipoproteins. In the early postprandial period, adipose LPL activity increases while muscle LPL activity decreases (Seip & Semenkovich, 1998), which is most likely due to the rise in post-meal insulin. Exercise is believed to increase muscle LPL activity via decreased circulating insulin levels and increased catecholamine levels (Seip & Semenkovich, 1998). In support of this, acute exercise was investigated with participants cycling for 60-90 min at 55-70% VO_{2max} (Seip et al., 1997). The investigators reported a significant increase in LPL activity at four and eight hours post-exercise, with a return to baseline values at 20 hours post-exercise. This increase corresponded with a significant decrease in triglycerides, an increase in norepinephrine and epinephrine, and a reduction in circulating insulin. Other investigators have noted an increase in LPL activity at 24 hours (Ferguson et al., 1998; Grandjean et al., 2000) and 48 hours (Grandjean et al., 2000) post-exercise, while triglycerides have been noted to be lower at 24 hours (Cullinane et al., 1982; Grandjean et al., 2000), 48 hours (Grandjean et al., 2000), and 66 hours (Ferguson et al., 1998) following exercise.

In addition to an increase in LPL activity following exercise, a decreased secretion of very low density lipoprotein (VLDL) may be another mechanism that results in lower circulating levels of triglycerides (Borsheim et al., 1999; Gill et al., 2001). With regards to VLDL, it appears that intensity plays a major role in decreasing secretion of VLDL. This is supported by the work of Borsheim et al. (Borsheim et al., 1999) who noted a decrease in VLDL at 4.5 hours after cycling for 90 minutes at ~58% VO_{2max}, while Magkos et al. (Magkos et al., 2008) reported no significant changes for 6 hours post-exercise when treadmill walking was performed for 90 minutes at intensity of ~30% VO_{2max}. One investigation reported no change in VLDL immediately and one hour following exhaustive cycling exercise performed at 115% VO_{2max} (Lira et al., 2010). One potential limitation to this study was that the sampling time course was only sustained for one hour post-exercise. This is considerably less than prior work demonstrating an effect of exercise on VLDL lowering when measured 4.5 hours post-exercise (Borsheim et al., 1999).

Resistance training has also been shown to have an effect on postprandial lipemia. Singhal et al. (Singhal et al., 2009) investigated the role of intensity on postprandial lipemia by performing 10 resistance exercises at either 50% of eight repetition maximum (RM) or at 100% of eight RM (the lower intensity group performed 16 repetitions and the higher intensity group performed eight repetitions, and both groups performed three sets). A high fat meal was administered 15.5 hours post-exercise and there was found to be no significant difference between intensities. Both exercise bouts resulted in a similar reduction in postprandial lipemia and increase in fat oxidation. Another investigation compared resistance exercise with aerobic exercise by matching energy expenditure between exercise type (Petitt et al., 2003). Resistance exercise was comprised of 10 exercises performed for three sets of 10 repetitions, at the participants' 10 RM, while the aerobic exercise involved walking for the same duration as resistance exercise, and at an intensity estimated to elicit an identical energy expenditure. The results indicated that resistance exercise more favorably impacted baseline triglyceride concentrations, as well as the total postprandial triglyceride response, as compared to aerobic exercise and control.

5.1.2 Glucose metabolism

Given that the hallmark characteristic of diabetes is elevated blood glucose, consumption of high caloric meals composed of processed carbohydrates should be cautioned, if not avoided completely. The post-meal hyperglycemia has been shown to elicit a subsequent rise in RONS (Fisher-Wellman & Bloomer, 2010; Mohanty et al., 2000; Monnier et al., 2006). While young, healthy, non-diabetic individuals may not be negatively affected by high "simple" carbohydrate meals (Bloomer, Kabir, Marshall et al., 2010), research has shown that obese and metabolically diseased populations (e.g., obese, diabetic) consuming such feedings may be at increased risk for postprandial oxidative stress (Bloomer & Fisher-Wellman, 2009).

Individuals with insulin resistance have noted improvements in glucose homeostasis following both acute exercise and chronic exercise training, resulting in numerous metabolic and hemodynamic changes that may contribute to improved glucose disposal. These adaptive responses include enhanced insulin action on the skeletal muscle glucose transport system, reduced hormonal stimulation of hepatic glucose production, improved blood flow to skeletal muscle, and normalization of an abnormal blood lipid profile (Henriksen, 2002).

There are two main mechanisms responsible for enhanced glucose disposal following an acute exercise bout. First, an observed stimulation of GLUT4 to the cell membrane is noted, which allows for glucose uptake into the cytosol from the vasculature. Second, an increase in insulin sensitivity within contracting skeletal muscle is noted, ultimately allowing for GLUT4 translocation. Both of these effects are welcome following the ingestion of a high carbohydrate meal in which blood glucose is elevated.

Under normal physiologic conditions, GLUT4 is translocated from the cytosol to the cell surface through an insulin signaling mechanism. This is accomplished when insulin binds to the insulin receptors of the cellular wall of the muscle, which in turn activates a cascade of protein kinases that eventually translocate GLUT4 (Rockl et al., 2008). However, muscular contraction also induces this translocation independently of the initial insulin signaling, possibly through calcium and/or AMP kinase (Henriksen, 2002). An immediate increase in plasma GLUT4 transport protein content following moderate (Kristiansen et al., 1999) and high (Green et al., 2008; Kristiansen et al., 1996) intensity aerobic exercise has been noted. The increase in GLUT4 translocation in response to exercise may be necessary to allow for adequate glycogen replenishment (Thompson et al., 2001).

In terms of improved insulin sensitivity in response to exercise, it has been reported that insulin transduction through insulin receptor IRS-1/2 and PI3-kinase is enhanced post-exercise (Peres et al., 2005). This increase in skeletal muscle insulin sensitivity has been shown to last for up to 16 hours post-exercise (Chibalin et al., 2000; Ren et al., 1994). The enhanced removal of excess glucose from within the vasculature may be in conjunction with insulin independent increases of GLUT4 translocation, which in turn may relate to both reduced RONS production and maintenance of endothelial function.

The majority of acute investigations related to increased glucose clearance have focused on moderate intensity aerobic exercise, with multiple studies reporting favorable effects, as reviewed elsewhere (Praet & van Loon, 2007). To our knowledge, only one investigation has focused on the effect of high intensity sprint exercise on glucose metabolism. Brestoff et al. (Brestoff et al., 2009) had subjects perform five 30 second sprints at 125% VO_{2peak} with four minutes rest between sprints or 45 minutes of continuous exercise at 75% VO_{2peak}. An oral glucose tolerance test (OGTT) was administered 12-16 hours after exercise, and blood samples were taken every 30 minutes for a two hour period following the OGTT. There was no significant effect of the sprint exercise with regards to blood glucose lowering; however, the endurance protocol significantly lowered the insulin response. One possible reason for the lack of significance regarding the sprint exercise bout may be due to the bout being performed 12-16 hours prior to the OGTT—a time that may have been too distant from exercise to elicit an effect. Kraniou et al. (G. N. Kraniou et al., 2006) also reported no significant differences in GLUT4 protein gene expression with higher intensity aerobic exercise (27 minutes at 83% VO_{2peak}) compared to lower intensity aerobic exercise (60 minutes at 39% VO_{2peak}). Despite no significant difference between trials, both intensities resulted in a significant increase in GLUT4 protein and gene expression immediately and three hours post-exercise. Collectively, improvements in GLUT4 translocation immediately post-exercise (Kristiansen et al., 1997; Thorell et al., 1999), with significant increases in both gene expression (G. N. Kraniou et al., 2006; Y. Kraniou et al., 2000) and insulin sensitivity (Thong et al., 2003) lasting up to three hours post-exercise, may provide evidence for exercise to be performed closer to the actual test meal.

In addition to aerobic and sprint exercise protocols, resistance exercise has also been used in an attempt to improve postprandial glucose metabolism. One investigation had subjects exercise 14 hours prior to consuming a carbohydrate-rich meal (Andersen & Hostmark, 2007). Resistance exercise consisted of seven exercises performed for three sets of 10 repetitions at an intensity of 50% 1RM. The authors reported that postprandial glucose response was significantly reduced in the exercise group when compared to the control group. Fluckey et al. (Fluckey et al., 1994) investigated the effects of resistance exercise on glucose tolerance in non-diabetic subjects and in those with non-insulin dependent diabetes mellitus (NIDDM) by performing three sets of 10 repetitions at 75% 1RM, 18 hours prior to an OGTT. It was concluded that a single resistance exercise session significantly enhanced insulin clearance, but not insulin secretion, in both control and NIDDM subjects.

5.1.3 Antioxidant capacity

Although both a lowering of circulating triglycerides and blood glucose are thought to lead to lower production of RONS, improved antioxidant capacity may also serve to minimize the potential harm of increased RONS postprandially. Besides including more global markers of total antioxidant status, such as TEAC and ORAC, performing assays for individual antioxidant enzymes is another method to assess oxidative stress (e.g., superoxide dismutase [SOD], glutathione peroxidase [GPx], catalase [CAT], or glutathione reductase [GR]), as these enzyme may be up-regulated by an acute bout of exercise or may be acutely lowered owing to their combating nature against RONS.

Many investigations have been performed to confirm the post-exercise change in antioxidant capacity. Although these investigations generally note a decrease in antioxidant status post-exercise (Di Massimo et al., 2004; Tozzi-Ciancarelli et al., 2002), this is usually transient, as defenses either return to, or exceed, their pre-exercise values shortly after exercise cessation (Alessio et al., 2000; Fatouros et al., 2004; Michailidis et al., 2007; Quindry et al., 2003; Steinberg et al., 2006; Vider et al., 2001; Watson et al., 2005). These findings confirm the short-term activity of antioxidants in handling RONS, as well as propose a hypothesis for the stimulatory effect of acute exercise on chronic antioxidant status. However, despite the increase in antioxidant status noted in some studies, other authors have reported no increase (Sen et al., 1994; H. K. Vincent et al., 2004), which may be attributed to sampling times related to the acute session.

When focusing specifically on individual antioxidant enzymes, investigations have reported increases in SOD (Buczynski et al., 1991; M. F. Chen et al., 1994; Elosua et al., 2003), GPx (Buczynski et al., 1991; Elosua et al., 2003; Fatouros et al., 2004; Laaksonen et al., 1999), and CAT (Buczynski et al., 1991; Michailidis et al., 2007; Vider et al., 2001) following exercise. This increase in antioxidant enzyme activity may function to combat any increase in RONS resulting from ingestion of dietary nutrients. Only a few studies have reported null findings for SOD (Tozzi-Ciancarelli et al., 2002), GPx (Akova et al., 2001), and GR (Elosua et al., 2003).

Although not directly considered to be an antioxidant, heat shock proteins (HSPs) have been shown to be important mediators of skeletal muscle insulin sensitivity, as well as aid in protection against oxidative stress (Geiger & Gupte, 2011). With acute exercise, HSPs have been shown to increase in response to body temperature variations, inflammation, and RONS production (K. L. Hamilton et al., 2003; Nishizawa et al., 1999; Smolka et al., 2000). Therefore, HSPs are sometimes considered as "complementary" to antioxidant function (Finaud, Lac, & Filaire, 2006; Smolka et al., 2000), due to protecting cells and intracellular proteins against RONS-induced damage (Fehrenbach & Northoff, 2001; K. L. Hamilton et al., 2003; Nishizawa et al., 1999). It's important to note that within certain disease states, especially those associated with insulin resistance and aging, HSPs are decreased. This becomes an unfavorable situation considering that HSPs have been shown to decrease oxidative stress, inhibit inflammatory pathways, and enhance metabolic characteristics in skeletal muscle (Geiger & Gupte, 2011). Therefore, methods of increasing HSP production should be considered, with exercise being one such method.

5.2 Chronic exercise

5.2.1 Triglyceride metabolism

As with acute exercise, chronic exercise training also results in beneficial changes in lipid metabolism and increased LPL activity (Peltonen et al., 1981); at least within a sample of non-diabetic subjects. However, when focusing on investigations using patients with T2DM, the results are mixed. Two investigations have reported that patients with T2DM experienced a decrease in total cholesterol and low-density lipoprotein-cholesterol (LDL-C), as well as elevations in high-density lipoprotein-cholesterol (HDL-C) with aerobic training (consisting of mainly walking or running on a treadmill, cycling and calisthenics involving the upper and lower limbs) (Kadoglou et al., 2007; Ronnemaa et al., 1988) or walking (Araiza et al., 2006). However, other investigations with T2DM participants have noted no effect on the blood lipid profile following a period of exercise training (Loimaala et al., 2009; Sigal et al., 2007; Tudor-Locke et al., 2004).

Some investigations have aimed to increase physical activity in an effort to attenuate triglyceride levels. Despite being successful in their objective to increase physical activity, this increase was not associated with any significant reductions in triglycerides (Loimaala et al., 2009; Sigal et al., 2007; Tudor-Locke et al., 2004). It is possible that exercise alone (particularly if low volume), without a concomitant change in dietary intake and decrease in weight loss, might not be adequate to significantly improve blood lipids in those with T2DM. For example, Barnard et al. (Barnard et al., 1982) completed a 26 day intervention involving exercise and dietary modification and noted that both total cholesterol and triglycerides were reduced compared to baseline. However, these changes appeared mediated by an average weight loss of 4.3 kg. Using a similar exercise and nutritional intervention, Barnard and colleagues (Barnard et al., 1992) later noted a reduction in total cholesterol, LDL-C, and the ratio of total cholesterol: HDL-C. However, like the earlier investigation, these effects may have been more mediated by the weight loss than by the exercise. These data highlight the potential role of combination treatment (i.e., exercise and weight reduction—possibly involving dietary modification) to improve blood lipids in those with T2DM.

5.2.2 Glucose metabolism

Aerobic exercise has been the primary mode prescribed for diabetes prevention and management. It has been shown that only one week of aerobic training can improve whole-body insulin sensitivity in individuals with T2DM (Winnick et al., 2008). Although only persisting for a period of hours to days, moderate and vigorous aerobic training has been shown to improve insulin sensitivity (Bajpeyi et al., 2009; Evans et al., 2005; Galbo et al., 2007; Houmard et al., 2004). The responsiveness of skeletal muscles to insulin has been shown to be enhanced with training due to the increases in expression and/or activity of proteins involved in glucose metabolism and insulin signaling (Christ-Roberts et al., 2004; Holten et al., 2004; O'Gorman et al., 2006; Y. Wang et al., 2009). Glycogen synthase activity and GLUT4 protein expression has been shown to increase from moderate training (Christ-Roberts et al., 2004). Another key aspect related to improved insulin action and glycemic control is mediated through fat oxidation, and chronic training induces increased lipid storage in muscle, as well as increased fat oxidation capacity (Duncan et al., 2003; Goodpaster et al., 2003; Kelley & Kelley, 2007; Pruchnic et al., 2004).

In addition to aerobic training, blood glucose control and insulin action has also been shown to be favorably impacted by resistance training (N. D. Cohen et al., 2008; Dunstan et al., 2002; Ibanez et al., 2005; Ibanez et al., 2008; Ishii et al., 1998). One investigation consisted of twice-weekly progressive resistance training for 16 weeks by older men with newly diagnosed T2DM (Ibanez et al., 2005). The authors reported a 46% increase in insulin action, 7% reduction in fasting blood glucose, and a significant loss of visceral fat. Muscle mass increases from resistance training may also aid in blood glucose uptake due to the actual increase in mass, and heavy resistance training may also help to reverse or prevent further loss of skeletal muscle due to disuse and aging (Castaneda et al., 2002; Willey & Singh, 2003).

5.2.3 Antioxidant capacity

Participating in regular physical activity has been shown to be an effective means of increasing antioxidant defense (Ji, 1999; Kojda & Hambrecht, 2005). Exercise, in particular of aerobic nature (Elosua et al., 2003; Marzatico et al., 1997; May et al., 1996; H. Miyazaki et al., 2001; Selamoglu et al., 2000), may lead to up-regulation in antioxidant enzymes that are situated at the muscular, plasmatic, hepatic, and cardiac levels (Chevion et al., 2003; Venditti & Di Meo, 1997). With regards to muscle, the effect may be strongest for tissue with high oxidative power (e.g., type I fibers) (Hollander et al., 1999; Inal et al., 2001; Leeuwenburgh et al., 1999). It should be noted that the absolute magnitude of change in antioxidant enzymes may differ, with SOD and GPx noted to increase more than CAT (Hollander et al., 1999; Leeuwenburgh et al., 1999; H. Miyazaki et al., 2001; Ohno et al., 1988; Powers et al., 1999).
There are less data pertaining to the impact of anaerobic exercise on antioxidant capacity. However, it has been reported that anaerobically trained individuals have lower oxidative stress and experience less muscular damage after exercise when compared with untrained individuals (Ortenblad et al., 1997; Selamoglu et al., 2000). Moreover, anaerobic trained participants have been reported to have higher antioxidant enzyme activity in blood and working muscle (Hellsten et al., 1996; Marzatico et al., 1997; Ortenblad et al., 1997; K. R. Vincent et al., 2002); however, exceptions to this finding exist (Selamoglu et al., 2000). Heat shock proteins have also been shown to increase as a result to chronic anaerobic training (Carmeli et al., 2010), suggesting that cellular protection is increased as an adaptation to this form of exercise.

5.3 Summary of exercise

Although exercise may elicit a transient increase in RONS, it is clear from multiple studies that both acute and chronic exercise may improve certain aspects of metabolic function—including enhanced triglyceride and glucose clearance, as well as increased antioxidant defense. Because elevated triglyceride and glucose (in particular in response to high fat and/or high carbohydrate feeding) is associated with increased production of RONS, any decrease in circulating triglyceride and glucose may be related to lower postprandial oxidative stress. Few studies have directly measured postprandial oxidative stress in association with acute or chronic exercise. Therefore results need to be inferred based on the observed changes in triglyceride and glucose. Further work is needed to provide more convincing evidence for such an effect.

6. Nutrients and postprandial oxidative stress

The multifaceted etiology of diabetes has given rise to a number of interventions in an attempt to minimize disease progression. Regular exercise (Praet & van Loon, 2007; Tucker et al., 2008), weight control (Mavian et al., 2010), pharmaceuticals (Nakajima, 2010; O'Keefe et al., 2011), and selected nutrients (Badimon et al., 2010; Davi et al., 2010; Nahas & Moher, 2009) have been scientifically supported to aid in diabetes management. Considering that inhabitants of the Western world spend up to 16 hours of the day in the postprandial state (de Koning & Rabelink, 2002), and that postprandial oxidative stress is hypothesized to be the pathogenic mechanism underlying diabetes and cardiovascular disease (Ceriello & Motz, 2004; Fisher-Wellman & Bloomer, 2009b), the use of selected nutrients as a therapeutic tool to help control diabetes should be considered. Of course, the fundamentals of optimal dietary intake inclusive of the consumption of a nutrient dense, moderate to low calorie diet, ideally consumed over multiple balanced meals throughout the day (Bloomer, Kabir, Marshall et al., 2010), and inclusive of fruits and vegetables (S. Liu et al., 2000), whole grains (S. Liu et al., 1999), and relatively low amounts of saturated fats should be considered first. However, beyond the foundational plan, there exist a number of nutraceuticals, functional foods, and dietary strategies that have been shown to attenuate the postprandial rise in triglycerides, glucose, and subsequent oxidative stress, as well as improve antioxidant status. Therefore, intake of selected nutrients may be considered as a preventive measure, as well as a treatment option, for individuals with impaired glucose tolerance (IGT).

The focus of this section is to highlight nutrients that have a potential influence on ameliorating the rise in postprandial oxidative stress. As mentioned previously in this chapter, postprandial oxidative stress appears contingent upon the magnitude and rate of postprandial glycemia and triglyceridemia (O'Keefe & Bell, 2007). Individuals who are obese or have metabolic or cardiovascular disease appear to be more susceptible to postprandial oxidative stress, and they typically experience more robust and prolonged periods of hyperglycemia (Y. Miyazaki et al., 2007; Schindhelm et al., 2007; Serin et al., 2007) and hypertriglyceridemia (Ceriello et al., 2002; Nappo et al., 2002) post-feeding, as compared to non-diseased individuals. Again, elevations in blood glucose and triglycerides are directly associated with superoxide production (Bae et al., 2001); hence, a greater increase in either blood glucose or triglyceride post-feeding may be associated with a greater increase in postprandial oxidative stress. This has been reported previously in patients with T2DM (Saxena et al., 2005), as well as in those with coronary artery disease (Graner et al., 2006).

The following sections are focused primarily on highlighting nutrients that enhance triglyceride and glucose clearance, are associated with lower biomarkers of oxidative stress, improve antioxidant status, and augment endothelial function. Specific attention is given to literature focused on outcomes in the postprandial period, given that fasting is not the usual physiological state of modern humans, especially in the Western world. It should be understood that due to the vast and increasing study in this area of investigation, the present chapter does not exhaust the literature pertaining to this line of work. However, several well-studied nutrients are included for discussion. Moreover, while we provide brief information pertaining to the potential mechanisms of actions for selected nutrients, a complete discussion is beyond the scope of this chapter. We refer readers to the individual manuscripts for more information on possible mechanisms of action.

6.1 Nutritional supplements

The use of nutrition supplements for purposes of aiding postprandial metabolism is widespread. Although a variety of ingredients and finished products have been studied, those with greatest interest appear to be antioxidants and insulin mimetic agents. The text below illustrates the varying effects of several antioxidants, in diabetic and healthy populations. Additional ingredients used primarily for purposes of altering glucose, and in some cases lipid, metabolism, are also presented. The mixed findings across studies extend to some longitudinal intervention studies (some of which may include the use of sub-optimal dosing of nutrients (Sesso et al., 2008)), indicating that more research is needed to elucidate the optimal dosage and duration of supplementation, as well as the population who might benefit most from supplementation.

6.1.1 Vitamin C

Vitamin C supplementation (800mg·day^{-1}) in T2DM patients with low plasma vitamin C for four weeks was found not to be effective at improving endothelial dysfunction and insulin sensitivity, despite increasing endogenous vitamin C levels (H. Chen et al., 2006). Similarly, 1.5g·day^{-1} of vitamin C for three weeks did not improve fasting plasma concentrations of oxidative stress biomarkers, blood glucose, lipid profile, or blood pressure, despite also increasing endogenous concentrations of vitamin C (Darko et al., 2002). In contrast to these null findings, 1g·day^{-1} of vitamin C for three days completely abolished the postprandial oxidative stress insult, and blunted the deterioration of endothelial function, to a high fat meal in patients with T2DM (R. A. Anderson et al., 2006). Moreover, pharmacological infusion with vitamin C has been found to acutely improve endothelial dysfunction in patients with insulin-dependent DM (Timimi et al., 1998), NIDDM (Ting et al., 1996), and healthy subjects (Beckman et al., 2001). Finally, intravenous infusion of vitamin C improved endothelial function and insulin sensitivity in patients with coronary spastic angina following an OGTT (Hirashima et al., 2000).

6.1.2 Vitamin E

Like vitamin C, vitamin E (α-tocopherol) supplementation has been similarly ambiguous with regards to improving biomarkers of oxidative stress and cardiovascular risk factors. On the one hand, vitamin E supplementation was associated with significant reduction in biomarkers of oxidative stress in NIDDM patients supplemented with 600mg·day^{-1} for two weeks (Davi et al., 1999). Additionally, 98 Korean patients with T2DM treated with continuous subcutaneous insulin infusion and 200mg·day^{-1} vitamin E for two months had significantly decreased red blood cell lipid peroxide concentrations (Park & Choi, 2002). However, Winterbone and colleagues (Winterbone et al., 2007) found that 1200IU·day^{-1} of vitamin E for four weeks in T2DM patients resulted in a significant prooxidant effect mediated through DNA damage to mononuclear cells after an OGTT, despite no changes in fasting oxidative measures. The ability of vitamin E to act as a pro-oxidant and increase the peroxidation of lipids has been established *in vitro* (Bowry et al., 1992; Santanam & Parthasarathy, 1995); while the work of Winterbone et al. (Winterbone et al., 2007) suggests the possibility that a high dose of vitamin E is also potentially damaging *in vivo* in patients with T2DM.

6.1.3 α-lipoic acid

The antioxidant α-lipoic acid (ALA) has illustrated efficacy when prescribed to patients with T2DM. Three weeks of treatment with ALA (600, 1200, or 1800 mg·day^{-1}) resulted in a significant increase in insulin-stimulated glucose disposal compared to placebo (Jacob et al., 1999). Three weeks of treatment with intravenous infusion of ALA (600mg·day^{-1}) in subjects with impaired fasting glucose (IFG) illustrated a significant increase in endothelium-dependent arterial dilation and a significant decrease in plasma TBARS (Xiang et al., 2011). Acutely, in patients with IGT, plasma glucose levels were similar between the ALA group (300mg) and placebo group during an OGTT. However, at 1 and 2 hours, flow mediated dilation was significantly elevated in the ALA group compared to the placebo group, and plasma glucose levels were negatively correlated with endothelial function. After supplementation with ALA, the power of this association decreased. Similarly, flow mediated dilation decreased in association with an increase in TBARS, and the strength of this association also decreased after supplementation with ALA (Xiang et al., 2008).

6.1.4 Coenzyme Q_{10}

Coenzyme Q_{10} (CoQ_{10}) is a critical intermediate of mitochondrial electron transport chain activity that regulates cytoplasmic redox potential and can inhibit superoxide generation by endothelial cells (Beyer, 1990; McCarty, 1999). Two separate human trials, one with hyperglycemic T2DM patients and one with statin-treated T2DM patients, elicited approximately parallel results. Specifically, twelve weeks of supplementation with 200mg of CoQ_{10} or placebo resulted in significant increases in plasma CoQ_{10}, respectively, and improved flow mediated dilation (S. J. Hamilton et al., 2009; Watts et al., 2002). However, neither trial found an alteration in biomarkers of oxidative stress or antioxidant capacity, lipid profiles, glycemic control, or blood pressure after supplementation.

6.1.5 Carnitine

Carnitine is an essential compound that assists in the transport of long-chain fatty acids into the mitochondrial matrix for subsequent oxidation. Additionally, *in vitro* and *in vivo* evidence supports the role of carnitine as an antioxidant (Calo et al., 2006). Endothelial function, assessed by flow mediated dilation in the brachial artery was improved after a high-fat meal consumed with 2g L-carnitine and preceded by three weeks of carnitine supplementation in healthy, young men and women (Volek et al., 2008). There was no significant postprandial differences in triglycerides, inflammatory markers, interleukin-6 (IL-6), TNF-α, or MDA between placebo and treatment. In pre-diabetics (fasting blood glucose: 100-125 $mg{\cdot}dL^{-1}$) $3g{\cdot}day^{-1}$ acetyl L-carnitine arginate resulted in a significant increase in fasting nitrate/nitrite, suggesting a possible impact on vascular function (although not specifically determined). However, little other effects were noted for a variety of oxidative stress biomarkers (Bloomer et al., 2009).

6.1.6 Lycopene

Lyopene is a highly unsaturated carotenoid found predominantly in tomato products (Clinton, 1998). Four weeks of lycopene supplementation (tomato-derived Lyc-O-Mato) at $30mg{\cdot}day^{-1}$ in obese patients was not found to favorably influence markers of inflammation and oxidation biomarkers, despite a significant increase in plasma cartenoids, and specifically lyopene (Markovits et al., 2009). One week of lyopene supplementation ($80mg{\cdot}day^{-1}$) was found again to increased endogenous capacity of plasma lipid-soluble antioxidants (lycopene, β-carotene, and α-tocopherol); however, biomarkers of vascular oxidative stress and inflammation were unaffected in the fasted state, as well as post consumption of a high fat meal, in young, healthy subjects (Denniss et al., 2008). Finally, both acute (24 hour) and long-term (seven day) tomato puree consumption had no effects on endothelial dysfunction after consumption of a meal, despite a significant increase in plasma lyopene levels in healthy postmenopausal women (Stangl et al., 2011).

6.1.7 Catechins

Tea is made from the leaves of the evergreen *Camellia sinensis*. Tea is a rich source polyphenolic compounds called catechins, especially epigallocatechin gallate (EGCG), which are hypothesized to have multiple health-promoting effects (Higdon & Frei, 2003), including a potential impact on T2DM (Thielecke & Boschmann, 2009). Chronic green tea supplementation has been shown to significantly decrease lipid peroxidation and a trend to lower LDL-C (non-significantly) when supplemented for eight weeks in obese subjects with metabolic syndrome (Basu et al., 2010). On the other hand, three months of supplementation with an extract of green and black tea was found to elicit non-significant differences in glycosylated hemoglobin (HbA_{1c}) between treatment groups in a placebo controlled multiple-dose study in patients with T2DM (Mackenzie et al., 2007).

Tea catechins consumed acutely have been shown to decrease incremental area under the curve (AUC) for triglycerides in a dose dependent manner in men with mild or borderline hypertriglyceridemia. Moreover, tea catechin supplementation resulted in a significant suppression of remnant-like particle cholesterol at an early postprandial stage, but this failed to achieve statistical significance for overall incremental AUC (Unno et al., 2005). In healthy subjects, 300mL of green tea was shown to have no glucose or insulin-lowering effects (Josic et al., 2010).

6.1.8 Red wine (polyphenols)

Consumption of 300mL of red wine taken in conjunction with an acute high fat meal was found to significantly preserve antioxidant defenses and reduce both LDL-C susceptibility to oxidation and thrombotic activation, in T2DM patients (Ceriello et al., 2001). Also, a trend was seen for decreased triglycerides across the 3 hour postprandial time period; however, glucose and insulin appeared to be unaffected. In healthy subjects, 250mL of red wine in conjunction with an acute high fat meal significantly reduced the oxidative insult (increased antioxidant capacity and decreased oxidative stress biomarkers), without significantly modifying lipid profile (Ventura et al., 2004). Finally, 300mg of grape seed proanthocyanidins was given to healthy volunteers before the consumption of a test meal. It was found that grape seed extract minimizes the postprandial oxidative stress by decreasing oxidants and increasing antioxidant levels, tending to protect LDL-C from oxidative modification (Natella et al., 2002).

In relation to the above, the consumption of red wine may be linked to the 'French Paradox' (Renaud & de Lorgeril, 1992): derived from an examination of World Health Organization (WHO) epidemiological data, identifying that subjects in France, despite of diet highly comprised of saturated fat, comparable cholesterol and similar risk factors, showed considerably lower incidence of death from coronary heart disease compared with other countries such as the USA. Further analysis suggests that alcohol consumption, in particular red wine, might provide superior protection compared with other nutrients and beverages. Although the specific mechanism behind the French paradox has not been identified, *in vitro* data has proposed that the flavonoid components in red wine have strong antioxidant properties (Demrow et al., 1995; Sun et al., 2009), possibly contributing to observed cardiovascular benefits.

Some subsequent applied human research has supported these claims. For example, moderate red wine consumption (118 $mL \cdot day^{-1}$) for 12 months, in subjects with T2DM who had sustained their first non-fatal myocardial infarction, was associated with significant improvements in oxidative stress, inflammatory response, and insulin sensitivity (Marfella et al., 2006). However, triglycerides and other markers of glycemic control were unaffected. Four weeks of grape seed extract (600mg·day^{-1}) in obese T2DM patients was associated with significantly improved markers of inflammation, glycemia, and the sole marker of oxidative stress (Kar et al., 2009). However, no significant changes were shown in endothelial function, insulin sensitivity, or total antioxidant status. Similarly, 360mL·day^{-1} of red wine showed no improvement in endothelial function after two weeks, in patients with T2DM (Napoli et al., 2005). In contrast, insulin-mediated whole body glucose disposal improved significantly. Finally, 400mL·day^{-1} of red wine for two weeks significantly increased total antioxidant status and significantly decreased MDA and reduced glutathione (GSH) of both young and old subjects, assumed to be healthy (Micallef et al., 2007). No significant effects were found for blood glucose or lipid parameters.

6.1.9 Combination antioxidant treatment

Combination treatments of antioxidants have been more efficacious in lowering oxidative stress biomarkers, most likely through a synergetic mechanism and their ability to function within different body compartments (e.g., aqueous for vitamin C vs. lipid for vitamin E). For example, vitamin C can assist in maintaining vitamin E in the reduced and active state (Packer et al., 1979). Neri et al. (Neri et al., 2005) investigated the effects of 15 days antioxidant supplementation with 600mg·day^{-1} N-acetylcysteine (NAC), 300mg·day^{-1} vitamin E, and 250mg·day^{-1} vitamin C on postprandial oxidative stress in patients with T2DM, IGT, and healthy volunteers. Antioxidant supplementation was associated with significant improvements in redox balance in all three groups, along with a reduced postprandial increase in biomarkers of oxidative stress, as well as plasma levels of von Willebrand factor (vWF), vascular cell adhesion molecule-1 (VCAM-1). Neri and colleagues (Neri et al., 2010) conducted a follow up investigation with an antioxidant cocktail of similar composition (600 mg·day^{-1} of NAC, 50 mg·day^{-1} of vitamin E, and 500 mg·day^{-1} of vitamin C) on postprandial oxidative stress. Again the trial was 15 days in duration with patients with T2DM, patients with IGT, and healthy controls. It was found that antioxidant supplementation lowered oxidative stress biomarkers in the control group and significantly decreased it in the IGT group after feeding. It was also noted that antioxidant supplementation was able to improve endothelial function, but only in healthy and IGT subjects. It should be noted that antioxidant supplementation did not alter any of the lipid variables in any of the groups. Finally, the acute intake of a combination vitamin C (2g) and vitamin E (800IU) was found to prevent the transient decrease in flow mediated dilation in healthy subjects following the OGTT, despite no significant effects being noted for biomarkers of oxidative stress (Title et al., 2000).

6.1.10 Omega-3 fatty acids

Evidence exists for the cardio-protective effects of the fatty acids found in fish (Cottin et al., 2011), which include the omega-3 fatty acids eicosapentanoic acid (EPA) and docosahexanoic acid (DHA). Therefore, fish oil supplementation has considerable potential for diabetic individuals. In a randomized, double-blinded, placebo controlled trial in treated, hypertensive T2DM patients, 4g·day^{-1} of purified EPA or DHA elicited a fall in urinary F2-isoprostane excretion following six weeks of supplementation (Mori et al., 2003). Moreover,

baseline urinary F2-isoprostanes were positively associated with indices of diabetic control and the changes in urinary F2-isoprostanes were positively associated with changes in TNF-α and HbA_{1c}. In another study with T2DM patients with treated hypertension, 4g·day^{-1} EPA, DHA, or olive oil for six weeks decreased serum triglycerides by 19% and 15% in the EPA and DHA groups respectively, but neither had significant effects on glycemic control (Woodman et al., 2002). Purified omega-3 fatty acids at 2g·day^{-1} for 10 weeks decreased fasting triglycerides relative to placebo, and ApoB-100, and MDA relative to baseline and placebo (Shidfar et al., 2008). Again, omega-3 fatty acids had no effect on glycemic control. Finally, 2g·day^{-1} of N-3 polyunsaturated fatty acids for 12 weeks in offspring of patients with T2DM, significantly improved flow mediated dilation that was accompanied by a significant decrease in triglycerides and TNF-α (Rizza et al., 2009).
Acute combination treatment of omega-3 fatty acids (400mg EPA and 200mg DHA) and isoflavones (150mg glycoside isoflavones) did not attenuate the postprandial rise in triglycerides after a high fat meal in obese hypertriglyceridemic men (Hanwell et al., 2009). Moreover, they did not induce any significant changes in oxidative stress biomarkers. On the other hand, 1g of EPA and DHA consumed by healthy subjects was able to preserve endothelial function following a high fat meal (Fahs et al., 2010).

6.1.11 Vitamin D

Investigations have shown that vitamin D helps to reduce the risk of bone fractures, falls, autoimmune diseases, cardiovascular disease and cancer (S. Wang, 2009), and has also been shown to be inversely associated with risk of T2DM (Pittas et al., 2006). Cholecalciferol (vitamin D_3) supplemented at 1332 IU·day^{-1} for one month in women with T2DM was shown to improve insulin secretion, with a tendency to decrease fasting plasma glucose (Borissova et al., 2003). On the other hand, supplementation with 40,000 IU·week^{-1} of cholecalciferol for six months in T2DM subjects treated with metformin and bed-time insulin had no significant effects on fasting glucose, insulin, C-peptide, fructosamine, and HbA_{1c} levels (Jorde & Figenschau, 2009). Finally, supplementation with 500mg·day^{-1} calcium citrate and 700IU·day^{-1} cholecalciferol in apparently healthy, older subjects (≥ 65 years), for three years, prevented increases in fasting plasma glucose and insulin resistance in the subgroup of participants with impaired fasting glucose at baseline. There was no effect among those with normal fasting glucose (Pittas et al., 2007).

6.1.12 Magnesium, Chromium, Vanadium

Certain elements have been proposed to have glucoregulatory effects, such as magnesium, chromium, and vanadium. In T2DM patients with low serum magnesium levels, 50mL·day^{-1} $MgCl_2$ solution given for 16 weeks was shown to improve fasting measures of insulin sensitivity, blood glucose, and HbA_{1c} (Rodriguez-Moran & Guerrero-Romero, 2003). Supplementation with 600mg·day^{-1} magnesium pidolate for 12 weeks in mildly-hypertensive patients was shown to have multiple benefits (Hadjistavri et al., 2010). Specifically, supplementation was shown to lower fasting insulin, heighten fasting insulin sensitivity, reduce postprandial measures of glucose and insulin AUC, ameliorate postprandial measures of insulin sensitivity, and improve total cholesterol, LDL-C, HDL-C, and triglycerides. Finally, chronic magnesium supplementation (2.5g·day^{-1} $MgCl_2$) for three months has been reported to result in improvements in fasting insulin sensitivity and the lipid profile in non-diabetic subjects with insulin resistance (Guerrero-Romero et al., 2004).

Opposite to the beneficial effects of magnesium, chronic supplementation with chromium picolinate has been relatively ineffective in improving metabolic features of patients with IGT (Ali et al., 2011; Iqbal et al., 2009), despite being commonly marketed as a hypoglycemic agent, and with efficacious data obtained in animals (Abdourahman & Edwards, 2008) and cell culture (Y. Q. Wang & Yao, 2009). It has been noted that the beneficial effects of chromium supplementation might be related to the severity of insulin resistance, with clinical response being more likely in individuals with more elevated fasting glucose and HbA_{1c} (Cefalu et al., 2010).

Finally, vanadium has been used with mixed success in prior trials in an attempt to lower blood glucose. The mechanism supporting vanadium supplementation is likely linked to its ability to promote increased insulin-mediated glucose disposal. Like chromium, vanadium efficacy appears to also depend on the degree of diabetic complications, with T2DM patients (N. Cohen et al., 1995; Cusi et al., 2001; Goldfine et al., 2000; Halberstam et al., 1996) reporting greater efficacy compared to non-diabetics (Halberstam et al., 1996; Jacques-Camarena et al., 2008; Jentjens & Jeukendrup, 2002).

6.1.13 Inositol phosphoglycans

Inositol phosphoglycans are potentially important post-receptor mediators of insulin action (Kelly et al., 1987; Larner et al., 1998). Pinitol (3-*O*-methyl-D-chiro-inositol) was identified in putative insulin mediator fractions that had hypoglycemic activity, and appears to mimic the effects of insulin by acting downstream in the insulin signaling pathway (Fonteles et al., 1996). After pinitol treatment ($20mg{\cdot}kg^{-1}{\cdot}day^{-1}$) in poorly controlled T2DM patients, fasting glucose, postprandial glucose, and HbA_{1c} were all significantly decreased. However, an effect on lipid profiles or adipocytokine levels was not noted (Kim et al., 2007). Acutely, pinitol supplemented at 1000mg 60 minutes before an OGTT was not shown to influence any indices of whole-body glucose tolerance and insulin sensitivity, or the activation of the skeletal insulin receptor in older, non-diabetic adults (Stull et al., 2009).

6.1.14 Cinnamon

Cinnamon is widely used as a spice, and research has suggested that it may have potential effects in improving not only glucose metabolism, but also lipid metabolism and antioxidant status. Kahn et al. (A. Khan et al., 2003) demonstrated that consumption of 1, 3, or $6g{\cdot}day^{-1}$ of cinnamon for 40 days reduces serum glucose, triglycerides, LDL-C, and total cholesterol in patients with T2DM. Moreover, lower serum glucose and lipid were maintained even when the individuals were not consuming cinnamon for 20 days. In a randomized, placebo-controlled double-blind clinical trial, intake of $2g{\cdot}day^{-1}$ of cinnamon for 12 weeks significantly reduces HbA_{1c} and systolic and diastolic blood pressure among poorly controlled T2DM patients compared to placebo (Akilen et al., 2010). Moreover, fasting blood glucose was significantly decreased compared to baseline. In opposition to these findings, Vanschoonbeek and colleagues (Vanschoonbeek et al., 2006) concluded that that cinnamon supplementation for 6-7 weeks at $1.5g{\cdot}day^{-1}$ does not improve fasting plasma glucose or insulin concentrations, whole body oral glucose tolerance, or lipid profiles in postmenopausal women with T2DM.

The antioxidant benefit of cinnamon has also been elucidated, suggesting a potential *in vivo* mechanism by which cinnamon acts. Subjects with impaired fasting glucose were assigned either 500mg·day^{-1} of an aqueous cinnamon extract or placebo for 12 weeks (Roussel et al., 2009). The cinnamon extract was shown to increase FRAP and plasma thiol groups, while decreasing MDA levels. In healthy humans, cinnamon supplementation at 3g·day^{-1} for 14 days reduced the glucose and insulin response to an OGTT (Solomon & Blannin, 2009). However, these effects were lost following cessation of cinnamon supplementation. Acutely, cinnamon ingestion reduced plasma glucose AUC and improved insulin sensitivity in inactive, healthy men (Solomon & Blannin, 2007).

6.1.15 Turmeric

Another spice proposed to have glucoregulatory effects is *Curcuma longa* (turmeric), due to its active component, curcumin. Curcumin is believed to have antioxidant and anti-inflammatory properties (Hsu & Cheng, 2007). A four week intervention study revealed no changes in fasting glucose or lipid profiles when 2.8g·day^{-1} turmeric was given to healthy subjects (Tang et al., 2008). However, acute ingestion of 6g *Curcuma longa* in healthy subjects had a significant effect on postprandial insulin levels, without influencing glucose (Wickenberg et al., 2010).

6.1.16 Banaba and Berberine

Lagerstroemia speciosa L. (banaba) standardized to 1% corosolic acid (Glucosol™) at daily dosages of 32 and 48mg·day^{-1} for two weeks showed a significant reduction in blood glucose in T2DM patients (Judy et al., 2003). Acutely, corosolic acid also attenuated the postprandial rise in blood glucose post-OGTT, in a mixed sample of IGT, IFG, and healthy subjects (Fukushima et al., 2006). Berberine is a natural plant alkaloid isolated from the Chinese herb, *Coptis chinensis* (Huanglian). Chronically supplemented at 1g·day^{-1} to dyslipidemic T2DM patients for three months, berberine was associated with significantly improved levels of fasting and postprandial blood glucose, HbA_{1c}, triglycerides, total cholesterol, LDL-C, blood pressure and IL-6, compared to placebo (Zhang et al., 2008). Moreover, markers of insulin sensitivity were improved in the berberine group, albeit, non-significantly. A similar investigation comprised of two components (study A and study B) also evaluated the efficacy of berberine in T2DM patients for 3 months (1.5g·day^{-1}) (Yin et al., 2008). Study A found that berberine had similar hypoglycemic effects to the anti-diabetic drug metformin. Significant decreases were noted in fasting and postprandial blood glucose, HbA_{1c}, and triglycerides were observed in the berberine group and in the metforin group (as expected). Study B consisted of the combination therapy, berberine (1.5g·day^{-1}) added to subjects' usual anti-diabetic medicine, again for 3 months. Significant reductions compared to baseline were found in fasting and postprandial blood glucose, HbA_{1c}, fasting insulin, insulin sensitivity, and lipid profile, including triglycerides, total cholesterol, and LDL-C. A proprietary blend of Phellodendron (which contains the active ingredient berberine) and Crape Myrtle (banaba; *Lagerstroemia speciosa* L.) has been shown to lower the postprandial glucose response to a modified OGTT, while resulting in a non-significant attenuation in insulin response, in a small sample of healthy, exercise-trained men (Canale et al., In Review). It is possible that a combination of nutrients may provide the most favorable effect on postprandial glucose response.

6.1.17 Fenugreek

Two months of supplementation with *Trigonella foenum graecum* (fenugreek) seeds in newly-diagnosed T2DM patients significantly attenuated incremental AUC of blood glucose and insulin, as well as demonstrating a trend to improve fasting and two hour postprandial glucose (Gupta et al., 2001). The rise in triglycerides and cholesterol were also significantly improved, along with insulin sensitivity and HDL-C after supplementation. Moreover, 12 weeks of supplementation with Fenugreek elicited significant decreases in fasting blood glucose, postprandial blood glucose, and HBA_{1c} (Lu et al., 2008). Acutely, Fenugreek added to two slices of bread (5% fenugreek), and fed to a small sample of T2DM patients, was shown to significantly reduce the AUC for insulin (Losso et al., 2009). Glucose AUC also tended to be improved.

6.1.18 Stevia

Steviol glycosides (or stevioside), isolated from the plant *Stevia rebaudiana Bertoni* and taken for three months ($250mg{\cdot}day^{-1}$) by patients with T1DM and T2DM, as well as by healthy controls, was not shown to elicit any significant differences in markers of glycemic control or blood pressure (Barriocanal et al., 2008). Acutely however, 1g of steviol glycosides reduced postprandial blood glucose levels in T2DM patients and increased the insulinogenic index ($AUC_{insulin}/AUC_{glucose}$) (Gregersen et al., 2004). The differences in dosages used in each respective study may be the reason for these conflicting results.

6.1.19 Gymnema sylvestre

Early intervention trials with *Gymnema sylvestre* ($400mg{\cdot}day^{-1}$) were associated with improved glycemic control in NIDDM patients (Baskaran et al., 1990) and insulin-dependent DM patients (Shanmugasundaram et al., 1990). Moreover, there was a significant improvement in terms of insulin response and lipid profiles, encompassing cholesterol, triglycerides, and free fatty acids. A more recent investigation, illustrated that $1g{\cdot}day^{-1}$ for 60 days of Om Santal Adivasi®, a novel high molecular weight *Gymnema sylvestre* extract, induced significant increases in circulating insulin and C-peptide, which were associated with significant reductions in fasting and postprandial blood glucose (Al-Romaiyan et al., 2010).

6.1.20 Cissus quadrangularis

Cissus quadrangularis is a relatively novel ingredient in the clinical setting; however, the few investigations that do exist exhibit a remarkable efficacy. In three clinical investigations (J. E. Oben et al., 2006; J. E. Oben et al., 2007; J. E. Oben et al., 2008), *cissus quadrangularis* supplemented to obese and overweight persons for 6-8 weeks has elicited significant net reductions in weight, body fat, fasting blood glucose, total cholesterol, LDL-C, triglycerides, C-reactive protein, biomarkers of oxidative stress, as well as a significant increase in HDL-C. As all work was conducted by the same group of investigators, additional studies performed by other research groups are needed to corroborate these findings.

6.1.21 Coccinia indica

Coccinia indica (*Coccinia cordifolia*) supplemented to T2DM patients for 90 days elicited a significant reduction in fasting and postprandial blood glucose and HbA_{1c}; however, there was no significant change in serum lipids, except for LDL-C (Kuriyan et al., 2008). In an earlier study, *Coccinia indica* powder, from crushed, dried leaves, significantly improved glycemic control following six weeks use in patients with poorly controlled or otherwise untreated T2DM (A. K. Khan et al., 1980). Moreover, animal data suggests that *Coccinia indica* has potentially beneficial antioxidant properties (Venkateswaran & Pari, 2003).

6.1.22 Nopal

The literature pertaining to *Opuntia Streptacantha* (Nopal or Prickly Pear Cactus) has been available for several years, and demonstrates efficacy in a dose-dependent manner, when its stems are broiled and provided to T2DM patients (Frati-Munari, Del Valle-Martinez et al., 1989). However in a follow up study, Nopal extract in encapsulated form did not reduce fasting glycemia in T2DM patients; however, the extract did diminish the increase of postprandial glucose following an OGTT (Frati-Munari, de Leon et al., 1989). Chronically, the efficacy of Nopal requires additional clarification (Frati Munari et al., 1992).

6.1.23 Ginseng

Ginseng has received considerable attention, dating back to ancient Chinese medicine (Y. Z. Xiang et al., 2008). Chronically, Korean red ginseng (*Panax ginseng*) supplemented for 12 weeks (6g·day^{-1}) in well controlled T2DM patients, significantly improved fasting insulin and insulin sensitivity, as well as postprandial glucose and insulin following an OGTT (Vuksan et al., 2008). However, supplementation did not significantly improve the primary endpoint HbA_{1c}. In healthy subjects, *Panax ginseng* supplemented for 57 days (200mg·day^{-1}), in a randomized crossover design, had no effect on fasting or postprandial measures of glucose regulation (Reay et al., 2009). Acutely, American ginseng (*panax quinquefolius* L.) has been shown to be beneficial in reducing postprandial glucose in T2DM patients irrespective of dose (3g, 6g, or 9g) (Vuksan, Stavro et al., 2000) or timing of consumption (40 minutes before a test meal or immediately preceding) (Vuksan, Sievenpiper et al., 2000). On the other hand, in healthy subjects, the postprandial response to supplementation was dependent on the timing of administration (Vuksan, Sievenpiper et al., 2000; Vuksan et al., 2001); however, like diabetic subjects, the dose did not influence the findings (1g, 2g, 3g) (Vuksan et al., 2001).

6.1.24 Russian tarragon

Russian tarragon (*Artemisia dracunculus* L.) is a relatively novel ingredient and to date only one reported investigation is available regarding its anti-diabetic effects in humans. An aqueous extract of Russian tarragon provided to a sample of healthy, exercise-trained men, did not significantly influence glucose or insulin response to an OGTT (Bloomer, Canale et al., 2011). However, approximately two-thirds of subjects ingesting the Russian tarragon did experience attenuation in both the glucose and insulin in response to the OGTT. It is possible that more favorable effects would be noted in a sample of diabetic subjects, as has been the case for animal (Zuberi, 2008) and cell culture (Z. Q. Wang et al., 2008) studies using Russian Tarragon.

6.1.25 Bitter Mellon

Despite being a frequently used ingredient within insulin mimetic and hypoglycemic agents sold as dietary supplements, *Momordica charantia* (bitter melon) has been shown to be relatively ineffective in attenuating measures of glycemia chronically in T2DM patients

(Dans et al., 2007) or acutely, following an OGTT (Kasbia, et al. 2009), in a sample of non-diabetic overweight men. Nonetheless, animal studies support its potential at ameliorating glycemic control, lipid profiles, and antioxidant status (Chaturvedi & George, 2010) and one recent human study supports a modest hypoglycemic effect at 2000 mg·day^{-1} for four weeks in T2DM patients (Fuangchan et al., 2011).

6.1.26 Garlic

Treatment with garlic (*Allium sativum*) has also elicited beneficial anti-diabetic effects. A garlic tablet taken at 600mg·day^{-1} for 12 weeks was shown to significantly reduce total cholesterol and LDL-C, and moderately raise HDL-C compared to placebo (Ashraf et al., 2005). In a later trial, a time-released garlic tablet, Allicor (600mg·day^{-1}), was investigated for four weeks using a double-blinded placebo controlled study with T2DM patients (Sobenin et al., 2008). Allicor was shown to significantly lower fasting blood glucose levels, serum fructosamine, and triglyceride levels.

6.1.27 Vinegar

Vinegar has been successfully added to feedings to ameliorate the glycemic response. In patients with T2DM, 20g of wine vinegar has been shown to reduce postprandial glucose and insulin AUC when added to a high, but not to a low, glycemic index meal (Liatis et al., 2010). In a four part investigation, the anti-glycemic properties of vinegar were investigated (Johnston et al., 2010). Pertinent for the present discussion, trial 4 examined whether a "vinegar pill" (i.e., the neutralized salt of acetic acid, sodium acetate) possessed anti-glycemic effect in individuals with T2DM, when compared to 20g of traditional vinegar (1g acetic acid), and placebo. Treatments were administered two minutes before a test meal and the results indicated that only acetic acid was effective at attenuating postprandial blood glucose. The other results from this overall investigation consisted of healthy subjects; however, trial 1 found that 10g of vinegar (0.5 acetic acid) was better at reducing postprandial blood glucose compared to 20g vinegar and 2g vinegar. Trial 2 indicated that vinegar (20g) ingested at meal time elicited a greater attenuation of postprandial glucose compared to five hours before the meal, albeit non-significantly. Finally, trial 3 indicated that the anti-glycemic effect of vinegar is best realized when ingested with food composed of complex carbohydrates and that vinegar may not attenuate postprandial glucose following the consumption of foods sweetened with dextrose, as is the case for many processed beverages and foods.

6.2 Macronutrients

6.2.1. Amino acids

The postprandial oxidative stress response to a macronutrient protein meal has been shown to be relatively diminutive in comparison to an isoenergetically comprised carbohydrate, lipid, and mixed composition meals (Fisher-Wellman & Bloomer, 2010). Moreover, endothelial dysfunction has been shown to be neutralized when proteins are added to a high fat meal (Westphal et al., 2006). Therefore, it is not surprising that amino acids, in particular L-arginine (one of the precursors to nitric oxide), have been investigated as a nutritional intervention for diabetes control. Amino acids (L-leucine; L-lysine; L-isoleucine; L-valine; L-threonine; L-cysteine; L-histidine; L-phenylalanine; L-methionine; L-thyrosine; and L-tryptophan) supplemented to elderly T2DM patients for 60 weeks (8g·day^{-1}) significantly decreased HbA_{1c}, fasting and postprandial blood glucose, fasting insulin, and insulin resistance (Solerte et al., 2008). Intravenous infusion of L-arginine (0.52mg·kg^{-1}· min^{-1}) in a mixed sample of NIDDM, obese, and healthy subjects restored the impaired insulin-mediated vasodilation observed in obese and NIDDM patients (Wascher et al., 1997). Moreover, insulin sensitivity was improved significantly in all three groups. In healthy subjects, an oral dose of L-arginine as low as 2.5g and as high as 15g, supplemented concomitantly with a high fat meal, has been shown to significantly improve endothelial function (Borucki et al., 2009; Lin et al., 2008) and favorably impact biomarkers of oxidative stress (Lin et al., 2008).

6.2.2 Nuts

The consumption of nuts could provide a benefit to those with T2DM given that nuts have an excellent nutritional profile, are high in monounsaturated fatty acids (MUFA) and polyunsaturated fatty acids (PUFA), contain polyphenols, and are a fair source of vegetable protein. However, results have been conflicting in diabetic and healthy populations with regards to the impact of nut intake on measures of glycemic regulation. In two studies (presented within one manuscript) Lovejoy et al. (Lovejoy et al., 2002) assessed the effect of almond-enriched diets on insulin sensitivity and lipids in patients with T2DM or healthy volunteers. Study one determined the effect of almonds on insulin sensitivity in healthy volunteers who received 100g·day^{-1} of almonds for four weeks. Results indicated that total cholesterol and LDL-C decreased significantly; however, there was no effect on insulin sensitivity. Study two was a randomized crossover design that compared 4 diets in T2DM patients, each diet being four weeks in duration. The high-fat, high-almond diet had the greatest decrease in total cholesterol; however, no diet impacted fasting glucose, postprandial glucose (following an OGTT), or HbA_{1c}. Tapsell et al. (Tapsell et al., 2004) found that a moderate-fat diet inclusive of walnuts for six months, significantly increased the plasma HDL-C: total cholesterol ratio and HDL-C, and significantly decreased plasma LDL-C in subjects with T2DM. Additionally, triglycerides showed a trend to be improved in the intervention group. However, there were no significant differences between treatment groups regarding total antioxidant capacity or HbA_{1c} levels. In subjects with metabolic syndrome, Davis et al. (Davis et al., 2007) noted non-significant effects in oxidative stress biomarkers after an 8 week walnut or cashew diet, despite ORAC being significantly higher compared to the control diet. Twelve weeks of mixed nut consumption (30g·day^{-1}) in 50 subjects also with metabolic syndrome was found to decrease DNA damage compared to the control group (Lopez-Uriarte et al., 2010). The nut group also tended to have less oxidative stress, as indicated by reductions, albeit non-significantly, in ox-LDL-C, conjugated diene formation, and 8-isoprostanes in urine. Null findings were reported for antioxidant capacity, endothelial function, and lipid profiles. Finally, in healthy subjects, walnut consumption for six weeks did not significantly change the plasma antioxidant capacity (McKay et al., 2010). Interestingly, plasma total cholesterol, LDL-C, and triglyceride levels decreased significantly compared to baseline in the lower dose group (21g·day^{-1}).

In healthy volunteers, acute almond intake has been shown to reduce glucose AUC after consuming 50g of white bread, in a dose dependent manner, as well as lowering total cholesterol levels (Josse et al., 2007). Moreover, almonds were shown to decrease the glycemic and insulinemic responses to white bread, and increase the serum protein thiol concentration, indicating less oxidative protein damage. Acute consumption of pecans by healthy subjects has been shown to significantly decrease ox-LDL-C, and increase the flavonoid EGCG (Hudthagosol et al., 2011). Additionally, the molar ratio of MDA: triglyceride was significantly lower as compared to baseline following the pecan meals (pooled data).

6.2.3 Fiber

Viscous fiber affects metabolism by its actions within the proximal digestive tube (Hunt et al., 1993). In the colon, soluble fibers bind, absorb, or sequester bile acids, products of fat digestion, fatty acids, and monglycerides during passage through the intestinal luman (Hunt et al., 1993). Moreover, soluble fibers delay gastric emptying and increase unstirred water in the small bowl producing satiety (Gray, 1995). These effects appear to make dietary fiber a beneficial intervention for patients with T2DM. Three doses of 5g·day^{-1} psyllium for six weeks was shown to significantly reduce fasting plasma glucose, total cholesterol, LDL-C, and triglycerides, as well as significantly increase HDL-C in patients with T2DM (Rodriguez-Moran et al., 1998). Similarly, 14g·day^{-1} of psyllium for six weeks significantly decreased postprandial glucose absorption, fructosamine, total cholesterol, and LDL-C cholesterol in T2DM patients (Sierra et al., 2002). Other markers of glycemic control also tended to be lower, albeit non-significantly. Guar gum for 48 weeks at 15g·day^{-1} in subjects with NIDDM has been shown to improve long-term glycemic control, postprandial glucose tolerance, and LDL-C (Groop et al., 1993). Finally, dietary assignment to food products that contained oat β-glucan in hypertensive subjects showed a favorable effects on postprandial glucose and insulin levels, as well as blood pressure, after 12 weeks of treatment. (Maki, Galant et al., 2007). However, these beneficial effects were independent of differences in oxidative stress biomarkers.

Acutely, high-viscosity hydroxypropylmethylcellulose (HV-HPMC) has been found to blunt postprandial glucose and insulin in a dose-dependent manner in subjects at risk for the development of T2DM (Maki et al., 2007; Maki et al., 2009). Moreover, triglyceride incremental AUC during the postprandial period was significantly lower after the consumption of 15g psyllium compared to 3g, and chylomicron levels were also influenced in this dose-dependent manner in overweight and obese men (Khossousi et al., 2008).

6.3 Whole food dietary intervention

Although supplementation with isolated ingredients provides unique insight into the beneficial effects of selected nutrients on human health, dietary interventions in which whole food intake is significantly altered in an attempt to improve health may have even more impact. One dietary approach that has received considerable attention is the Mediterranean diet—a plan rich in the intake of olive oil.

Acutely, extra virgin olive oil has been shown decrease postprandial inflammatory markers and up-regulate antioxidant capacity (Bogani et al., 2007). As a consequence of proposed benefit of olive oil, coupled with the supporting evidence for the consumption of red wine, the Mediterranean diet has been met with a good degree of success. For example, in overweight men followed for 24 months, the Mediterranean diet, with or without caloric restriction, resulted in improved fasting measures of glucose, insulin, oxidative stress, total cholesterol, blood pressure, and adiponectin (Esposito et al., 2010). In elderly subjects, consumption of the Mediterranean diet for four weeks was shown to induce a reduction in endothelial dysfunction and improve the regenerative capacity of the endothelium (Marin et al., 2011). Specifically it was found that the Mediterranean diet led to lower total microparticle, activated endothelial microparticle, and apoptotic endothelial microparticle concentrations, and a higher number of endothelial progenitor cells compared to the other diets. Moreover, the Mediterranean diet was associated with lower oxidative stress and elevated β-carotene concentrations. Finally, in an elderly population, the Mediterranean diet alone for four weeks was found to improve postprandial oxidative stress with a higher increase in capillary flow and nitric oxide levels, lower lipid peroxidation products, and a lower postprandial decrease in HDL-C compared to a diet rich in saturated fat (Yubero-Serrano et al., 2010). Moreover, CoQ_{10} supplemented to the Mediterranean diet further improved postprandial levels of oxidative stress and elicited a superior increase in capillary flow and nitric oxide levels, with respect to the other diets.

We have recently demonstrated the beneficial metabolic and cardiovascular effects of a dietary restriction model known as the Daniel Fast. The Daniel Fast involves a 21 day *ad libitum* food intake period, devoid of animal products and preservatives, and inclusive of fruits, vegetables, whole grains, legumes, nuts, and seeds. In our first study, the Daniel Fast elicited a significant lowering of total cholesterol, LDL-C, HDL-C, SBP, and DBP. Moreover, insulin, HOMA-IR, and C-reactive protein all showed a trend for improvement (Bloomer, Kabir, Canale et al., 2010). Improvements were also noted in several measures of oxidative stress and antioxidant capacity (Bloomer, Kabir, Trepanowski et al., 2011). In a follow-up study involving this model, both resting and postprandial biomarkers were favorably impacted (unpublished findings), suggesting that this form of eating (e.g., stringent vegan diet) may be associated with multiple favorable effects on metabolic and cardiovascular health. Longer term studies are needed to determine the potential impact of the acute changes on health and disease over time.

Other dietary interventions exist that have been investigated and proposed to have beneficial effects on metabolic and cardiovascular risk factors. The Portfolio Diet developed by Jenkins et al. (Jenkins et al., 2007) consists of using combinations of cholesterol-lowering foods within one diet, rather than single foods, to achieve more favorable effects on serum cholesterol. The dietary portfolio currently contains four main elements with proven cholesterol lowering efficacy, some of which have been highlighted in the preceding text. These include soy, viscous fibers, plant sterols, and nuts. In a similar manner as the Daniel Fast, the Portfolio Diet encourages the consumption of foods that are traditionally found in a vegetarian/vegan plan, which may prove beneficial for controlling and preventing T2DM (Tonstad et al., 2009). Readers are referred to the following papers for more information on such diets (Jenkins et al., 2003; Key et al., 2006).

Finally, although emphasis in this section is on specific nutrients and types of dietary approaches to improve metabolic health, it should be noted that a reduction in dietary energy and modification of portion sizes should be considered. Indeed, the literature pertaining to caloric restriction is lengthy, with multiple known benefits with a reduction in normal dietary energy intake (Civitarese et al., 2007; Redman et al., 2009).

6.4 Summary of nutrients

As illustrated above, results for improvement in selected markers of cardiovascular and metabolic health through dietary manipulation in individuals with T2DM have been mixed. Some potential reasons for conflicting findings across studies include the degree of diabetic complication, the timing and dosage of dietary supplement or food, the duration of treatment, and the fact that some individuals are noted "responders" and others are "non-

Exercise	**What to Include**	**What to Consider**
Aerobic	• Walking, Jogging, Cycling, Stepping, Swimming, etc. • (Most or all days of week; 30-60 minutes; 50-80% of VO_{2max})	• Interval training – light running (50-60% of VO_{2max}) combined with short, fast bursts of running (1-2 days per week; 20-40min) • Sports and physical activities (e.g., soccer, basketball)
Anaerobic	• Resistance exercise: free weights and/or machines • (2-3 days per week; 30-45 minutes; 50-80% 1RM)	• Maximal-intensity repetition training (1 day per week; 80-100% 1RM—focus on development of muscular strength)

Whole Food Intake	**What to Include**	**What to Consider**	**What to Avoid**
	Whole grains, fruits, vegetables, beans, nuts, seeds, low fat or fat free dairy, lean poultry, fish, olive oil, vinegar	Red wine (in moderation), tea (green or black)	Saturated fat, processed carbohydrate, packaged foods, sugar-rich carbonated beverages

Nutritional Supplements	**What to Consider (Suggested Dosage)**	**What Requires More Research***

	• Amino acids ($8.0g{\cdot}day^{-1}$)
	  • L-arginine ($2.5\text{-}15g{\cdot}day^{-1}$)
	• Antioxidants
	  • α-Lipoic acid ($0.3\text{-}1.8g{\cdot}day^{-1}$)
	  • Vitamin C ($1.0\text{-}2.0g{\cdot}day^{-1}$)
	  • Vitamin E ($0.6\text{-}0.9g{\cdot}day^{-1}$)
	• Banaba/corosolic acid (*Lagerstroemia speciosa* L.) ($0.1\text{-}0.5g{\cdot}day^{-1}$)
	• Berberine ($1.0\text{-}1.5g{\cdot}day^{-1}$)
	• Cinnamon ($0.5\text{-}6.0g{\cdot}day^{-1}$)
	• Fenugreek (*Trigonella foenum graecum*) ($8.0\text{-}10.0g{\cdot}day^{-1}$)
	• Fish oil (omega-3 fatty acids; EPA, DHA) ($1.0\text{-}4.0g{\cdot}day^{-1}$)
	• Ginseng (*Panax ginseng* or *Panax quinquefolius* L.) ($1.0\text{-}6.0g{\cdot}day^{-1}$)
	• Garlic extracts ($0.6g{\cdot}day^{-1}$)
	• Magnesium ($0.6\text{-}2.5g{\cdot}day^{-1}$)
	• Multi-vitamins ($\geq 1.0g{\cdot}day^{-1}$)
	• Tea catechins ($0.6\text{-}1.0g{\cdot}day^{-1}$)
	• Vitamin D ($\geq 700IU{\cdot}day^{-1}$)
		• Coenzyme Q_{10}
		  • Lycopene
		  • Bitter melon (Momordica charantia)
		• Carnitine
		• Chromium
		• Cissus quadrangularis
		• Coccinia indica
		• Gymnema sylvestre
		• Inositol phosphoglycans (pinitol)
		• Nopal or Prickly Pear Cactus (*Opuntia Streptacantha*)
		• Russian tarragon (Artemisia dracunculus L.)
		• Selenium
		• Steviol glycosides (Stevia rebaudiana Bertoni)
		• Turmeric (Curcuma longa)
		• Vanadium

*Current concerns exist regarding efficacy—especially in diabetic populations, paucity of data, dosage, or safety.

Table 1. Lifestyle approach to improving metabolic health at rest and in response to feeding

responders" to treatment (in the same manner as certain individuals respond better to certain drugs than do others). Additional, well-controlled investigations are needed to clarify which nutrients and which dietary models may be most conducive to improving the metabolic profile at rest and in response to feeding—in particular as related to oxidative stress.

7. Conclusions and practical application

As there currently exists no cure for diabetes, lifestyle factors should be strongly considered as the first line treatment for this disease—as these activities may improve fasting and postprandial lipid and glucose metabolism, as well as antioxidant capacity. Collectively these effects may help to minimize postprandial oxidative stress. The rationale for regular and structured exercise (Praet & van Loon, 2007; Tucker et al., 2008), coupled with the intake of a nutrient dense, macronutrient balanced, and portion controlled eating plan (Bloomer, Kabir, Canale et al., 2010; Bloomer, Kabir, Trepanowski et al., 2011; Jenkins et al., 2007), complete with use of selected nutrients to aid in both glucose and triglyceride processing (Badimon et al., 2010; Davi et al., 2010; Nahas & Moher, 2009), appears well supported. Suggestions are provided in Table 1. Adherence to these guidelines, or those which are similar, may be associated with improved metabolic control in both the fasting and fed state. This may be met with a reduction in RONS production and ensuing oxidative stress, which may be correlated to improved health and quality of life (Frisard & Ravussin, 2006), and a reduction in disease progression over time (Ceriello & Motz, 2004).

8. References

Abdourahman, A., & Edwards, J. G. (2008). Chromium supplementation improves glucose tolerance in diabetic goto-kakizaki rats. *IUBMB Life, 60*(8), 541-548.

Akilen, R., Tsiami, A., Devendra, D., & Robinson, N. (2010). Glycated haemoglobin and blood pressure-lowering effect of cinnamon in multi-ethnic type 2 diabetic patients in the UK: A randomized, placebo-controlled, double-blind clinical trial. *Diabetic Medicine : A Journal of the British Diabetic Association, 27*(10), 1159-1167.

Akova, B., Surmen-Gur, E., Gur, H., Dirican, M., Sarandol, E., & Kucukoglu, S. (2001). Exercise-induced oxidative stress and muscle performance in healthy women: Role of vitamin E supplementation and endogenous oestradiol. *European Journal of Applied Physiology, 84*(1-2), 141-147.

Alessio, H. M., Hagerman, A. E., Fulkerson, B. K., Ambrose, J., Rice, R. E., & Wiley, R. L. (2000). Generation of reactive oxygen species after exhaustive aerobic and isometric exercise. *Medicine and Science in Sports and Exercise, 32*(9), 1576-1581.

Ali, A., Ma, Y., Reynolds, J., Wise, J. P., Inzucchi, S. E., & Katz, D. L. (2011). Chromium effects on glucose tolerance and insulin sensitivity in persons at risk for diabetes mellitus. *Endocrine Practice : Official Journal of the American College of Endocrinology and the American Association of Clinical Endocrinologists, 17*(1), 16-25.

Aljada, A., Friedman, J., Ghanim, H., Mohanty, P., Hofmeyer, D., Chaudhuri, A., et al. (2006). Glucose ingestion induces an increase in intranuclear nuclear factor kappaB, a fall in cellular inhibitor kappaB, and an increase in tumor necrosis factor alpha messenger RNA by mononuclear cells in healthy human subjects. *Metabolism: Clinical and Experimental, 55*(9), 1177-1185.

Al-Romaiyan, A., Liu, B., Asare-Anane, H., Maity, C. R., Chatterjee, S. K., Koley, N., et al. (2010). A novel gymnema sylvestre extract stimulates insulin secretion from human islets in vivo and in vitro. *Phytotherapy Research : PTR, 24*(9), 1370-1376.

Andersen, E., & Hostmark, A. T. (2007). Effect of a single bout of resistance exercise on postprandial glucose and insulin response the next day in healthy, strength-trained men. *Journal of Strength and Conditioning Research / National Strength & Conditioning Association, 21*(2), 487-491.

Anderson, E. J., Lustig, M. E., Boyle, K. E., Woodlief, T. L., Kane, D. A., Lin, C. T., et al. (2009). Mitochondrial H2O2 emission and cellular redox state link excess fat intake to insulin resistance in both rodents and humans. *The Journal of Clinical Investigation,*

Anderson, R. A., Evans, L. M., Ellis, G. R., Khan, N., Morris, K., Jackson, S. K., et al. (2006). Prolonged deterioration of endothelial dysfunction in response to postprandial lipaemia is attenuated by vitamin C in type 2 diabetes. *Diabetic Medicine : A Journal of the British Diabetic Association, 23*(3), 258-264.

Araiza, P., Hewes, H., Gashetewa, C., Vella, C. A., & Burge, M. R. (2006). Efficacy of a pedometer-based physical activity program on parameters of diabetes control in type 2 diabetes mellitus. *Metabolism: Clinical and Experimental, 55*(10), 1382-1387.

Ashraf, R., Aamir, K., Shaikh, A. R., & Ahmed, T. (2005). Effects of garlic on dyslipidemia in patients with type 2 diabetes mellitus. *Journal of Ayub Medical College, Abbottabad : JAMC, 17*(3), 60-64.

Badimon, L., Vilahur, G., & Padro, T. (2010). Nutraceuticals and atherosclerosis: Human trials. *Cardiovascular Therapeutics, 28*(4), 202-215.

Bae, J. H., Bassenge, E., Kim, K. B., Kim, Y. N., Kim, K. S., Lee, H. J., et al. (2001). Postprandial hypertriglyceridemia impairs endothelial function by enhanced oxidant stress. *Atherosclerosis, 155*(2), 517-523.

Bajpeyi, S., Tanner, C. J., Slentz, C. A., Duscha, B. D., McCartney, J. S., Hickner, R. C., et al. (2009). Effect of exercise intensity and volume on persistence of insulin sensitivity during training cessation. *Journal of Applied Physiology (Bethesda, Md.: 1985), 106*(4), 1079-1085.

Barnard, R. J., Lattimore, L., Holly, R. G., Cherny, S., & Pritikin, N. (1982). Response of non-insulin-dependent diabetic patients to an intensive program of diet and exercise. *Diabetes Care, 5*(4), 370-374.

Barnard, R. J., Ugianskis, E. J., & Martin, D. A. (1992). The effects of an intensive diet and exercise program on patients with non-insulin-dependent diabetes mellitus and hypertension. *Journal of Cardiopulmonary Rehabilitation and Prevention, 12*(3), 194-201.

Barriocanal, L. A., Palacios, M., Benitez, G., Benitez, S., Jimenez, J. T., Jimenez, N., et al. (2008). Apparent lack of pharmacological effect of steviol glycosides used as sweeteners in humans. A pilot study of repeated exposures in some normotensive and hypotensive individuals and in type 1 and type 2 diabetics. *Regulatory Toxicology and Pharmacology : RTP, 51*(1), 37-41.

Baskaran, K., Kizar Ahamath, B., Radha Shanmugasundaram, K., & Shanmugasundaram, E. R. (1990). Antidiabetic effect of a leaf extract from gymnema sylvestre in non-insulin-dependent diabetes mellitus patients. *Journal of Ethnopharmacology, 30*(3), 295-300.

Basu, A., Sanchez, K., Leyva, M. J., Wu, M., Betts, N. M., Aston, C. E., et al. (2010). Green tea supplementation affects body weight, lipids, and lipid peroxidation in obese subjects with metabolic syndrome. *Journal of the American College of Nutrition, 29*(1), 31-40.

Baynes, J. W., & Thorpe, S. R. (1999). Role of oxidative stress in diabetic complications: A new perspective on an old paradigm. *Diabetes, 48*(1), 1-9.

Beckman, J. A., Goldfine, A. B., Gordon, M. B., & Creager, M. A. (2001). Ascorbate restores endothelium-dependent vasodilation impaired by acute hyperglycemia in humans. *Circulation, 103*(12), 1618-1623.

Beyer, R. E. (1990). The participation of coenzyme Q in free radical production and antioxidation. *Free Radical Biology & Medicine, 8*(6), 545-565.

Bloomer, R. J. (2008). Effect of exercise on oxidative stress biomarkers. *Advances in Clinical Chemistry, 46*, 1-50.

Bloomer, R. J., Canale, R. E., & Pischel, I. (2011). Effect of an aqueous russian tarragon extract on glucose tolerance in response to an oral dextrose load in non-diabetic men. *Nutrition and Dietary Supplements, 3*, 43-49.

Bloomer, R. J., Cole, B., & Fisher-Wellman, K. H. (2009). Racial differences in postprandial oxidative stress with and without acute exercise. *International Journal of Sport Nutrition and Exercise Metabolism, 19*(5), 457-472.

Bloomer, R. J., Ferebee, D. E., Fisher-Wellman, K. H., Quindry, J. C., & Schilling, B. K. (2009). Postprandial oxidative stress: Influence of sex and exercise training status. *Medicine and Science in Sports and Exercise, 41*(12), 2111-2119.

Bloomer, R. J., & Fisher-Wellman, K. H. (2009). Systemic oxidative stress is increased to a greater degree in young, obese women following consumption of a high fat meal. *Oxid Med Cell Longev., 2*, 19-25.

Bloomer, R. J., & Fisher-Wellman, K. H. (2010). Lower postprandial oxidative stress in women compared with men. *Gender Medicine, 7*(4), 340-349.

Bloomer, R. J., Fisher-Wellman, K. H., & Tucker, P. S. (2009). Effect of oral acetyl L-carnitine arginate on resting and postprandial blood biomarkers in pre-diabetics. *Nutrition & Metabolism, 6*, 25.

Bloomer, R. J., Kabir, M. M., Canale, R. E., Trepanowski, J. F., Marshall, K. E., Farney, T. M., et al. (2010). Effect of a 21 day daniel fast on metabolic and cardiovascular disease risk factors in men and women. *Lipids in Health and Disease, 9*, 94.

Bloomer, R. J., Kabir, M. M., Marshall, K. E., Canale, R. E., & Farney, T. M. (2010). Postprandial oxidative stress in response to dextrose and lipid meals of differing size. *Lipids in Health and Disease, 9*(1), 79.

Bloomer, R. J., Kabir, M. M., Trepanowski, J. F., Canale, R. E., & Farney, T. M. (2011). A 21 day daniel fast improves selected biomarkers of antioxidant status and oxidative stress in men and women. *Nutrition & Metabolism, 8*, 17.

Bocci, V., Borrelli, E., Travagli, V., & Zanardi, I. (2009). The ozone paradox: Ozone is a strong oxidant as well as a medical drug. *Medicinal Research Reviews, 29*(4), 646-682.

Bogani, P., Galli, C., Villa, M., & Visioli, F. (2007). Postprandial anti-inflammatory and antioxidant effects of extra virgin olive oil. *Atherosclerosis, 190*(1), 181-186.

Borissova, A. M., Tankova, T., Kirilov, G., Dakovska, L., & Kovacheva, R. (2003). The effect of vitamin D3 on insulin secretion and peripheral insulin sensitivity in type 2 diabetic patients. *International Journal of Clinical Practice, 57*(4), 258-261.

Borsheim, E., Knardahl, S., & Hostmark, A. T. (1999). Short-term effects of exercise on plasma very low density lipoproteins (VLDL) and fatty acids. *Medicine and Science in Sports and Exercise, 31*(4), 522-530.

Borucki, K., Aronica, S., Starke, I., Luley, C., & Westphal, S. (2009). Addition of 2.5 g L-arginine in a fatty meal prevents the lipemia-induced endothelial dysfunction in healthy volunteers. *Atherosclerosis, 205*(1), 251-254.

Bowry, V. W., Ingold, K. U., & Stocker, R. (1992). Vitamin E in human low-density lipoprotein. when and how this antioxidant becomes a pro-oxidant. *The Biochemical Journal, 288 (Pt 2)*(Pt 2), 341-344.

Brestoff, J. R., Clippinger, B., Spinella, T., von Duvillard, S. P., Nindl, B. C., & Arciero, P. J. (2009). An acute bout of endurance exercise but not sprint interval exercise enhances insulin sensitivity. *Applied Physiology, Nutrition, and Metabolism = Physiologie Appliquee, Nutrition Et Metabolisme, 34*(1), 25-32.

Brownlee, M. (2005). The pathobiology of diabetic complications: A unifying mechanism. *Diabetes, 54*(6), 1615-1625.

Buczynski, A., Kedziora, J., Tkaczewski, W., & Wachowicz, B. (1991). Effect of submaximal physical exercise on antioxidative protection of human blood platelets. *International Journal of Sports Medicine, 12*(1), 52-54.

Calo, L. A., Pagnin, E., Davis, P. A., Semplicini, A., Nicolai, R., Calvani, M., et al. (2006). Antioxidant effect of L-carnitine and its short chain esters: Relevance for the protection from oxidative stress related cardiovascular damage. *International Journal of Cardiology, 107*(1), 54-60.

Canale, R. E., Farney, T. M., McCarthy, C. G., & Bloomer, R. J. (In Review). A proprietary blend of phellodendron and crape myrtle improves glucose tolerance in response to an oral dextrose load in exercise-trained non-diabetic men. *Journal of Nutrition and Metabolic Insights*

Carmeli, E., Beiker, R., Maor, M., & Kodesh, E. (2010). Increased iNOS, MMP-2, and HSP-72 in skeletal muscle following high-intensity exercise training. *Journal of Basic and Clinical Physiology and Pharmacology, 21*(2), 127-146.

Castaneda, C., Layne, J. E., Munoz-Orians, L., Gordon, P. L., Walsmith, J., Foldvari, M., et al. (2002). A randomized controlled trial of resistance exercise training to improve glycemic control in older adults with type 2 diabetes. *Diabetes Care, 25*(12), 2335-2341.

Cefalu, W. T., Rood, J., Pinsonat, P., Qin, J., Sereda, O., Levitan, L., et al. (2010). Characterization of the metabolic and physiologic response to chromium supplementation in subjects with type 2 diabetes mellitus. *Metabolism: Clinical and Experimental, 59*(5), 755-762.

Ceriello, A. (2004). Impaired glucose tolerance and cardiovascular disease: The possible role of post-prandial hyperglycemia. *American Heart Journal, 147*(5), 803-807.

Ceriello, A., Bortolotti, N., Motz, E., Lizzio, S., Catone, B., Assaloni, R., et al. (2001). Red wine protects diabetic patients from meal-induced oxidative stress and thrombosis activation: A pleasant approach to the prevention of cardiovascular disease in diabetes. *European Journal of Clinical Investigation, 31*(4), 322-328.

Ceriello, A., & Motz, E. (2004). Is oxidative stress the pathogenic mechanism underlying insulin resistance, diabetes, and cardiovascular disease? the common soil hypothesis revisited. *Arteriosclerosis, Thrombosis, and Vascular Biology, 24*(5), 816-823.

Ceriello, A., Quagliaro, L., Piconi, L., Assaloni, R., Da Ros, R., Maier, A., et al. (2004). Effect of postprandial hypertriglyceridemia and hyperglycemia on circulating adhesion molecules and oxidative stress generation and the possible role of simvastatin treatment. *Diabetes, 53*(3), 701-710.

Ceriello, A., Taboga, C., Tonutti, L., Quagliaro, L., Piconi, L., Bais, B., et al. (2002). Evidence for an independent and cumulative effect of postprandial hypertriglyceridemia and hyperglycemia on endothelial dysfunction and oxidative stress generation: Effects of short- and long-term simvastatin treatment. *Circulation, 106*(10), 1211-1218.

Chaturvedi, P., & George, S. (2010). Momordica charantia maintains normal glucose levels and lipid profiles and prevents oxidative stress in diabetic rats subjected to chronic sucrose load. *Journal of Medicinal Food, 13*(3), 520-527.

Chen, H., Karne, R. J., Hall, G., Campia, U., Panza, J. A., Cannon, R. O.,3rd, et al. (2006). High-dose oral vitamin C partially replenishes vitamin C levels in patients with type 2 diabetes and low vitamin C levels but does not improve endothelial dysfunction or insulin resistance. *American Journal of Physiology.Heart and Circulatory Physiology, 290*(1), H137-45.

Chen, M. F., Hsu, H. C., & Lee, Y. T. (1994). Effects of acute exercise on the changes of lipid profiles and peroxides, prostanoids, and platelet activation in hypercholesterolemic patients before and after treatment. *Prostaglandins, 48*(3), 157-174.

Chevion, S., Moran, D. S., Heled, Y., Shani, Y., Regev, G., Abbou, B., et al. (2003). Plasma antioxidant status and cell injury after severe physical exercise. *Proceedings of the National Academy of Sciences of the United States of America, 100*(9), 5119-5123.

Chibalin, A. V., Yu, M., Ryder, J. W., Song, X. M., Galuska, D., Krook, A., et al. (2000). Exercise-induced changes in expression and activity of proteins involved in insulin signal transduction in skeletal muscle: Differential effects on insulin-receptor substrates 1 and 2. *Proceedings of the National Academy of Sciences of the United States of America, 97*(1), 38-43.

Christ-Roberts, C. Y., Pratipanawatr, T., Pratipanawatr, W., Berria, R., Belfort, R., Kashyap, S., et al. (2004). Exercise training increases glycogen synthase activity and GLUT4 expression but not insulin signaling in overweight nondiabetic and type 2 diabetic subjects. *Metabolism: Clinical and Experimental, 53*(9), 1233-1242.

Civitarese, A. E., Carling, S., Heilbronn, L. K., Hulver, M. H., Ukropcova, B., Deutsch, W. A., et al. (2007). Calorie restriction increases muscle mitochondrial biogenesis in healthy humans. *PLoS Medicine, 4*(3), e76.

Clegg, M., McClean, C., Davison, W. G., Murphy, H. M., Trinick, T., Duly, E., et al. (2007). Exercise and postprandial lipaemia: Effects on peripheral vascular function, oxidative stress and gastrointestinal transit. *Lipids in Health and Disease, 6*, 30.

Clinton, S. K. (1998). Lycopene: Chemistry, biology, and implications for human health and disease. *Nutrition Reviews, 56*(2 Pt 1), 35-51.

Cohen, J. C., Noakes, T. D., & Benade, A. J. (1989). Postprandial lipemia and chylomicron clearance in athletes and in sedentary men. *The American Journal of Clinical Nutrition, 49*(3), 443-447.

Cohen, N., Halberstam, M., Shlimovich, P., Chang, C. J., Shamoon, H., & Rossetti, L. (1995). Oral vanadyl sulfate improves hepatic and peripheral insulin sensitivity in patients with non-insulin-dependent diabetes mellitus. *The Journal of Clinical Investigation, 95*(6), 2501-2509.

Cohen, N. D., Dunstan, D. W., Robinson, C., Vulikh, E., Zimmet, P. Z., & Shaw, J. E. (2008). Improved endothelial function following a 14-month resistance exercise training program in adults with type 2 diabetes. *Diabetes Research and Clinical Practice, 79*(3), 405-411.

Cottin, S. C., Sanders, T. A., & Hall, W. L. (2011). The differential effects of EPA and DHA on cardiovascular risk factors. *The Proceedings of the Nutrition Society*, , 1-17.

Cullinane, E., Siconolfi, S., Saritelli, A., & Thompson, P. D. (1982). Acute decrease in serum triglycerides with exercise: Is there a threshold for an exercise effect? *Metabolism: Clinical and Experimental, 31*(8), 844-847.

Cusi, K., Cukier, S., DeFronzo, R. A., Torres, M., Puchulu, F. M., & Redondo, J. C. (2001). Vanadyl sulfate improves hepatic and muscle insulin sensitivity in type 2 diabetes. *The Journal of Clinical Endocrinology and Metabolism, 86*(3), 1410-1417.

Dalle-Donne, I., Rossi, R., Colombo, R., Giustarini, D., & Milzani, A. (2006). Biomarkers of oxidative damage in human disease. *Clinical Chemistry, 52*(4), 601-623.

Dans, A. M., Villarruz, M. V., Jimeno, C. A., Javelosa, M. A., Chua, J., Bautista, R., et al. (2007). The effect of momordica charantia capsule preparation on glycemic control in type 2 diabetes mellitus needs further studies. *Journal of Clinical Epidemiology, 60*(6), 554-559.

Darko, D., Dornhorst, A., Kelly, F. J., Ritter, J. M., & Chowienczyk, P. J. (2002). Lack of effect of oral vitamin C on blood pressure, oxidative stress and endothelial function in type II diabetes. *Clinical Science (London, England : 1979), 103*(4), 339-344.

Davi, G., Ciabattoni, G., Consoli, A., Mezzetti, A., Falco, A., Santarone, S., et al. (1999). In vivo formation of 8-iso-prostaglandin f2alpha and platelet activation in diabetes mellitus: Effects of improved metabolic control and vitamin E supplementation. *Circulation, 99*(2), 224-229.

Davi, G., Santilli, F., & Patrono, C. (2010). Nutraceuticals in diabetes and metabolic syndrome. *Cardiovascular Therapeutics, 28*(4), 216-226.

Davis, L., Stonehouse, W., Loots du, T., Mukuddem-Petersen, J., van der Westhuizen, F. H., Hanekom, S. M., et al. (2007). The effects of high walnut and cashew nut diets on the antioxidant status of subjects with metabolic syndrome. *European Journal of Nutrition, 46*(3), 155-164.

de Koning, E. J., & Rabelink, T. J. (2002). Endothelial function in the post-prandial state. *Atherosclerosis.Supplements, 3*(1), 11-16.

Demrow, H. S., Slane, P. R., & Folts, J. D. (1995). Administration of wine and grape juice inhibits in vivo platelet activity and thrombosis in stenosed canine coronary arteries. *Circulation, 91*(4), 1182-1188.

Denniss, S. G., Haffner, T. D., Kroetsch, J. T., Davidson, S. R., Rush, J. W., & Hughson, R. L. (2008). Effect of short-term lycopene supplementation and postprandial dyslipidemia on plasma antioxidants and biomarkers of endothelial health in young, healthy individuals. *Vascular Health and Risk Management, 4*(1), 213-222.

Di Massimo, C., Scarpelli, P., & Tozzi-Ciancarelli, M. G. (2004). Possible involvement of oxidative stress in exercise-mediated platelet activation. *Clinical Hemorheology and Microcirculation, 30*(3-4), 313-316.

Drewnowski, A. (2007). The real contribution of added sugars and fats to obesity. *Epidemiologic Reviews, 29*, 160-171.

Duncan, G. E., Perri, M. G., Theriaque, D. W., Hutson, A. D., Eckel, R. H., & Stacpoole, P. W. (2003). Exercise training, without weight loss, increases insulin sensitivity and postheparin plasma lipase activity in previously sedentary adults. *Diabetes Care, 26*(3), 557-562.

Dunstan, D. W., Daly, R. M., Owen, N., Jolley, D., De Courten, M., Shaw, J., et al. (2002). High-intensity resistance training improves glycemic control in older patients with type 2 diabetes. *Diabetes Care, 25*(10), 1729-1736.

Edirisinghe, I., & Rahman, I. (2010). Cigarette smoke-mediated oxidative stress, shear stress, and endothelial dysfunction: Role of VEGFR2. *Annals of the New York Academy of Sciences, 1203*, 66-72.

Elosua, R., Molina, L., Fito, M., Arquer, A., Sanchez-Quesada, J. L., Covas, M. I., et al. (2003). Response of oxidative stress biomarkers to a 16-week aerobic physical activity program, and to acute physical activity, in healthy young men and women. *Atherosclerosis, 167*(2), 327-334.

Esposito, K., Di Palo, C., Maiorino, M. I., Petrizzo, M., Bellastella, G., Siniscalchi, I., et al. (2010). Long-term effect of mediterranean-style diet and calorie restriction on biomarkers of longevity and oxidative stress in overweight men. *Cardiology Research and Practice, 2011*, 293916.

Evans, E. M., Racette, S. B., Peterson, L. R., Villareal, D. T., Greiwe, J. S., & Holloszy, J. O. (2005). Aerobic power and insulin action improve in response to endurance exercise training in healthy 77-87 yr olds. *Journal of Applied Physiology (Bethesda, Md.: 1985), 98*(1), 40-45.

Fahs, C. A., Yan, H., Ranadive, S., Rossow, L. M., Agiovlasitis, S., Wilund, K. R., et al. (2010). The effect of acute fish-oil supplementation on endothelial function and arterial stiffness following a high-fat meal. *Applied Physiology, Nutrition, and Metabolism = Physiologie Appliquee, Nutrition Et Metabolisme, 35*(3), 294-302.

Fatouros, I. G., Jamurtas, A. Z., Villiotou, V., Pouliopoulou, S., Fotinakis, P., Taxildaris, K., et al. (2004). Oxidative stress responses in older men during endurance training and detraining. *Medicine and Science in Sports and Exercise, 36*(12), 2065-2072.

Fehrenbach, E., & Northoff, H. (2001). Free radicals, exercise, apoptosis, and heat shock proteins. *Exercise Immunology Review, 7*, 66-89.

Ferguson, M. A., Alderson, N. L., Trost, S. G., Essig, D. A., Burke, J. R., & Durstine, J. L. (1998). Effects of four different single exercise sessions on lipids, lipoproteins, and lipoprotein lipase. *Journal of Applied Physiology (Bethesda, Md.: 1985), 85*(3), 1169-1174.

Fialkow, L., Wang, Y., & Downey, G. P. (2007). Reactive oxygen and nitrogen species as signaling molecules regulating neutrophil function. *Free Radical Biology & Medicine, 42*(2), 153-164.

Finaud, J., Lac, G., & Filaire, E. (2006). Oxidative stress : Relationship with exercise and training. *Sports Medicine (Auckland, N.Z.), 36*(4), 327-358.

Fisher-Wellman, K. H., & Bloomer, R. J. (2009a). Acute exercise and oxidative stress: A 30 year history. *Dynamic Medicine : DM, 8*, 1.

Fisher-Wellman, K. H., & Bloomer, R. J. (2009b). Macronutrient specific postprandial oxidative stress: Relevance to the development of insulin resistance. *Current Diabetes Reviews, 5*(4), 228-238.

Fisher-Wellman, K. H., & Bloomer, R. J. (2010). Exacerbated postprandial oxidative stress induced by the acute intake of a lipid meal compared to isoenergetically administered carbohydrate, protein, and mixed meals in young, healthy men. *Journal of the American College of Nutrition, 29*(4), 373-381.

Fluckey, J. D., Hickey, M. S., Brambrink, J. K., Hart, K. K., Alexander, K., & Craig, B. W. (1994). Effects of resistance exercise on glucose tolerance in normal and glucose-intolerant subjects. *Journal of Applied Physiology (Bethesda, Md.: 1985), 77*(3), 1087-1092.

Fonteles, M. C., Huang, L. C., & Larner, J. (1996). Infusion of pH 2.0 D-chiro-inositol glycan insulin putative mediator normalizes plasma glucose in streptozotocin diabetic rats at a dose equivalent to insulin without inducing hypoglycaemia. *Diabetologia, 39*(6), 731-734.

Frati Munari, A. C., Vera Lastra, O., & Ariza Andraca, C. R. (1992). Evaluation of nopal capsules in diabetes mellitus]. [Evaluacion de capsulas de nopal en diabetes mellitus] *Gaceta Medica De Mexico, 128*(4), 431-436.

Frati-Munari, A. C., de Leon, C., Ariza-Andraca, R., Banales-Ham, M. B., Lopez-Ledesma, R., & Lozoya, X. (1989). Effect of a dehydrated extract of nopal (opuntia ficus indica mill.) on blood glucose]. [Influencia de un extracto deshidratado de nopal (Opuntia ficus-indica mill.) en la glucemia] *Archivos De Investigacion Medica, 20*(3), 211-216.

Frati-Munari, A. C., Del Valle-Martinez, L. M., Ariza-Andraca, C. R., Islas-Andrade, S., & Chavez-Negrete, A. (1989). Hypoglycemic action of different doses of nopal (opuntia streptacantha lemaire) in patients with type II diabetes mellitus]. [Accion hipoglucemiante de diferentes dosis de nopal (Opuntia streptacantha Lemaire) en pacientes con diabetes mellitus tipo II] *Archivos De Investigacion Medica, 20*(2), 197-201.

Frisard, M., & Ravussin, E. (2006). Energy metabolism and oxidative stress: Impact on the metabolic syndrome and the aging process. *Endocrine, 29*(1), 27-32.

Fuangchan, A., Sonthisombat, P., Seubnukarn, T., Chanouan, R., Chotchaisuwat, P., Sirigulsatien, V., et al. (2011). Hypoglycemic effect of bitter melon compared with metformin in newly diagnosed type 2 diabetes patients. *Journal of Ethnopharmacology, 134*(2), 422-428.

Fukushima, M., Matsuyama, F., Ueda, N., Egawa, K., Takemoto, J., Kajimoto, Y., et al. (2006). Effect of corosolic acid on postchallenge plasma glucose levels. *Diabetes Research and Clinical Practice, 73*(2), 174-177.

Galbo, H., Tobin, L., & van Loon, L. J. (2007). Responses to acute exercise in type 2 diabetes, with an emphasis on metabolism and interaction with oral hypoglycemic agents and food intake. *Applied Physiology, Nutrition, and Metabolism = Physiologie Appliquee, Nutrition Et Metabolisme, 32*(3), 567-575.

Geiger, P. C., & Gupte, A. A. (2011). Heat shock proteins are important mediators of skeletal muscle insulin sensitivity. *Exercise and Sport Sciences Reviews, 39*(1), 34-42.

Giacco, F., & Brownlee, M. (2010). Oxidative stress and diabetic complications. *Circulation Research, 107*(9), 1058-1070.

Gill, J. M., Frayn, K. N., Wootton, S. A., Miller, G. J., & Hardman, A. E. (2001). Effects of prior moderate exercise on exogenous and endogenous lipid metabolism and plasma factor VII activity. *Clinical Science (London, England : 1979), 100*(5), 517-527.

Goldfine, A. B., Patti, M. E., Zuberi, L., Goldstein, B. J., LeBlanc, R., Landaker, E. J., et al. (2000). Metabolic effects of vanadyl sulfate in humans with non-insulin-dependent diabetes mellitus: In vivo and in vitro studies. *Metabolism: Clinical and Experimental, 49*(3), 400-410.

Goodpaster, B. H., Katsiaras, A., & Kelley, D. E. (2003). Enhanced fat oxidation through physical activity is associated with improvements in insulin sensitivity in obesity. *Diabetes, 52*(9), 2191-2197.

Grandjean, P. W., Crouse, S. F., & Rohack, J. J. (2000). Influence of cholesterol status on blood lipid and lipoprotein enzyme responses to aerobic exercise. *Journal of Applied Physiology (Bethesda, Md.: 1985), 89*(2), 472-480.

Graner, M., Kahri, J., Nakano, T., Sarna, S. J., Nieminen, M. S., Syvanne, M., et al. (2006). Impact of postprandial lipaemia on low-density lipoprotein (LDL) size and oxidized LDL in patients with coronary artery disease. *European Journal of Clinical Investigation, 36*(11), 764-770.

Gray, D. S. (1995). The clinical uses of dietary fiber. *American Family Physician, 51*(2), 419-426.

Green, H. J., Duhamel, T. A., Holloway, G. P., Moule, J. W., Ranney, D. W., Tupling, A. R., et al. (2008). Rapid upregulation of GLUT-4 and MCT-4 expression during 16 h of heavy intermittent cycle exercise. *American Journal of Physiology.Regulatory, Integrative and Comparative Physiology, 294*(2), R594-600.

Gregersen, S., Jeppesen, P. B., Holst, J. J., & Hermansen, K. (2004). Antihyperglycemic effects of stevioside in type 2 diabetic subjects. *Metabolism: Clinical and Experimental, 53*(1), 73-76.

Groop, P. H., Aro, A., Stenman, S., & Groop, L. (1993). Long-term effects of guar gum in subjects with non-insulin-dependent diabetes mellitus. *The American Journal of Clinical Nutrition, 58*(4), 513-518.

Guerrero-Romero, F., Tamez-Perez, H. E., Gonzalez-Gonzalez, G., Salinas-Martinez, A. M., Montes-Villarreal, J., Trevino-Ortiz, J. H., et al. (2004). Oral magnesium supplementation improves insulin sensitivity in non-diabetic subjects with insulin resistance. A double-blind placebo-controlled randomized trial. *Diabetes & Metabolism, 30*(3), 253-258.

Gupta, A., Gupta, R., & Lal, B. (2001). Effect of trigonella foenum-graecum (fenugreek) seeds on glycaemic control and insulin resistance in type 2 diabetes mellitus: A double blind placebo controlled study. *The Journal of the Association of Physicians of India, 49*, 1057-1061.

Haddad, J. J. (2002). Antioxidant and prooxidant mechanisms in the regulation of redox(y)-sensitive transcription factors. *Cellular Signalling, 14*(11), 879-897.

Hadjistavri, L. S., Sarafidis, P. A., Georgianos, P. I., Tziolas, I. M., Aroditis, C. P., Hitoglou-Makedou, A., et al. (2010). Beneficial effects of oral magnesium supplementation on insulin sensitivity and serum lipid profile. *Medical Science Monitor : International Medical Journal of Experimental and Clinical Research, 16*(6), CR307-312.

Halberstam, M., Cohen, N., Shlimovich, P., Rossetti, L., & Shamoon, H. (1996). Oral vanadyl sulfate improves insulin sensitivity in NIDDM but not in obese nondiabetic subjects. *Diabetes, 45*(5), 659-666.

Halliwell, B. (1991). Reactive oxygen species in living systems: Source, biochemistry, and role in human disease. *The American Journal of Medicine, 91*(3C), 14S-22S.

Halliwell, B., & Cross, C. E. (1994). Oxygen-derived species: Their relation to human disease and environmental stress. *Environmental Health Perspectives, 102 Suppl 10*, 5-12.

Hamilton, K. L., Staib, J. L., Phillips, T., Hess, A., Lennon, S. L., & Powers, S. K. (2003). Exercise, antioxidants, and HSP72: Protection against myocardial ischemia/reperfusion. *Free Radical Biology & Medicine, 34*(7), 800-809.

Hamilton, S. J., Chew, G. T., & Watts, G. F. (2009). Coenzyme Q10 improves endothelial dysfunction in statin-treated type 2 diabetic patients. *Diabetes Care, 32*(5), 810-812.

Hanwell, H. E., Kay, C. D., Lampe, J. W., Holub, B. J., & Duncan, A. M. (2009). Acute fish oil and soy isoflavone supplementation increase postprandial serum (n-3) polyunsaturated fatty acids and isoflavones but do not affect triacylglycerols or biomarkers of oxidative stress in overweight and obese hypertriglyceridemic men. *The Journal of Nutrition, 139*(6), 1128-1134.

Hellsten, Y., Apple, F. S., & Sjodin, B. (1996). Effect of sprint cycle training on activities of antioxidant enzymes in human skeletal muscle. *Journal of Applied Physiology (Bethesda, Md.: 1985), 81*(4), 1484-1487.

Henriksen, E. J. (2002). Invited review: Effects of acute exercise and exercise training on insulin resistance. *Journal of Applied Physiology (Bethesda, Md.: 1985), 93*(2), 788-796.

Higdon, J. V., & Frei, B. (2003). Tea catechins and polyphenols: Health effects, metabolism, and antioxidant functions. *Critical Reviews in Food Science and Nutrition, 43*(1), 89-143.

Hirashima, O., Kawano, H., Motoyama, T., Hirai, N., Ohgushi, M., Kugiyama, K., et al. (2000). Improvement of endothelial function and insulin sensitivity with vitamin C in patients with coronary spastic angina: Possible role of reactive oxygen species. *Journal of the American College of Cardiology, 35*(7), 1860-1866.

Hollander, J., Fiebig, R., Gore, M., Bejma, J., Ookawara, T., Ohno, H., et al. (1999). Superoxide dismutase gene expression in skeletal muscle: Fiber-specific adaptation to endurance training. *The American Journal of Physiology, 277*(3 Pt 2), R856-62.

Holten, M. K., Zacho, M., Gaster, M., Juel, C., Wojtaszewski, J. F., & Dela, F. (2004). Strength training increases insulin-mediated glucose uptake, GLUT4 content, and insulin signaling in skeletal muscle in patients with type 2 diabetes. *Diabetes, 53*(2), 294-305.

Houmard, J. A., Tanner, C. J., Slentz, C. A., Duscha, B. D., McCartney, J. S., & Kraus, W. E. (2004). Effect of the volume and intensity of exercise training on insulin sensitivity. *Journal of Applied Physiology (Bethesda, Md.: 1985), 96*(1), 101-106.

Hsu, C. H., & Cheng, A. L. (2007). Clinical studies with curcumin. *Advances in Experimental Medicine and Biology, 595*, 471-480.

Hudthagosol, C., Haddad, E. H., McCarthy, K., Wang, P., Oda, K., & Sabate, J. (2011). Pecans acutely increase plasma postprandial antioxidant capacity and catechins and decrease LDL oxidation in humans. *The Journal of Nutrition, 141*(1), 56-62.

Hunt, R., Fedorak, R., Frohlich, J., McLennan, C., & Pavilanis, A. (1993). Therapeutic role of dietary fibre. *Canadian Family Physician Medecin De Famille Canadien, 39*, 897-900, 903-10.

Ibanez, J., Gorostiaga, E. M., Alonso, A. M., Forga, L., Arguelles, I., Larrion, J. L., et al. (2008). Lower muscle strength gains in older men with type 2 diabetes after resistance training. *Journal of Diabetes and its Complications, 22*(2), 112-118.

Ibanez, J., Izquierdo, M., Arguelles, I., Forga, L., Larrion, J. L., Garcia-Unciti, M., et al. (2005). Twice-weekly progressive resistance training decreases abdominal fat and improves insulin sensitivity in older men with type 2 diabetes. *Diabetes Care, 28*(3), 662-667.

Inal, M., Akyuz, F., Turgut, A., & Getsfrid, W. M. (2001). Effect of aerobic and anaerobic metabolism on free radical generation swimmers. *Medicine and Science in Sports and Exercise, 33*(4), 564-567.

Iqbal, N., Cardillo, S., Volger, S., Bloedon, L. T., Anderson, R. A., Boston, R., et al. (2009). Chromium picolinate does not improve key features of metabolic syndrome in obese nondiabetic adults. *Metabolic Syndrome and Related Disorders, 7*(2), 143-150.

Ishii, T., Yamakita, T., Sato, T., Tanaka, S., & Fujii, S. (1998). Resistance training improves insulin sensitivity in NIDDM subjects without altering maximal oxygen uptake. *Diabetes Care, 21*(8), 1353-1355.

Jackson, M. J., Pye, D., & Palomero, J. (2007). The production of reactive oxygen and nitrogen species by skeletal muscle. *Journal of Applied Physiology (Bethesda, Md.: 1985), 102*(4), 1664-1670.

Jacob, S., Ruus, P., Hermann, R., Tritschler, H. J., Maerker, E., Renn, W., et al. (1999). Oral administration of RAC-alpha-lipoic acid modulates insulin sensitivity in patients with type-2 diabetes mellitus: A placebo-controlled pilot trial. *Free Radical Biology & Medicine, 27*(3-4), 309-314.

Jacques-Camarena, O., Gonzalez-Ortiz, M., Martinez-Abundis, E., Lopez-Madrueno, J. F., & Medina-Santillan, R. (2008). Effect of vanadium on insulin sensitivity in patients with impaired glucose tolerance. *Annals of Nutrition & Metabolism, 53*(3-4), 195-198.

Jenkins, D. J., Josse, A. R., Wong, J. M., Nguyen, T. H., & Kendall, C. W. (2007). The portfolio diet for cardiovascular risk reduction. *Current Atherosclerosis Reports, 9*(6), 501-507.

Jenkins, D. J., Kendall, C. W., Marchie, A., Jenkins, A. L., Augustin, L. S., Ludwig, D. S., et al. (2003). Type 2 diabetes and the vegetarian diet. *The American Journal of Clinical Nutrition, 78*(3 Suppl), 610S-616S.

Jentjens, R. L., & Jeukendrup, A. E. (2002). Effect of acute and short-term administration of vanadyl sulphate on insulin sensitivity in healthy active humans. *International Journal of Sport Nutrition and Exercise Metabolism, 12*(4), 470-479.

Ji, L. L. (1999). Antioxidants and oxidative stress in exercise. *Proceedings of the Society for Experimental Biology and Medicine.Society for Experimental Biology and Medicine (New York, N.Y.), 222*(3), 283-292.

Johnston, C. S., Steplewska, I., Long, C. A., Harris, L. N., & Ryals, R. H. (2010). Examination of the antiglycemic properties of vinegar in healthy adults. *Annals of Nutrition & Metabolism, 56*(1), 74-79.

Jorde, R., & Figenschau, Y. (2009). Supplementation with cholecalciferol does not improve glycaemic control in diabetic subjects with normal serum 25-hydroxyvitamin D levels. *European Journal of Nutrition, 48*(6), 349-354.

Josic, J., Olsson, A. T., Wickeberg, J., Lindstedt, S., & Hlebowicz, J. (2010). Does green tea affect postprandial glucose, insulin and satiety in healthy subjects: A randomized controlled trial. *Nutrition Journal, 9*, 63.

Josse, A. R., Kendall, C. W., Augustin, L. S., Ellis, P. R., & Jenkins, D. J. (2007). Almonds and postprandial glycemia--a dose-response study. *Metabolism: Clinical and Experimental, 56*(3), 400-404.

Judy, W. V., Hari, S. P., Stogsdill, W. W., Judy, J. S., Naguib, Y. M., & Passwater, R. (2003). Antidiabetic activity of a standardized extract (glucosol) from lagerstroemia speciosa leaves in type II diabetics. A dose-dependence study. *Journal of Ethnopharmacology, 87*(1), 115-117.

Kadoglou, N. P., Iliadis, F., Angelopoulou, N., Perrea, D., Ampatzidis, G., Liapis, C. D., et al. (2007). The anti-inflammatory effects of exercise training in patients with type 2 diabetes mellitus. *European Journal of Cardiovascular Prevention and Rehabilitation : Official Journal of the European Society of Cardiology, Working Groups on Epidemiology & Prevention and Cardiac Rehabilitation and Exercise Physiology, 14*(6), 837-843.

Kar, P., Laight, D., Rooprai, H. K., Shaw, K. M., & Cummings, M. (2009). Effects of grape seed extract in type 2 diabetic subjects at high cardiovascular risk: A double blind randomized placebo controlled trial examining metabolic markers, vascular tone, inflammation, oxidative stress and insulin sensitivity. *Diabetic Medicine : A Journal of the British Diabetic Association, 26*(5), 526-531.

Kasbia, G. S., Arnason, J. T., & Imbeault, P. (2009). No effect of acute, single dose oral administration of momordica charantia linn., on glycemia, energy expenditure and appetite: A pilot study in non-diabetic overweight men. *Journal of Ethnopharmacology, 126*(1), 127-133.

Katsanos, C. S. (2006). Prescribing aerobic exercise for the regulation of postprandial lipid metabolism : Current research and recommendations. *Sports Medicine (Auckland, N.Z.), 36*(7), 547-560.

Kelley, G. A., & Kelley, K. S. (2007). Effects of aerobic exercise on lipids and lipoproteins in adults with type 2 diabetes: A meta-analysis of randomized-controlled trials. *Public Health, 121*(9), 643-655.

Kelly, K. L., Mato, J. M., Merida, I., & Jarett, L. (1987). Glucose transport and antilipolysis are differentially regulated by the polar head group of an insulin-sensitive glycophospholipid. *Proceedings of the National Academy of Sciences of the United States of America, 84*(18), 6404-6407.

Key, T. J., Appleby, P. N., & Rosell, M. S. (2006). Health effects of vegetarian and vegan diets. *The Proceedings of the Nutrition Society, 65*(1), 35-41.

Khan, A., Safdar, M., Ali Khan, M. M., Khattak, K. N., & Anderson, R. A. (2003). Cinnamon improves glucose and lipids of people with type 2 diabetes. *Diabetes Care, 26*(12), 3215-3218.

Khan, A. K., AKhtar, S., & Mahtab, H. (1980). Treatment of diabetes mellitus with coccinia indica. *British Medical Journal, 280*(6220), 1044.

Khossousi, A., Binns, C. W., Dhaliwal, S. S., & Pal, S. (2008). The acute effects of psyllium on postprandial lipaemia and thermogenesis in overweight and obese men. *The British Journal of Nutrition, 99*(5), 1068-1075.

Kim, M. J., Yoo, K. H., Kim, J. H., Seo, Y. T., Ha, B. W., Kho, J. H., et al. (2007). Effect of pinitol on glucose metabolism and adipocytokines in uncontrolled type 2 diabetes. *Diabetes Research and Clinical Practice, 77 Suppl 1*, S247-51.

Knight, J. A. (1999). *Free radicals, antioxidants, aging, and disease*. Washington: American Association for Clinical Chemistry Press.

Kojda, G., & Hambrecht, R. (2005). Molecular mechanisms of vascular adaptations to exercise. physical activity as an effective antioxidant therapy? *Cardiovascular Research, 67*(2), 187-197.

Koves, T. R., Ussher, J. R., Noland, R. C., Slentz, D., Mosedale, M., Ilkayeva, O., et al. (2008). Mitochondrial overload and incomplete fatty acid oxidation contribute to skeletal muscle insulin resistance. *Cell Metabolism, 7*(1), 45-56.

Kraniou, G. N., Cameron-Smith, D., & Hargreaves, M. (2006). Acute exercise and GLUT4 expression in human skeletal muscle: Influence of exercise intensity. *Journal of Applied Physiology (Bethesda, Md.: 1985), 101*(3), 934-937.

Kraniou, Y., Cameron-Smith, D., Misso, M., Collier, G., & Hargreaves, M. (2000). Effects of exercise on GLUT-4 and glycogenin gene expression in human skeletal muscle. *Journal of Applied Physiology (Bethesda, Md.: 1985), 88*(2), 794-796.

Kristiansen, S., Hargreaves, M., & Richter, E. A. (1996). Exercise-induced increase in glucose transport, GLUT-4, and VAMP-2 in plasma membrane from human muscle. *The American Journal of Physiology, 270*(1 Pt 1), E197-201.

Kristiansen, S., Hargreaves, M., & Richter, E. A. (1997). Progressive increase in glucose transport and GLUT-4 in human sarcolemmal vesicles during moderate exercise. *The American Journal of Physiology, 272*(3 Pt 1), E385-9.

Kuriyan, R., Rajendran, R., Bantwal, G., & Kurpad, A. V. (2008). Effect of supplementation of coccinia cordifolia extract on newly detected diabetic patients. *Diabetes Care, 31*(2), 216-220.

Laaksonen, D. E., Atalay, M., Niskanen, L., Uusitupa, M., Hanninen, O., & Sen, C. K. (1999). Blood glutathione homeostasis as a determinant of resting and exercise-induced oxidative stress in young men. *Redox Report : Communications in Free Radical Research, 4*(1-2), 53-59.

Larner, J., Allan, G., Kessler, C., Reamer, P., Gunn, R., & Huang, L. C. (1998). Phosphoinositol glycan derived mediators and insulin resistance. prospects for diagnosis and therapy. *Journal of Basic and Clinical Physiology and Pharmacology, 9*(2-4), 127-137.

Lee, H. C., & Wei, Y. H. (2007). Oxidative stress, mitochondrial DNA mutation, and apoptosis in aging. *Experimental Biology and Medicine (Maywood, N.J.), 232*(5), 592-606.

Leeuwenburgh, C., Hansen, P. A., Holloszy, J. O., & Heinecke, J. W. (1999). Hydroxyl radical generation during exercise increases mitochondrial protein oxidation and levels of urinary dityrosine. *Free Radical Biology & Medicine, 27*(1-2), 186-192.

Liatis, S., Grammatikou, S., Poulia, K. A., Perrea, D., Makrilakis, K., Diakoumopoulou, E., et al. (2010). Vinegar reduces postprandial hyperglycaemia in patients with type II diabetes when added to a high, but not to a low, glycaemic index meal. *European Journal of Clinical Nutrition, 64*(7), 727-732.

Lin, C. C., Tsai, W. C., Chen, J. Y., Li, Y. H., Lin, L. J., & Chen, J. H. (2008). Supplements of L-arginine attenuate the effects of high-fat meal on endothelial function and oxidative stress. *International Journal of Cardiology, 127*(3), 337-341.

Lira, F. S., Zanchi, N. E., Lima-Silva, A. E., Pires, F. O., Bertuzzi, R. C., Caperuto, E. C., et al. (2010). Is acute supramaximal exercise capable of modulating lipoprotein profile in healthy men? *European Journal of Clinical Investigation, 40*(8), 759-765.

Liu, H., Colavitti, R., Rovira, I. I., & Finkel, T. (2005). Redox-dependent transcriptional regulation. *Circulation Research, 97*(10), 967-974.

Liu, S., Manson, J. E., Lee, I. M., Cole, S. R., Hennekens, C. H., Willett, W. C., et al. (2000). Fruit and vegetable intake and risk of cardiovascular disease: The women's health study. *The American Journal of Clinical Nutrition, 72*(4), 922-928.

Liu, S., Stampfer, M. J., Hu, F. B., Giovannucci, E., Rimm, E., Manson, J. E., et al. (1999). Whole-grain consumption and risk of coronary heart disease: Results from the nurses' health study. *The American Journal of Clinical Nutrition, 70*(3), 412-419.

Livesey, G., Taylor, R., Hulshof, T., & Howlett, J. (2008). Glycemic response and health--a systematic review and meta-analysis: Relations between dietary glycemic properties and health outcomes. *The American Journal of Clinical Nutrition, 87*(1), 258S-268S.

Loimaala, A., Groundstroem, K., Rinne, M., Nenonen, A., Huhtala, H., Parkkari, J., et al. (2009). Effect of long-term endurance and strength training on metabolic control and arterial elasticity in patients with type 2 diabetes mellitus. *The American Journal of Cardiology, 103*(7), 972-977.

Lopez-Uriarte, P., Nogues, R., Saez, G., Bullo, M., Romeu, M., Masana, L., et al. (2010). Effect of nut consumption on oxidative stress and the endothelial function in metabolic syndrome. *Clinical Nutrition (Edinburgh, Scotland), 29*(3), 373-380.

Losso, J. N., Holliday, D. L., Finley, J. W., Martin, R. J., Rood, J. C., Yu, Y., et al. (2009). Fenugreek bread: A treatment for diabetes mellitus. *Journal of Medicinal Food, 12*(5), 1046-1049.

Lovejoy, J. C., Most, M. M., Lefevre, M., Greenway, F. L., & Rood, J. C. (2002). Effect of diets enriched in almonds on insulin action and serum lipids in adults with normal glucose tolerance or type 2 diabetes. *The American Journal of Clinical Nutrition, 76*(5), 1000-1006.

Lu, F. R., Shen, L., Qin, Y., Gao, L., Li, H., & Dai, Y. (2008). Clinical observation on trigonella foenum-graecum L. total saponins in combination with sulfonylureas in the treatment of type 2 diabetes mellitus. *Chinese Journal of Integrative Medicine, 14*(1), 56-60.

Mackenzie, T., Leary, L., & Brooks, W. B. (2007). The effect of an extract of green and black tea on glucose control in adults with type 2 diabetes mellitus: Double-blind randomized study. *Metabolism: Clinical and Experimental, 56*(10), 1340-1344.

Magkos, F., Tsekouras, Y. E., Prentzas, K. I., Basioukas, K. N., Matsama, S. G., Yanni, A. E., et al. (2008). Acute exercise-induced changes in basal VLDL-triglyceride kinetics leading to hypotriglyceridemia manifest more readily after resistance than endurance exercise. *Journal of Applied Physiology (Bethesda, Md.: 1985), 105*(4), 1228-1236.

Maiese, K., Morhan, S. D., & Chong, Z. Z. (2007). Oxidative stress biology and cell injury during type 1 and type 2 diabetes mellitus. *Current Neurovascular Research, 4*(1), 63-71.

Maki, K. C., Carson, M. L., Miller, M. P., Turowski, M., Bell, M., Wilder, D. M., et al. (2007). High-viscosity hydroxypropylmethylcellulose blunts postprandial glucose and insulin responses. *Diabetes Care, 30*(5), 1039-1043.

Maki, K. C., Galant, R., Samuel, P., Tesser, J., Witchger, M. S., Ribaya-Mercado, J. D., et al. (2007). Effects of consuming foods containing oat beta-glucan on blood pressure, carbohydrate metabolism and biomarkers of oxidative stress in men and women with elevated blood pressure. *European Journal of Clinical Nutrition, 61*(6), 786-795.

Maki, K. C., Reeves, M. S., Carson, M. L., Miller, M. P., Turowski, M., Rains, T. M., et al. (2009). Dose-response characteristics of high-viscosity hydroxypropylmethylcellulose in subjects at risk for the development of type 2 diabetes mellitus. *Diabetes Technology & Therapeutics, 11*(2), 119-125.

Marfella, R., Cacciapuoti, F., Siniscalchi, M., Sasso, F. C., Marchese, F., Cinone, F., et al. (2006). Effect of moderate red wine intake on cardiac prognosis after recent acute myocardial infarction of subjects with type 2 diabetes mellitus. *Diabetic Medicine : A Journal of the British Diabetic Association, 23*(9), 974-981.

Marin, C., Ramirez, R., Delgado-Lista, J., Yubero-Serrano, E. M., Perez-Martinez, P., Carracedo, J., et al. (2011). Mediterranean diet reduces endothelial damage and improves the regenerative capacity of endothelium. *The American Journal of Clinical Nutrition, 93*(2), 267-274.

Markovits, N., Ben Amotz, A., & Levy, Y. (2009). The effect of tomato-derived lycopene on low carotenoids and enhanced systemic inflammation and oxidation in severe obesity. *The Israel Medical Association Journal : IMAJ, 11*(10), 598-601.

Marzatico, F., Pansarasa, O., Bertorelli, L., Somenzini, L., & Della Valle, G. (1997). Blood free radical antioxidant enzymes and lipid peroxides following long-distance and lactacidemic performances in highly trained aerobic and sprint athletes. *The Journal of Sports Medicine and Physical Fitness, 37*(4), 235-239.

Matsuoka, T., Takaki, A., Ohtaki, H., & Shioda, S. (2010). Early changes to oxidative stress levels following exposure to formaldehyde in ICR mice. *The Journal of Toxicological Sciences, 35*(5), 721-730.

Mavian, A. A., Miller, S., & Henry, R. R. (2010). Managing type 2 diabetes: Balancing HbA1c and body weight. *Postgraduate Medicine, 122*(3), 106-117.

May, J. M., Qu, Z. C., Whitesell, R. R., & Cobb, C. E. (1996). Ascorbate recycling in human erythrocytes: Role of GSH in reducing dehydroascorbate. *Free Radical Biology & Medicine, 20*(4), 543-551.

McCarty, M. F. (1999). Coenzyme Q versus hypertension: Does CoQ decrease endothelial superoxide generation? *Medical Hypotheses, 53*(4), 300-304.

McClean, C. M., Clegg, M., Shafat, A., Murphy, M. H., Trinick, T., Duly, E., et al. (2011). The impact of acute moderate intensity exercise on arterial regional stiffness, lipid peroxidation, and antioxidant status in healthy males. *Research in Sports Medicine (Print), 19*(1), 1-13.

McClean, C. M., Mc Laughlin, J., Burke, G., Murphy, M. H., Trinick, T., Duly, E., et al. (2007). The effect of acute aerobic exercise on pulse wave velocity and oxidative stress following postprandial hypertriglyceridemia in healthy men. *European Journal of Applied Physiology, 100*(2), 225-234.

McGee, S. L., & Hargreaves, M. (2006). Exercise and skeletal muscle glucose transporter 4 expression: Molecular mechanisms. *Clinical and Experimental Pharmacology & Physiology, 33*(4), 395-399.

McKay, D. L., Chen, C. Y., Yeum, K. J., Matthan, N. R., Lichtenstein, A. H., & Blumberg, J. B. (2010). Chronic and acute effects of walnuts on antioxidant capacity and nutritional status in humans: A randomized, cross-over pilot study. *Nutrition Journal, 9*, 21.

Melton, C. E., Tucker, P. S., Fisher-Wellman, K. H., Schilling, B. K., & Bloomer, R. J. (2009). Acute exercise does not attenuate postprandial oxidative stress in prediabetic women. *Phys Sportsmed., 36*

Micallef, M., Lexis, L., & Lewandowski, P. (2007). Red wine consumption increases antioxidant status and decreases oxidative stress in the circulation of both young and old humans. *Nutrition Journal, 6*, 27.

Michailidis, Y., Jamurtas, A. Z., Nikolaidis, M. G., Fatouros, I. G., Koutedakis, Y., Papassotiriou, I., et al. (2007). Sampling time is crucial for measurement of aerobic exercise-induced oxidative stress. *Medicine and Science in Sports and Exercise, 39*(7), 1107-1113.

Miyazaki, H., Oh-ishi, S., Ookawara, T., Kizaki, T., Toshinai, K., Ha, S., et al. (2001). Strenuous endurance training in humans reduces oxidative stress following exhausting exercise. *European Journal of Applied Physiology, 84*(1-2), 1-6.

Miyazaki, Y., Kawano, H., Yoshida, T., Miyamoto, S., Hokamaki, J., Nagayoshi, Y., et al. (2007). Pancreatic B-cell function is altered by oxidative stress induced by acute hyperglycaemia. *Diabetic Medicine : A Journal of the British Diabetic Association, 24*(2), 154-160.

Mohanty, P., Ghanim, H., Hamouda, W., Aljada, A., Garg, R., & Dandona, P. (2002). Both lipid and protein intakes stimulate increased generation of reactive oxygen species by polymorphonuclear leukocytes and mononuclear cells. *The American Journal of Clinical Nutrition, 75*(4), 767-772.

Mohanty, P., Hamouda, W., Garg, R., Aljada, A., Ghanim, H., & Dandona, P. (2000). Glucose challenge stimulates reactive oxygen species (ROS) generation by leucocytes. *The Journal of Clinical Endocrinology and Metabolism, 85*(8), 2970-2973.

Monnier, L., Mas, E., Ginet, C., Michel, F., Villon, L., Cristol, J. P., et al. (2006). Activation of oxidative stress by acute glucose fluctuations compared with sustained chronic hyperglycemia in patients with type 2 diabetes. *JAMA : The Journal of the American Medical Association, 295*(14), 1681-1687.

Mori, T. A., Woodman, R. J., Burke, V., Puddey, I. B., Croft, K. D., & Beilin, L. J. (2003). Effect of eicosapentaenoic acid and docosahexaenoic acid on oxidative stress and inflammatory markers in treated-hypertensive type 2 diabetic subjects. *Free Radical Biology & Medicine, 35*(7), 772-781.

Nahas, R., & Moher, M. (2009). Complementary and alternative medicine for the treatment of type 2 diabetes. *Canadian Family Physician Medecin De Famille Canadien, 55*(6), 591-596.

Nakajima, K. (2010). Pharmacotherapy of mixed dyslipidemia in the metabolic syndrome. *Current Clinical Pharmacology, 5*(2), 133-139.

Napoli, R., Cozzolino, D., Guardasole, V., Angelini, V., Zarra, E., Matarazzo, M., et al. (2005). Red wine consumption improves insulin resistance but not endothelial function in type 2 diabetic patients. *Metabolism: Clinical and Experimental, 54*(3), 306-313.

Nappo, F., Esposito, K., Cioffi, M., Giugliano, G., Molinari, A. M., Paolisso, G., et al. (2002). Postprandial endothelial activation in healthy subjects and in type 2 diabetic patients: Role of fat and carbohydrate meals. *Journal of the American College of Cardiology, 39*(7), 1145-1150.

Natella, F., Belelli, F., Gentili, V., Ursini, F., & Scaccini, C. (2002). Grape seed proanthocyanidins prevent plasma postprandial oxidative stress in humans. *Journal of Agricultural and Food Chemistry, 50*(26), 7720-7725.

Neri, S., Calvagno, S., Mauceri, B., Misseri, M., Tsami, A., Vecchio, C., et al. (2010). Effects of antioxidants on postprandial oxidative stress and endothelial dysfunction in subjects with impaired glucose tolerance and type 2 diabetes. *European Journal of Nutrition, 49*(7), 409-416.

Neri, S., Signorelli, S. S., Torrisi, B., Pulvirenti, D., Mauceri, B., Abate, G., et al. (2005). Effects of antioxidant supplementation on postprandial oxidative stress and endothelial dysfunction: A single-blind, 15-day clinical trial in patients with untreated type 2 diabetes, subjects with impaired glucose tolerance, and healthy controls. *Clinical Therapeutics, 27*(11), 1764-1773.

Nishikawa, T., Edelstein, D., Du, X. L., Yamagishi, S., Matsumura, T., Kaneda, Y., et al. (2000). Normalizing mitochondrial superoxide production blocks three pathways of hyperglycaemic damage. *Nature, 404*(6779), 787-790.

Nishizawa, J., Nakai, A., Matsuda, K., Komeda, M., Ban, T., & Nagata, K. (1999). Reactive oxygen species play an important role in the activation of heat shock factor 1 in ischemic-reperfused heart. *Circulation, 99*(7), 934-941.

Oben, J. E., Kuate, D., Agbor, G., Momo, C., & Talla, X. (2006). The use of a cissus quadrangularis formulation in the management of weight loss and metabolic syndrome. *Lipids in Health and Disease, 5*, 24.

Oben, J. E., Enyegue, D. M., Fomekong, G. I., Soukontoua, Y. B., & Agbor, G. A. (2007). The effect of cissus quadrangularis (CQR-300) and a cissus formulation (CORE) on obesity and obesity-induced oxidative stress. *Lipids in Health and Disease, 6*, 4.

Oben, J. E., Ngondi, J. L., Momo, C. N., Agbor, G. A., & Sobgui, C. S. (2008). The use of a cissus quadrangularis/Irvingia gabonensis combination in the management of weight loss: A double-blind placebo-controlled study. *Lipids in Health and Disease, 7*, 12.

O'Gorman, D. J., Karlsson, H. K., McQuaid, S., Yousif, O., Rahman, Y., Gasparro, D., et al. (2006). Exercise training increases insulin-stimulated glucose disposal and GLUT4 (SLC2A4) protein content in patients with type 2 diabetes. *Diabetologia, 49*(12), 2983-2992.

Ohno, H., Yahata, T., Sato, Y., Yamamura, K., & Taniguchi, N. (1988). Physical training and fasting erythrocyte activities of free radical scavenging enzyme systems in sedentary men. *European Journal of Applied Physiology and Occupational Physiology, 57*(2), 173-176.

O'Keefe, J. H., Abuannadi, M., Lavie, C. J., & Bell, D. S. (2011). Strategies for optimizing glycemic control and cardiovascular prognosis in patients with type 2 diabetes mellitus. *Mayo Clinic Proceedings.Mayo Clinic, 86*(2), 128-138.

O'Keefe, J. H., & Bell, D. S. (2007). Postprandial hyperglycemia/hyperlipidemia (postprandial dysmetabolism) is a cardiovascular risk factor. *The American Journal of Cardiology, 100*(5), 899-904.

Ortenblad, N., Madsen, K., & Djurhuus, M. S. (1997). Antioxidant status and lipid peroxidation after short-term maximal exercise in trained and untrained humans. *The American Journal of Physiology, 272*(4 Pt 2), R1258-63.

Packer, J. E., Slater, T. F., & Willson, R. L. (1979). Direct observation of a free radical interaction between vitamin E and vitamin C. *Nature, 278*(5706), 737-738.

Park, S., & Choi, S. B. (2002). Effects of alpha-tocopherol supplementation and continuous subcutaneous insulin infusion on oxidative stress in korean patients with type 2 diabetes. *The American Journal of Clinical Nutrition, 75*(4), 728-733.

Pastromas, S., Terzi, A. B., Tousoulis, D., & Koulouris, S. (2008). Postprandial lipemia: An under-recognized atherogenic factor in patients with diabetes mellitus. *International Journal of Cardiology, 126*(1), 3-12.

Peltonen, P., Marniemi, J., Hietanen, E., Vuori, I., & Ehnholm, C. (1981). Changes in serum lipids, lipoproteins, and heparin releasable lipolytic enzymes during moderate physical training in man: A longitudinal study. *Metabolism: Clinical and Experimental, 30*(5), 518-526.

Peres, S. B., de Moraes, S. M., Costa, C. E., Brito, L. C., Takada, J., Andreotti, S., et al. (2005). Endurance exercise training increases insulin responsiveness in isolated adipocytes through IRS/PI3-kinase/Akt pathway. *Journal of Applied Physiology (Bethesda, Md.: 1985), 98*(3), 1037-1043.

Petitt, D. S., Arngrimsson, S. A., & Cureton, K. J. (2003). Effect of resistance exercise on postprandial lipemia. *Journal of Applied Physiology (Bethesda, Md.: 1985), 94*(2), 694-700.

Pittas, A. G., Dawson-Hughes, B., Li, T., Van Dam, R. M., Willett, W. C., Manson, J. E., et al. (2006). Vitamin D and calcium intake in relation to type 2 diabetes in women. *Diabetes Care, 29*(3), 650-656.

Pittas, A. G., Harris, S. S., Stark, P. C., & Dawson-Hughes, B. (2007). The effects of calcium and vitamin D supplementation on blood glucose and markers of inflammation in nondiabetic adults. *Diabetes Care, 30*(4), 980-986.

Powers, S. K., Ji, L. L., & Leeuwenburgh, C. (1999). Exercise training-induced alterations in skeletal muscle antioxidant capacity: A brief review. *Medicine and Science in Sports and Exercise, 31*(7), 987-997.

Praet, S. F., & van Loon, L. J. (2007). Optimizing the therapeutic benefits of exercise in type 2 diabetes. *Journal of Applied Physiology (Bethesda, Md.: 1985), 103*(4), 1113-1120.

Pronk, N. P. (1993). Short term effects of exercise on plasma lipids and lipoproteins in humans. *Sports Medicine (Auckland, N.Z.), 16*(6), 431-448.

Pruchnic, R., Katsiaras, A., He, J., Kelley, D. E., Winters, C., & Goodpaster, B. H. (2004). Exercise training increases intramyocellular lipid and oxidative capacity in older adults. *American Journal of Physiology.Endocrinology and Metabolism, 287*(5), E857-62.

Quindry, J. C., Stone, W. L., King, J., & Broeder, C. E. (2003). The effects of acute exercise on neutrophils and plasma oxidative stress. *Medicine and Science in Sports and Exercise, 35*(7), 1139-1145.

Radak, Z., Chung, H. Y., Koltai, E., Taylor, A. W., & Goto, S. (2008). Exercise, oxidative stress and hormesis. *Ageing Research Reviews, 7*(1), 34-42.

Reay, J. L., Scholey, A. B., Milne, A., Fenwick, J., & Kennedy, D. O. (2009). Panax ginseng has no effect on indices of glucose regulation following acute or chronic ingestion in healthy volunteers. *The British Journal of Nutrition, 101*(11), 1673-1678.

Redman, L. M., Heilbronn, L. K., Martin, C. K., de Jonge, L., Williamson, D. A., Delany, J. P., et al. (2009). Metabolic and behavioral compensations in response to caloric restriction: Implications for the maintenance of weight loss. *PloS One, 4*(2), e4377.

Ren, J. M., Semenkovich, C. F., Gulve, E. A., Gao, J., & Holloszy, J. O. (1994). Exercise induces rapid increases in GLUT4 expression, glucose transport capacity, and insulin-stimulated glycogen storage in muscle. *The Journal of Biological Chemistry, 269*(20), 14396-14401.

Renaud, S., & de Lorgeril, M. (1992). Wine, alcohol, platelets, and the french paradox for coronary heart disease. *Lancet, 339*(8808), 1523-1526.

Rimbach, G., Hohler, D., Fischer, A., Roy, S., Virgili, F., Pallauf, J., et al. (1999). Methods to assess free radicals and oxidative stress in biological systems. *Archiv Fur Tierernahrung, 52*(3), 203-222.

Rizza, S., Tesauro, M., Cardillo, C., Galli, A., Iantorno, M., Gigli, F., et al. (2009). Fish oil supplementation improves endothelial function in normoglycemic offspring of patients with type 2 diabetes. *Atherosclerosis, 206*(2), 569-574.

Rockl, K. S., Witczak, C. A., & Goodyear, L. J. (2008). Signaling mechanisms in skeletal muscle: Acute responses and chronic adaptations to exercise. *IUBMB Life, 60*(3), 145-153.

Rodriguez-Moran, M., & Guerrero-Romero, F. (2003). Oral magnesium supplementation improves insulin sensitivity and metabolic control in type 2 diabetic subjects: A randomized double-blind controlled trial. *Diabetes Care, 26*(4), 1147-1152.

Rodriguez-Moran, M., Guerrero-Romero, F., & Lazcano-Burciaga, G. (1998). Lipid- and glucose-lowering efficacy of plantago psyllium in type II diabetes. *Journal of Diabetes and its Complications, 12*(5), 273-278.

Ronnemaa, T., Marniemi, J., Puukka, P., & Kuusi, T. (1988). Effects of long-term physical exercise on serum lipids, lipoproteins and lipid metabolizing enzymes in type 2 (non-insulin-dependent) diabetic patients. *Diabetes Research (Edinburgh, Scotland), 7*(2), 79-84.

Roussel, A. M., Hininger, I., Benaraba, R., Ziegenfuss, T. N., & Anderson, R. A. (2009). Antioxidant effects of a cinnamon extract in people with impaired fasting glucose that are overweight or obese. *Journal of the American College of Nutrition, 28*(1), 16-21.

Rubin, D., Claas, S., Pfeuffer, M., Nothnagel, M., Foelsch, U. R., & Schrezenmeir, J. (2008). s-ICAM-1 and s-VCAM-1 in healthy men are strongly associated with traits of the metabolic syndrome, becoming evident in the postprandial response to a lipid-rich meal. *Lipids in Health and Disease, 7*, 32.

Santanam, N., & Parthasarathy, S. (1995). Paradoxical actions of antioxidants in the oxidation of low density lipoprotein by peroxidases. *The Journal of Clinical Investigation, 95*(6), 2594-2600.

Saxena, R., Madhu, S. V., Shukla, R., Prabhu, K. M., & Gambhir, J. K. (2005). Postprandial hypertriglyceridemia and oxidative stress in patients of type 2 diabetes mellitus with macrovascular complications. *Clinica Chimica Acta; International Journal of Clinical Chemistry, 359*(1-2), 101-108.

Schindhelm, R. K., Alssema, M., Scheffer, P. G., Diamant, M., Dekker, J. M., Barto, R., et al. (2007). Fasting and postprandial glycoxidative and lipoxidative stress are increased in women with type 2 diabetes. *Diabetes Care, 30*(7), 1789-1794.

Seip, R. L., Mair, K., Cole, T. G., & Semenkovich, C. F. (1997). Induction of human skeletal muscle lipoprotein lipase gene expression by short-term exercise is transient. *The American Journal of Physiology, 272*(2 Pt 1), E255-61.

Seip, R. L., & Semenkovich, C. F. (1998). Skeletal muscle lipoprotein lipase: Molecular regulation and physiological effects in relation to exercise. *Exercise and Sport Sciences Reviews, 26*, 191-218.

Selamoglu, S., Turgay, F., Kayatekin, B. M., Gonenc, S., & Yslegen, C. (2000). Aerobic and anaerobic training effects on the antioxidant enzymes of the blood. *Acta Physiologica Hungarica, 87*(3), 267-273.

Sen, C. K., Rankinen, T., Vaisanen, S., & Rauramaa, R. (1994). Oxidative stress after human exercise: Effect of N-acetylcysteine supplementation. *Journal of Applied Physiology (Bethesda, Md.: 1985), 76*(6), 2570-2577.

Serin, O., Konukoglu, D., Firtina, S., & Mavis, O. (2007). Serum oxidized low density lipoprotein, paraoxonase 1 and lipid peroxidation levels during oral glucose tolerance test. *Hormone and Metabolic Research = Hormon- Und Stoffwechselforschung = Hormones Et Metabolisme, 39*(3), 207-211.

Sesso, H. D., Buring, J. E., Christen, W. G., Kurth, T., Belanger, C., MacFadyen, J., et al. (2008). Vitamins E and C in the prevention of cardiovascular disease in men: The physicians' health study II randomized controlled trial. *JAMA : The Journal of the American Medical Association, 300*(18), 2123-2133.

Shanmugasundaram, E. R., Rajeswari, G., Baskaran, K., Rajesh Kumar, B. R., Radha Shanmugasundaram, K., & Kizar Ahmath, B. (1990). Use of gymnema sylvestre leaf extract in the control of blood glucose in insulin-dependent diabetes mellitus. *Journal of Ethnopharmacology, 30*(3), 281-294.

Shidfar, F., Keshavarz, A., Hosseyni, S., Ameri, A., & Yarahmadi, S. (2008). Effects of omega-3 fatty acid supplements on serum lipids, apolipoproteins and malondialdehyde in type 2 diabetes patients. *Eastern Mediterranean Health Journal = La Revue De Sante De*

La Mediterranee Orientale = Al-Majallah Al-Sihhiyah Li-Sharq Al-Mutawassit, 14(2), 305-313.

Sierra, M., Garcia, J. J., Fernandez, N., Diez, M. J., & Calle, A. P. (2002). Therapeutic effects of psyllium in type 2 diabetic patients. *European Journal of Clinical Nutrition, 56*(9), 830-842.

Sies, H., Stahl, W., & Sevanian, A. (2005). Nutritional, dietary and postprandial oxidative stress. *The Journal of Nutrition, 135*(5), 969-972.

Sigal, R. J., Kenny, G. P., Boule, N. G., Wells, G. A., Prud'homme, D., Fortier, M., et al. (2007). Effects of aerobic training, resistance training, or both on glycemic control in type 2 diabetes: A randomized trial. *Annals of Internal Medicine, 147*(6), 357-369.

Singhal, A., Trilk, J. L., Jenkins, N. T., Bigelman, K. A., & Cureton, K. J. (2009). Effect of intensity of resistance exercise on postprandial lipemia. *Journal of Applied Physiology (Bethesda, Md.: 1985), 106*(3), 823-829.

Sinha, S., Perdomo, G., Brown, N. F., & O'Doherty, R. M. (2004). Fatty acid-induced insulin resistance in L6 myotubes is prevented by inhibition of activation and nuclear localization of nuclear factor kappa B. *The Journal of Biological Chemistry, 279*(40), 41294-41301.

Smolka, M. B., Zoppi, C. C., Alves, A. A., Silveira, L. R., Marangoni, S., Pereira-Da-Silva, L., et al. (2000). HSP72 as a complementary protection against oxidative stress induced by exercise in the soleus muscle of rats. *American Journal of Physiology.Regulatory, Integrative and Comparative Physiology, 279*(5), R1539-45.

Sobenin, I. A., Nedosugova, L. V., Filatova, L. V., Balabolkin, M. I., Gorchakova, T. V., & Orekhov, A. N. (2008). Metabolic effects of time-released garlic powder tablets in type 2 diabetes mellitus: The results of double-blinded placebo-controlled study. *Acta Diabetologica, 45*(1), 1-6.

Solerte, S. B., Fioravanti, M., Locatelli, E., Bonacasa, R., Zamboni, M., Basso, C., et al. (2008). Improvement of blood glucose control and insulin sensitivity during a long-term (60 weeks) randomized study with amino acid dietary supplements in elderly subjects with type 2 diabetes mellitus. *The American Journal of Cardiology, 101*(11A), 82E-88E.

Solomon, T. P., & Blannin, A. K. (2007). Effects of short-term cinnamon ingestion on in vivo glucose tolerance. *Diabetes, Obesity & Metabolism, 9*(6), 895-901.

Solomon, T. P., & Blannin, A. K. (2009). Changes in glucose tolerance and insulin sensitivity following 2 weeks of daily cinnamon ingestion in healthy humans. *European Journal of Applied Physiology, 105*(6), 969-976.

Stangl, V., Kuhn, C., Hentschel, S., Jochmann, N., Jacob, C., Bohm, V., et al. (2011). Lack of effects of tomato products on endothelial function in human subjects: Results of a randomised, placebo-controlled cross-over study. *The British Journal of Nutrition, 105*(2), 263-267.

Steinberg, J. G., Delliaux, S., & Jammes, Y. (2006). Reliability of different blood indices to explore the oxidative stress in response to maximal cycling and static exercises. *Clinical Physiology and Functional Imaging, 26*(2), 106-112.

Stull, A. J., Wood, K. V., Thyfault, J. P., & Campbell, W. W. (2009). Effects of acute pinitol supplementation on plasma pinitol concentration, whole body glucose tolerance, and activation of the skeletal muscle insulin receptor in older humans. *Hormone and Metabolic Research = Hormon- Und Stoffwechselforschung = Hormones Et Metabolisme, 41*(5), 381-386.

Sun, B., Spranger, I., Yang, J., Leandro, C., Guo, L., Canario, S., et al. (2009). Red wine phenolic complexes and their in vitro antioxidant activity. *Journal of Agricultural and Food Chemistry, 57*(18), 8623-8627.

Tang, M., Larson-Meyer, D. E., & Liebman, M. (2008). Effect of cinnamon and turmeric on urinary oxalate excretion, plasma lipids, and plasma glucose in healthy subjects. *The American Journal of Clinical Nutrition, 87*(5), 1262-1267.

Tapsell, L. C., Gillen, L. J., Patch, C. S., Batterham, M., Owen, A., Bare, M., et al. (2004). Including walnuts in a low-fat/modified-fat diet improves HDL cholesterol-to-total cholesterol ratios in patients with type 2 diabetes. *Diabetes Care, 27*(12), 2777-2783.

Thielecke, F., & Boschmann, M. (2009). The potential role of green tea catechins in the prevention of the metabolic syndrome - a review. *Phytochemistry, 70*(1), 11-24.

Thompson, P. D., Crouse, S. F., Goodpaster, B., Kelley, D., Moyna, N., & Pescatello, L. (2001). The acute versus the chronic response to exercise. *Medicine and Science in Sports and Exercise, 33*(6 Suppl), S438-45; discussion S452-3.

Thong, F. S., Derave, W., Urso, B., Kiens, B., & Richter, E. A. (2003). Prior exercise increases basal and insulin-induced p38 mitogen-activated protein kinase phosphorylation in human skeletal muscle. *Journal of Applied Physiology (Bethesda, Md.: 1985), 94*(6), 2337-2341.

Thorell, A., Hirshman, M. F., Nygren, J., Jorfeldt, L., Wojtaszewski, J. F., Dufresne, S. D., et al. (1999). Exercise and insulin cause GLUT-4 translocation in human skeletal muscle. *The American Journal of Physiology, 277*(4 Pt 1), E733-41.

Timimi, F. K., Ting, H. H., Haley, E. A., Roddy, M. A., Ganz, P., & Creager, M. A. (1998). Vitamin C improves endothelium-dependent vasodilation in patients with insulin-dependent diabetes mellitus. *Journal of the American College of Cardiology, 31*(3), 552-557.

Ting, H. H., Timimi, F. K., Boles, K. S., Creager, S. J., Ganz, P., & Creager, M. A. (1996). Vitamin C improves endothelium-dependent vasodilation in patients with non-insulin-dependent diabetes mellitus. *The Journal of Clinical Investigation, 97*(1), 22-28.

Title, L. M., Cummings, P. M., Giddens, K., & Nassar, B. A. (2000). Oral glucose loading acutely attenuates endothelium-dependent vasodilation in healthy adults without diabetes: An effect prevented by vitamins C and E. *Journal of the American College of Cardiology, 36*(7), 2185-2191.

Tonstad, S., Butler, T., Yan, R., & Fraser, G. E. (2009). Type of vegetarian diet, body weight, and prevalence of type 2 diabetes. *Diabetes Care, 32*(5), 791-796.

Tozzi-Ciancarelli, M. G., Penco, M., & Di Massimo, C. (2002). Influence of acute exercise on human platelet responsiveness: Possible involvement of exercise-induced oxidative stress. *European Journal of Applied Physiology, 86*(3), 266-272.

Tsimikas, S. (2006). Oxidative biomarkers in the diagnosis and prognosis of cardiovascular disease. *The American Journal of Cardiology, 98*(11A), 9P-17P.

Tucker, P. S., Fisher-Wellman, K. H., & Bloomer, R. J. (2008). Can exercise minimize postprandial oxidative stress in patients with type 2 diabetes? *Current Diabetes Reviews, 4*(4), 309-319.

Tudor-Locke, C., Bell, R. C., Myers, A. M., Harris, S. B., Ecclestone, N. A., Lauzon, N., et al. (2004). Controlled outcome evaluation of the first step program: A daily physical activity intervention for individuals with type II diabetes. *International Journal of Obesity and Related Metabolic Disorders : Journal of the International Association for the Study of Obesity, 28*(1), 113-119.

Unno, T., Tago, M., Suzuki, Y., Nozawa, A., Sagesaka, Y. M., Kakuda, T., et al. (2005). Effect of tea catechins on postprandial plasma lipid responses in human subjects. *The British Journal of Nutrition, 93*(4), 543-547.

Van Oostrom, A. J., Sijmonsma, T. P., Rabelink, T. J., Van Asbeck, B. S., & Cabezas, M. C. (2003). Postprandial leukocyte increase in healthy subjects. *Metabolism: Clinical and Experimental, 52*(2), 199-202.

Vanschoonbeek, K., Thomassen, B. J., Senden, J. M., Wodzig, W. K., & van Loon, L. J. (2006). Cinnamon supplementation does not improve glycemic control in postmenopausal type 2 diabetes patients. *The Journal of Nutrition, 136*(4), 977-980.

Venditti, P., & Di Meo, S. (1997). Effect of training on antioxidant capacity, tissue damage, and endurance of adult male rats. *International Journal of Sports Medicine, 18*(7), 497-502.

Venkateswaran, S., & Pari, L. (2003). Effect of coccinia indica leaves on antioxidant status in streptozotocin-induced diabetic rats. *Journal of Ethnopharmacology, 84*(2-3), 163-168.

Ventura, P., Bini, A., Panini, R., Marri, L., Tomasi, A., & Salvioli, G. (2004). Red wine consumption prevents vascular oxidative stress induced by a high-fat meal in healthy volunteers. *International Journal for Vitamin and Nutrition Research.Internationale Zeitschrift Fur Vitamin- Und Ernahrungsforschung.Journal International De Vitaminologie Et De Nutrition, 74*(2), 137-143.

Vider, J., Lehtmaa, J., Kullisaar, T., Vihalemm, T., Zilmer, K., Kairane, C., et al. (2001). Acute immune response in respect to exercise-induced oxidative stress. *Pathophysiology : The Official Journal of the International Society for Pathophysiology / ISP, 7*(4), 263-270.

Vincent, H. K., Morgan, J. W., & Vincent, K. R. (2004). Obesity exacerbates oxidative stress levels after acute exercise. *Medicine and Science in Sports and Exercise, 36*(5), 772-779.

Vincent, K. R., Vincent, H. K., Braith, R. W., Lennon, S. L., & Lowenthal, D. T. (2002). Resistance exercise training attenuates exercise-induced lipid peroxidation in the elderly. *European Journal of Applied Physiology, 87*(4-5), 416-423.

Volek, J. S., Judelson, D. A., Silvestre, R., Yamamoto, L. M., Spiering, B. A., Hatfield, D. L., et al. (2008). Effects of carnitine supplementation on flow-mediated dilation and vascular inflammatory responses to a high-fat meal in healthy young adults. *The American Journal of Cardiology, 102*(10), 1413-1417.

Vuksan, V., Sievenpiper, J. L., Koo, V. Y., Francis, T., Beljan-Zdravkovic, U., Xu, Z., et al. (2000). American ginseng (panax quinquefolius L) reduces postprandial glycemia in nondiabetic subjects and subjects with type 2 diabetes mellitus. *Archives of Internal Medicine, 160*(7), 1009-1013.

Vuksan, V., Sievenpiper, J. L., Wong, J., Xu, Z., Beljan-Zdravkovic, U., Arnason, J. T., et al. (2001). American ginseng (panax quinquefolius L.) attenuates postprandial glycemia in a time-dependent but not dose-dependent manner in healthy individuals. *The American Journal of Clinical Nutrition, 73*(4), 753-758.

Vuksan, V., Stavro, M. P., Sievenpiper, J. L., Beljan-Zdravkovic, U., Leiter, L. A., Josse, R. G., et al. (2000). Similar postprandial glycemic reductions with escalation of dose and administration time of american ginseng in type 2 diabetes. *Diabetes Care, 23*(9), 1221-1226.

Vuksan, V., Sung, M. K., Sievenpiper, J. L., Stavro, P. M., Jenkins, A. L., Di Buono, M., et al. (2008). Korean red ginseng (panax ginseng) improves glucose and insulin regulation in well-controlled, type 2 diabetes: Results of a randomized, double-blind, placebo-controlled study of efficacy and safety. *Nutrition, Metabolism, and Cardiovascular Diseases : NMCD, 18*(1), 46-56.

Wang, S. (2009). Epidemiology of vitamin D in health and disease. *Nutrition Research Reviews, 22*(2), 188-203.

Wang, Y., Simar, D., & Fiatarone Singh, M. A. (2009). Adaptations to exercise training within skeletal muscle in adults with type 2 diabetes or impaired glucose tolerance: A systematic review. *Diabetes/metabolism Research and Reviews, 25*(1), 13-40.

Wang, Y. Q., & Yao, M. H. (2009). Effects of chromium picolinate on glucose uptake in insulin-resistant 3T3-L1 adipocytes involve activation of p38 MAPK. *The Journal of Nutritional Biochemistry, 20*(12), 982-991.

Wang, Z. Q., Ribnicky, D., Zhang, X. H., Raskin, I., Yu, Y., & Cefalu, W. T. (2008). Bioactives of artemisia dracunculus L enhance cellular insulin signaling in primary human skeletal muscle culture. *Metabolism: Clinical and Experimental, 57*(7 Suppl 1), S58-64.

Wascher, T. C., Graier, W. F., Dittrich, P., Hussain, M. A., Bahadori, B., Wallner, S., et al. (1997). Effects of low-dose L-arginine on insulin-mediated vasodilatation and insulin sensitivity. *European Journal of Clinical Investigation, 27*(8), 690-695.

Watson, T. A., Callister, R., Taylor, R. D., Sibbritt, D. W., MacDonald-Wicks, L. K., & Garg, M. L. (2005). Antioxidant restriction and oxidative stress in short-duration exhaustive exercise. *Medicine and Science in Sports and Exercise, 37*(1), 63-71.

Watts, G. F., Playford, D. A., Croft, K. D., Ward, N. C., Mori, T. A., & Burke, V. (2002). Coenzyme Q(10) improves endothelial dysfunction of the brachial artery in type II diabetes mellitus. *Diabetologia, 45*(3), 420-426.

Westphal, S., Taneva, E., Kastner, S., Martens-Lobenhoffer, J., Bode-Boger, S., Kropf, S., et al. (2006). Endothelial dysfunction induced by postprandial lipemia is neutralized by addition of proteins to the fatty meal. *Atherosclerosis, 185*(2), 313-319.

Wickenberg, J., Ingemansson, S. L., & Hlebowicz, J. (2010). Effects of curcuma longa (turmeric) on postprandial plasma glucose and insulin in healthy subjects. *Nutrition Journal, 9*, 43.

Willey, K. A., & Singh, M. A. (2003). Battling insulin resistance in elderly obese people with type 2 diabetes: Bring on the heavy weights. *Diabetes Care, 26*(5), 1580-1588.

Winnick, J. J., Sherman, W. M., Habash, D. L., Stout, M. B., Failla, M. L., Belury, M. A., et al. (2008). Short-term aerobic exercise training in obese humans with type 2 diabetes mellitus improves whole-body insulin sensitivity through gains in peripheral, not hepatic insulin sensitivity. *The Journal of Clinical Endocrinology and Metabolism, 93*(3), 771-778.

Winterbone, M. S., Sampson, M. J., Saha, S., Hughes, J. C., & Hughes, D. A. (2007). Pro-oxidant effect of alpha-tocopherol in patients with type 2 diabetes after an oral glucose tolerance test--a randomised controlled trial. *Cardiovascular Diabetology, 6*, 8.

Woodman, R. J., Mori, T. A., Burke, V., Puddey, I. B., Watts, G. F., & Beilin, L. J. (2002). Effects of purified eicosapentaenoic and docosahexaenoic acids on glycemic control, blood pressure, and serum lipids in type 2 diabetic patients with treated hypertension. *The American Journal of Clinical Nutrition, 76*(5), 1007-1015.

World Health Organization. (2011). *Diabetes fact sheet number 312*

Wright, E.,Jr, Scism-Bacon, J. L., & Glass, L. C. (2006). Oxidative stress in type 2 diabetes: The role of fasting and postprandial glycaemia. *International Journal of Clinical Practice, 60*(3), 308-314.

Wu, J. H., Ward, N. C., Indrawan, A. P., Almeida, C. A., Hodgson, J. M., Proudfoot, J. M., et al. (2007). Effects of alpha-tocopherol and mixed tocopherol supplementation on markers of oxidative stress and inflammation in type 2 diabetes. *Clinical Chemistry, 53*(3), 511-519.

Xiang, G. D., Pu, J., Yue, L., Hou, J., & Sun, H. (2011). Alpha-lipoic acid can improve endothelial dysfunction in subjects with impaired fasting glucose. *Metabolism: Clinical and Experimental,*

Xiang, G. D., Sun, H. L., Zhao, L. S., Hou, J., Yue, L., & Xu, L. (2008). The antioxidant alpha-lipoic acid improves endothelial dysfunction induced by acute hyperglycaemia during OGTT in impaired glucose tolerance. *Clinical Endocrinology, 68*(5), 716-723.

Xiang, Y. Z., Shang, H. C., Gao, X. M., & Zhang, B. L. (2008). A comparison of the ancient use of ginseng in traditional chinese medicine with modern pharmacological experiments and clinical trials. *Phytotherapy Research : PTR, 22*(7), 851-858.

Yang, W., & Omaye, S. T. (2009). Air pollutants, oxidative stress and human health. *Mutation Research, 674*(1-2), 45-54.

Yin, J., Xing, H., & Ye, J. (2008). Efficacy of berberine in patients with type 2 diabetes mellitus. *Metabolism: Clinical and Experimental, 57*(5), 712-717.

Yubero-Serrano, E. M., Delgado-Casado, N., Delgado-Lista, J., Perez-Martinez, P., Tasset-Cuevas, I., Santos-Gonzalez, M., et al. (2010). Postprandial antioxidant effect of the mediterranean diet supplemented with coenzyme Q(10) in elderly men and women. *Age (Dordrecht, Netherlands),*

Zhang, Y., Li, X., Zou, D., Liu, W., Yang, J., Zhu, N., et al. (2008). Treatment of type 2 diabetes and dyslipidemia with the natural plant alkaloid berberine. *The Journal of Clinical Endocrinology and Metabolism, 93*(7), 2559-2565.

Zilversmit, D. B. (1979). Atherogenesis: A postprandial phenomenon. *Circulation, 60*(3), 473-485.

Zuberi, A. R. (2008). Strategies for assessment of botanical action on metabolic syndrome in the mouse and evidence for a genotype-specific effect of russian tarragon in the regulation of insulin sensitivity. *Metabolism: Clinical and Experimental, 57*(7 Suppl 1), S10-5.